Caring for the
Hospitalized
Child

A Handbook of Inpatient Pediatrics

2nd Edition

Author
American Academy of Pediatrics Section on Hospital Medicine

Editors
Jeffrey C. Gershel, MD, FAAP
Daniel A. Rauch, MD, FAAP, FHM

American Academy of Pediatrics
DEDICATED TO THE HEALTH OF ALL CHILDREN®

American Academy of Pediatrics Publishing Staff

Mark Grimes, *Director, Department of Publishing*

Chris Wiberg, *Senior Editor, Professional/Clinical Publishing*

Theresa Wiener, *Production Manager, Clinical and Professional Publications*

Heather Babiar, *Medical Copy Editor*

Peg Mulcahy, *Manager, Art Direction and Production*

Mary Lou White, *Chief Product and Services Officer/SVP, Membership, Marketing, and Publishing*

Mary Louise Carr, MBA, *Marketing Manager, Clinical Publications*

141 Northwest Point Blvd
Elk Grove Village, IL 60007-1019
Telephone: 847/434-4000
Facsimile: 847/434-8000
www.aap.org

The recommendations in this publication do not indicate an exclusive course of treatment or serve as a standard of medical care. Variations, taking into account individual circumstances, may be appropriate. Listing of resources does not imply an endorsement by the American Academy of Pediatrics (AAP). The AAP is not responsible for the content of external resources. Information was current at the time of publication.

Brand names are furnished for identification purposes only. No endorsement of the manufacturers or products mentioned is implied.

Every effort has been made to ensure that the drug selection and dosages set forth in this text are in accordance with the current recommendations and practice at the time of publication. It is the responsibility of the health care professional to check the package insert of each drug for any change in indications and dosages and for added warnings and precautions.

The publishers have made every effort to trace the copyright holders for borrowed material. If they have inadvertently overlooked any, they will be pleased to make the necessary arrangements at the first opportunity.

This publication has been developed by the American Academy of Pediatrics. The authors, editors, and contributors are expert authorities in the field of pediatrics. No commercial involvement of any kind has been solicited or accepted in the development of the content of this publication. Disclosures: Dr Walley indicated stock ownership in Gilead Sciences and Atea Pharmaceuticals.

Every effort is made to keep *Caring for the Hospitalized Child: A Handbook of Inpatient Pediatrics,* 2nd Edition, consistent with the most recent advice and information available from the American Academy of Pediatrics.

Special discounts are available for bulk purchases of this publication. E-mail our Special Sales Department at aapsales@aap.org for more information.

Printed in the United States of America
9-382/0917

MA0840
ISBN: 978-1-61002-114-2
eBook: 978-1-61002-115-9
Library of Congress Control Number: 2016959829

1 2 3 4 5 6 7 8 9 10

American Academy of Pediatrics
Section on Hospital Medicine
2017–2018

Executive Committee

Brian Alverson, MD, FAAP, *Chairperson*
Matthew Garber, MD, FAAP, *Chairperson-Elect*
Eric A. Biondi, MD, FAAP
Lindsay Chase, MD, FAAP
Barrett Fromme, MD, FAAP
Rachel Marek, MD, FAAP, *Community Hospitalist Member*
Kevin Powell, MD, PhD, FAAP
Geeta Singhal, MD, MEd, FAAP
Ricardo Quinonez, MD, FAAP, *Immediate Past Chairperson*
Neha Joshi, MD, *Section on Pediatric Trainees Liaison*

Staff

S. Niccole Alexander, MPP, *Manager, Division of Hospital and Surgical Services*

Contributors/Reviewers

Editors

Jeffrey C. Gershel, MD, FAAP
Vice Chairman, Department of Pediatrics
Jacobi Medical Center
Professor of Clinical Pediatrics
Albert Einstein College of Medicine
Bronx, NY

Daniel A. Rauch, MD, FAAP, FHM
Visiting Associate Professor of Pediatrics
Tufts University School of Medicine
Chief of Pediatric Hospital Medicine
Floating Hospital for Children at Tufts
    Medical Center
Boston, MA

Chapter Authors

Oloruntosin Adeyanju, MD, FAAP
Fellow, Pediatric Hospital Medicine
Cleveland Clinic Children's
Cleveland, OH
Ch 65: Fever in the International Traveler

David Amrol, MD
Associate Professor of Clinical Internal
    Medicine
Division Director, Allergy and Clinical
    Immunology
University of South Carolina School
    of Medicine
Columbia, SC
Ch 63: Immunodeficiency

Justen Aprile, MD, FAAP
Assistant Professor of Pediatrics
Penn State Milton S. Hershey Medical
    Center
Penn State College of Medicine
Division of Pediatric Inpatient Medicine
Hershey, PA
Ch 27: Hypoglycemia

Moises Auron, MD, FACP, SFHM, FAAP
Associate Professor of Medicine and
    Pediatrics
Cleveland Clinic Lerner College of
    Medicine
Case Western Reserve University
Staff, Department of Hospital Medicine
    and Pediatric Hospital Medicine
Cleveland Clinic
Cleveland, OH
Ch 76: Nephrotic Syndrome

Khyzer Aziz, MD
Pediatric Chief Resident
Lewis M. Fraad Department of Pediatrics
Albert Einstein College of Medicine
Bronx, NY
Ch 96: Fractures

Gabriella C. Azzarone, MD
Assistant Professor of Pediatrics
Albert Einstein College of Medicine
Attending Physician, Pediatric Hospital
    Medicine
Children's Hospital at Montefiore
Bronx, NY
Ch 73: Hemolytic Uremic Syndrome

Ara Balkian, MD, MBA, FAAP
Chief Medical Director, Inpatient
    Operations
Children's Hospital Los Angeles
Associate Professor of Pediatrics
Keck School of Medicine at the University
    of Southern California
Los Angeles, CA
Ch 38: Gastrointestinal Bleeding

Meital Barzideh, MD
Assistant Professor of Pediatrics
Associate Program Director, Department
    of Pediatrics
Jacobi Medical Center
Albert Einstein College of Medicine
Bronx, NY
Ch 72: Neonatal Hyperbilirubinemia

Julia Beauchamp-Walters, MD, FAAP
Clinical Professors of Pediatrics
University of California San Diego
Division of Pediatric Hospital Medicine
Rady Children's Hospital
San Diego, CA
Ch 42: Genetics

Sheldon Berkowitz, MD, FAAP
Pediatrician and Physician Advisor
Children's Hospitals and Clinics of
    Minnesota
Assistant Professor of Pediatrics
University of Minnesota
Minneapolis, MN
Ch 34: Do Not Resuscitate/Do Not
    Intubate
Ch 35: Informed Consent, Assent, and
    Confidentiality
Ch 57: Microeconomics

Laurie Bernard Stover, MD, FAAP
Clinical Professor of Pediatrics
University of California, San Diego
Division of Hospital Medicine and
    Pediatrics
Rady Children's Hospital
San Diego, CA
Ch 11: Erythema Multiforme and Stevens-
    Johnson Syndrome/Toxic Epidermal
    Necrolysis

Eric A. Biondi, MD, MS, FAAP
Assistant Professor of Pediatrics
Division of Pediatric Hospital Medicine
University of Rochester Medical Center
Rochester, NY
Ch 64: Fever in Infants Younger Than
    60 Days

J. Auxford Burks, MD, FAAP
Assistant Professor of Pediatrics
Director, Residency Training Program
The Lewis M. Fraad Department of
    Pediatrics
Jacobi Medical Center, Albert Einstein
    College of Medicine
Bronx, NY
Ch 18: Orbital and Periorbital Cellulitis
Ch 88: Fluids and Electrolytes

Genevieve Buser, MDCM, MSHP, FAAP
Pediatric Infectious Diseases
Providence St Vincent Medical Center
Portland, OR
Ch 97: Osteomyelitis
Ch 98: Septic Arthritis

Brendan T. Campbell, MD, MPH, FAAP
Donald W. Hight Endowed Chair in
    Pediatric Surgery
Associate Professor of Surgery and
    Pediatrics
Connecticut Children's Medical Center
University of Connecticut School of
    Medicine
Hartford, CT
Ch 45: Ovarian Torsion

Douglas W. Carlson, MD, FAAP
Professor of Pediatrics and Emergency
    Medicine
Chair, Department of Pediatrics
Southern Illinois University School of
    Medicine
Medical Director
St John's Children's Hospital
Springfield, IL
Ch 30: Noninvasive Monitoring
Ch 116: Sedation

Scott Carney, MD, FAAP
Assistant Professor of Pediatrics
Director, Pediatric Hospitalists
Medical Director, COMPASS
Assistant Program Director
University of South Carolina School of
    Medicine
Palmetto Health Richland Pediatric
    Residency
Columbia, SC
Ch 66: Fever of Unknown Origin

Jennifer Casatelli, MD, FAAP
Pediatric Hospitalist
University of South Florida
Tampa, FL
Ch 71: Acute Liver Failure

Julie Cernanec, MD, FAAP
Staff Physician, Pediatric Hospital Medicine
Cleveland Clinic Children's
Cleveland, OH
Ch 75: Nephrolithiasis

Lindsay Chase, MD, FAAP
Associate Professor of Pediatrics
Director of the Section of Hospital
    Pediatrics
Division of General Pediatrics and
    Adolescent Medicine
University of North Carolina
Chapel Hill, NC
Ch 13: Skin and Soft-Tissue Infections
Ch 17: Neck Masses
Ch 19: Parotitis
Ch 91: Acute Vision Loss
Ch 95: White Eye (Leukocoria)

Daxa P. Clarke, MD, FAAP
Program Director, Pediatric Hospitalist
    Fellowship
Medical Director, Coding and
    Documentation and Utilization
    Management
Phoenix Children's Hospital
Phoenix, AZ
Ch 61: Transition to Adult Care

Daniel T. Coghlin, MD, FAAP
Associate Professor of Pediatrics, Clinical
Division of Pediatric Hospital Medicine
The Warren Alpert Medical School of
    Brown University
Providence, RI
Ch 78: Urinary Tract Infection

Eyal Cohen, MD, MSc, FRCP(C)
Associate Professor of Pediatrics
The Hospital for Sick Children
University of Toronto
Toronto, Ontario, Canada
Ch 87: Feeding Tubes and Enteral
    Nutrition

Laurie S. Conklin, MD
Children's National Health System
Assistant Professor of Pediatrics
The George Washington University School
    of Medicine
Washington, DC
Ch 39: Inflammatory Bowel Disease

Yong-Sing Da Silva, MD
Assistant Professor of Pediatrics
New York Medical College
Valhalla, NY
Ch 85: Seizures

Sharon Dabrow, MD, FAAP
Professor of Pediatrics
Program Director, Residency Program
University of South Florida
Tampa, FL
Ch 119: Pyloric Stenosis

Elizabeth N. Davis, MD, FAAP
Assistant Professor of Pediatrics
Division of Pediatric Hospital Medicine
Associate Director, Pediatric Hospital
    Medicine Fellowship
Baylor College of Medicine
The Children's Hospital of San Antonio
San Antonio, TX
Ch 37: Gastroenteritis

Paola Dees, MD, FAAP
Pediatric Hospitalist
Johns Hopkins All Children's Hospital
St Petersburg, FL
Ch 119: Pyloric Stenosis

Marcella Donaruma-Kwoh, MD, FAAP
Assistant Professor of Pediatrics
Director, Child Abuse Fellowship Program
Section of Public Health Pediatrics
Baylor College of Medicine
Texas Children's Hospital
Houston, TX
Ch 102: Child Abuse and Neglect
Ch 103: Sexual Abuse

Lindsey C. Douglas, MD, MS, FAAP
Assistant Professor of Pediatrics
Division of Hospital Medicine
The Children's Hospital at Montefiore
Albert Einstein College of Medicine
Bronx, NY
Ch 7: Endocarditis

Carla Falco, MD, FAAP
Assistant Professor of Pediatrics
Baylor College of Medicine
Texas Children's Hospital
Houston, TX
Ch 54: Family-Centered Rounds
Ch 102: Child Abuse and Neglect
Ch 103: Sexual Abuse

Bryan R. Fine, MD, MPH, FAAP
Chief, Division of Pediatric Hospital
    Medicine
Children's Hospital of the King's Daughter
Associate Professor of Pediatrics
Eastern Virginia Medical School
Norfolk, VA
Ch 56: Macroeconomics
Ch 62: Transport
Ch 87: Feeding Tubes and Enteral
    Nutrition

Darren Fiore, MD, FAAP
Associate Professor of Pediatrics
Division of Pediatric Hospital Medicine
University of California San Francisco
San Francisco, CA
Ch 112: Foreign-Body Aspiration

Brock Fisher, MD
Department of Critical Care and
    Anesthesia
Rady Children's Hospital San Diego
San Diego, CA
Ch 106: Airway Management and
    Respiratory Support

Erin Ragan-Stucky Fisher, MD, MHM, FAAP

Division Director and Fellowship Director, Pediatric Hospital Medicine Program
Medical Director Quality Management
Rady Children's Hospital San Diego
Professor of Clinical Pediatrics
Department of Pediatrics
University of California San Diego
San Diego, CA
Ch 59: Patient Safety
Ch 68: Sepsis
Ch 106: Airway Management and Respiratory Support

Dana Foradori, MD, FAAP

Assistant Professor of Pediatrics
Section of Pediatric Hospital Medicine
Baylor College of Medicine
Texas Children's Hospital
Houston, TX
Ch 113: Juvenile Idiopathic Arthritis

Jason L. Freedman, MD, MSCE

Inpatient Medical Director, Oncology/BMT
Assistant Professor of Clinical Pediatrics
Division of Oncology
The Children's Hospital of Philadelphia
Department of Pediatrics
Perelman School of Medicine
University of Pennsylvania
Philadelphia, PA
Ch 48: Complications of Cancer Therapy

Jason A. French, MD, FAAP

Senior Instructor
Section of Pediatric Hospital Medicine
Department of Pediatrics
University of Colorado School of Medicine
Children's Hospital Colorado
Aurora, CO
Ch 84: Headache

Blake Froberg, MD

Assistant Professor of Pediatrics and Emergency Medicine
Indiana University School of Medicine
Indianapolis, IN
Ch 70: Toxic Exposures

Jennifer Fuchs, MD, FAAP

Assistant Professor of Pediatrics
Section of Hospital Medicine
University of Texas Southwestern
Dallas Children's Hospital
Dallas, TX
Ch 114: Systemic Lupus Erythematosus

Sandra Gage, MD, PhD, FAAP, SFHM

Associate Professor of Pediatrics
Division of Hospital Medicine
Medical College of Wisconsin
Milwaukee, WI
Ch 79: Acute Ataxia

Matthew Garber, MD, FAAP

Professor of Pediatrics
Division of Hospital Medicine
Woldson Children's Hospital
University of Florida College of Medicine—Jacksonville
Jacksonville, FL
Ch 66: Fever of Unknown Origin

Brian Gin, MD, PhD

Assistant Clinical Professor of Pediatrics
Department of Pediatrics, Division of Hospital Medicine
University of California, San Francisco
San Francisco, CA
Ch 112: Foreign-Body Aspiration

Laurie Gordon, MD, MA, FAAP

Associate Clinical Professor of Pediatrics
Weill Cornell Medical College, New York, NY
Director, Pediatric Inpatient Unit, Queens, NY
Site Director, Pediatric Resident Training
New York Presbyterian/Queens, Flushing, NY
Ch 12: Rashes Associated With Serious Underlying Disease

Elizabeth Halvorson, MD, FAAP

Assistant Professor of Pediatrics
Wake Forest School of Medicine
Winston-Salem, NC
Ch 117: Abdominal Masses

Daniel Hershey, MD, SFHM, FAAP
Associate Professor of Pediatrics
University of California, San Diego
Rady Children's Hospital
San Diego, CA
Ch 118: Acute Abdomen

Samantha House, DO, MPH, FAAP
Assistant Professor of Pediatrics
Children's Hospital at Dartmouth
Lebanon, NH
Ch 109: Bronchiolitis

Maria Z. Huang, MD, FAAP
Fellow, Pediatric Hospital Medicine
University of California San Diego
Rady Children's Hospital San Diego
San Diego, CA
Ch 42: Genetics

Rebecca Ivancie, MD, FAAP
Clinical Instructor of Pediatrics
Stanford University School of Medicine
Division of Hospital Medicine
Lucile Packard Children's Hospital
Stanford, CA
Ch 68: Sepsis

Stephanie Jennings, MD, FAAP
Regional Director
Department of Pediatric Hospital Medicine
Cleveland Clinic
Cleveland, OH
Ch 2: Anaphylaxis
Ch 14: Cervical Lymphadenopathy
Ch 16: Mastoiditis
Ch 18: Orbital and Periorbital Cellulitis
Ch 22: Sinusitis

Valerie Jurgens, MD, FAAP
Assistant Professor of Pediatrics
University of Texas at Austin
Dell Medical School
Austin, TX
Ch 37: Gastroenteritis

Daran Kaufman, MD, FAAP
Assistant Professor, Department of
   Pediatrics
Albert Einstein College of Medicine
Bronx, NY
Ch 115: Pain Management

Brent D. Kaziny, MD, MA, FAAP
Assistant Professor of Pediatrics
Section of Emergency Medicine
Department of Pediatrics
Baylor College of Medicine
Texas Children's Hospital
Houston, TX
Ch 53: Disaster Preparedness

Caryn Kerman, MD
Clinical Assistant Professor of Pediatrics
Perelman School of Medicine, University
   of Pennsylvania
Division of General Pediatrics
Children's Hospital of Philadelphia
Philadelphia, PA
Ch 48: Complications of Cancer Therapy

Sangeeta Krishna, MD, FAAP
Adviser, Peru Health Outreach Project
Co-Director, Pediatrics Clerkship
Fellowship Director, Pediatric Hospital
   Medicine
Cleveland Clinic
Cleveland, OH
Ch 23: Acute Adrenal Insufficiency
Ch 26: Hyperthyroidism
Ch 65: Fever in the International Traveler

Deepa Kulkarni, MD, FAAP
Assistant Clinical Professor of Pediatrics
David Geffen School of Medicine at UCLA
Mattel Children's Hospital at UCLA
Division of Pediatric Hospital Medicine
Los Angeles, CA
Ch 49: Neutropenia

Jacquelyn Kuzminski, MD, FAAP
Assistant Professor of Pediatrics
Section of Hospital Medicine
Medical College of Wisconsin
Milwaukee, WI
Ch 47: Anemia

Kyle A. Lamphier, MD
Assistant Professor of Clinical Pediatrics
Division of Hospital Medicine
Children's Hospital Los Angeles
University of Southern California Keck
   School of Medicine
Los Angeles, CA
Ch 38: Gastrointestinal Bleeding

Vivian Lee, MD, FAAP
Assistant Professor of Clinical Pediatrics
University of Southern California Keck
    School of Medicine
Division of Hospital Medicine
Children's Hospital Los Angeles
Los Angeles, CA
Ch 77: Postinfectious Glomerulonephritis

Carly Levy, MD, FAAP
Clinical Assistant Professor of Pediatrics
Division of Palliative Medicine
Sidney Kimmel Medical College at
    Thomas Jefferson University
Nemours/Alfred I. duPont Hospital for
    Children
Wilmington, DE
Ch 64: Fever in Infants Younger Than
    60 Days

Jonathan Lewis, MD, FAAP
Assistant Professor of Pediatrics
Baylor College of Medicine
Section of Emergency Medicine
Texas Children's Hospital
Houston, TX
Ch 10: Shock

Jamie Librizzi, MD, MSHS, FAAP
Assistant Professor of Pediatrics
Division of Pediatric Hospital Medicine
Phoenix Children's Hospital
Phoenix, AZ
Ch 1: Eating Disorders

Sheila K. Liewehr, MD, FAAP
Pediatric Hospitalist Attending
Cohen Children's Northwell Health
Assistant Professor of Pediatrics
Hofstra Northwell School of Medicine
New Hyde Park, NY
Ch 73: Hemolytic Uremic Syndrome

Huay-ying Lo, MD, FAAP
Assistant Professor of Pediatrics
Division of Pediatric Hospital Medicine
Baylor College of Medicine
Houston, TX
Ch 41: Pancreatitis

Michelle A. Lopez, MD, MPH, FAAP
Assistant Professor of Pediatrics
Section of Hospital Medicine
Baylor College of Medicine
Texas Children's Hospital
Houston, TX
Ch 13: Skin and Soft-Tissue Infections
Ch 52: Cultural Effectiveness

Cara G. Lye, MD, FAAP
Baylor College of Medicine
Division of Pediatric Hospital Medicine
Houston, TX
Ch 19: Parotitis

Tamara Maginot, PhD
University of California, San Diego
UCSD Eating Disorders Treatment and
    Research Center
Rady Children's Hospital San Diego
San Diego, CA
Ch 101: Suicide

Sanjay Mahant, MD, FRCPC, MSc
Associate Professor
Department of Pediatrics
University of Toronto
Hospital for Sick Children
Toronto, Ontario, Canada
Ch 87: Feeding Tubes and Enteral
    Nutrition

Kiranvir Mangat, MD, FAAP
Pediatric Hospitalist
Phoenix Children's Hospital
Phoenix, AZ
Ch 1: Eating Disorders

Jennifer Maniscalco, MD, MPH, FAAP
Vice Chair, Education, Department of
    Pediatrics
Associate Professor of Clinical Pediatrics
USC Keck School of Medicine
Director, Pediatric Hospital Medicine
    Fellowship
Children's Hospital Los Angeles
Los Angeles, CA
Ch 77: Postinfectious Glomerulonephritis

Kristie Manning, MD, FAAP
Pediatric Hospitalist
Kaiser Santa Clara Medical Center
Santa Clara, CA
Ch 62: Transport

Rachel Marek, MD, FAAP
Medical Director, Pediatric Hospital
    Medicine
Texas Children's Hospital Woodlands
Assistant Professor of Pediatrics
Baylor College of Medicine
The Woodlands, TX
Ch 53: Disaster Preparedness

Michelle Marks, DO, FAAP, SFHM
Chair, Department of Pediatric Hospital
    Medicine
Medical Director, Inpatient Pediatrics
Cleveland Clinic Children's
Cleveland, OH
Ch 111: Complications of Cystic Fibrosis

Erich Maul, DO, MPH, FAAP
Associate Professor of Pediatrics
Division of Hospital Pediatrics
University of Kentucky
Lexington, KY
Ch 3: Arrhythmias
Ch 6: Electrocardiogram Interpretation

Sonaly Rao McClymont, MD, FAAP
Assistant Professor of Pediatrics
Hospital Medicine Division, Children's
    National Health System
The George Washington University School
    of Medicine
Washington, DC
Ch 4: Congestive Heart Failure

Jerry McLaughlin, MD
Clinical Assistant Professor
Pediatrics—Critical Care
Stanford University
Palo Alto, CA
Ch 105: Acute Respiratory Failure

Scott Miller, MD
Co-Director of Inpatient Pediatrics
Jacobi Medical Center
Assistant Professor of Pediatrics
Albert Einstein College of Medicine
Bronx, NY
Ch 67: Kawasaki Disease
Ch 100: Depression

Brent Mothner, MD, FAAP
Assistant Professor of Pediatrics
Baylor College of Medicine
Houston, TX
Ch 41: Pancreatitis

Meaghan Mungekar, MD, FAAP
Assistant Clinical Professor of Pediatrics
Icahn School of Medicine at Mount Sinai
New York, NY
Ch 82: Altered Mental Status

Steve Narang, MD, MHCM
CEO, Banner-University Medical Center
Phoenix Banner Health
Phoenix, AZ
Ch 60: Quality Improvement

Sridaran Narayanan, MD, FAAP
Director, Hospital Medicine Fellowship
Assistant Professor, Department of
    Pediatrics
Division of Hospital Medicine
University of Alabama at Birmingham
Birmingham, AL
Ch 43: Inborn Errors of Metabolism

Joanne M. Nazif, MD, FAAP
Assistant Professor of Pediatrics
Albert Einstein College of Medicine
Attending Physician, Pediatric Hospital
    Medicine
Children's Hospital at Montefiore
Bronx, NY
Ch 8: Myocarditis
Ch 9: Pericarditis

Jennifer A. Nead, MD, FAAP
Assistant Professor of Pediatrics
Division of Pediatric Inpatient Medicine
SUNY Upstate Medical University
Upstate Golisano Children's Hospital
Syracuse, NY
Ch 15: Infectious Croup
Ch 17: Neck Masses

Roger Nicome, MD, FAAP
Assistant Professor of Pediatrics
Section of Pediatric Hospital Medicine
Baylor College of Medicine
Texas Children's Hospital
Houston, TX
Ch 24: Diabetes Insipidus
Ch 25: Diabetic Ketoacidosis

Katherine M. O'Connor, MD
Assistant Professor of Pediatrics
Associate Division Director, Pediatric
    Hospital Medicine
Albert Einstein College of Medicine
The Children's Hospital at Montefiore
Bronx, NY
Ch 36: Gallbladder Disease

Ololade Okito, MD, FAAP
Chief Resident, Department of Pediatrics
Jacobi Medical Center
Albert Einstein College of Medicine
Bronx, NY
Ch 22: Sinusitis

Snezana Nena Osorio, MD, MS
Associate Professor of Clinical Pediatrics
Director, Quality and Patient Safety
Chair, Quality and Patient Safety
Weill Cornell Medicine
New York, NY
Ch 44: Dysfunctional Uterine Bleeding
Ch 46: Sexually Transmitted Infections

Mary C. Ottolini, MD, MPH, FAAP
Professor of Pediatrics
George Washington University School
    of Medicine
Vice Chair Medical Education
DIO Children's National Medical Center
Washington, DC
Ch 37: Gastroenteritis

Philip Overby, MD, MA
Director, Inpatient Neurology
Maria Fareri Children's Hospital
Assistant Professor of Pediatrics
Division of Pediatric Neurology
New York Medical College
Valhalla, NY
Ch 80: Acute Hemiparesis
Ch 85: Seizures

Nancy Palumbo, MD, FAAP
Division Director, Pediatric Hospital
    Medicine
Hofstra Northwell School of Medicine
New Hyde Park, NY
Ch 31: Suprapubic Bladder Aspiration
Ch 33: Urinary Bladder Catheterization

Rita M. Pappas, MD, FHM, FAAP
Staff, Pediatric Hospital Medicine
Cleveland Clinic Children's
Cleveland, OH
Ch 107: Bacterial Tracheitis

Binita Patel, MD, FAAP
Associate Professor, Pediatrics
Section of Pediatric Emergency Medicine
Baylor College of Medicine
Texas Children's Hospital
Houston, TX
Ch 10: Shock

Lina Patel, MD, FAAP
Fellow, Pediatric Hospitalist Medicine
Mattel Children's Hospital at UCLA
Los Angeles, CA
Ch 49: Neutropenia

Jack M. Percelay, MD, MPH, FAAP, MHM
Clinical Professor of Pediatrics
Associate Division Chief, Hospital
    Medicine, Regional Program
Division of General Pediatrics and
    Hospital Medicine
Seattle Children's
Seattle, WA
Ch 29: Lumbar Puncture

Katie Pestak, DO
Staff, Pediatric Hospital Medicine
Associate Program Director, Pediatric
  Residency Program
Cleveland Clinic Children's
Cleveland, OH
Ch 94: Red Eye

Sarah M. Phillips, MS, RD
Clinical Instructor of Pediatrics
Baylor College of Medicine
Texas Children's Hospital
Houston, TX
Ch 90: Parenteral Nutrition

Stacy B. Pierson, MD, FAAP
Assistant Professor of Pediatrics
Baylor College of Medicine
Attending, Section of Pediatric Hospital
  Medicine
Texas Children's Hospital
Houston, TX
Ch 74: Henoch-Schönlein Purpura

Gregory Plemmons, MD
Associate Professor
Division of Hospital Medicine
Monroe Carell Jr Children's Hospital
Vanderbilt University Medical Center
Nashville, TN
Ch 89: Obesity

Kevin Powell, MD, PhD, FAAP
Saint Louis, MO
Ch 34: Do Not Resuscitate/Do Not Intubate
Ch 35: Informed Consent, Assent, and
  Confidentiality

Ricardo Quinonez, MD, FAAP
Associate Professor of Pediatrics
Section Chief, Pediatric Hospital Medicine
Baylor College of Medicine
Texas Children's Hospital
Houston, TX
Ch 110: Community-Acquired Pneumonia

Prabi Rajbhandari, MD, FAAP
Department of Hospital Medicine
Akron Children's Hospital
Akron, OH
Ch 23: Acute Adrenal Insufficiency
Ch 27: Hypoglycemia

Shawn L. Ralston, MD, MS, FAAP
Vice Chair for Clinical Affairs
Children's Hospital at Dartmouth
Associate Professor of Pediatrics
Geisel School of Medicine at Dartmouth
Lebanon, NH
Ch 109: Bronchiolitis

David I. Rappaport, MD, FAAP
Hospitalist and Associate Residency
  Program Director
Nemours/Alfred I. duPont Hospital for
  Children
Wilmington, DE
Associate Professor of Pediatrics
Sidney Kimmel Medical College at
  Thomas Jefferson University
Philadelphia, PA
Ch 51: Comanagement

Kyung E. Rhee, MD, MSc, MA, FAAP
Associate Professor of Pediatrics
Medical Director, Medical Behavioral Unit
Rady Children's Hospital San Diego
Director of Research, Division of Hospital
  Medicine
University of California San Diego, School
  of Medicine
San Diego, CA
Ch 101: Suicide

Hai Jung Helen Rhim, MD, MPH
Director, Pediatric Hospital Medicine
  Fellowship Program
Children's Hospital at Montefiore
Assistant Professor of Pediatrics
Division of Pediatric Hospital Medicine
Albert Einstein College of Medicine
Bronx, NY
Ch 69: Esophageal Foreign Body

Jay Riva-Cambrin, MD, MSc, FRCS(C)
Associate Professor, Neurosurgery
Department of Clinical Neurosciences
Department of Community Health
University of Calgary
Calgary, Alberta, Canada
Ch 83: Cerebrospinal Fluid Shunt
  Complications

W. LeGrande Rives, MD
Assistant Professor of Pediatrics
Division of Pediatric Hospitalist Medicine
Washington University School of Medicine
St Louis, MO
Ch 30: Noninvasive Monitoring

Kenneth Rivlin, MD, PhD
Chief, Division of Pediatric Hematology/
    Oncology
Jacobi Medical Center
Assistant Professor of Pediatrics
Albert Einstein College of Medicine
Bronx, NY
Ch 50: Sickle Cell Disease

Mary E. M. Rocha, MD, MPH, FAAP
Associate Professor of Pediatrics
Section of Pediatric Hospital Medicine
Baylor College of Medicine
Texas Children's Hospital
Houston, TX
Ch 32: Tracheostomies
Ch 55: Leading a Team
Ch 113: Juvenile Idiopathic Arthritis
Ch 114: Systemic Lupus Erythematosus

Camille Rodriguez, MD
Pediatric Chief Resident
Lewis M. Fraad Department of Pediatrics
Albert Einstein College of Medicine
Bronx, NY
Ch 96: Fractures

Daniel Rodriguez, MD
Fellow, Allergy Immunology Program
Louisiana State University
New Orleans, LA
Ch 2: Anaphylaxis

Noé D. Romo, MD, MSc
Assistant Professor of Pediatrics
The Albert Einstein College of Medicine
Co-Director, Pediatrics Inpatient Service
NYC Health + Hospitals Jacobi—Lewis M.
    Fraad Department of Pediatrics
Bronx, NY
Ch 5: Deep Venous Thrombosis
Ch 50: Sickle Cell Disease

Rebecca E. Rosenberg, MD, MPH, FAAP
Assistant Professor of Pediatrics
NYU School of Medicine
Hassenfeld Children's Hospital of New
    York at NYU Langone
New York, NY
Ch 51: Comanagement

Colleen Schelzig, MD, FAAP
Medical Director, Pediatric Hospital
    Medicine
Cleveland Clinic Children's
Cleveland, OH
Ch 92: Ocular Trauma

Helen Maliagros Scott, MD
Assistant Professor of Pediatrics
Northwell Health School of Medicine at
    Hofstra University
Pediatric Hospitalist
Steven and Alexandra Cohen Children's
    Medical Center of New York
New Hyde Park, NY
Ch 28: Intravenous Line Placement

Anand Sekaran, MD, FAAP
Associate Professor of Pediatrics
University of Connecticut School of
    Medicine
Medical Director, Inpatient Services
Connecticut Children's Medical Center
Hartford, CT
Ch 45: Ovarian Torsion

Samir S. Shah, MD, MSCE
Professor, Department of Pediatrics
University of Cincinnati College of
    Medicine
Director, Division of Hospital Medicine
James M. Ewell Endowed Chair
Attending Physician in Hospital Medicine
    and Infectious Diseases
Cincinnati Children's Hospital Medical
    Center
Cincinnati, OH
Ch 97: Osteomyelitis
Ch 98: Septic Arthritis

Anjali Sharma, MD, FAAP
Department of Pediatrics, Section of
  Hospital Medicine
Medical College of Wisconsin
Milwaukee, WI
Ch 81: Acute Weakness

Jacqueline Shiels, PsyD
Psychology Fellow
University of San Diego
San Diego, CA
Ch 101: Suicide

Alyssa Silver, MD, FAAP
Assistant Professor of Pediatrics
Division of Pediatric Hospital Medicine
Children's Hospital at Montefiore
Albert Einstein College of Medicine
Bronx, NY
Ch 8: Myocarditis
Ch 9: Pericarditis

Tamara D. Simon, MD, MSPH, FAAP
Associate Professor of Pediatrics
Divisions of Hospital Medicine and
  General Pediatrics
Department of Pediatrics
University of Washington and Seattle
  Children's Hospital
Associate Program Director, Quality of
  Care Research Fellow
Center for Clinical and Translational
  Research, Seattle Children's
  Research Institute
Seattle, WA
Ch 83: Cerebrospinal Fluid Shunt
  Complications

Geeta Singhal, MD, MEd, FAAP
Associate Professor of Pediatrics
Section of Pediatric Hospital Medicine
Baylor College of Medicine
Houston, TX
Ch 54: Family-Centered Rounds

Jasmine Smith, MD, MBA, FAAP
Clinical Assistant Professor
Department of Child Health
University of Arizona College of Medicine
Phoenix Children's Hospital
Phoenix, AZ
Ch 61: Transition to Adult Care

Loretta Sonnier, MD, FAAP
Assistant Professor
Department of Psychiatry and Behavioral
  Sciences
Tulane University
New Orleans, LA
Ch 99: Acute Agitation

Damani Taylor, MD, FAAP
Staff, Pediatric Pain & Palliative Care Team
  (PACT)
Department of Pediatrics
Memorial Sloan Kettering Cancer Center
New York, NY
Ch 58: Palliative Care

Joel S. Tieder, MD, MPH
Associate Professor of Pediatrics
Division of Hospital Medicine and.
  General Pediatrics
Seattle Children's Hospital
University of Washington School
  of Medicine
Seattle, WA
Ch 108: Brief, Resolved, Unexplained
  Events (Formerly Apparent Life-
  Threatening Events)

Jayne S. Truckenbrod, DO, FAAP
Assistant Professor of Pediatrics
Dell Medical School at the University
  of Texas
Austin, TX
Ch 4: Congestive Heart Failure

Joyee Goswami Vachani, MD, MEd
Assistant Professor of Pediatrics
Section of Pediatric Hospital Medicine
Baylor College of Medicine
Texas Children's Hospital
Houston, TX
Ch 86: Failure to Thrive

Wendy Van Ittersum, MD, FAAP
Assistant Professor of Pediatrics, College
  of Medicine
Division of Pediatric Hospital Medicine
Northeast Ohio Medical University
Akron, OH
Ch 40: Meckel Diverticulum

Contributors/Reviewers

Sindy Villacres, DO, FAAP
Assistant Professor of Pediatrics
Attending Physician, Division of Pediatric
  Critical Care Medicine
Jacobi Medical Center—Albert Einstein
  College of Medicine
Bronx, NY
Ch 115: Pain Management

Colleen M. Wallace, MD, FAAP
Assistant Professor of Pediatrics
Division of Hospital Medicine
Co-Director, Pediatrics Clerkship
Director, Program for Humanities in
  Medicine
Washington University School of Medicine
St Louis, MO
Ch 116: Sedation

Susan C. Walley, MD, CTTS, FAAP
Associate Professor of Pediatrics
Division of Pediatric Hospital Medicine
University of Alabama at Birmingham/
  Children's of Alabama
Birmingham, AL
Ch 104: Acute Asthma Exacerbation

Stephen E. Whitney, MD, MBA, FAAP
Director, MD, MBA Dual Degree Program
Baylor College of Medicine
Texas Children's Hospital
Houston, TX
Ch 55: Leading a Team

Arnaldo Zayas-Santiago, MD, FAAP
Associate Staff
Department of Pediatric Hospital
  Medicine
Cleveland Clinic
Cleveland, OH
Ch 93: Ophthalmoplegia

Derek Zhorne, MD
Assistant Professor of Pediatrics
Division of General Pediatrics and
  Adolescent Medicine
University of Iowa
Iowa City, IA
Ch 20: Peritonsillar Abscess
Ch 21: Retropharyngeal Abscess

Eric Zwemer, MD
Assistant Professor of Pediatrics
University of North Carolina Children's
  Hospital
Chapel Hill, NC
Ch 91: Acute Vision Loss
Ch 95: White Eye (Leukocoria)

American Academy of Pediatrics Reviewers

Board of Directors Reviewer
Warren M. Seigel, MD, MBA, FAAP

Committees, Councils, and Sections
Clinical Practice Guideline Subcommittee
  on Fluid and Electrolyte Therapy
  in Children
Clinical Practice Guideline Subcommittee
  on Urinary Tract Infections
Committee on Adolescence
Committee on Bioethics
Committee on Child Abuse and Neglect
Committee on Child Health Financing
Committee on Drugs
Committee on Medical Liability and
  Risk Management
Committee on Native American Child
  Health
Committee on Nutrition
Committee on Pediatric Emergency
  Medicine
Committee on Psychosocial Aspects of
  Child and Family Health
Council on Children With Disabilities
Council on Genetics
Council on Injury, Violence, and Poison
  Prevention
Council on Quality Improvement and
  Patient Safety
Medical Home Implementation Program
  Advisory Committee
Section on Adolescent Health
Section on Bioethics
Section on Breastfeeding
Section on Cardiology and Cardiac Surgery
Section on Clinical Pharmacology and
  Therapeutics
Section on Critical Care

Section on Developmental and
   Behavioral Pediatrics
Section on Early Career Physicians
Section on Emergency Medicine
Section on Endocrinology
Section on Epidemiology, Public Health,
   and Evidence
Section on Gastroenterology, Hepatology,
   and Nutrition
Section on Hematology/Oncology
Section on Home Care
Section on Hospice and Palliative
   Medicine

Section on Infectious Diseases
Section on Nephrology
Section on Ophthalmology
Section on Otolaryngology/Head and
   Neck Surgery
Section on Pediatric Pulmonology and
   Sleep Medicine
Section on Pediatric Trainees
Section on Surgery
Section on Tobacco Control
Section on Urology

Contents

Adolescent Medicine

Jamie Librizzi, MD, MSHS, FAAP, and Kiranvir Mangat, MD, FAAP

Allergy

Stephanie Jennings, MD, FAAP, and Daniel Rodriguez, MD

Cardiology

Erich Maul, DO, MPH, FAAP

Sonaly Rao McClymont, MD, FAAP, and Jayne S. Truckenbrod, DO, FAAP

Noé D. Romo, MD, MSc

Erich Maul, DO, MPH, FAAP

Lindsey C. Douglas, MD, MS, FAAP

Alyssa Silver, MD, FAAP, and Joanne M. Nazif, MD, FAAP

Joanne M. Nazif, MD, FAAP, and Alyssa Silver, MD, FAAP

Jonathan Lewis, MD, FAAP, and Binita Patel, MD, FAAP

Dermatology

Laurie Bernard Stover, MD, FAAP

Laurie Gordon, MD, MA, FAAP

Equipment and Procedures

Ethics

Gastroenterology

Genetics and Metabolism

Gynecology

Hematology

Hospitalist Practice

Immunology

Infectious Diseases

Ingestions

Liver Diseases

Nephrology

Neurology

Nutrition

Ophthalmology

Orthopedics

Psychiatry

Psychosocial Issues

Pulmonology

Rheumatology

Sedation and Analgesia

Surgery

Preface

Care for the hospitalized child has evolved significantly since the term "hospitalist" was first used over 20 years ago. In most pediatric teaching services, hospitalists care for general pediatric inpatients, but the scope of practice often extends to comanagement of subspecialty and surgical patients, as well as coverage in intensive care units and newborn nurseries. Community hospitals are also employing hospitalists to improve the quality and efficiency of care while expediting admissions from ambulatory physicians who are not able to care for inpatients.

Today's hospitalized children tend to be sicker than before, and care can be more complicated. As a result of pressures from payers, previously well patients must now be more seriously ill to justify admission, while children who require complex care and those who are technology dependent represent an ever-increasing percentage of inpatients. Furthermore, decreasing hospitalization days and lengths of stay have become priorities for both hospitals and insurance companies. At the same time, all parties insist on care that is safe, efficient, timely, cost-effective, patient centered, and equitable. The net result is that providing care for the hospitalized child has become increasingly challenging.

The treatment of pediatric inpatients is addressed in many available resources, including textbooks, handbooks, and online resources. However, very few provide concise, specific, point-of-care recommendations about the most common diagnoses encountered, and none have relied solely on hospitalists as contributors. This book was conceived as a resource written and edited by experts in the field of pediatric hospital medicine, whose primary focus is the care of hospitalized children. The authors all have hands-on experience with their topics and represent leaders in the field. Their practice settings vary from children's hospitals to private community hospitals to general pediatric services in public hospitals, so that their recommendations can be used in any of these settings. The clinical chapters are meant to be directive in immediate care and specific about when to either escalate care or begin discharge planning.

Written specifically for the hospitalist, this book includes chapters beyond just clinical care to address the "whole" of a hospitalist's work. We have included discussions about activities such as leadership, economics, consent, and management of the inpatient service and have incorporated other facets of patient care beyond laboratory tests and treatments. Comprehensive care for hospitalized children must include attention to medical systems, procedures, and ethics, because no sick child exists in a vacuum, and non-bedside activities can have a profound effect on patient outcomes.

No clinical manual, textbook, or online resource can be all-encompassing, and this one is no exception. Every child is unique. Although this book gives specific direction for most cases, no one resource can account for every clinical possibility. We all learn very early in our careers that there are many ways to address a given clinical issue. We present the approaches of our contributors while recognizing that there are many equally satisfactory alternatives.

This second edition includes updates to all chapters and 20 new topics, such as abdominal masses, eating disorders, juvenile idiopathic arthritis, sepsis, and transition to adult care, among others. We are very appreciative of all the comments we received on the first edition. We update the eBook edition as we are made aware of the need, and all prior corrections have been made in this text. Many of the additions were based on reader feedback. We also eliminated coding tips for this edition because of the change from the *International Statistical Classification of Diseases, Ninth Revision (ICD-9)* to the *10th Revision (ICD-10)*. Please continue to let us know your feedback and corrections.

> *Jeffrey C. Gershel, MD, FAAP*
> *Daniel A. Rauch, MD, FAAP, FHM*

Adolescent Medicine

Eating Disorders

Introduction

Most patients admitted to the hospital for an eating disorder have anorexia nervosa (AN), which is a refusal to maintain body weight at or above a minimally normal weight for a person's age and height. The patient may also experience an intense fear of gaining weight or "becoming fat" while being underweight, a disturbance in the way body weight or shape is experienced, self-evaluation that is overly influenced by body shape and weight, and denial of the significance of the current abnormal weight. There are 2 types of anorexia: the restrictive type and the binge-eating and purging type. In the restrictive type, the patient has not engaged in binge-eating or purging during the previous 3 months, whereas in the binge-eating and purging type, the behavior is recurrent in that period. The peak onset of AN occurs at 13 to 18 years of age, with a mortality rate of 5% to 6%.

A newly recognized category of AN is atypical AN. A patient with atypical AN meets all of the criteria for AN but, despite significant weight loss, remains at or above the ideal body weight. As a result of the rapid weight loss, the patient may have the same physical and psychiatric issues as someone who is extremely underweight.

Bulimia nervosa (BN) is recurrent binge eating and recurrent inappropriate compensatory behavior undertaken to prevent weight gain, with both behaviors occurring at least once a week for 3 months. As with AN, self-evaluation is unduly influenced by body shape and weight. Binge eating is defined as eating an amount of food that is significantly larger than what most people would typically ingest in a 2-hour period and is associated with a lack of control over consumption during the episode. Compensatory behavior includes self-induced vomiting; use of laxatives, diuretics, and enemas; fasting; and excessive exercise. BN may be classified as purging (the patient regularly engages in self-induced vomiting or misuse of laxatives, diuretics, or enemas) or non-purging (the patient engages in excessive exercise or fasting, without regular purging behaviors). The peak onset of BN occurs at 16 to 17 years of age, with a mortality rate of 3%.

Clinical Presentation

The clinical presentation and physical examination findings of an eating disorder are a result of 2 factors: the degree of malnutrition and the extent of inappropriate compensatory behaviors. The patient may present with some combination of amenorrhea, irregular menses, weight loss, refusal to eat, weakness, syncope, seizure, edema, hematemesis, constipation, low-impact fracture, and attempted suicide. If the patient also has type 1 diabetes, she may intentionally restrict or omit insulin doses to augment weight loss, potentially leading to diabetic ketoacidosis.

History

Obtain the patient's history with and without the presence of the family or guardian, and then interview the parents separately. Ask about the patient's minimum and maximum weight levels and corresponding height levels. Assess the patient's perception of her ideal weight and her understanding of what a healthy weight is. Note whether she feels guilt when eating and counting calories. Compile a 24-hour diet recall and inquire about any dietary restrictions, portion sizes, caffeine and/or fluid intake, eating rituals, and vegetarianism. Investigate exercise patterns, such as exercising alone in a room or having feelings of stress if an exercise session is missed. Look for secretive behaviors, such as hoarding food; using diuretics, laxatives, diet pills, or enemas; or visiting pro-anorexia or bulimia Web sites. When conducting the patient's social history, probe for sexual or physical abuse, suicidality, and substance use disorder. Elicit any family history of eating disorder, obesity, mental illness, or substance use disorder.

Ask about associated symptoms, such as fatigue, weakness, muscle cramps, dizziness, syncope, chest pain, palpitations, exercise intolerance, fullness, bloating, epigastric pain, abdominal pain, nausea, emesis, reflux, pallor, easy bruising, bleeding, poor wound healing, and intolerance to cold temperatures.

Physical Examination

Perform a thorough physical examination, including plotting the patient's height, weight (in a gown only), and body mass index on growth curves and evaluating the patient for sexual maturity. Assess the patient's vital signs, noting any orthostatic changes. Other evaluation priorities include

- Affect (flat, anxious)
- Body habitus, possibly cachectic with obvious prominences of bone
- Facial wasting
- Thin hair on the scalp
- Signs of induced emesis (scleral hemorrhage, periorbital or palatal petechiae, oral ulcers, dental erosion, loss of gag reflex, calluses on knuckles [Russell sign], and enlarged parotid gland)
- Abdominal shape (scaphoid, distended)
- Abdominal distention from constipation or bloating because of delayed gastric emptying

- Signs of cutting on areas such as the wrists, hips, thighs, and stomach
- Cool extremities and bluish nail beds
- Edema

Laboratory Workup

The goal of the laboratory workup is to identify complications and exclude other differential diagnoses. No test is diagnostic for an eating disorder, and normal laboratory results do not exclude serious illness or medical instability. Order a complete blood cell count to look for anemia, leukopenia, or thrombocytopenia, which can result from bone marrow hypoplasia. Assess magnesium and phosphorous levels and obtain a comprehensive metabolic panel, paying attention to aspartate aminotransferase, alanine aminotransferase, and albumin levels.

In the setting of laxative abuse, hyperchloremic metabolic acidosis, hyperuricemia, hypocalcemia, and elevated transaminase levels can occur. With persistent emesis, a hypokalemic, hypochloremic metabolic alkalosis can be present. Assess thyrotropin and free thyroxine levels to evaluate the presence of euthyroid sick syndrome (low free thyroxine level and normal thyrotropin level). Obtain an electrocardiogram if there are any electrolyte abnormalities, cardiac symptoms, significant purging, or weight loss. Electrocardiographic findings may include bradycardia, low-voltage changes, prolonged corrected QT interval, ST depression, and T-wave inversion.

Perform a urine pregnancy test, and, if the patient is amenorrheic, test prolactin, luteinizing hormone, follicle-stimulating hormone, and estradiol levels. If the patient has been amenorrheic for more than 6 months or if there is a history of recurrent low-impact fractures, order a bone mineral density scan. Osteopenia is considered a bone mineral density level greater than 1.0 SD below normal; osteoporosis is indicated by 2.5 SDs below normal.

The following studies should not be ordered for routine screening, although they may be helpful if the patient's history is not conclusive for an eating disorder: upper gastrointestinal series with small-bowel follow-through, neuroimaging, and celiac blood panel.

Differential Diagnosis

The differential diagnosis of eating disorders is summarized in Table 1-1.

Complications

The most common complications of eating disorders are summarized in Table 1-2. Heart failure and suicide are the most common causes of death.

Table 1-1. Differential Diagnosis of Eating Disorders	
Vomiting	
Diagnosis	**Clinical Features**
Central nervous system lesion	Headache, seizure, visual disturbances
Chronic cholecystitis	Constant right upper quadrant pain
Pancreatitis	Persistent, severe epigastric abdominal pain
Pregnancy	Amenorrhea, fatigue, (+) pregnancy test result
Superior mesenteric artery syndrome	Postprandial epigastric pain with early satiety, bilious emesis
Weight Loss	
Diagnosis	**Clinical Features**
Adrenal insufficiency	Postural dizziness, hypotension, hyperkalemia, hyponatremia, hypercalcemia
Celiac disease	Chronic diarrhea with foul-smelling and/or floating stools, constipation with abdominal distention
Depression	Anhedonia, ↓ appetite, sleep disturbance, feelings of worthlessness or guilt, impaired concentration
Diabetes mellitus	Polyuria, polydipsia, hyperglycemia
HIV	Fever, lymphadenopathy, sore throat, mucocutaneous ulcer, rash, myalgia, night sweats, diarrhea
Hyperthyroidism	Anxiety, emotional lability, weakness, tremor, palpitations, heat intolerance, ↑ perspiration
Inflammatory bowel disease	Bloody diarrhea, colicky abdominal pain, urgency, tenesmus, incontinence, and hypotension
Substance abuse	Needle marks, skin infections, unexplained burns, atrophy of nasal mucosa

"+" indicates a positive finding.

Refeeding Syndrome

Refeeding syndrome is primarily caused by total body phosphorous depletion during the starving state, leading to hypophosphatemia, hypokalemia, and hypomagnesemia. With reintroduction of carbohydrates into the diet, insulin is released, which facilitates uptake of phosphorous, potassium, and magnesium and causes a shift of the oxygen dissociation curve to the right with subsequent tissue hypoxia. This compromises cardiac and respiratory function because of decreased contractility. If refeeding syndrome is not diagnosed and managed expeditiously, it may lead to potentially fatal congestive heart failure and respiratory failure.

Treatment

The goals of hospitalization include vital sign and electrolyte stabilization, reversal of medical complications, monitoring for refeeding syndrome,

Table 1-2. Common Complications of Eating Disorders	
Organ System	**Complications**
Cardiac	Bradycardia Conduction abnormalities Mitral valve prolapse Pericardial effusion Congestive heart failure
Electrolyte	Refeeding syndrome: ↓ potassium, phosphate, magnesium levels ↓ or ↑ sodium level ↓ potassium level
Endocrine	Anovulation Growth retardation Euthyroid sick syndrome Vitamin D deficiency
Gastrointestinal	Esophagitis, Mallory-Weiss tear Constipation Delayed gastric emptying, leading to bloating Superior mesenteric artery syndrome Rectal prolapse
Hematologic	Bone marrow hypoplasia
Neurologic	Peripheral neuropathy Seizures In AN: cortical atrophy, ventriculomegaly, white/gray matter loss
Orthopedic	Osteopenia
Psychiatric	Suicidal ideation Comorbid disorders include anxiety, depression, and substance abuse.
Pulmonary	In BN: pneumomediastinum and aspiration pneumonia
Renal	Nephrolithiasis In AN: concentrating defect (polyuria) In BN: sodium and water retention (edema)

Abbreviations: AN, anorexia nervosa; BN, bulimia nervosa.

initiation of weight gain, and reintroducing healthy eating behaviors. These goals require a multidisciplinary approach, with involvement of the medical team, nutritionist, social worker, therapist, and psychiatrist, and typically requires 7 to 10 days of inpatient treatment. Nutritional rehabilitation is the key to management of reversible complications. Basic steps in treatment include the following:

- Consult with the appropriate specialists (in nutrition, gastroenterology, adolescent medicine, and endocrinology) to develop and implement an eating disorder protocol with a behavior plan and contract.
- Search the patient's belongings for laxatives, diuretics, diet pills, chewing gum, and exercise weights. Do not allow the patient Internet and cell phone access.

- Perform suicidality screening and arrange for the patient to have a one-on-one sitter or nurse.
- Insert an intravenous catheter for emergency access in case of complications.
- Initially, keep the patient on bed rest; then, upgrade the patient's activity level according to stability of vital signs—but do not permit exercise.
- Obtain the patient's weight in the morning (in a gown only), after voiding; if being weighed heightens the patient's anxiety level, this can be performed with the patient blinded to the result.
- Limit meals to 30 minutes in the patient's room, with no visitors present.
- Restrict bathroom access for 1 hour after meals and instruct the patient to not flush the toilet after use, so the staff can evaluate the toilet for signs of purging.

If the patient is refusing to be fed orally, nasogastric (NG) tube placement is necessary. A nasal bridle may be placed with the NG tube to secure it from dislodgement if there is concern that the patient will remove it. Rarely, if the patient is not tolerating feedings, central line placement and total parenteral nutrition should to be initiated. Address the patient's hydration status and monitor fluid intake, if inadequate. Unless medically necessary, limit rapid fluid infusion because it can cause cardiac compromise. Cardiac monitoring with telemetry is necessary for patients with bradycardia or other forms of dysrhythmia.

Refeeding syndrome most commonly manifests in the first week of nutritional rehabilitation and can last for 2 weeks. Check daily phosphorous, magnesium, and potassium levels; monitor strict fluid intake and output; assess the patient for edema; and order continuous cardiorespiratory monitoring. Address nutritional deficiencies, such as thiamine or phosphorous levels, with the appropriate supplementation.

Do not order pharmacotherapy routinely; however, medication may be indicated for a patient with a comorbid psychiatric diagnosis. Oral contraceptives and bisphosphonates do not help to restore bone mineral density.

Disposition

- **Intensive care unit monitoring:** Dysrhythmia, severe bradycardia, severe electrolyte abnormality, congestive heart failure.
- **Discharge criteria:** Once the patient is medically stable, disposition is variable and depends on the appropriate resources available to the patient. Options include an intensive outpatient program, partial hospitalization programs (6 hours a day), and residential programs that provide intense therapy and nutritional counseling with an in-house physician.

Follow-up

- **Primary care:** Weekly for weight checks and monitoring for refeeding syndrome. Refer the patient to an adolescent medicine specialist if the primary care physician is not comfortable coordinating care.
- **Psychotherapy:** As recommended by the treating psychologist or psychiatrist.

Pearls and Pitfalls

- Amenorrhea is no longer part of the diagnostic criteria for anorexia.
- Fluid retention can occur after laxative cessation, with up to a 4.5-kg (10-lb) weight gain in 24 hours.
- Edema can last up to 3 weeks.
- Refeeding syndrome most commonly manifests in the first week of nutritional rehabilitation and can last for 2 weeks.
- Identify comorbid psychiatric illness (including suicidal ideation) or substance abuse.
- Do not order selective serotonin reuptake inhibitors for anorexia alone.
- Heart failure and suicide are the most common causes of death.
- It can be a challenge to obtain inpatient and outpatient services.
- Avoid discharging the patient on Fridays or weekends to ensure that adequate follow-up occurs.

Bibliography

Academy for Eating Disorders. Eating disorders: critical points for early recognition and medical risk management in the care of individuals with eating disorders. 2nd ed. Updated 2012. http://www.aedweb.org/downloads/Guide-English.pdf. Accessed January 18, 2017

American Psychiatric Association. *Feeding and Eating Disorders: DSM-5 Selections.* Arlington, VA: American Psychiatric Publishing; 2015

Campbell K, Peebles R. Eating disorders in children and adolescents: state of the art review. *Pediatrics.* 2014;134(3):582–592

Goldstein MA, Dechant EJ, Beresin EV. Eating disorders. *Pediatr Rev.* 2011;32(12): 508–521

Rosen DS; American Academy of Pediatrics Committee on Adolescence. Clinical report—identification and management of eating disorders in children and adolescents. *Pediatrics.* 2010;126(6):1240–1253

Allergy

Anaphylaxis

Introduction

The term *anaphylaxis* applies to anaphylactic (immunoglobulin E [IgE]–mediated) and anaphylactoid (non–IgE-mediated) release of immune mediators from basophils and mast cells. It is a severe, potentially fatal, multi–organ system allergic reaction. Therefore, it is imperative to recognize the signs and symptoms of anaphylaxis and treat it rapidly. The most common triggers are peanuts, tree nuts, and shellfish, although anaphylaxis in an inpatient may be triggered by exposure to latex, radiocontrast material, medications, or foods (Table 2-1).

As many as 15% to 20% of patients will have a biphasic response, with most occurring within 1 to 8 hours after the initial reaction has abated. Risk factors for a biphasic reaction are age of 6 to 9 years, a delay of more than 90 minutes in the initial presentation of symptoms, and widened pulse pressure at presentation, as well as acute treatment that requires more than 1 dose of epinephrine and albuterol. Protracted anaphylaxis (occurring for up to 72 hours) is rare and usually occurs when there is continued exposure to the trigger.

Table 2-1. Agents That Can Trigger Anaphylaxis in the Inpatient Setting

Trigger	Examples
Medication	Antibiotics (β-lactam antibiotics, sulfonamides), neuromuscular blocking agents, nonsteroidal anti-inflammatory drugs, opioids
Food	Egg whites, fish and shellfish, milk, peanuts, sesame, soy, tree nuts (pecans, pistachios, walnuts), mammalian meat
Hormone	Estrogen, progesterone
Infusion	Blood transfusion; infusion of dextran, infliximab, intravenous immunoglobulin, radiocontrast material
Latex	Balloons, gloves
Physiological factor	Cold, exercise, heat, pressure, sunlight

Clinical Presentation

History

The patient usually presents with some combination of flushing, pruritus, urticaria and/or angioedema, tightness of the throat, respiratory distress, vomiting and/or diarrhea, and a sense of impending doom (Table 2-2). Ask the patient about possible triggers, location and timing of events that led up to the anaphylaxis, and history of atopy or prior episodes of anaphylaxis, as well

Table 2-2. Presentation of Anaphylaxis	
Organ System	**Presentation**
Cardiovascular	Hypotension, syncope, arrhythmias, chest pain
Central nervous	Confusion, dizziness, light-headedness, behavior changes, headache, seizures
Gastrointestinal	Nausea, abdominal pain, vomiting, diarrhea
Mucocutaneous	Urticaria, angioedema, flushing, pruritus without rash, diaphoresis
Respiratory	Cough, stridor, dyspnea, wheezing, rhinitis
Other	Sense of impending doom, rhinitis, metallic taste in the mouth

as treatment administered (especially use of an epinephrine auto-injector) and whether the patient is taking any chronic medications—particularly a β-blocker—which can worsen symptoms and decrease response to epinephrine.

Physical Examination

Perform a rapid examination to assess vital signs, airway patency, respiratory sufficiency, cardiac rhythm, and mental status. The most frequently involved organ system is the skin, followed by the respiratory system and the gastro-intestinal tract (including the oral mucosa).

Differential Diagnosis

By definition, the diagnosis of anaphylaxis is based on specific signs and symptoms of the involvement of at least 2 organ systems (Table 2-3). If any of the following 3 criteria are present, the diagnosis of anaphylaxis is likely:

- Rapid onset of illness that involves hives and/or mucosal changes, along with any of the following conditions:
  — Respiratory compromise
  — Cardiovascular involvement
  — Evidence of end-organ dysfunction
- Two or more organ systems involved after a known allergen exposure
- Hypotension that occurs minutes to hours after an allergen exposure

Treatment

Anaphylaxis is a medical emergency and requires immediate care and atten-tion. Address the CABs—chest compressions, airway, and breathing—and provide oxygen as needed, discontinue all in-going intravenous (IV) anti-biotics or contrast material infusions, avoid any latex products, remove any indwelling latex catheters, and begin continuous cardiorespiratory monitoring and pulse oximetry. If the patient has stridor at rest or respiratory compromise despite the administration of epinephrine (see the following section), prepare

Table 2-3. Differential Diagnosis of Anaphylaxis	
Diagnosis	**Clinical Features**
Angioedema	Swelling of the face, neck, and extremities without pruritus No acute respiratory or cardiovascular symptoms
Asthma	Patient may have had previous similar episodes No acute dermatologic, GI, or cardiovascular symptoms
Cardiac tamponade	Muffled heart sounds and presence of pericardial friction rub No acute dermatologic or GI symptoms
Cholinergic urticaria	Urticaria and wheezing occurring within 30 min of vigorous exercise
Croup	Barking cough, stridor, fever No acute dermatologic, GI, or cardiovascular symptoms
Food poisoning and scombroid poisoning	Vomiting, diarrhea, possible flushing No acute dermatologic, respiratory, or cardiovascular symptoms
Mastocytosis	Most often involves the skin Patient may have bone marrow and solid organ infiltration
Neuroendocrine tumor	Predominantly GI symptoms with intermittent flushing ↑ Catecholamine levels, vasoactive intestinal polypeptide levels, neurokinin levels
Panic attack	Feeling of impending doom No acute dermatologic symptoms
Red man syndrome	Infusion with vancomycin may mimic anaphylaxis Slowing the rate of infusion decreases symptoms
Urticaria	No acute GI, respiratory, or cardiovascular symptoms

Abbreviation: GI, gastrointestinal.

to intubate. Place a hypotensive patient in the supine position, with elevation of the lower extremities. Note that treatment may prove especially challenging if the patient is taking a β-blocker.

Epinephrine

Epinephrine is the first and most important treatment for anaphylaxis; there are no contraindications. It will reverse peripheral vasodilatation and bronchoconstriction, decrease angioedema and urticaria, decrease upper airway edema, enhance myocardial contractility, and suppress further release of immune mediators from mast cells and basophils.

Normotensive patient: Administer 0.01 mL per kilogram of body weight (0.5-mL maximum) of *1:1,000* epinephrine *intramuscularly* into the lateral thigh. Repeat the dose every 5 to 15 minutes, as needed.

Hypotensive patient: Arrange for transfer of the patient to an intensive care unit and administer 0.01 mg/kg (0.1 mL/kg, 10-mL maximum) of *1:10,000* epinephrine *intravenously*. Repeat every 3 to 5 minutes. In the absence of IV access, administer 0.01 mg/kg of *1:1,000* epinephrine *intramuscularly* (0.1 mL/kg, 3-mL maximum). If the patient remains hypotensive, initiate an IV drip, starting with 0.1 µg/kg/min (1.5-µg/kg/min maximum).

Vasopressor Infusion

If the patient remains hypotensive despite epinephrine administration and volume repletion, start a dopamine drip (2–20 µg/kg/min).

Antihistamines

H_1- and H_2-antihistamines block the effect of circulating histamines but do not exert an immediate effect or decrease further mediator release. Antihistamines are therefore secondary treatment, and epinephrine administration is still necessary. Administer *(a)* IV or oral diphenhydramine ([H_1-antihistamine] 1–2 mg/kg, every 6 hours; maximum, 100 mg per dose) *or* oral hydroxyzine ([H1-antihistamine] 2 mg/kg/d, divided into doses administered every 6–8 hours, 100-mg/d maximum) *(b) plus* IV or oral ranitidine ([H_2-antihistamine] 2 mg/kg, administered every 6–8 hours, 50-mg maximum).

Albuterol

If the patient continues to experience bronchospasm after epinephrine administration, treat with nebulized albuterol (0.15 mg/kg per dose, 2.5-mg minimum, 10-mg maximum), hourly or continuously.

Corticosteroids

Administer either IV or oral methylprednisolone or oral prednisone (1–2 mg/kg/d divided into doses administered every 6 hours, 80-mg/d maximum) for 3 days. This will decrease the risk of recurrent or protracted anaphylaxis but has no effect on the immediate reaction.

Glucagon

A patient taking β-blockers will have a limited response to epinephrine, which increases the risk for bronchospasm, hypotension, and paradoxical bradycardia. Administer an IV loading dose of 20 to 30 µg/kg (1-mg maximum) over 5 minutes, followed by a continuous infusion of 5 to 15 µg/min by titrating the dose to the ideal blood pressure. Glucagon may cause emesis, with subsequent risk of aspiration in a drowsy or obtunded patient, which necessitates airway protection.

Indications for Consultation

Allergist: First or severe episode of anaphylaxis, recurrent anaphylaxis, unknown anaphylaxis origin or allergen exposure, systemic reaction to hymenoptera venom.

Disposition

- **Intensive care unit transfer:** Severe respiratory distress requiring intubation, continuous epinephrine drip needed, hypotension requiring vasopressor infusion, patient has taken a β-blocker.
- **Discharge criteria**
  — The patient is normotensive, without respiratory distress or end-organ dysfunction, and is taking oral therapy after a 24-hour observation period.
  — The patient and/or family has a prescription for an epinephrine auto-injector and is educated about its use (carry 2 injectors stored at room temperature, administer through the clothing at the anterolateral aspect of the thigh, and avoid holding the thumb over the tip of the applicator).
  — The patient and/or family is aware of the importance of avoiding triggers, including cross-reacting substances.
  — The patient and/or family has been instructed on how to order a MedicAlert bracelet (888/633-4298 or www.medicalert.org).

Discharge Management

- Continue the H_1- and H_2-antihistamines for 2 to 3 days after discharge.
- Stop the administration of glucocorticoids after 3 days, without a taper.

Follow-up

- **Allergist:** 2 to 3 weeks
- **Primary care:** 2 to 3 days

Pearls and Pitfalls

- Resuscitation will be challenging if the patient is taking a β-blocker.
- Anaphylaxis can be triggered by exposure to foods or medications during an inpatient service.
- Response may be seen as late as 72 hours after allergen exposure.
- A biphasic response occurs most commonly within 8 hours after resolution of initial symptoms.

Bibliography

Alqurashi W, Stiell I, Chan K, Neto G, Alsadoon A, Wells G. Epidemiology and clinical predictors of biphasic reactions in children. *Ann Allergy Asthma Immunol.* 2015;115(3):217–223

Golden DB. Anaphylaxis to insect stings. *Immunol Allergy Clin North Am.* 2015;35(2):287–302

Greenhawt M. The Learning Early About Peanut Allergy study: the benefits of early peanut introduction, and a new horizon in fighting the food allergy epidemic. *Pediatr Clin North Am.* 2015;62(6):1509–1521

Sicherer SH, Leung DY. Advances in allergic skin disease, anaphylaxis, and hypersensitivity reactions to foods, drugs, and insects in 2014. *J Allergy Clin Immunol.* 2015;135(2):357–367

Sicherer SH, Sampson HA. Food allergy: epidemiology, pathogenesis, diagnosis, and treatment. *J Allergy Clin Immunol.* 2014;133(2):291–307

Cardiology

Arrhythmias

Introduction

Arrhythmias are encountered in 2 types of inpatients. One is the patient with a history of known or recently diagnosed heart disease who is admitted for medical or surgical treatment or for management of a complication from the heart disease or its treatment. In the second type of patient, the arrhythmia either is an incidental finding or is related to a non–cardiac disease process, such as hyperthyroidism, fever, electrolyte abnormality, toxic ingestion, or medication side effect.

Clinical Presentation

When a child presents with a suspected arrhythmia (Table 3-1), it is critical to focus on the history and physical examination findings. The amount of detail obtained depends on how stable the patient is. In an unstable patient, perform a directed history and examination, so as not to delay the administration of lifesaving treatment.

History

A patient with an arrhythmia can present in a variety of ways, depending on his or her age and underlying heart rhythm and/or heart disease. An infant may have nonspecific signs and symptoms, such as tachypnea, diaphoresis and/or cyanosis during feeding, irritability, and inconsolability. An older patient may complain of chest pain, nausea, palpitations, syncope or near syncope, or shortness of breath. A patient of any age may present with cardio-vascular collapse.

Have the patient or family describe the current episode and any previous similar episodes. Assess the patient for other symptoms, including chest pain, light-headedness, dyspnea, palpitations, fatigue, irritability, and altered mental status. Ask about recent illnesses and review any medications or possible ingestions. Determine the patient's medical history, especially if there are any chronic illnesses or a family history of heart disease or sudden or unexplained death.

Physical Examination

Perform a directed physical examination, focusing on the vital signs and CABs—chest compressions, airway, and breathing—to determine if the patient is hemodynamically stable. A stable patient has a maintainable airway,

Chapter 3: Arrhythmias

Table 3-1. Electrocardiographic Findings in Arrhythmias

Heart Rate (bpm)	Heart Rhythm	PR Interval	QRS Interval	Causes
Asystole				
0	None	Absent	Absent	See Box 3-1
Atrial fibrillation				
Atrial, 350–600; ventricular, variable	Irregularly irregular	Absent; fibrillation waves present	Normal	Cardiac surgery, valvular or ischemic disease, idiopathic origin, WPW
Atrial flutter				
Atrial, 240–360; ventricular, depends on degree of block (2:1–4:1)	Saw-toothed flutter waves with regular ventricular conduction at a fixed ratio (2:1–4:1)	Absent	Normal	Same as atrial fibrillation
First-degree AV block				
Normal for age	Regular	Prolonged for age	Normal	Normal variant, ARF, CM, CHD, digitalis toxicity, CTD
Second-degree AV block type I				
Normal for age	Progressive lengthening of PR interval until nonconduction of a QRS	Progressively lengthening	Normal	Normal variant, myocarditis, CM, CHD, AMI, SLE, Lyme disease, digitalis or β-blocker toxicity
Second-degree AV block type II				
Normal to bradycardic for age	AV conduction cycles between normal and complete block, resulting in dropped QRS (blocked P wave)	Normal, fixed duration	Normal	Same as type I
Third-degree AV block				
Dissociation between atrial and ventricular heart rates; heart rate of P wave > QRS	Heart rate of P waves and QRSs are regular but independent of each other	Variable	Normal in congenital cases; prolonged in acquired cases	Congenital causes include (a) maternal SLE or CTD and (b) CHD; acquired causes include ARF, myocarditis, Lyme disease, CM, AMI, and digitalis toxicity

Table 3-1. Electrocardiographic Findings in Arrhythmias, continued

Heart Rate (bpm)	Heart Rhythm	PR Interval	QRS Interval	Causes
Long QT syndrome				
Normal for age	Regular; prolonged QTc interval >0.45; can lead to ventricular ectopy or TdP	Normal	Normal	Acquired causes include drug toxicity, and ↓potassium, ↓calcium, and ↓magnesium levels; congenital causes include JLNS, RWS, various channelopathies
Sinus arrhythmia				
Normal for age	Regularly irregular; rhythm changes with respirations	Normal	Normal	Normal respiration
Sinus bradycardia				
Infant, <80; child, <60	Regular	Normal	Normal	Normal in athletes; ↑ ICP; see Box 3-1
Sinus tachycardia				
Infant, 140–200; child, 120–180	Regular	Normal	Normal	Shock, sepsis, pain, fever, anxiety, AMI, drug toxicity
Supraventricular tachycardia				
Infant, >220; child, >180	Regular, does not vary	Masked by tachycardia	Normal	Idiopathic origin, CHD, postoperative origin
Ventricular fibrillation				
150–300	Chaotic, no organized electric activity	Absent	Absent	See Box 3-1
Ventricular tachycardia				
120–200, with ≥3 consecutive PVCs	Regular, beat-to-beat variability	Masked by tachycardia	Widened	Myocarditis, AMI, CM, LQTS, CHD, drug toxicity; see Box 3-1

Abbreviations: AMI, acute myocardial infarction; ARF, acute rheumatic fever; AV, atrioventricular; bpm, beats per minute; CHD, congenital heart disease; CM, cardiomyopathy; CTD, connective tissue disease; ICP, intracranial pressure; JLNS, Jervell and Lange-Nielsen syndrome; LQTS, long QT syndrome; PVC, premature ventricular contractions; QTc, corrected QT interval; RWS, Romano-Ward syndrome; SLE, systemic lupus erythematosus; TdP, torsades de pointes; WPW, Wolff-Parkinson-White syndrome.

minimal to no respiratory distress, and adequate perfusion. *Adequate perfusion* is defined as appropriate mental status, capillary refill test time of less than 2 seconds, appropriate blood pressure for the patient's age, normal oxygen saturation, and adequate urine output. Auscultate for breath sounds, as well as heart rate, rhythm, murmur, and additional sounds, such as clicks or gallops. Check for hepatosplenomegaly, jugular venous distention, and peripheral edema.

Treatment of Specific Arrhythmias

If the patient is stable, there is time to systematically evaluate the situation. Many arrhythmias have underlying reversible causes, for which the American Heart Association has coined the mnemonic of "H's and T's" (Box 3-1). It is imperative that these conditions are diagnosed and treated.

Box 3-1. The "H's and T's" of the Reversible Causes of Arrhythmias	
Hypovolemia	**T**ension pneumothorax
Hypoxia	**T**amponade (cardiac)
Hydrogen ion (acidosis)	**T**oxins
Hypoglycemia	**T**hrombosis, pulmonary
Hypokalemia, **H**yperkalemia	**T**hrombosis, coronary
Hypothermia	

From Neumar RW, Otto CW, Link MS, et al. 2010 American Heart Association guidelines for cardiopulmonary resuscitation and emergency cardiovascular care. Part 8: adult advanced cardiovascular life support. *Circulation*. 2010;122(18 Suppl 3):S729–S767.

Asystole

Confirm that the monitor leads are properly attached to the patient's chest and the monitor; then, change the monitor lead setting and confirm asystole with a second lead. Initiate cardiopulmonary resuscitation (CPR), secure an airway, obtain intravenous (IV) or intraosseous (IO) access, and provide oxygen and adequate ventilation.

Administer 0.01 mg/kg (1-mg maximum) of *1:10,000* epinephrine intravenously or via IO infusion, followed by 5 to 10 mL of normal saline. If there is no IV or IO access, use 0.1 mg/kg (3-mg maximum) of *1:1,000* epinephrine, followed by 5 to 10 mL of physiological (normal) saline solution via the endotracheal tube every 3 to 5 minutes until vascular access is achieved.

Atrial Fibrillation and Atrial Flutter

Investigate whether underlying medical conditions are present. The goals are to convert the atrial rhythm, control the ventricular response, and prevent recurrences. The approach varies, depending on the patient's clinical status.

In an acute, life-threatening situation, attempt cardioversion (0.5–1.0 J/kg). Consult with a pediatric cardiologist to initiate anticoagulation with heparin and ventricular rate control with digoxin, a β-blocker, or a calcium channel blocker. If the patient is stable with atrial fibrillation or flutter of unknown duration, consult with a pediatric cardiologist and delay cardioversion until adequate anticoagulation has been achieved.

First-degree Atrioventricular Block

In cases of first-degree atrioventricular (AV) block, no treatment is needed except in the setting of structural heart disease and drug toxicity.

Second-degree AV Block, Type I

In cases of second-degree AV block, type I, treat the underlying disease that is causing the arrhythmia.

Second-degree AV Block, Type II

In cases of second-degree AV block, type II, treat the underlying disorder. Be aware that this arrhythmia has a high risk for progression to third-degree AV block. Consult a pediatric cardiologist for potential pacemaker placement.

Third-degree AV Block

In cases of third-degree AV block, treat the patient with IV atropine at a dose of 0.02 mg/kg every 5 minutes for 2 to 3 doses (minimum single dose, 0.1 mg; maximum single dose, 0.5 mg in children and 1 mg in adolescents; maximum total dose, 1 mg for children and 2 mg for adolescents). Use this intervention to increase the heart rate while arranging for transcutaneous or transvenous cardiac pacing until a permanent pacemaker can be placed. Indications for pacemaker therapy include

- Signs and symptoms of congestive heart failure
- Infants with a structurally normal heart and a ventricular rate less than 50 beats per minute (bpm)
- Infants with structural heart disease and a ventricular rate less than 70 bpm
- Patients with a wide QRS escape rhythm, ventricular ectopy, or ventricular dysfunction

Long QT Syndrome

If the patient presents with ventricular ectopy or torsades de pointes, begin basic life support, evaluate serum electrolyte levels, and begin administration of IV magnesium sulfate at a dose of 25 to 50 mg/kg (2-g maximum). Contact a pediatric cardiologist and monitor the patient closely, because further resuscitation may be required.

If the long QT interval is an incidental finding or is discovered during the evaluation for syncope, investigate reversible causes, such as medications (most commonly macrolides, azole antifungal agents, antipsychotic agents, or fluoroquinolones). A comprehensive list can be found at www.crediblemeds. org. Refer the patient to a pediatric cardiologist if the QT interval does not normalize.

If congenital long QT syndrome is suspected, refer the patient to a pediatric cardiologist and arrange for all first-degree relatives to undergo screening. Coordinate long-term therapies with the cardiology staff.

Symptomatic Sinus Bradycardia

Initiate basic life support, obtain IV or IO access, provide oxygen, and place the patient on a monitor. Assess the patient for reversible causes (H's and T's) and treat the underlying disease. Start transcutaneous pacing, if readily available. Otherwise, treat the patient with epinephrine, as described for asystole.

If there is increased vagal tone or if the patient has an AV block, administer atropine, as described earlier for third-degree AV block. Situations where increased vagal tone is encountered include myocardial disease, hypoglycemia, hypothyroidism, increased intracranial pressure, sick sinus syndrome, and potassium abnormalities. Numerous drugs, such as digoxin and β-blockers, can also cause increased vagal tone.

Supraventricular Tachycardia

In the event of supraventricular tachycardia (SVT), initiate basic life support, obtain IV or IO access, provide oxygen, and place the patient on a monitor. Assess the patient for reversible causes (H's and T's) and treat the underlying disease. Initial treatment depends on whether or not the patient is well perfused.

If the patient is well perfused, initially attempt vagal maneuvers, such as covering the face with a bag of slushy ice water or attempting a Valsalva maneuver. If unsuccessful, administer adenosine as a 0.1-mg/kg rapid IV push (6-mg maximum), with the syringe as close to the IV site as possible, followed by a rapid IV push of 5 to 10 mL of normal saline. A stopcock can be used to facilitate the rapid infusion of the adenosine and the flush. If the first dose is not successful, repeat as a 0.2-mg/kg rapid IV push (12-mg maximum). If the second dose of adenosine does not convert the rhythm, administer another 0.2-mg/kg rapid IV push (12-mg maximum). If the SVT persists, consult a pediatric cardiologist to discuss the next step (administration of additional antiarrhythmic agents or synchronized cardioversion).

If the patient is poorly perfused, perform synchronized cardioversion at 0.5 to 1.0 J/kg. If unsuccessful, increase to 2.0 J/kg. If cardioversion is unsuccessful or if SVT recurs, consult with a cardiologist whenever possible and administer either IV amiodarone at 5 mg/kg over 20 to 60 minutes or IV procainamide at 15 mg/kg over 30 to 60 minutes. Be prepared to treat bradycardia or other dysrhythmias that may result after amiodarone or procainamide administration.

Ventricular Fibrillation

In the event of ventricular fibrillation (VF), initiate basic life support, obtain IV or IO access, provide oxygen, ensure adequate ventilation, and place the patient on a monitor. Once VF is noted, proceed to immediate defibrillation. Administer a single shock of 2 J/kg, followed by 2 minutes of CPR; a second shock of 4 J/kg should be followed by 2 minutes of CPR; subsequent shocks of 4 J/kg or greater to a maximum of 10 J/kg or adult levels of energy can be further administered. After the second defibrillation attempt, administer epinephrine every 3 to 5 minutes, as for asystole. After the third defibrillation attempt, start administration of an antiarrhythmic agent, either amiodarone (5-mg/kg IV or IO bolus; may be repeated twice for refractory VF or pulseless VT) or lidocaine as a 1-mg/kg IV or IO bolus. Continue cycles of the "CPR shock drug" until there is return of spontaneous circulation, a rhythm change, or termination of resuscitative efforts.

Ventricular Tachycardia

If ventricular tachycardia (VT) occurs, initiate basic life support, obtain IV or IO access, provide oxygen, ensure adequate ventilation, and place the patient on a monitor. If the patient is pulseless, treat with an approach identical to that used for VF. If the patient has a pulse and poor perfusion, use synchronized cardioversion, as for SVT. Consult a pediatric cardiologist or intensivist to assist with further management (including possible procainamide infusion or synchronized cardioversion).

If the patient has a pulse and good perfusion, administer IV amiodarone (5 mg/kg over 20 minutes) or consult a pediatric cardiologist to assist with further management (including possible procainamide infusion or synchronized cardioversion).

Disposition

- **Intensive care unit transfer:** Life-threatening arrhythmias (VF, VT, sustained SVT, symptomatic bradycardia, AV block of second-degree type II and higher, atrial flutter or fibrillation, asystole).
- **Discharge criteria:** Hemodynamically stable and placed on a regimen that can be managed at home.

Indications for Consultation

Pediatric cardiology: Life-threatening arrhythmias (as discussed earlier), long QT interval, SVT, heart block

Pearls and Pitfalls

- The stability of the patient determines how rapidly the arrhythmia should be treated.
- Always confirm asystole with 2 different leads.
- Symptomatic bradycardia of less than 60 bpm in any age group requires initiation of CPR.
- Suspect SVT when age-specific rate criteria are exceeded and there is no beat-to-beat variability of the rhythm. Signs and symptoms of SVT can be very nonspecific in infants.
- Second-degree AV block, type II, has a high risk of progression to complete AV block. Be prepared to pace the patient's heart, should this deterioration occur.

Bibliography

Biondi EA. Focus on diagnosis: cardiac arrhythmias in children. *Pediatr Rev.* 2010;31(9): 375–379

de Caen AR, Berg MD, Chameides L, et al. Part 12: Pediatric Advanced Life Support: 2015 American Heart Association Guidelines Update for Cardiopulmonary Resuscitation and Emergency Cardiovascular Care. *Circulation.* 2015;132(18 Suppl 2):S526–S542

Marzuillo P, Benettoni A, Germani C, Ferrara G, D'Agata B, Barbi E. Acquired long QT syndrome: a focus for the general pediatrician. *Pediatr Emerg Care.* 2014;30(4):257–261

Park M. Cardiac arrhythmias. In: *Park's Pediatric Cardiology for Practitioners.* 6th ed. Philadelphia, PA: Mosby Elsevier; 2014:407–435

Park M. Disturbances of atrioventricular conduction. In: *Park's Pediatric Cardiology for Practitioners.* 6th ed. Philadelphia, PA: Mosby Elsevier; 2014:436–439

CHAPTER 4

Congestive Heart Failure

Introduction

Congestive heart failure (CHF) is the inability of the heart to meet the metabolic demands of the body. Rather than a single disease entity, CHF represents a constellation of signs and symptoms that arise from a number of origins. The most common causes of CHF in children are congenital heart disease (CHD), cardiomyopathies (genetic, acquired, and inherited metabolic or muscle disorders; infectious diseases; drugs; toxins; Kawasaki disease; and autoimmune diseases), and myocardial dysfunction after surgical repair of heart defects. Other causes include arrhythmias and cardiac valve disease. Regardless of the origins of CHF, the resulting pathophysiological syndrome requires immediate attention, supportive care, and prompt cardiologist consultation.

Clinical Presentation

History

Infants

Feeding difficulty is the most prominent symptom and is often associated with tachycardia, tachypnea, and diaphoresis. Poor feeding ultimately leads to failure to thrive.

Children/Adolescents

Toddlers and older children often exhibit fatigue; exercise intolerance; poor appetite; abdominal complaints, such as nausea and vomiting; and growth failure. Adolescents may have additional symptoms that are similar to those of adults, including shortness of breath, orthopnea, nocturnal dyspnea, abdominal pain, and chronic cough.

Physical Examination

All age groups typically present with tachycardia and tachypnea. Hepatomegaly is an early finding, and if the enlargement is relatively acute, there may be flank pain or tenderness due to stretching of the liver capsule. Mild to moderate disease may appear with no distress at presentation, while a patient with severe disease may be dyspneic at rest. With an acute onset, the patient may appear anxious but well nourished, versus calm yet malnourished with chronic CHF.

An infant with severe disease may have nasal flaring, retractions, grunting, and—occasionally—wheezing. Rales are rare in an infant unless there is coexisting pneumonia. An infant with low cardiac output may have cool and/ or mottled extremities, a weakly palpable pulse, a narrow pulse pressure, and delayed capillary refill.

While uncommon in an infant, signs of increased systemic venous pressure may be exhibited in an older child, including distention of neck veins (venous pulsations visible above the clavicle while the patient is sitting) and peripheral edema (particularly in the face and dependent parts of the body). Low cardiac output may cause peripheral vasoconstriction that leads to cool extremities, pallor, cyanosis, and delayed capillary refill. With more advanced disease, pulmonary edema and rales are more likely.

The cardiac examination findings can be variable, depending on the etiology of disease. In cardiomyopathy, there is usually a quiet precordium. Shunt lesions (ventricular septal defect, patent ductus arteriosus) usually cause a hyperdynamic precordium. Obstructive lesions (aortic stenosis, coarctation of the aorta) may have a systolic thrill. A third heart sound in mid-diastole can be a normal finding in children but is noted more frequently in those with heart disease. Regardless of the etiology of heart failure, a holosystolic murmur of mitral regurgitation is often present with advanced disease.

Laboratory Workup

Standard testing to determine the etiology of CHF includes chest radiography, electrocardiography (ECG), and echocardiography. Chest radiographs will usually show cardiac enlargement, with or without evidence of pulmonary venous congestion. The presence of pulmonary congestion depends on the etiology of disease. It is less likely in early cardiomyopathy but more common with a left-to-right shunt or advanced disease. Echocardiography is the primary diagnostic modality for confirming the etiology of CHF (ie, ventricular dysfunction, anatomic abnormality). In contrast, ECG, while almost always yielding an abnormal finding, is generally not useful in the diagnosis of heart failure but may provide clues to the etiology.

If it is difficult to determine whether a patient is exhibiting signs of a primary respiratory process versus cardiac-induced respiratory symptoms, perform a brain natriuretic peptide test. Brain natriuretic peptide is a hormone secreted by the heart in response to volume and pressure overload and is a sensitive marker of cardiac filling pressure and diastolic dysfunction. It will be increased in heart failure and normal in a primarily respiratory process.

Once a diagnosis of CHF has been established, the remainder of the laboratory testing depends on the age of the patient, the presence or absence of CHD, and coexistent systemic disorders. Obtain a complete blood cell count (CBC), determine electrolyte levels, and perform liver function tests, renal function tests, a blood gas assessment, and a lactate test. The CBC may reveal a leukocytosis secondary to an infection, anemia as an etiology, thrombocytopenia in disseminated intravascular coagulation, or pancytopenia caused by viral suppression. A patient with CHF may have electrolyte abnormalities, including hyponatremia (fluid overload) and metabolic acidosis (poor perfusion). Renal failure may be a consequence or a cause of CHF, and increased liver function test levels occur with end-organ damage or a viral illness. The blood gas assessment provides objective evidence of impending respiratory failure, while an abnormal lactate test finding can be a sign of poor tissue perfusion or a clue to a metabolic cause of illness.

Differential Diagnosis

It is important to differentiate CHF from possible respiratory and/or infectious illnesses, in which case the patient is unlikely to have hepatomegaly, cardiomegaly, or failure to thrive (Table 4-1). If a patient has a history of structural heart disease and presents with new signs and symptoms of CHF, it may be caused by an aggravating condition, such as fever, anemia, or arrhythmia. In a patient without structural heart disease, there are many possible etiologies of CHF, some of which are listed in Box 4-1.

Treatment

If CHF is suspected, immediately consult with a cardiologist for recommendations regarding appropriate management. Initial stabilization includes intravenous (IV) or intraosseous access (essential), cardiorespiratory monitoring (with telemetry if available), and judicious fluid administration. Volume overload is almost always present, so use smaller 5- to 10-mL/kg boluses in place of the typical 20 mL/kg bolus, as well as a slower administration rate

Table 4-1. Differential Diagnosis of CHF	
Diagnosis	**Clinical Features[a]**
Asthma	Previous episodes Wheezing, tachypnea, retractions On chest radiograph: hyperinflation without cardiomegaly or pulmonary congestion
Bronchiolitis	Rales with or without wheezing, tachypnea, retractions On chest radiograph: atelectasis and hyperinflation without cardiomegaly
Pneumonia	Fever, rales, tachypnea On chest radiograph: focal consolidation
Sepsis	Fever, ill appearance, poor perfusion Tachypnea, tachycardia

Abbreviation: CHF, congestive heart failure.

[a] Note the absence of hepatomegaly, cardiomegaly, failure to thrive, and increased brain natriuretic peptide level in all features.

Box 4-1. Etiologies of Heart Failure in a Previously Structurally Normal Heart	
Acquired valvular disease (rheumatic heart disease)	Kawasaki disease
Anemia	Muscular dystrophy
Arrhythmia (bradycardia or tachycardia)	Myocardial infarction
Atrioventricular fistula	Myocarditis (usually viral: adenovirus, coxsackievirus, parvovirus)
Cardiomyopathy (acquired or genetic)	
Chemotherapy (anthracyclines)	Pulmonary disease
Collagen vascular disease	Renal failure
Eating disorders or caloric deficiency	Sepsis
Hypertension (systemic or pulmonary)	Systemic lupus erythematosus
Hypocalcemia	Thyroid disease (hypothyroidism, thyrotoxicosis)
Hypoglycemia	
Inborn errors of metabolism (disorders of fatty acid oxidation, mitochondria, glycogen storage)	

while continuously monitoring the patient for signs of pulmonary and hepatic congestion. The overall goals of medical management are decreasing afterload, increasing contractility, and reducing preload volume. The most commonly used medications are diuretics, typically IV or oral furosemide (1 mg/kg) to decrease preload.

The cardiologist may recommend administration of vasoactive or inotropic medications (dopamine, milrinone, or epinephrine) for acute management instead of further IV fluid administration. Other commonly used medications include digoxin to improve contractility and systolic ventricular function, and angiotensin-converting enzyme inhibitors to decrease afterload.

If structural heart disease is suspected, use oxygen cautiously and only in consultation with a cardiologist. This is critical because oxygen, by lowering pulmonary vascular resistance, shunts blood from the systemic circulation to the pulmonary circulation, potentially causing rapid deterioration in certain ductal-dependent or mixing lesions (hypoplastic left heart syndrome, transposition of the great arteries, and large ventricular septal defects). Once these etiologies have been ruled out, it is safe to administer oxygen to supplement tissue oxygenation and alleviate respiratory distress. If further respiratory support is required, use a high fraction of inspired oxygen bag and mask, followed by noninvasive positive pressure ventilation, because the required sedation and vagal effects of endotracheal intubation can be detrimental to cardiac function.

After initiating cardiovascular stabilization, consider noncardiac causes of heart failure and treat these accordingly before initiating further intervention. Once a cardiac etiology is confirmed, treatment options are varied on the basis of etiology and severity and may include medical management, cardiac catheterization, and surgical intervention. Transfer a patient with severe or unresponsive heart failure to an intensive care unit (ICU), where additional modalities, such as extracorporeal membrane oxygenation or left ventricular assist devices, may be available. Regardless of intervention or severity, proper nutrition and growth must be addressed in continued management, along with general health measures, such as vaccinations and exercise parameters.

Disposition
- **ICU transfer:** Impending respiratory failure, poor perfusion, hypotension, severe electrolyte abnormalities, metabolic acidosis, lethargy, or any other evidence of cardiovascular compromise or end-organ damage.
- **Interinstitutional transfer:** Diagnostic and treatment modalities or a pediatric cardiologist and/or intensivist are not immediately available at the current location.
- **Discharge criteria:** Breathing easily without respiratory distress, maintaining adequate fluid and nutrition intake, demonstrating normal electrolyte levels, and, usually, requiring no supplemental oxygen. Discharge ultimately depends on the specific etiology of disease and the cardiologist's plan of care.

Follow-up
- **Primary care:** 1 week
- **Cardiology:** 2 to 3 days, depending on etiology and severity

Pearls and Pitfalls
- Family members or caretakers who see a patient on a regular basis may not notice subtle changes in the patient's appearance or behavior in the presence of CHF. For example, edema may be mistaken for normal weight gain, and exercise intolerance may be mistaken for lack of interest in activities.
- A patient may present with primarily abdominal symptoms (nausea, vomiting, abdominal pain) without respiratory complaints. These can then be mistaken for acute gastroenteritis or another gastrointestinal process, leading to an excessive fluid resuscitation in a fluid-overloaded patient.
- Supplemental oxygen may worsen the status of a patient with structural disease and a left-to-right shunt.

Bibliography

Cantinotti M, Law Y, Vittorini S, et al. The potential and limitations of plasma BNP measurement in the diagnosis, prognosis, and management of children with heart failure due to congenital cardiac disease: an update. *Heart Fail Rev*. 2014 Nov;19(6):727–742

Kantor PF, Lougheed J, Dancea A, et al. Children's Heart Failure Study Group. Presentation, diagnosis, and medical management of heart failure in children: Canadian Cardiovascular Society guidelines. *Can J Cardiol*. 2013 Dec;29(12):1535–1552

Park MK. Congestive heart failure. In: *Park's Pediatric Cardiology for Practitioners*. 6th ed. Philadelphia, PA: Elsevier Saunders; 2014:451–464

Rossano JW, Cabrera AG, Jefferies JL, Naim MP, Humlicek T. Pediatric Cardiac Intensive Care Society 2014 Consensus Statement: Pharmacotherapies in Cardiac Critical Care Chronic Heart Failure. *Pediatr Crit Care Med*. 2016 Mar;17(3 Suppl 1):S20–S34

Rossano JW, Shaddy RE. Heart failure in children: etiology and treatment. *J Pediatr*. 2014 Aug;165(2):228–233

CHAPTER 5

Deep Venous Thrombosis

Introduction

Deep venous thrombosis (DVT) is rare in children, although the incidence has recently increased to 60 to 70 cases per 10,000 hospital admissions. Prompt diagnosis is critical because an undiagnosed and untreated DVT can lead to a fatal pulmonary embolism (PE) or cause serious long-term morbidity. The most important risk factors for a DVT are a venous central line, altered mobility (for >48 hours), local infection (osteomyelitis and skin and soft-tissue infections), and a family history of DVT (Box 5-1).

DVT primarily affects the lower extremities and is subdivided into 2 groups: distal (calf veins) and proximal (thigh veins) thrombosis. Up to 90% of PEs originate from a dislodged thrombus from one of the proximal lower-extremity veins. Involvement of the upper extremities is much less common and is almost always associated with a central line, total parenteral nutrition, dialysis, a hypercoagulable state, or chemotherapy. Although a PE can be found in up to 60% of patients with DVTs, most PEs are clinically silent. Nonetheless, maintain a high clinical suspicion for PE, because the mortality rate from clinically apparent PEs approaches 30%.

Box 5-1. Risk Factors for DVT	
Acquired Conditions	
Acute osteomyelitis	Nephrotic syndrome
Diabetes mellitus	Obesity (BMI >95th percentile for age)
Family or personal history of DVT	Oncologic diagnosis
Hyperosmolality >320 mmol/kg (>320 serum mOsm/kg)	Pregnancy
Immobilization (postsurgery, posttrauma)	Prosthetic cardiac valves
Indwelling venous catheter (central, PICCs)	Serious infections (sepsis)
Inflammatory diseases (SLE, IBD, RA)	Sickle cell disease
Malignancy	Spinal cord injury
Medications (estrogen use in the past 2 mo)	Trauma: >1 lower-extremity fracture or a complex pelvic fracture
Inherited Hypercoagulable Conditions	
Antiphospholipid antibody syndrome	Protein S and C deficiency
Antithrombin deficiency	Prothrombin gene mutation
Factor V Leiden mutation	

Abbreviations: BMI, body mass index; DVT, deep venous thrombosis; IBD, inflammatory bowel syndrome; PICC, peripherally inserted central catheter; RA, rheumatoid arthritis; SLE, systemic lupus erythematosus.

Clinical Presentation

History

Ask about a personal or family history of the risk factors and predisposing conditions listed in Box 5-1. The patient may complain of some combination of leg pain and swelling, pitting edema, warmth and erythema, dilated superficial veins, and, on occasion, a palpable cord in the calf, caused by a thrombosed vein. The pain may result in a limp or a limitation of activity, and it may be worse during activity or when the affected limb is dependent because of swelling.

The most common symptoms of PE are dyspnea and pleuritic chest pain. Less frequently, the patient may complain of fever, cough, and hemoptysis.

Physical Examination

Carefully inspect the extremity, looking for swelling, erythema, tenderness, and dilated superficial veins. Palpate for a cord, which represents subcutaneous venous clots. Measure the circumference of the mid-portion of the affected limb segment (usually 10 cm below the tibial plateau) and compare it to that of the unaffected side. A difference greater than 3 cm is concerning for a DVT. Attempt to elicit the Homans sign, which is popliteal calf pain that occurs with forceful and abrupt dorsiflexion of the ankle while the knee is held in the flexed position. However, these findings are neither sensitive nor specific for DVT. If a lower-extremity DVT is a possibility, determine the Wells score (Table 5-1) based on signs, symptoms, and risk factors.

Table 5-1. The Wells Score[a]	
Clinical Feature	**Score**
Entire leg swollen	1
Calf swelling >3 cm compared to other calf (measured 10 cm below the tibial tuberosity)	1
Localized tenderness along the distribution of the deep venous system	1
Pitting edema, greater in the symptomatic leg	1
Collateral superficial veins, not varicose	1
Active cancer, treatment ongoing or within previous 6 months of palliative treatment	1
Paralysis, paresis, or recent plaster immobilization of the lower extremity	1
Patient recently bedridden for more than 3 d or major surgery performed within 4 wk	1
Alternative diagnosis as likely as or likelier than DVT	Subtract 2 points

Abbreviation: DVT, deep venous thrombosis.

[a] Interpretation: High probability, score ≥3; moderate probability, score of 1 or 2; low probability, score ≤0.

Complications

Pulmonary embolism is the major complication of DVT and presents with tachypnea, dyspnea, fever, tachycardia, and hemoptysis. Rales and/or an S3 or S4 gallop rhythm may be detected.

Laboratory Workup

If a DVT is suspected, obtain a complete blood cell count (CBC), prothrombin time (PT), activated partial thromboplastin time (aPTT), fibrinogen level, and quantitative D-dimer level. If an inherited hypercoagulable condition is a concern in a patient with either no evident risk factors or recurrent DVTs, consult with a hematologist to determine if further testing is indicated (antithrombin III, protein C deficiency, protein S deficiency, factor V Leiden mutation, antiphospholipid antibodies, lupus anticoagulant, homocysteine, α2-antitrypsin, and prothrombin 20210 mutation).

Radiology Examinations

Doppler ultrasonography (US) (US with Doppler imaging and compression of the major veins) of the affected limb is the noninvasive test of choice. It is highly sensitive (89%–96%) and specific (94%–99%) for lower-extremity symptomatic proximal DVT. It is much less sensitive in the upper extremity but remains the initial study of choice. If the Doppler US finding is negative but the clinical suspicion of DVT remains high, perform computed tomographic (CT) angiography or magnetic resonance venography of the limb. If PE is suspected, immediately order CT angiography.

Differential Diagnosis

A clotting activation marker, such as quantitative D-dimer, has a high sensitivity and negative predictive value but a low specificity. The combination of low pretest probability or clinical decision rule (Wells score) and a negative D-dimer result has an extremely high negative predictive value for venous thromboembolism (about 99%). However, a positive D-dimer result does not confirm the diagnosis of DVT. False-positive levels occur with malignancies, trauma, recent surgery, infections, pregnancy, and acute bleeding.

The differential diagnosis of suspected DVT (Table 5-2) includes a variety of disorders that present in a similar fashion. It is essential to assign the correct diagnosis because an untreated DVT may have serious sequelae.

Table 5-2. Differential Diagnosis of DVT[a]	
Diagnosis	**Clinical Features**
Muscle strain/sprain	History of trauma Localized tenderness Bruising and/or hematoma
Cellulitis	Local area of skin with redness/warmth Clear demarcation between involved/uninvolved areas Constitutional symptoms (fever, malaise)
Baker cyst	Prior history of knee swelling and/or pain Palpable fluid-filled mass behind the knee
Lymphedema	Insidious onset Cutaneous and subcutaneous thickening
Venous insufficiency	Visible dilated veins Chronic skin changes with possible ulceration Muscle cramping, numbness, tingling, or itching
Superficial thrombophlebitis	Palpable superficial veins

Abbreviation: DVT, deep venous thrombosis.

[a] In each case, the Homans sign will be negative, except with a calf muscle strain.

Treatment

If DVT is suspected, consult a hematologist. To decrease the chance of embolization, order strict bed rest until the Doppler US examination is performed. Also, discontinue the use of any sequential compression device (SCD). The goals of treating DVT are to prevent local extension of the thrombus and embolization (usually PE), reduce the risk of recurrent thrombosis, and minimize long-term complications (chronic venous insufficiency, postthrombotic syndrome, or chronic thromboembolic pulmonary hypertension). There is no consensus on DVT management for children, so the treatment of choice is individualized to the specific circumstances of the patient and the preference of the consultants. Options include thrombolytic therapy for a massive PE, administration of anticoagulation therapy for at least 3 months, placement of a vena cava filter to prevent PE, surgical thrombectomy, and supportive care, including compressive stockings, use of a venous compressing pump, and management of skin ulcers.

Low–Molecular Weight Heparin

In contrast to unfractionated heparin (UFH), low–molecular weight heparin (LMWH) has high specific activity against factor Xa and less activity against thrombin. DVT treatment dosing is twice that for prophylaxis (<2 months of age, 1.5 mg/kg delivered subcutaneously every 12 hours; >2 months of age, 1 mg/kg delivered subcutaneously every 12 hours). Monitor LMWH with anti-factor Xa levels obtained 4 hours after the dose. The goal is 0.5 to 1.0 units/mL

4 hours after the last subcutaneous injection. Once this is achieved, follow the anti-factor Xa level weekly. For a DVT, treat with LMWH for up to 3 months.

LMWH offers several advantages over UFH, including superior bioavailability with a longer half-life and dose-independent clearance, which results in a more predictable anticoagulation response. It can be administered subcutaneously, with minimal laboratory monitoring and dose adjustment. Prior to the institution of LMWH therapy, obtain a CBC, PT, aPTT, and platelet count. Do not give the patient salicylates and avoid administration of intramuscular injections and arterial punctures while the patient is receiving LMWH. Withhold LMWH for 24 hours prior to an invasive procedure, especially lumbar puncture; resume the therapeutic dose *(a)* 24 hours later for minor surgery or an invasive procedure or *(b)* 48 to 72 hours later for a major surgery.

Unfractionated Heparin

Use UFH specifically in a neurosurgical patient and as an option in all other children. The loading dose is 75 units/kg delivered intravenously (IV) over 10 minutes, followed immediately by an infusion of 28 units/kg/h if younger than 1 year of age or 20 units/kg/h if older than 1 year of age. Use the aPTT to closely monitor therapy and always obtain the sample from a different limb than that used for the infusion site. Alternatively, monitor anti-factor Xa levels, aiming for a therapeutic range of 0.3 to 0.7 units/mL (laboratory dependent).

Obtain the aPTT 4 hours after administration of the UFH loading dose. When the aPTT is 2 to 3 times the mean control value, repeat a CBC with platelet count. If the platelet count is less than $100,000/mm^3$ $(100 \times 10^9/L)$, consider the discontinuation of heparin and institution of an alternative therapy. The risk of heparin-induced thrombocytopenia is greatest after 5 to 7 days of treatment, so recheck the CBC after a week of therapy. Because UFH has a short half-life, excessive levels can usually be controlled by stopping the infusion. Treat a symptomatic overdose with protamine (1 mg for each 100 units of UFH).

The duration of UFH therapy for DVT is 5 to 7 days. Institute warfarin therapy on day 1 or 2 (see the next section on warfarin) to facilitate the transition to long-term oral treatment. If the patient has a PE, administer the heparin therapy for 7 to 14 days and start the warfarin on day 5.

Warfarin

Use warfarin (oral vitamin K antagonist) to transition from IV heparin administration to oral treatment for outpatient management. It is significantly less costly than LMWH but requires more frequent monitoring. The loading and maintenance dose is 0.1 to 0.2 mg/kg (10-mg maximum), delivered as single daily oral doses over 3 to 5 days. Base subsequent doses on the international normalized ratio (INR) response, measured every 3 to 5 days. When 2 INRs obtained 24 hours apart are between 2 and 3, discontinue the heparin. Continue to measure the INR weekly until stable, as well as after *any medication change*. The diet also must be stable. Prior to any surgery, consult with a hematologist to determine appropriate warfarin management.

DVT Prophylaxis

Consider DVT prophylaxis for a patient with identifiable risk factors for DVT (Box 5-1). One of the major risk factors is altered mobility, which is defined as a patient who requires complete bed rest or is unable to move an extremity freely. Although there are no consensus pediatric protocols, do not initiate thromboprophylaxis in a patient under 14 years of age, unless the child is at significantly high risk (>4 DVT risk factors)—particularly a trauma patient (Box 5-1). Treat an adolescent over 14 years of age according to risk level (Table 5-3). Mobilization, in the form of early ambulation in coordination with physical therapy, is preferred for all risk categories. This is in addition to mechanical prophylaxis (use of compression stockings and sequential SCDs) for a moderate-risk patient and medical prophylaxis for a high-risk patient (Table 5-3). Mechanical methods decrease venous stasis, but the effectiveness of an SCD is related to duration of use, with a goal of 18 hours per day.

Consult with a pediatric hematologist to initiate prophylactic anticoagulation with LMWH in a high-risk patient (Table 5-3). Use half the DVT treatment dose (<2 months of age, 0.75 mg/kg administered subcutaneously every

Table 5-3. DVT Categorization and Prophylaxis According to Risk		
Risk Level	**Criteria**	**Intervention**
Low risk	Altered mobility[a] <48 h No DVT risk factors	Encourage early ambulation
Moderate risk	Altered mobility[a] <48 h *plus* ≥1 DVT risk factors *or* Altered mobility[a] >48 h *plus* 0–1 DVT risk factor	Encourage early ambulation Mechanical prophylaxis: SCD (preferred) or compression stockings Goal of 18 h/d use
High risk	Altered mobility[a] >48 h *plus* ≥2 DVT risk factors	Encourage early ambulation Mechanical prophylaxis: SCD (preferred) or compression stockings Goal of 18 h/d use Consult with hematologist for medical prophylaxis

Abbreviations: DVT, deep venous thrombosis; SCD, sequential compression device.
[a] Altered mobility definition: Patient requires complete bed rest or is unable to move an extremity freely.

12 hours; >2 months of age, 0.5 mg/kg administered subcutaneously every 12 hours). For UFH, titrate the dose to an aPTT of 1.2 to 1.5 times the control. Absolute contraindications to medical DVT prophylaxis include a known bleeding disorder, high risk of hemorrhage or active hemorrhage, and a platelet count not sustained at >50,000/mm^3 (50×10^9/L).

Indications for Consultation

- **Hematologist:** All patients
- **Vascular surgeon:** Extensive thrombosis above the knee or elbow and involvement of any vessels of the chest or abdomen

Disposition

- **Intensive care unit transfer:** Pulmonary embolism
- **Discharge criteria:** Therapeutic range of INR or anti-factor Xa achieved, parent/patient education completed (for DVT, anticoagulants, PE, and diet if the patient is taking warfarin), and patient stable

Follow-up

- **Primary care:** 1 week
- **Hematologist (depending on the outpatient anticoagulant choice):** Within 3 days if taking warfarin or after 1 week if taking LMWH
- **Vascular surgeon:** If involved, per the surgeon's request

Pearls and Pitfalls

- A positive D-dimer result does not confirm the diagnosis of DVT.
- Tailor the treatment to the clinical picture, because there is no consensus on pediatric DVT management.
- Do not initiate thromboprophylaxis in a patient under 14 years of age.

Bibliography

Bates SM, Jaeschke R, Stevens SM, et al. Diagnosis of DVT: Antithrombotic Therapy and Prevention of Thrombosis, 9th ed: American College of Chest Physicians evidence-based clinical practice guidelines. *Chest.* 2012;141(2 suppl):e351S–e418S

Cincinnati Children's Hospital Medical Center. Venous thromboembolism (VTE) prophylaxis in children and adolescents—best evidence statement. http://www.cincinnatichildrens.org/service/j/anderson-center/evidence-based-care/recommendations/default/. Accessed January 23, 2017

Falck-Ytter Y, Francis CW, Johanson NA, et al. Prevention of VTE in orthopedic surgery patients: Antithrombotic Therapy and Prevention of Thrombosis, 9th ed: American College of Chest Physicians Evidence-Based Clinical Practice Guidelines. *Chest.* 2012;141(2 suppl):e278S–e325S

Gould MK, Garcia DA, Wren SM, et al; and American College of Chest Physicians. Prevention of VTE in nonorthopedic surgical patients: Antithrombotic Therapy and Prevention of Thrombosis, 9th ed: American College of Chest Physicians Evidence-Based Clinical Practice Guidelines. *Chest.* 2012;141(2 Suppl):e227S–e277S

Hanson SJ, Punzalan RC, Arca MJ, et al. Effectiveness of clinical guidelines for deep vein thrombosis prophylaxis in reducing the incidence of venous thromboembolism in critically ill children after trauma. *J Trauma Acute Care Surg.* 2012;72(5):1292–1297

Monagle P, Chan AK, Goldenberg NA, Ichord RN, et al; and American College of Chest Physicians. Antithrombotic therapy in neonates and children: Antithrombotic Therapy and Prevention of Thrombosis, 9th ed: American College of Chest Physicians Evidence-Based Clinical Practice Guidelines. *Chest.* 2012;141(2 Suppl):e737S–e801S

Electrocardiogram Interpretation

Introduction

An electrocardiogram (ECG) is a graphic representation of the progression of electric activity through the heart. It is often used as a screening test in situations such as suspected congenital heart disease, arrhythmias, chest pain, syncope, acquired heart disease, hypertension, and medication monitoring.

Systematic Interpretation of ECGs

1. **Patient identification:** Always confirm that the ECG was obtained in the correct patient.
2. **Standardization:** Check the bottom of the ECG for the paper speed, which is typically 25 mm/s. This makes the x-axis time 0.04 seconds per small box or 0.2 seconds for each large box on the tracing paper. Also note the calibration marker, which is usually 10 mm high by 5 mm wide. This is called *full standard,* but a common variation is to have a stair-step pattern to the calibration, with a 10-mm block followed by a 5-mm step-down. This means that the limb leads (I, II, III, aVR, aVL, and aVF) are at full standard, while the precordial leads (V_1–V_6) are at half standard. When this is the case, remember to multiply the precordial voltage values by 2 for accurate interpretation.
3. **Rate, rhythm, and axis**
   a. Rate: Interpret the heart rate in beats per minute (bpm) directly from the computer interpretation or use one of the following methods (Table 6-1):
      i.   60/R-R interval = heart rate (in bpm)
      ii. (number of R waves in 6 large boxes) × 50 = heart rate (in bpm)
   b. Rhythm
      i.   Regular vs irregular
      ii. Sinus or nonsinus: Sinus rhythm *always* has a P wave before every QRS, a normal PR interval for the patient's age, and a normal P wave axis
   c. Axis: This refers to the vector of electric force. Calculate the axis for P waves, QRS complexes, and T waves by using leads I and aVF. To determine the axis of any wave:
      i.   Look at the wave voltage in leads I and aVF and determine if the wave is positive or negative (ie, most of the wave is above [positive] or below [negative] the isoelectric line). Then, determine the quadrant of the axis.

Chapter 6: Electrocardiogram Interpretation

Table 6-1. ECG Reference Values[a]

Age	Parameter				Lead V$_1$			Lead V$_6$		
	Heart rate (bpm)[b]	QRS axis[b]	PR interval (s)[b]	QRS duration (s)[c]	R wave amplitude (mm)[c]	S wave amplitude (mm)[c]	R/S ratio	R wave amplitude (mm)[c]	S wave amplitude (mm)[c]	R/S ratio
0–7 d	95–160 (125)	30–180 (110)	0.08–0.12 (0.10)	0.05 (0.07)	13.3 (25.5)	7.7 (18.8)	2.5	4.8 (11.8)	3.2 (9.6)	2.2
1–3 wk	105–180 (145)	30–180 (110)	0.08–0.12 (0.10)	0.05 (0.07)	10.6 (20.8)	4.2 (10.8)	2.9	7.6 (16.4)	3.4 (9.8)	3.3
1–6 mo	110–180 (145)	10–125 (70)	0.08–0.13 (0.11)	0.05 (0.07)	9.7 (19)	5.4 (15)	2.3	12.4 (22)	2.8 (8.3)	5.6
6–12 mo	110–170 (135)	10–125 (60)	0.10–0.14 (0.12)	0.05 (0.07)	9.4 (20.3)	6.4 (18.1)	1.6	12.6 (22.7)	2.1 (7.2)	7.6
1–3 y	90–150 (120)	10–125 (60)	0.10–0.14 (0.12)	0.06 (0.07)	8.5 (18)	9 (21)	1.2	14 (23.3)	1.7 (6)	10
4–5 y	65–135 (110)	0–110 (60)	0.11–0.15 (0.13)	0.07 (0.08)	7.6 (16)	11 (22.5)	0.8	15.6 (25)	1.4 (4.7)	11.2
6–8 y	60–130 (100)	–15 to 110 (60)	0.12–0.16 (0.14)	0.07 (0.08)	6 (13)	12 (24.5)	0.6	16.3 (26)	1.1 (3.9)	13
9–11 y	60–110 (85)	–15 to 110 (60)	0.12–0.17 (0.15)	0.07 (0.09)	5.4 (12.1)	11.9 (25.4)	0.5	16.3 (25.4)	1 (3.9)	14.3
12–16 y	60–110 (85)	–15 to 110 (60)	0.12–0.17 (0.14)	0.07 (0.10)	4.1 (9.9)	10.8 (21.2)	0.5	14.3 (23)	0.8 (3.7)	14.7
>16 y	60–100 (80)	–15 to 110 (60)	0.12–0.20 (0.15)	0.08 (0.10)	3 (9)	10 (20)	0.3	10 (20)	0.8 (3.7)	12

[a] From Engorn B, Flerlage J, eds. *The Harriet Lane Handbook*. 20th ed. Philadelphia, PA: Saunders Elsevier; 2015. Adapted with permission from Elsevier.

[b] Data are ranges, with mean values in parentheses.

[c] Data are means, with 98th percentiles in parentheses.

Lead I[a]	aVF Lead[a]	Axis
+	+	0–90 (normal)
+	−	0 to -90 (left)
−	+	90–180 (right)
−	−	-90 to 180 (superior)

[a] "+" indicates a positive wave (most of the wave is above the isoelectric line), and "−" indicates a negative wave (most of the wave is below the isoelectric line).

    ii. P wave axis: An upright P wave in leads I and aVF is normal. All other configurations are abnormal (nonsinus).

    iii. QRS axis: Always interpret the QRS axis relative to the patient's age, because normality will vary. Newborns typically have a right axis, while the normal adult ECG form is present by 3 years of age, with most of the changes occurring in the first 3 to 6 months of life.

    iv. T wave axis: An upright T wave in leads I and aVF is normal, except on the first day of life, when lead I waves may be negative.

4. Waves and intervals

  a. P wave morphology: Check the height and duration; look for notched or biphasic waves or changing morphologies.

  b. QRS morphology: Assess the amplitude, duration, and presence of Q waves, R/S progression, and R/S ratio.

  c. ST-T wave morphology: Look for elevated or depressed ST segments, alternating polarity, and notched T waves; note the amplitude.

  d. PR interval: Determine whether it is prolonged or short for the patient's age or varying over time.

  e. QTc interval: Calculate by using the Bazett formula: $QTc = \dfrac{QT}{\sqrt{R\text{-}R \text{ interval}}}$ Although the QTc varies with age, consider any QTc of 0.45 and greater to be abnormal.

5. Chamber hypertrophy

  a. Right atrial hypertrophy

    i. Tall P waves greater than 3 mm in any lead, most commonly leads II, V_1, and V_2

  b. Left atrial hypertrophy

    i. Prolonged P wave duration (>0.1 seconds) in any lead

    ii. Notched or biphasic P wave in lead V_1

  c. Biatrial hypertrophy

    i. Combination of P wave prolongation and increased P wave amplitude

   d. Right ventricular hypertrophy (RVH)

      i. Right axis deviation

      ii. R wave in lead V_1 or S wave in lead V_6 greater than the 98th percentile for the patient's age

      iii. Upright T wave in lead V_1 after the third day of life

      iv. R/S ratio greater than the reference in lead V_1 or less than the reference in lead V_6

      v. Q wave in lead V_1 (qR or qRs pattern) also suggests RVH

      vi. Voltage criteria for RVH with abnormal T wave axis indicates strain pattern

   e. Left ventricular hypertrophy (LVH)

      i. Left axis deviation

      ii. R wave in lead V_6 or S wave in lead V_1 greater than the 98th percentile for the patient's age

      iii. R/S ratio less than the reference in lead V_1 or greater than the reference in lead V_6

      iv. Q wave of 5 mm and greater in lead V_5 or V_6, with tall T waves in those leads

      v. Voltage criteria for LVH with abnormal T wave axis indicates strain pattern

   f. Biventricular hypertrophy

      i. Voltage criteria for LVH and RVH in the absence of a bundle branch block or pre-excitation (see "Conduction disturbances")

      ii. Voltage criteria for RVH or LVH and relatively large voltages for the other ventricle

      iii. Large, equiphasic QRS complexes in 2 or more limb leads and in leads V_2–V_5

6. **Conduction disturbances**

   a. Right bundle branch block (RBBB): This is the most common conduction disturbance seen in children. The differential diagnosis includes status after open heart surgery, right ventricular volume overload, Ebstein anomaly, coarctation of the aorta, cardiomyopathy, myocarditis, heart failure, muscular dystrophy, Kearns-Sayre syndrome, Brugada syndrome, arrhythmogenic right ventricular dysplasia, and congenital hereditary RBBB. Criteria for RBBB include

      i. Right axis deviation

      ii. Prolonged QRS duration for the patient's age

      iii. Terminal slurring of the QRS complex

         1. Wide, slurred S wave in leads I, V_5, and V_6

         2. Terminal, slurred R' wave in leads aVR, V_4R, V_1, and V_2

iv. ST depression and T wave inversion (not common in children)

b. Left bundle branch block (LBBB): This is uncommon in children but can be seen after cardiac surgery and in hypertrophic cardiomyopathy and myocarditis. Criteria for LBBB include

   i. Left axis deviation

   ii. Prolonged QRS duration for the patient's age

   iii. Loss of Q wave in leads V_5 and V_6

   iv. QS pattern in lead V_1

   v. Slurred QRS complex

      1. Slurred, wide R wave in leads I, aVL, V_5, and V_6

      2. Wide S wave in leads V_1 and V_2

   vi. ST depression and T wave inversion in leads V_4 through V_6

c. Pre-excitation: This occurs when there is accelerated atrioventricular conduction to 1 ventricle via an accessory pathway, such as in Wolff-Parkinson-White syndrome. Criteria are

   i. Short PR interval for the patient's age

   ii. Delta wave

   iii. Wide QRS complex for the patient's age

Common ECG Patterns in Clinical Diseases

1. **Innocent murmurs:** No abnormal ECG changes

2. **Pathologic murmurs** (associated with structural heart disease): See Table 6-2.

Table 6-2. ECG Findings in Structural Heart Disease	
Heart Condition	**ECG Findings**
Aortic regurgitation	Normal to LVH, LAH
Aortic valve stenosis	Normal to LVH; strain pattern
Atrial septal defect	RAD, RVH, RBBB
Coarctation of the aorta	LVH; infants may have RBBB or RVH
Endocardial cushion defect	Superior QRS axis, LVH or BVH
Hypertrophic obstructive cardiomyopathy	LVH, deep Q waves in leads V_5 and V_6
Patent ductus arteriosus	Normal to LVH or BVH
Pulmonary stenosis	Normal to RAD, RVH (RAH in severe cases)
Tetralogy of Fallot	RAD, RVH or BVH, possibly RAH
Ventricular septal defect	Normal to LVH or BVH

Abbreviations: BVH, biventricular hypertrophy; ECG, electrocardiogram; LAH, left atrial hypertrophy; LVH, left ventricular hypertrophy; RAD, right axis deviation; RAH, right atrial hypertrophy; RBBB, right bundle branch block; RVH, right ventricular hypertrophy.

3. **Chest pain/ischemia**
   a. The etiology of 96% of the cases of pediatric chest pain is noncardiac, so most ECG findings will be normal. Clinical manifestations more concerning for underlying cardiac chest pain include chest pain with exertion; diaphoresis; pallor; anxiety; shortness of breath; nausea and/or vomiting; radiation of pain to the arm, jaw, neck, or back; and syncope.
   b. The adult pattern of ECG changes of ST segment elevation with deep, wide Q waves evolving to wide Q waves with T wave inversion is not always seen. Frequent findings in pediatric ischemia include wide Q waves (>0.035 seconds), ST segment elevation >2 mm, and a prolonged QTc with pathologic Q waves.
   c. Serial ECGs become important when ischemia is suspected, because 40% to 65% of initial ECG findings in the setting of myocardial infarction are normal.

4. **Myocarditis**
   a. ECG findings are variable in myocarditis. Any of the following may be seen:
      i. Low-voltage QRS
      ii. Nonspecific ST segment changes, T wave inversion possible
      iii. Long QT interval
      iv. Arrhythmias, especially premature atrial or ventricular contractions

5. **Pericarditis**
   a. Low-voltage QRS caused by pericardial effusion
   b. ST-T changes follow a time-dependent progression
      i. Patient initially has ST segment elevation
      ii. Elevation returns to normal levels over 2 to 3 days
      iii. T wave inversion occurs 2 to 4 weeks after the onset of disease

6. **Long QT syndrome**
   a. QTc varies with age; the rule of thumb is that any QTc greater than 0.45 is abnormal and requires evaluation by a cardiologist
   b. In addition to prolonged QTc, the following can also be seen: abnormal T wave morphology, bradycardia, second-degree atrioventricular block, multifocal premature ventricular contractions, and ventricular tachycardia
   c. Screen all first-degree relatives of the patient to look for familial long QT syndromes, such as
      i. Jervell and Lange-Nielsen syndrome: congenital deafness, syncope, and family history of sudden death

    ii. Romano-Ward syndrome: The same findings are seen as with Jervell and Lange-Nielsen syndrome, but with normal hearing

    iii. Timothy syndrome: Webbed fingers and toes

    iv. Andersen-Tawil syndrome: Muscle weakness, periodic paralysis, ventricular arrhythmias, and developmental delays

7. **Electrolyte disorders**
   a. Hyperkalemia: ECG changes vary with the level of hyperkalemia
      i. Potassium level greater than 6 mEq/L (6 mmol/L): tall, peaked T waves
      ii. Potassium level greater than 7.5 mEq/L (7.5 mmol/L): widened QRS complex, PR prolongation, tall T waves
      iii. Potassium level greater than 9 mEq/L (9 mmol/L): disappearance of P waves and sinusoidal QRS; ultimately leads to asystole
   b. Hypokalemia: Changes not apparent until potassium level is 2.5 mEq/L (2.5 mmol/L)
      i. Depressed ST segments, biphasic T waves, prolonged QTc, possible appearance of U waves
   c. Hypercalcemia: Serum calcium level greater than 11 mg/dL (2.75 mmol/L) or ionized calcium level greater than 5 mg/dL (1.25 mmol/L)
      i. Shortened ST segment without changing the T wave morphologic appearance
      ii. Shortened QTc interval
   d. Hypocalcemia: Infant serum calcium level greater than 11 mg/dL (2.75 mmol/L) or ionized calcium level greater than 5 mg/dL (1.25 mmol/L); child serum calcium level less than 8.5 mg/dL (2.13 mmol/L) or ionized calcium level less than 4.5 mg/dL (1.13 mmol/L)
      i. Prolonged ST segment without changing T wave morphologic appearance
      ii. Prolonged QTc interval

8. **Kawasaki disease**
   a. Up to 60% of patients have prolonged PR interval during acute presentation
   b. May see arrhythmias, nonspecific ST-T wave changes, or ischemic changes with severe disease

9. **Lyme carditis**
   a. PR interval prolongation

10. **Acute rheumatic fever**
    a. PR interval prolongation is seen, after accounting for age and variability

Ambulatory Monitoring

1. **Ambulatory monitors,** which can be initiated either in the inpatient setting or at the time of discharge, are indicated in the following situations:
    a. Determine if chest pain, palpitation, or syncope are arrhythmic in origin.
    b. Evaluate the effectiveness of antiarrhythmic therapy.
    c. Screen high-risk cardiac patients (with cardiomyopathies or postoperative status).
    d. Evaluate implanted pacemaker dysfunction.
    e. Determine the effects of sleep on arrhythmias.
2. **Holter monitors** are for short-duration use (24–72 hours).
3. **Event recorders** can be used to monitor the patient for longer periods. When the patient senses the onset of symptoms, he or she is expected to press a button. This records the current ECG activity, as well as a time-limited amount of the ECG activity that precedes and follows the event trigger.

Pearls and Pitfalls

- The only way to interpret an ECG correctly is within the context of the clinical history, medical factors, and age-appropriate reference values.
- Verify that the correct settings are used: paper speed of 25 mm/s and voltage at full standard.
- Use the same interpretation system and calipers for every ECG acquisition.
- The only way to recognize abnormal ECG findings is to look at many normal ones.
- Leads may be cut lengthwise to ensure proper placement on an infant's chest.
- If something doesn't seem right, discuss it with a pediatric cardiologist.

Bibliography

Gewitz MH, Baltimore RS, Tani LY, et al; and American Heart Association Committee on Rheumatic Fever, Endocarditis, and Kawasaki Disease of the Council on Cardiovascular Disease in the Young. Revision of the Jones Criteria for the diagnosis of acute rheumatic fever in the era of Doppler echocardiography: a scientific statement from the American Heart Association. *Circulation*. 2015 May 19;131(20):1806–1818

Gretchen CB, Rayannavar AS. Cardiology. In: Enghorn B, Flerlage J, eds. *The Harriet Lane Handbook*. 20th ed. Philadelphia, PA: Elsevier; 2015:127–171

Park MK. Electrocardiography. In: *Park's Pediatric Cardiology for Practitioners*. 6th ed. Philadelphia, PA: Mosby Elsevier; 2014:41–66

Park M, Guntheroth W. *How to Read Pediatric ECGs*. 4th ed. Philadelphia, PA: Mosby Elsevier; 2006

Endocarditis

Introduction

Infective endocarditis (IE) is an infection of the endothelium of the heart initiated by endothelial damage, leading to the adherence of bacteria or fungi and ultimately the entrapment of organisms that evade host defenses. The incidence ranges from 1 in 1,300 to 1 in 20,000 pediatric admissions a year. However, the incidence rate is increasing as a result of the survival of children with congenital heart disease (CHD) and the more frequent use of indwelling central venous catheters (CVCs), especially in premature infants. Although IE is rare in children, there is significant morbidity and mortality associated with the condition.

The most common organisms that cause IE are *Staphylococcus aureus* (especially for acute IE), *Streptococcus viridans*, coagulase-negative staphylococci, pneumococcus, "HACEK" organisms (*Haemophilus* species, *Aggregatibacter actinomycetemcomitans*, *Cardiobacterium hominis*, *Eikenella corrodens*, and *Kingella kingae*), enterococcus, and *Candida* spp (especially in newborns). However, blood culture findings are negative in 5% to 7% of cases.

Clinical Presentation

History

IE can be a subacute or acute process. Subacute IE is caused by less virulent organisms and usually presents with nonspecific signs and symptoms, such as prolonged fever, fatigue, weakness, arthralgia, myalgia, and weight loss. Acute IE is a fulminant disease that presents with high fever, shock, and a toxic-appearing patient. *S aureus* is more often associated with acute IE. There can be a history of CHD (especially cyanotic), cardiac surgery, indwelling catheter placement, prematurity, or previous endocarditis.

Physical Examination

There are rarely any abnormal physical findings in subacute IE, so a new heart murmur is neither necessary nor sufficient to assign the diagnosis. Extracardiac manifestations (Osler nodes, Roth spots, Janeway lesions, petechiae, hemorrhages, splenomegaly, glomerulonephritis) are rare in children, although emboli to the abdominal viscera, lung, or brain are more common.

At presentation, acute IE can demonstrate the physical findings associated with shock, including hypotension, tachycardia, tachypnea, and low oxygen saturation (in CHD graft infection), along with high fever and signs of congestive heart failure (CHF).

Laboratory Workup

If IE is suspected, obtain a complete blood cell count (the patient may be anemic secondary to hemolysis or chronic disease), erythrocyte sedimentation rate or C-reactive protein level (usually increased), rheumatoid factor levels (often increased), and urinalysis results (an immune complex glomerulonephritis can lead to red blood cell casts and proteinuria).

Perform 3 blood cultures from separate venipunctures on the first day, then perform 2 to 3 more cultures if the first ones have no growth at 48 hours. If acute IE is suspected, perform 3 separate venipunctures for culture in a 1- to 2-hour time span. Ensure that the sample size is sufficient (1–3 mL in an infant, 5–7 mL in a young child). If there is difficulty obtaining an adequate sample, inoculate the aerobic culture only. Culture of arterial blood does not increase yield but constitutes an acceptable sample.

Radiology Examinations

Obtain a transthoracic echocardiogram (TTE) when IE is suspected. Although a TTE is sufficient for most patients younger than 10 years of age and less than 60 kg, obtain a transesophageal echocardiogram for a patient with obesity, previous heart surgery, anomalies of the thoracic cage, or chronic lung disease.

Differential Diagnosis

The diagnosis of IE can be challenging, but the modified Duke criteria have been validated for use in children (Table 7-1 and Box 7-1). Consider the diagnosis of IE for a patient with fever of unknown origin, new murmur, history of cardiac disease (especially after cardiac surgery), or history of CVC placement (Table 7-2).

Treatment

Consult both a cardiologist and an infectious diseases specialist. While antibiotics are the mainstay of treatment for IE, they can be withheld for 48 hours until culture findings are positive in a patient with stable, subacute IE. The antibiotic therapy for IE is complex. Choose a regimen in consultation with an infectious diseases specialist, taking into account the organism, sensitivities, and minimum inhibitory concentration and whether the patient has native or

Table 7-1. Modified Duke IE Criteria

Major Criteria

(+) Blood culture finding	>2 Blood cultures with a microorganism consistent with infective endocarditis (*Streptococcus viridans, Streptococcus bovis, Staphylococcus aureus,* HACEK organisms, enterococci) ≥2 (+) Blood cultures performed >12 h apart ≥3 (+) Blood cultures performed >1 h apart (+) Blood culture finding for *Coxiella burnetii* or anti–phase I IgG antibody titer >1:800
Endocardial involvement	(+) Echocardiographic findings: oscillating mass (vegetation), abscess, new dehiscence of prosthetic valve *or* New valvular regurgitation

Minor Criteria

Vascular phenomena	Arterial emboli, intracranial or conjunctival hemorrhages, septic pulmonary infarcts, mycotic aneurysms, Janeway lesions
Immunologic phenomena	Glomerulonephritis, Osler nodes, Roth spots, (+) rheumatoid factor test result
Microbiological evidence	(+) Blood culture finding not meeting major criteria *or* Serologic evidence of infection
Predisposition	Heart condition Intravenous drug use
Fever	≥38.0°C (≥100.4°F)

Abbreviations: HACEK, *Haemophilus* species, *Aggregatibacter actinomycetemcomitans, Cardiobacterium hominis, Eikenella corrodens,* and *Kingella kingae*; IE, infective endocarditis; IgG, immunoglobulin G; +, positive finding.

Box 7-1. Identifying IE by Using Modified Duke Criteria

Definite Criteria

Pathologic criteria: microorganism detection according to culture or histologic finding of vegetation or abscess
2 major criteria
1 major criterion and 3 minor criteria
5 minor criteria

Possible Criterion

Findings consistent with IE that fall short of "definite" but not "rejected"

Rejected Criteria

Resolution in ≤4 d of treatment with antibiotics
No pathologic evidence of IE at surgery or autopsy with ≤4 d of treatment with antibiotics
Firm alternate diagnosis

Abbreviation: IE, infective endocarditis.

Table 7-2. Differential Diagnosis of IE	
Sign/Symptom	**Diagnoses**
Prolonged fever	Infection caused by Bartonella species
	Collagen vascular disease
	Inflammatory bowel disease
	Kawasaki disease
	Malignancy
	Occult abscess
	Osteoarticular infections
New murmur	Anemia
	Fever
	Innocent murmur
	Previously undiagnosed cardiac anomaly
(+) Blood culture finding	Bacteremia or sepsis without IE
	Contaminated specimen

Abbreviations: IE, infective endocarditis; +, positive finding.

prosthetic cardiac material. Treat intravenously (IV) rather than intramuscularly, with bactericidal rather than bacteriostatic antibiotics.

For specific antibiotic treatment regimens once the organism is known, refer to the American Heart Association scientific statement "Infective Endocarditis in Childhood: 2015 Update." In general, treat streptococcal IE with penicillin G or ampicillin IV for 4 weeks. Extend treatment to 6 weeks if the patient has a prosthetic valve, and add gentamicin IV for synergy for 1 to 2 weeks. For staphylococcal IE secondary to a methicillin-susceptible strain, use nafcillin or oxacillin IV for 4 to 6 weeks and add gentamicin IV for the first 3 to 5 days. For methicillin-resistant *Staphylococcus*, use vancomycin IV for 6 weeks and evaluate whether surgical intervention is warranted. Treat HACEK organisms with ceftriaxone IV or ampicillin IV for 4 weeks. Fungal infections often require surgery in addition to amphotericin B treatment.

If the patient is unstable and antibiotics cannot be withheld for 48 hours or if antibiotics are being initiated for a case of culture-negative endocarditis at 48 hours, treat empirically with ampicillin/sulbactam IV plus gentamycin IV with or without vancomycin IV. If a prosthetic valve is in place, add rifampin IV.

Indications for surgery for IE include large vegetations (>1 cm), anterior mitral valve leaflet vegetation, growing vegetation after therapy, extension of abscess after therapy, valvular dysfunction, heart failure, heart block, embolic events after therapy, fungal endocarditis, and mycotic aneurysm.

Prophylactic antibiotics are currently recommended only for a limited number of patients in the highest-risk groups before certain dental procedures. There has been a shift toward emphasizing optimal oral hygiene in lieu of prophylactic administration of antibiotics for most patients. Educate a patient at risk for IE about the importance of good oral hygiene, including dental cleaning every 6 months and daily tooth brushing.

Indications for Consultation

- **Cardiology:** All patients (echocardiographic interpretation)
- **Infectious disease:** All patients, especially for treatment-resistant or unusual organisms
- **Cardiothoracic surgery:** If surgery is indicated

Disposition

- **Intensive care unit transfer:** Shock, extracardiac embolic events (especially with organ dysfunction), unstable vegetation, CHF, cardio-thoracic surgery required
- **Interinstitutional transfer:** For cardiology or cardiothoracic surgery consult, if not available locally
- **Discharge criteria:** Afebrile, negative blood culture findings, completed IV antibiotic course or patient is a suitable candidate for outpatient antibiotics (condition is stable, afebrile, at low risk for embolism; peripherally inserted central catheter is placed; home nursing is arranged; family is willing; there is prompt access to medical/surgical care if complications arise)

Follow-up

- **Primary care:** 1 to 2 weeks
- **Cardiology:** 1 week
- **Repeat echocardiogram:** Clinical deterioration during treatment in a patient with abnormal echocardiographic findings and also at the completion of treatment

Pearls and Pitfalls

- Include IE in the workup of fever of unknown origin.
- Antibiotic therapy can be delayed until cultures are positive in a stable patient with subacute IE.
- IE can be diagnosed in the setting of negative blood culture findings and/or negative echocardiographic findings.

Bibliography

Baltimore RS, Gewitz M, Baddour LM, et al; and Kawasaki Committee of the Council on Cardiovascular Disease in the Young and the Council on Cardiovascular and Stroke Nursing. Infective endocarditis in childhood: 2015 update: a scientific statement from the American Heart Association. *Circulation.* 2015;132(15):1487–1515

Day MD, Gauvreau K, Shulman S, Newburger JW. Characteristics of children hospitalized with infective endocarditis. *Circulation.* 2009;119:865–870

Knirsch W, Nadal D. Infective endocarditis in congenital heart disease. *Eur J Pediatr.* 2011;170(9):1111–1127

Tissières P, Gervaix A, Beghetti M, Jaeggi ET. Value and limitations of the von Reyn, Duke, and modified Duke criteria for the diagnosis of infective endocarditis in children. *Pediatrics.* 2003;112(6):e467–e471

Myocarditis

Introduction

Acute myocarditis is inflammation of the muscular wall of the heart, which may also extend to involve the endocardium and pericardium. Most cases in the United States are caused by viruses—historically, coxsackievirus and adenovirus. More recently, parvovirus B19, human herpesvirus 6, cyto-megalovirus (CMV), Epstein-Barr virus (EBV), and novel H1N1 influenza have been diagnosed more frequently. Other less common infectious causes include bacteria (meningococcus, *Streptococcus, Staphylococcus, Listeria,* and *Mycobacterium* species), spirochetes (*Borrelia burgdorferi*), *Rickettsia* species (especially scrub typhus), and protozoa (*Trypanosoma cruzi*). Medications can also cause myocardial inflammation by means of direct toxic effect (chemo-therapeutic agents) or by inducing hypersensitivity reactions (anticonvulsants, antipsychotics, antibiotics). Often, the specific causative agent is not identified.

The presentation of myocarditis ranges from subclinical or mild disease with spontaneous resolution to fulminant disease with cardiogenic shock. Recently, the prognosis has improved, and the mortality rate has decreased to 10%. About 70% of patients experience full cardiac recovery, and 20% develop cardiac sequelae, including dilated cardiomyopathy that ultimately necessi-tates cardiac transplantation. However, a patient who presents with fulminant myocarditis and survives is more likely to experience complete cardiac recov-ery than someone with a less severe presentation.

Clinical Presentation

History

Clinical presentation varies according to age and severity of disease. An infant often presents with nonspecific symptoms, including poor feeding, fever, tachypnea, irritability, listlessness, pallor, diaphoresis, vomiting without diarrhea, and episodic cyanosis. Additionally, infants are more likely to have a fulminant presentation that requires early, advanced cardiorespiratory support. An older child can present with a nonspecific flulike illness or gastro-enteritis. In more severe cases, there may be symptoms of congestive heart failure (CHF), including malaise, decreased appetite, shortness of breath, and exercise intolerance.

An adolescent may complain of chest pain similar to ischemia, with anterior chest pressure radiating to the neck and arms, in addition to other symptoms noted previously. Older patients may also present with palpitations, syncope, and, rarely, sudden death. Patients with pancarditis (myocarditis and pericarditis) present with precordial pain that varies with respiration and position.

Physical Examination

Look for signs of heart failure or cardiogenic shock, including hypotension, tachypnea, hepatomegaly, abnormal heart sounds (including an S_3 or S_4 gallop), a murmur associated with mitral or tricuspid insufficiency, abnormal lung examination findings with evidence of pulmonary venous congestion (rales), and poor perfusion (weak pulse and prolonged capillary refill time). Tachycardia out of proportion to the fever or the hydration status is a frequent, but not universal, finding.

Laboratory Workup

Obtain a complete blood cell count and either a C-reactive protein level or erythrocyte sedimentation rate, which are often increased in acute myocarditis. To identify a possible pathogen, perform a blood culture, a polymerase chain reaction of nasal or tracheal aspirates for viruses, and further viral testing as suggested by the clinical picture (viral titers [CMV, EBV, parvovirus], nasal and rectal viral cultures, Lyme titer). Evaluate cardiac enzyme levels, cardiac troponin T (cTnT) levels, and B-type natriuretic peptide levels, which are often increased at the time of acute presentation. Increased troponin levels help confirm the diagnosis, and in patients without pre-existing cardiac disease, a cTnT cutoff value of 0.01 ng/mL (0.01 µg/L) has a high sensitivity and negative predictive value.

Obtain a chest radiograph, which frequently demonstrates cardiomegaly. Other findings include pulmonary venous congestion, interstitial infiltrates, and pleural effusions. Also obtain a 12-lead electrocardiogram (ECG), which most commonly shows sinus tachycardia, low-voltage QRS complexes, and nonspecific T wave changes. Other ECG changes can mimic those of myocardial infarction or pericarditis, including ST segment changes and pathologic Q waves. Arrhythmias, such as supraventricular or ventricular tachycardia or varying degrees of atrioventricular block, can also be present.

Obtain a transthoracic echocardiogram to help rule out other causes of cardiac dysfunction, including vegetation (endocarditis) and pericardial effusion (pericarditis). Findings in myocarditis are variable and can include left ventricular or biventricular dysfunction, dilatation, wall motion abnormalities, and mitral and tricuspid valve regurgitation. Loss of right ventricular function is the best predictor of death or need for cardiac transplant. Pericardial effusion, if present, is typically limited.

The standard of reference for the diagnosis of myocarditis has been endomyocardial biopsy. However, it has fallen out of favor as a result of its low sensitivity and the risks associated with the procedure. Cardiac magnetic resonance (CMR) imaging has become more widely used to identify patients with myocarditis because it helps to localize affected areas of the myocardium. The use of late gadolinium-based contrast material enhancement increases specificity. CMR imaging is also useful as a noninvasive means to follow a patient's progress over time.

Differential Diagnosis

The presentation of myocarditis is variable, depending on disease severity. Because it can be subtle, a high index of suspicion is needed to diagnose a nonfulminant case. Consider myocarditis in any patient with vomiting without diarrhea, respiratory distress, tachycardia out of proportion to the patient's fever or hydration status, new-onset CHF or arrhythmia, or ischemic chest pain. Myocarditis can often be initially mistaken for an acute viral illness or a respiratory disorder. Other entities to consider include myocardial ischemia or infarction, pericarditis with or without myocarditis, endocarditis, other causes of CHF (see Chapter 4, Congestive Heart Failure), dilated cardiomyopathy, and pulmonary embolism. Inflammatory processes, such as systemic lupus erythematosus, rheumatic fever, and Kawasaki disease, can also occur with myocarditis at presentation.

Treatment

If myocarditis is suspected, immediately consult a cardiologist who can direct further workup and management. However, the treatment for myocarditis remains largely supportive. If a treatable infectious pathogen is identified, administer appropriate therapy. Closely monitor hemodynamic status for signs of worsening cardiac function or shock. Observe a patient who presents with mild disease for developing signs of heart failure. Depending on disease severity, recommend bed rest to reduce the patient's metabolic needs.

With the guidance of a pediatric cardiologist, treat heart failure with traditional therapy, such as diuretics, angiotensin-converting enzyme inhibitors, angiotensin II receptor antagonists, and β-blockers (see Chapter 4, Congestive Heart Failure). Manage arrhythmias with appropriate medications (see Chapter 3, Arrhythmias), although a persistent arrhythmia may require temporary or permanent pacing and possibly an implantable cardioverter-defibrillator.

Defer the decision about administering steroids and/or intravenous immunoglobulins to the cardiologist.

A patient presenting with profound shock may require mechanical ventilation (to reduce metabolic demand), cardiac afterload reduction, and/or inotropic support. Other potential treatment modalities include circulatory support via extracorporeal membrane oxygenation (ECMO) and, if the clinical picture deteriorates despite medical management, a ventricular assist device (VAD). If the patient is refractory to both medical and mechanical circulatory efforts, transfer the patient to a center that performs cardiac transplantation.

Indications for Consultation
- **Cardiology:** Suspected myocarditis
- **Infectious disease:** Myocarditis secondary to sepsis, spirochetes, or protozoa

Disposition
- **Intensive care unit transfer:** Symptomatic myocarditis
- **Interinstitutional transfer:** Patient requires technology or management options not available locally (echocardiogram, pediatric intensive care unit, ECMO, VAD, transplantation), or a pediatric cardiologist is not immediately available
- **Discharge criteria:** Stable or improving cardiac function, managed with oral medication; advise the patient to refrain from competitive sports and vigorous exercise until cleared by a pediatric cardiologist

Follow-up
- **Cardiology:** 2 days to 2 weeks, depending on the severity of the illness
- **Primary care:** 3 to 5 days

Pearls and Pitfalls
- Given the often subtle, nonspecific, and variable presentations of a patient with myocarditis, prompt diagnosis requires a high index of suspicion.
- Suspect myocarditis when a patient with presumed gastroenteritis and/or dehydration with unopposed vomiting worsens after the administration of fluid boluses.
- Suspect myocarditis in any patient with unexplained CHF or arrhythmia, especially after an acute viral illness.

Bibliography

Banka P, Robinson JD, Uppu SC, et al. Cardiovascular magnetic resonance techniques and findings in children with myocarditis: a multicenter retrospective study. *J Cardiovasc Magn Reson.* 2015;17:96–103

Canter CE, Simpson KE. Diagnosis and treatment of myocarditis in children in the current era. *Circulation.* 2014;129(1):115–128

Eisenberg et al. Cardiac troponin T as a screening test for myocarditis in children. *Pediatr Emerg Care.* 2012;28:1173–1178

Petit MA, Koyfman A, Foran M. Myocarditis. *Pediatr Emerg Care.* 2014;30(11):832–838

Shauer A, Gotsman I, Keren A, at al. Acute viral myocarditis: current concepts in diagnosis and treatment. *Isr Med Assoc J.* 2013;15(3):180–185

Towbin JA, Lorts A, Jefferies JL. Myocarditis. In: Allen HD, Driscoll DJ, Shaddy RE, Feltes TF, eds. *Moss and Adams' Heart Disease in Infants, Children, and Adolescents.* 8th ed. Philadelphia, PA: Lippincott Williams & Wilkins; 2012:1247–1266

Pericarditis

Introduction

Acute pericarditis is an inflammatory condition of the fibrous pericardium that surrounds the heart, often accompanied by an effusion in the pericardial cavity. It may be isolated or part of a systemic disease, although most cases are considered idiopathic because no source can be identified. Specific etiologies include viral infection (most often enteroviruses), bacterial infection (purulent pericarditis), tuberculosis, connective tissue or collagen vascular diseases, metabolic diseases, uremia, neoplasms, drug reactions, trauma, and post-pericardiotomy syndrome.

Purulent pericarditis is often associated with infection at another site, with hematogenous or direct spread. The most common causative organisms are *Staphylococcus aureus*, group A β-hemolytic streptococcus, pneumococcus, and meningococcus. Complications of pericarditis include pericardial constriction and cardiac tamponade (acute compression of the heart from increased intrapericardial pressure caused by pericardial effusion).

Clinical Presentation

History

The classic presentation of acute pericarditis is sudden onset of chest pain that is pleuritic in nature (exacerbated by inspiration), worse when recumbent, and alleviated by sitting upright and leaning forward. The pain can radiate to the neck, arms, back, or shoulders. In a younger child, however, chest pain may be absent. A young patient may present solely with tachycardia, tachypnea, and fever. A child with viral pericarditis may have a history of a recent upper respiratory infection or gastroenteritis, while bacterial pericarditis is generally more acute in onset, with symptoms developing over a few days.

Physical Examination

A pericardial friction rub is diagnostic but not always present. Auscultate while the patient is leaning forward. With large effusions, the heart sounds may be muffled.

A patient with cardiac tamponade has an ill appearance, with signs of right-sided heart failure (lower-extremity edema, hepatomegaly) and poor systemic perfusion (weak pulse, cool extremities, delayed capillary refill) because of decreased cardiac output. Other findings suggestive of tamponade include pulsus paradoxus (a decrease in systolic blood pressure of more than

10 mm Hg with inspiration) and Beck triad (systemic hypotension, increased jugular venous pressure, and muffled heart sounds).

Laboratory Workup

Obtain a complete blood cell count and either a C-reactive protein level or erythrocyte sedimentation rate, which are often increased in acute pericarditis. A markedly increased white blood cell count can suggest bacterial pericarditis. Perform a blood culture when sepsis is suspected (fever, tachycardia, toxic appearance). Order serologic testing, including antinuclear antibody and rheumatoid factor, in patients with suggestive signs and symptoms, such as arthritis, rash, or weight loss. Evaluate cardiac enzyme levels when the diagnosis is unclear. Cardiac troponin T levels may be mildly increased in pericarditis, while creatine kinase–MB increase occurs in myopericarditis.

Obtain a chest radiograph, which may have normal findings or show an enlarged cardiac silhouette with a characteristic globular ("water bottle") appearance if a large effusion is present.

Obtain a 12-lead electrocardiogram (ECG). The ECG may progress through 4 stages: Diffuse ST elevation and PR depression (the classic finding), normalization of ST and PR segments, diffuse T wave inversion, and normalization of T waves (Figure 9-1).

If pericardial tamponade is suspected, obtain an urgent transthoracic echocardiogram. The presence of a pericardial effusion on an echocardiogram can support the diagnosis, although absence of an effusion does not exclude pericarditis.

Figure 9-1. Twelve-lead electrocardiogram from a patient with acute pericarditis demonstrates diffuse ST elevation and PR depression.

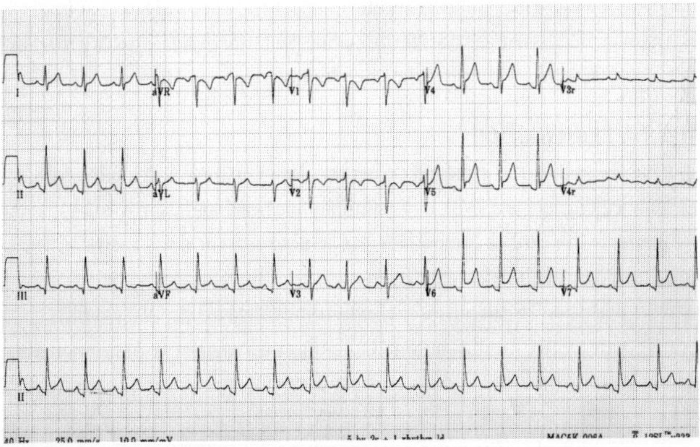

Differential Diagnosis

Pediatric chest pain is usually a benign complaint. The most common etiologies are either idiopathic or musculoskeletal. See Table 9-1 for a differential diagnosis.

Treatment

Closely monitor the patient's hemodynamic status. If tamponade is suspected, administer volume resuscitation (a 20-mL/kg bolus of normal saline delivered over 15 minutes) until the diagnosis is confirmed with an echocardiogram and/or an urgent pericardiocentesis can be performed. Other indications for pericardiocentesis include suspected purulent, tuberculous, or neoplastic pericarditis or a large pericardial effusion. Send the fluid for a blood cell count, evaluation of glucose and protein levels, Gram stain and cultures, acid-fast bacilli stain, viral polymerase chain reaction (most commonly for enterovirus), evaluation for triglyceride levels (to evaluate the presence of chylous

Table 9-1. Differential Diagnosis of Pericarditis	
Diagnosis	**Clinical Features**
Costochondritis	Chest pain reproducible by palpation at the costochondral junction Chest radiography and ECG findings normal
Endocarditis	Chest pain rare Echocardiogram findings may be (+) Osler nodes, Janeway lesions, Roth spots, splinter hemorrhages
Myocardial ischemia or infarction	Nonpleuritic chest pain Friction rub absent PR depression rare T wave inversion accompanies localized ST elevation
Myocarditis	Chest pain rare Friction rub absent Signs of congestive heart failure Low QRS voltages and occasional dysrhythmias Enlarged chambers, impaired left ventricular function on the echocardiogram
Pneumonia	↓ Breath sounds or other focal findings (rales) ECG findings normal Chest radiography findings are usually diagnostic
Pneumothorax	↓ Breath sounds on the affected side ↓ QRS voltages, possible right shift of QRS axis Chest radiography findings are usually diagnostic
Pulmonary embolism	Nonpleuritic chest pain Friction rub rare No PR depression ST elevation, with T wave inversion only in leads III, aVF, and V_1

Abbreviations: ECG, electrocardiogram; +, positive finding.

effusion in a patient with a history of cardiac surgery), and, if indicated, cytologic examination.

If the clinical picture suggests purulent pericarditis, start empirical parenteral antibiotic therapy and arrange drainage via pericardiocentesis, a pericardial catheter, or an open procedure. Start with vancomycin (60 mg/kg/d divided into doses administered every 8 hours, with a 4-g/d maximum) combined with a third-generation cephalosporin (ceftriaxone, 100 mg/kg/d divided into doses administered every 12 hours with a 4-g/d maximum) until an organism is identified. Consult with an infectious diseases specialist to tailor the duration of antibiotic therapy, which averages 3 to 4 weeks. At a minimum, continue antibiotics until clinical resolution (no effusion present, patient is afebrile, white blood cell count has normalized).

If the patient is well appearing with an idiopathic or presumed viral peri-carditis and a limited or midsized effusion, treat with rest and a nonsteroidal anti-inflammatory agent for relief of chest pain and inflammation. Administer high-dose ibuprofen (30–50 mg/kg/d divided into doses delivered every 8 hours, with a 2.4-g/d maximum) until symptoms resolve, typically within 1 to 2 weeks. Add ranitidine (2–4 mg/kg/d divided into doses administered every 12 hours, with a 300-mg/d maximum) for gastroprotection while ibuprofen is administered. Add colchicine for recurrent pericarditis (<5 years of age, 0.5 mg/d; >5 years of age, 1.0–1.5 mg/d administered in 2–3 divided doses). Do not administer steroids routinely; prescribe only for a patient with collagen vascular disease, an immune-mediated process, or an idiopathic effusion that is refractory to treatment with ibuprofen. If steroids are indicated, then use low-dose prednisone (0.2–0.5 mg/kg/d, with a 60-mg/d maximum for 4 weeks with subsequent taper).

Indications for Consultation

- **Cardiology:** Suspected pericarditis
- **Infectious disease:** Purulent or tuberculous pericarditis
- **Rheumatology:** Known or suspected collagen vascular disease

Disposition

- **Intensive care unit transfer:** Suspected or confirmed cardiac tamponade
- **Interinstitutional transfer:** For cardiac consultation or drainage, if either is not available on-site

Discharge Criteria

- **Pericarditis:** Asymptomatic (no fever or chest pain)
- **Pericardial effusion:** Effusion is resolved or stable
- **Patient has undergone a drainage procedure:** No fluid reaccumulation during 1 week of observation

Follow-up

- **Primary care:** 1 week
- **Patient with effusion:** Follow-up echocardiogram obtained within 1 week to document resolution of effusion
- **Patient with purulent pericarditis:** Cardiology follow-up within 1 to 2 weeks

Pearls and Pitfalls

- The patient may not have the "classic" signs and symptoms of pericarditis, such as a friction rub and pleuritic chest pain that change with position.
- A chest radiograph and echocardiogram may only be useful if an effusion accompanies pericardial inflammation.
- The most reliable study for assigning the diagnosis of pericarditis is an ECG with characteristic ST and PR segment changes.

Bibliography

Adler Y, Charron P, Imazio M, et al. 2015 ESC Guidelines for the diagnosis and management of pericardial diseases: The Task Force for the Diagnosis and Management of Pericardial Diseases of the European Society of Cardiology (ESC). *Eur Heart J.* 2015;36(42):2921–2964

Bergmann KR, Kharbanda A, Haveman L. Myocarditis and pericarditis in the pediatric patient: validated management strategies. *Pediatr Emerg Med Pract.* 2015;12(7):1–22

Imazio M, Gaita F, LeWinter M. Evaluation and treatment of pericarditis: a systematic review. *JAMA.* 2015;314(14):1498–1506

Johnson JN, Cetta F. Pericardial diseases. In: Allen HD, Driscoll DJ, Shaddy RE, Feltes TF, eds. *Moss and Adams' Heart Disease in Infants, Children, and Adolescents.* 8th ed. Philadelphia, PA: Lippincott Williams & Wilkins; 2012:1350–1362

Shock

Introduction

Shock is a state of systemic hypoperfusion. It represents a final common pathway for several derangements in volume status, vascular tone, venous return to the heart, and cardiac pump physiology. Septic shock, which is the most common type in children, often has a progression through signs and symptoms of compensation until overt hypotension and cardiovascular collapse ensue (*decompensated shock*). Other types of shock are classified by etiology (anaphylactic, neurogenic, cardiogenic) or physiology (distributive, low cardiac output, obstructive, hypovolemic), with considerable overlap in clinical presentation. The key to successful shock treatment is early recognition of shock in its *compensated* stages.

Management of shock (along with respiratory failure, cardiac dysrhythmia, and arrest) is a core portion of the American Heart Association's Pediatric Advanced Life Support (PALS) program. The American College of Critical Care Medicine's (ACCM) frequently updated pediatric septic shock guidelines have become the standard evidence-based practice regarding shock management. The ACCM septic shock algorithm has become a part of PALS and is featured on the PALS pocket-reference card.

Clinical Presentation

History

Ask about fever, difficulty breathing, skin color (from the caregiver's knowledge of baseline appearance), changes in mental status and behavior, and urine output, as well as history of trauma and potential sources of infection and fluid loss (cough, congestion, vomiting, diarrhea, abdominal pain, bleeding). In addition, confirm that the patient has normal immune status and no history of hemodynamically significant heart disease. If the child is currently an inpatient, review the vital signs from the prior 6 to 12 hours, intake-output flow sheets, and observations made by bedside nurses, respiratory therapists, and parents.

Physical Examination

The patient typically presents in compensated shock with fever (or hypothermia), tachycardia (persistent and out of proportion to the fever), widened pulse pressure (indicating low systemic vascular resistance), difficulty breathing, and signs of altered perfusion (pallor, mottled skin, delayed capillary refill, weak pulse, altered mental status, oliguria), but with a *normal, age-appropriate blood pressure*. There are a number of trendable, validated measures of ongoing decompensation. One is the Monaghan/Brighton early warning score, which uses 3 domains: behavioral, cardiovascular, and respiratory (Table 10-1). An ongoing score of 5 or higher indicates the need for intervention, rapid-response team notification, and, if the patient is not readily improving, transfer to the intensive care unit (ICU).

Laboratory Workup

Obtain a bedside glucose level, a complete blood cell count with differential, a comprehensive chemistry panel (end-organ hypoperfusion leads to acute renal and hepatic injury, as well as electrolyte abnormalities), and a blood culture. If sepsis is of particular concern, order a disseminated intravascular coagulation panel, type, and screen. Obtain additional cultures (eg, urine, spinal fluid, cutaneous abscess, joint), depending on the patient's history, physical examination findings, and ability to tolerate the procedure. Perform blood gas analysis with measurement of serum lactate levels (variably increased

Table 10-1. Monaghan/Brighton Early Warning Score				
Domain	**0**	**1**	**2**	**3**
Behavior	Playing Appropriate	Sleeping	Irritable	Lethargic/confused *or* ↓ Response to pain
Cardiovascular	Pink appearance *or* Capillary refill time of 1–2 s	Pale/dusky appearance *or* Capillary refill time of 3 s	Gray/cyanotic appearance *or* Capillary refill time of 4 s *or* Pulse >20 beats/min above normal	Gray/cyanotic/mottled appearance *or* Capillary refill time ≥5 s *or* Pulse >30 beats/min above normal *or* Bradycardia
Respiratory	Within normal limits No retractions	>10 breaths/min above normal *or* Accessory muscle use *or* >30% FiO$_2$ or >3 L/min	>20 breaths/min above normal *or* Retractions *or* >40% FiO$_2$ or >6 L/min	≥5 breaths/min below normal parameters with retractions/ grunting *or* >50% FiO$_2$ or >8 L/min
Score 2 extra for nebulizer treatments every 15 minutes or persistent vomiting after surgery.				

Abbreviation: FiO$_2$, fraction of inspired oxygen.

Adapted from Monaghan A. Detecting and managing deterioration in children. *Paediatr Nurs.* 2005;17(1):32–35.

with tissue hypoperfusion) and ionized calcium levels (decreased in some cases of sepsis, can lead to refractory shock). In general, venous specimens are adequate. Obtain a chest radiograph, which may reveal infiltrates, cardiomegaly, or findings of acute respiratory distress syndrome.

Differential Diagnosis

The priority is recognizing shock early, while it is in the compensated stage. Viral, bacterial, and other infectious agents may cause fever and tachycardia in the absence of actual shock. In general, the pulse increases by approximately 9 beats per degree Celsius of temperature increase. The differential diagnosis for categories of shock is summarized in Table 10-2.

Volume Loss

Vomiting and diarrhea, along with inadequate oral intake, are common symptoms of hypovolemic shock (hypovolemia is a component of other forms of shock, as well). Hemorrhage, including hemorrhage from accidental or inflicted trauma, is another important etiology. Typical signs include decreased pulse, dry mucosal surfaces, delayed capillary refill time, decreased skin turgor, and late tachycardia and hypotension.

Sepsis

The patient will present with fever (or hypothermia) and signs and symptoms of infection (cough, congestion, vomiting, diarrhea, rash, etc). Because sepsis may manifest hypovolemic and distributive components (low vascular tone),

Table 10-2. Differential Diagnosis for Types of Shock	
Diagnosis	**Clinical Features**
Sepsis	Fever Widened pulse pressure (warm shock) Poor response to fluid administration
Hypovolemia	History of fluid loss, poor oral intake, bleeding (including internal intravascular loss) Delayed capillary refill time Dry mucosal surfaces Vital signs responsive to fluid bolus(es)
Cardiogenic shock	Rales, worsening with fluid bolus(es) Hepatomegaly Cardiac gallop Cardiomegaly on radiographs
Other shock types (ie, neurogenic, obstructive, anaphylactic)	History of trauma with paralysis: neurogenic shock History of blunt trauma with dyspnea: obstructive shock History of exposure with rash: anaphylactic shock

as well as myocardial depression, a complex mix of phenotypes is seen. These are described as *cold shock* (*vasoconstricted*) and *warm shock* (*vasodilated*). In general, the patient with warm shock presents with bounding pulses and flash capillary refill, with wide pulse pressure reflecting low systemic vascular resistance. The patient with cold shock presents with capillary refill time delayed more than 2 seconds, cool extremities, and diminished peripheral pulse.

Cardiogenic Shock

The typical findings of cardiogenic shock are tachypnea, dyspnea, tachycardia, rales, hepatomegaly, jugular venous distention, and cardiac murmurs and gallops. Cardiomegaly and poor or delayed pulse may also be seen. Causes include congenital heart lesions, myocarditis, persistent dysrhythmias, and high-outflow conditions (anemia, vascular malformations).

Anaphylactic Shock

The patient with anaphylactic shock presents with difficulty breathing, adventitious sounds, and poor aeration, with or without an urticarial eruption, often in the setting of a suspected allergen.

Neurogenic Shock

Neurogenic shock involves a spinal cord injury, which leads to sympathetic denervation of the vascular bed. Warm extremities from vasodilation and relative or absolute bradycardia accompany hypotension refractory to the delivery of fluid boluses. If seen, start vasopressor support early.

Obstructive Shock

Obstructive shock is caused by impeded venous return secondary to pneumothorax, hemothorax, pericardial tamponade, or left ventricular outflow obstructive lesions. Heart and/or lung sounds may be diminished, low voltages may be seen on the electrocardiogram, and pulsus paradoxus may be noted. Distended neck veins and tracheal deviation away from the side of tension pneumothorax may also be seen.

Treatment

Early in the care process, consult with a critical care specialist or initiate transfer of the patient to a tertiary care center. For all forms of shock, initial management includes the CABs (chest compressions, airway, and breathing), including establishing and maintaining an airway, providing oxygen and ventilatory support, and securing 2 sites of vascular access (peripheral venous, intraosseous [IO], central venous). If there is any concern for sepsis, administer broad-spectrum intravenous (IV) antibiotics, such as vancomycin

(15 mg/kg every 8 hours or every 6 hours if meningitis is suspected, with a 4-g/d maximum) *and* ceftriaxone (50 mg/kg; or 75 mg/kg if meningitis is suspected, by administering a dose every 8 to 12 hours, with a 12-g/d maximum). However, do not delay the administration of antibiotics if the patient is too unstable to have all indicated cultures obtained (ie, lumbar puncture). See Chapter 68, Sepsis, for the antibiotic coverage for an immunocompromised patient.

Hypovolemic, Septic, and Other Etiologies With the Component of Hypovolemia

Administer prompt, rapid volume resuscitation with crystalloid fluids (normal saline, lactated Ringer solution). Deliver boluses of 20 mL/kg over 5 to 10 minutes by using a push-pull technique or rapid infuser systems, because IV infusion pumps cannot achieve the needed rate for patients in shock. Try to achieve resuscitation by using a "golden hour" approach, minimizing delays between fluid boluses and reassessments. This is associated with decreased mortality and involves the delivery of rapid volume boluses, followed by rapid reassessment. Attempt to normalize capillary refill time, pulse, mental status, and blood pressure, but maintain ongoing monitoring for signs of volume overload (rales, jugular venous distention, hepatomegaly). Control the patient's temperature with antipyretics when possible.

If hypotension persists or develops, in the absence of ongoing losses, despite the infusion of 60 mL/kg of crystalloid fluids, the patient may benefit from further crystalloid resuscitation because 80 mL/kg and even 100 mL/kg are at times necessary to reverse shock, particularly in a patient with septic shock. Also, consider the need for steroids, even in a patient without chronic steroid use or history of adrenal insufficiency. Administer IV hydrocortisone as follows for fluid refractory shock: 0 to 3 years of age, 25 mg; ≥3 to 12 years of age, 50 mg; and ≥12 years of age, 100 mg (100-mg maximum).

When pressors are necessary, administer epinephrine via a peripheral or central line, but do not delay administration pending central access. Start at 0.04 μg/kg/min and titrate upward in increments of 0.02 μg/kg/min every 5 minutes (0.1-μg/kg/min maximum). However, in the case of warm shock, local protocols may recommend the use of other pressors, such as norepinephrine (initial dose of 0.05–0.10 μg/kg/min, titrate to effect; 1–2-μg/kg/min maximum).

If the hemoglobin level is lower than 10 g/dL (100 g/L), consider blood product transfusion support to increase the oxygen-carrying capacity. Indications for intubation and mechanical ventilation include respiratory failure, poor airway protection in an obtunded patient, and unreversed shock despite the administration of fluid boluses and peripheral epinephrine infusion. Correct hypoglycemia, hypocalcemia, and disturbances in the patient's temperature.

Cardiogenic Shock

See Chapter 3, Arrhythmias; Chapter 4, Congestive Heart Failure; Chapter 8, Myocarditis; and Chapter 9, Pericarditis, for specific therapies for cardiogenic shock. Consult with a cardiologist or intensivist, who may recommend afterload-reducing inotropic support, such as milrinone (50–75-µg/kg infused over 10–60 minutes, followed by delivery of 0.50–0.75 µg/kg/min). For a neonate with ductal-dependent congenital heart lesions or undifferentiated shock, administer a prostaglandin E infusion (alprostadil, 0.05–0.10 µg/kg/min delivered initially, followed by 0.01–0.05 µg/kg/min). The patient is at risk for apnea, so prepare for potential intubation.

Anaphylactic Shock

If anaphylaxis is suspected, immediately administer intramuscular epinephrine (see Chapter 2, Anaphylaxis, for the treatment of anaphylaxis) into the lateral quadriceps. Repeat the dose every 10 to 15 minutes, as needed, or start a continuous epinephrine infusion as detailed earlier for hypovolemic shock.

Obstructive Shock

Do not delay therapy while awaiting chest radiography. Perform lifesaving needle thoracentesis, evacuation of pericardial tamponade, or prostaglandin E infusion. Treat a pneumothorax with placement of an 18- or 20-gauge angiocatheter in the midclavicular line, second intercostal space (over the top of the third rib), followed by tube thoracostomy. Treat pericardial tamponade with volume support to increase preload, and if the patient is unresponsive to fluid administration, pericardiocentesis should be performed by a qualified physician.

Indications for Consultation

- **Cardiology:** Cardiogenic shock or obstructive shock from cardiac tamponade and need for urgent pericardiocentesis
- **Critical care specialist:** Fluid refractory shock
- **Infectious diseases:** Resistant or complex infections
- **Surgeon, intensivist, other qualified physician:** If central venous access is needed or if reliable IV access cannot be obtained promptly

Disposition

- **ICU transfer:** Fluid refractory shock, ongoing increased early warning score
- **Institutional transfer:** Need for ICU or specialist consultation not available locally
- **Discharge criteria:** Normal vital signs and adequate oral intake

Follow-up

- **Primary care:** 2 to 3 days
- **Infectious diseases:** 1 week if long-term antibiotic therapy is initiated

Pearls and Pitfalls

- Inadequate recognition of compensated forms of shock (persistent tachycardia being a prime example) is associated with time-dependent mortality. Early goal-directed therapy saves lives.
- Remain vigilant for tachycardia that is persistent and out of proportion to the patient's fever temperature as a sign of continued shock and need for prompt treatment.
- A patient with persistently abnormal vital signs (tachycardia, wide pulse pressure) or impaired perfusion, even in the absence of hypotension or vasoactive infusion requirement, may require ICU transfer for close monitoring and additional resuscitation.
- Resuscitations that require multiple boluses of 20 mL/kg of crystalloid IV fluids are common. Do not hesitate to provide adequate resuscitation (even to 80–100 mL/kg), but re-evaluate the vital signs and physical examination between boluses.
- Administer hydrocortisone with or without pressors for fluid refractory shock.
- Promptly attempt IO line placement if securing IV access is a problem.

Bibliography

Akre M, Finkelstein M, Erickson M, Liu M, Vanderbilt L, Billman G. Sensitivity of the Pediatric Early Warning Score to identify patient deterioration. *Pediatrics.* 2010;125(4):e763–e769

Brierley J, Carcillo JA, Choong K, et al. Clinical practice parameters for hemodynamic support of pediatric and neonatal septic shock: 2007 update from the American College of Critical Care Medicine. *Crit Care Med.* 2009;37(2):666–688

Carcillo JA, Kuch BA, Han YY, et al. Mortality and functional morbidity after use of PALS/APLS by community physicians. *Pediatrics.* 2009;124(2):500–508

Kissoon N, Orr RA, Carcillo JA. Updated American College of Critical Care Medicine—pediatric advanced life support guidelines for management of pediatric and neonatal septic shock: relevance to the emergency care clinician. *Pediatr Emerg Care.* 2010;26(11):867–869

Singer M, Deutschman CS, Seymour CW, et al. The Third International Consensus Definitions for Sepsis and Septic Shock (Sepsis-3). *JAMA.* 2016;315(8):801–810

Dermatology

CHAPTER 11

Erythema Multiforme and Stevens-Johnson Syndrome/ Toxic Epidermal Necrolysis

Introduction

Erythema multiforme (EM) and Stevens-Johnson syndrome (SJS) are relatively uncommon disorders of the skin and mucous membranes. The previous terminology of "EM minor" and "EM major" has fallen out of favor, as recent evidence suggests that EM and SJS/toxic epidermal necrolysis (TEN) have distinct precipitating factors and clinical features and are therefore separate entities.

Classic EM involves the skin only, whereas SJS always affects the skin and mucous membranes. EM is thought to be a postinfectious process, with herpes simplex virus (HSV) being the most well-documented trigger. Both SJS and TEN are considered variants of the same hypersensitivity disorder, with epidermal detachment of less than 10% of the body surface area (BSA) defined as SJS, more than 30% of the BSA defined as TEN, and between 10% and 30% of the BSA defined as SJS/TEN.

Drugs are the cause of most nonidiopathic SJS/TEN cases, although infections and autoimmune diseases may also be triggers. Many drugs have been implicated, but the most common are sulfonamides, anticonvulsants, β-lactam antibiotics, and nonsteroidal anti-inflammatory drugs. The most frequently identified infectious etiology is *Mycoplasma pneumonia;* this may be a distinct entity.

SJS/TEN typically resolves over a 4- to 6-week period, but the mortality rate remains high at 5% to 30%, with many more patients experiencing long-term morbidities. Early recognition and prompt withdrawal of the causative agent increase patient survival.

Clinical Presentation

History

A patient with EM typically presents with a mildly pruritic rash in association with a prodrome of mild, nonspecific systemic symptoms, such as fever, cough, and rhinorrhea.

A patient with SJS/TEN will present with pronounced constitutional symptoms, such as high fever and malaise, along with cutaneous rash and discomfort or poor oral intake related to mucous membrane lesions. The disease typically develops within 2 to 8 weeks of exposure to the offending agent.

Physical Examination

The prototypic EM lesion is a 1- to 3-cm erythematous, edematous plaque that develops a dusky vesicular, purpuric, or necrotic center. Often there is also an edematous ring of pallor surrounded by an erythematous outer ring (the target lesion). In many cases the typical target is not seen, and only the first 2 zones are present. The lesions are typically distributed symmetrically and acrally, predominantly on extensor surfaces. They may also be present on the trunk, palms, soles, and face. The patient may have a low-grade fever, as well as mild extremity and/or facial edema.

A patient with SJS/TEN is typically highly febrile and ill appearing. The cutaneous lesions are more likely to occur on the face and trunk than in classic EM, and they are more often reported as painful or burning. They also tend to be macular and predominate on the trunk, and they may be coalescent and often exhibit the Nikolsky sign, which is positive when slight rubbing of the skin causes exfoliation of the outermost layer. Epidermal detachment may occur but does not typically involve more than 10% of the BSA. If more than 10% of the BSA is involved, then SJS/TEN is likely. Mucosal lesions (≥2 sites) are requisite for a diagnosis of SJS/TEN and are characterized by erythema and bullae that become confluent with pseudomembrane formation. The mucous membrane lesions are typically hemorrhagic in appearance, which is not the case in EM. Oral lesions may extend to the respiratory mucosa, and complications may include pneumonitis and respiratory failure. Ophthalmologic findings include conjunctivitis, keratitis, and uveitis. Less commonly, urethritis may be seen. Mycoplasma-associated disease has been shown to be more common in male subjects, with more prominent mucositis but sparse cutaneous involvement.

Laboratory Workup

Both EM and SJS/TEN are clinical diagnoses. If SJS/TEN is suspected, obtain a complete blood cell count, erythrocyte sedimentation rate and/or C-reactive protein level, and comprehensive metabolic panel. The patient may have a leukocytosis or leukopenia and thrombocytosis, while eosinophilia is common in drug-related cases. Chemical abnormalities include hypoalbuminemia, increased liver transaminase levels (in 75% of patients), and electrolyte imbalances, including hypernatremia, hyponatremia, acidosis, and increased blood urea nitrogen and creatinine levels. The clinical picture is usually clear, but if there is diagnostic uncertainty, perform a skin biopsy to rule out other diagnoses. In EM, there is more dermal inflammation and individual keratinocyte necrosis when compared to SJS/TEN, which has minimal inflammation and sheets of epidermal necrosis. Conduct serologic testing for *Mycoplasma* if that is a likely organism.

Differential Diagnosis

EM is most often confused with urticaria. Other common diagnostic possibilities include drug eruptions, urticarial vasculitis, and viral exanthems. The diagnosis of SJS/TEN is usually evident and not confused with other entities. SJS/TEN may be confused with DRESS (drug reaction with eosinophilia and systemic symptoms), although a patient with DRESS often has dramatic facial edema and more internal organ involvement (liver, kidney, lungs), without significant mucous membrane involvement. Other entities to consider in the differential diagnosis include Kawasaki disease, bullous pemphigoid, bullous drug eruption, linear immunoglobulin A dermatosis, erythema annulare centrifugum, staphylococcal scalded skin syndrome, serum sickness, herpetic gingivostomatitis, and Behçet syndrome (Table 11-1).

Treatment

Treatment of EM is supportive, and its course is usually self-limited over 1 to 2 weeks. Treat the underlying cause (if identified) and discontinue nonessential medications. Topical treatments are typically not helpful. Recurrences may occur, particularly with HSV-associated EM.

Table 11-1. Differential Diagnosis of SJS	
Diagnosis	**Clinical Features**
Behçet syndrome	Uncommon in children Discrete genital ulcers Recurrences common
Bullous drug eruption	No systemic symptoms
DRESS	Facial edema Limited mucous membrane involvement Eosinophilia Lesions predominate on extremities and face
Herpetic gingivostomatitis	Fever and oral lesions only No cutaneous eruption
Kawasaki disease	Discrete oral lesions uncommon Nonexudative conjunctivitis, strawberry tongue Edema of the hands and feet
Serum sickness	Arthralgia common No bullae or Nikolsky sign
Staphylococcal scalded skin syndrome	Diffuse, painful erythroderma No discrete oral lesions Fissuring and crusting of the perioral area

Abbreviations: DRESS, drug reaction with eosinophilia and systemic symptoms; SJS, Stevens-Johnson syndrome.

The treatment of SJS/TEN is also primarily supportive, including meticulous skin care, intravenous (IV) hydration and nutrition, provision of adequate analgesia, and monitoring for complications, such as fluid or electrolyte abnormalities, secondary bacterial infection, severe hepatitis, and ocular and/or airway involvement. Provision of adequate nutrition in the form of enteral feedings and/or total parenteral nutrition can prevent a catabolic state and may improve outcome. Clear treatment guidelines are lacking. However, the only aspects of treatment that have been proven to improve outcome are rapid withdrawal of the offending agent(s) and optimal management of nutrition and denuded skin areas. Therefore, early recognition of the disease is critical. Systemic corticosteroids, IV immune globulin, plasmapheresis, cyclosporine, and immunomodulators have all been used, but their effectiveness has not been proven and their use remains controversial. Consult a dermatologist to determine if any medication is indicated. Reserve antibiotics for identified infections.

Indications for Consultation

- **Dermatology:** Suspected SJS, SJS/TEN, or TEN
- **Ophthalmology:** Suspected SJS, SJS/TEN, or TEN
- **Burn specialist:** Extensive disease or more than 10% epidermal detachment

Disposition

- **Intensive care unit transfer:** Extensive amount of BSA affected, respiratory mucosa involvement (risk of respiratory failure and loss of airway)
- **Burn unit:** Extensive disease or more than 10% BSA epidermal detachment
- **Discharge criteria:** Improving clinical condition, adequate oral intake

Follow-up

- **Dermatology:** 3 to 5 days
- **Primary care:** 1 to 2 weeks
- **Ophthalmology:** 3 to 5 days (if ocular involvement present)

Pearls and Pitfalls

- Discontinue any suspected etiologic agent immediately and avoid known precipitants while the patient is hospitalized (eg, nonsteroidal anti-inflammatory drugs).
- Use of specific treatment agents remains controversial and must be administered in consultation with a dermatologist.

- Consult a burn specialist and/or pediatric intensivist for severe disease.
- A patient with SJS/TEN is at risk for long-term, severe ophthalmic sequelae (corneal ulceration and blindness). Involve an ophthalmologist at the time of admission for all patients with SJS/TEN.

Bibliography

Canavan TN, Mathes EF, Frieden I, Shinkai K. Mycoplasma pneumoniae-induced rash and mucositis as a syndrome distinct from Stevens-Johnson syndrome and erythema mutiforme: a systematic review. *J Am Acad Dermatol.* 2015;72(2):239–245

Ferrandiz-Pulido C, Garcia-Patos V. A review of causes of Stevens-Johnson syndrome and toxic epidermal necrolysis in children. *Arch Dis Child.* 2013;98(12):998–1003

Mockenhaupt M. Stevens-Johnson syndrome and toxic epidermal necrolysis: clinical patterns, diagnostic considerations, etiology, and therapeutic management. *Semin Cutan Med Surg.* 2014;33(1):10–16

Moreau JF, Watson RS, Hartman ME, Linde-Zwirble WT, Ferris LK. Epidemiology of ophthalmologic disease associated with erythema multiforme, Stevens-Johnson syndrome, and toxic epidermal necrolysis in hospitalized children in the United States. *Pediatr Dermatol.* 2014;31(2):163–168

Quirke KP, Beck A, Gamelli RL, Mosier MJ. A 15-year review of pediatric toxic epidermal necrolysis. *J Burn Care Res.* 2015;36(1):130–136

Rashes Associated With Serious Underlying Disease

Introduction

Rashes associated with acute illnesses are common in children. However, there are a few that can be associated with serious diseases that can have significant morbidity and mortality. These include erythroderma, some cases of cellulitis, petechiae/purpura, target lesions, and vesicles/bullae.

Clinical Presentation

History

Obtain a thorough description of the evolution of the rash. Determine when and where it started, the initial appearance and any change, and the pattern of spread (eg, from head to trunk or from hands to trunk). Note if the rash is painful or pruritic.

Ask about associated symptoms, such as the duration and intensity of any fever, fatigue, irritability, headache, sore throat, myalgia, arthralgia, abdominal pain, vomiting, and diarrhea. Document whether the patient is currently taking or was recently taking any medication and whether there has been any travel or any contact with sick persons.

Physical Examination

Determine the size and morphology of the rash. Flat lesions smaller than 0.5 cm are called *macules;* raised lesions of similar size are *papules.* Vesicles are lesions filled with fluid; if the fluid is purulent, the lesions are *pustules.* Lesions that do not blanch suggest bleeding into the skin and are called *petechiae, purpura,* or *ecchymoses,* depending on the size.

Document the distribution of the rash. Assess the patient for desquamation and the Nikolsky sign (separation of the epidermis from the dermis with light pressure), which occurs in staphylococcal scalded skin syndrome (SSSS), toxic epidermal necrolysis (TEN), Stevens-Johnson syndrome (SJS), and various bullous disorders.

Examine all of the mucous membranes (throat, lips, buccal mucosa, conjunctiva, urethra, and anus) and look for vesicles, crusting, erythema, or other abnormalities. Note if there is any eye involvement, such as conjunctival injection, purulent discharge, and abnormalities of the cornea or iris.

Look for edema of the face and/or extremities and check for lymphadenopathy and hepatosplenomegaly.

Laboratory Workup

Obtain a complete blood cell count (CBC) with differential, as well as a complete metabolic panel to assess renal and liver function. A urinalysis is helpful to look for hematuria, pyuria, and proteinuria, if suspected. In an ill-appearing patient, obtain a C-reactive protein level and/or erythrocyte sedimentation rate, blood culture, coagulation panel, D-dimer level, and fibrinogen level. In addition, collect cultures from any suspected sites of infection, such as skin, cerebrospinal fluid, and urine. Further bacterial or viral testing may be necessary, depending on the clinical picture. If lupus is suspected, order a rheumatologic panel that includes antinuclear antibodies, anti–double-stranded DNA, anti–Smith antibodies, and antiphospholipid antibodies.

In some cases, a skin biopsy finding can be diagnostic.

Radiology Examinations

If Kawasaki disease (see Chapter 67) is suspected, order an echocardiogram.

Differential Diagnosis

Classify the rash according to its morphologic appearance and distribution (Table 12-1).

The differential diagnosis includes infectious exanthems, which often have characteristic features. For example, measles typically presents with a red maculopapular rash that begins on the face and moves down the body, becoming confluent (or *morbilliform*—ie, measles-like), in association with fever, cough, coryza, and conjunctivitis. Scarlet fever is characterized by a red, diffuse, sandpapery rash with accentuation in the flexion creases (Pastia lines), fever, and pharyngitis. Epstein-Barr virus may cause a maculopapular rash that is predominantly truncal, along with fever, lymphadenopathy, pharyngitis, and splenomegaly. The differential diagnosis is summarized in Table 12-2.

Treatment

Institute contact and/or droplet precautions if an infectious etiology is being considered in an ill-appearing patient.

The treatment of erythema multiforme (Chapter 11), Henoch-Schönlein purpura (HSP) (Chapter 74), Kawasaki disease (Chapter 67), and SJS (Chapter 11) is detailed elsewhere.

Table 12-1. Serious Rash Morphologic Appearances		
Rash Type	**Description**	**Possible Diagnoses**
Erythema: areas of significant redness		
Erythroderma	Diffuse erythema (looks like sunburn) Pruritus, desquamation Large portion of body surface involved	TSS Drug reaction Viral or bacterial sepsis Kawasaki disease
Painful erythema	Localized erythema that spreads rapidly Severe pain	Necrotizing fasciitis
Bleeding into the skin		
Petechiae	Pinpoint (<2-mm), nonblanching, round macules Not palpable	*Infectious:* sepsis (meningo-coccal, staphylococcal, strep-tococcal), RMSF, other viral, bacterial and fungal causes
Purpura	2-mm to 1-cm nonblanching spots May be palpable	*Vasculitis:* HSP, SLE *Trauma:* Accidental, inflicted
Ecchymoses	>1-cm nonblanching spots May be palpable	*Hematologic/oncologic:* ITP, leukemia
Target lesions: round or oval macules with red edges and clearing or dusky centers		
	Circular/ovoid macules with erythematous periphery and clearing centers, which can become vesicular or dusky Symmetrical eruption Can involve the palms of the hands and soles of the feet Minimal epidermal detachment (<10% BSA)	EM
Vesicobullous lesions: blisters filled with clear, nonpurulent fluid **Vesicle, <1-cm diameter; bullae, >1-cm diameter**		
	Characteristically on the face and/or trunk Mucosal involvement of the lips, mouth, nose, conjunctiva, genitals, and rectum (+) Nikolsky sign May become pustular	SJS TEN
	Initial erythema progressing to fragile bullae Prominent on flexural surfaces No mucosal involvement (+) Nikolsky sign May become pustular	SSSS
	Erythroderma or morbilliform rash, progressing to vesicles, bullae, and/or purpura Head-to-toe progression May involve the mucous membranes Prominent facial and periorbital edema	DRESS
	Similarly sized, clustered vesicles on an erythematous base Vesicles become hemorrhagic erosions and/or pustules History of eczema	Eczema herpeticum

Abbreviations: BSA, body surface area; DRESS, drug reaction with eosinophilia and systemic symptoms; EM, erythema multiforme; HSP, Henoch-Schönlein purpura; ITP, idiopathic thrombocytopenic purpura; RMSF, Rocky Mountain spotted fever; SJS, Stevens-Johnson syndrome; SLE, systemic lupus erythematosus; SSSS, staphylococcal scalded skin syndrome; TEN, toxic epidermal necrolysis; TSS, toxic shock syndrome; +, positive finding.

Chapter 12: Rashes Associated With Serious Underlying Disease

Table 12-2. Differential Diagnosis of Serious Rashes	
Clinical Features	**Differential Diagnosis**
DRESS syndrome	
Eruption begins 2–6 wk after starting the inciting drug (eg, anti-epileptics, sulfonamides) Symmetrical erythroderma or morbilliform rash becomes vesicular and/or purpuric Triad of fever, rash, and internal organ involvement May have lymphadenopathy, pharyngitis, and/or facial swelling Eosinophilia, atypical lymphocytosis May have abnormal LFT and TFT results and abnormal renal function	Infectious mononucleosis Reactivation of HHV-6 Leukemia Lymphoma Viral syndrome
Eczema herpeticum	
History of eczema or other skin disease Fever Uniform-sized papulovesicles on an erythematous base, which progress to erosions and crusting Laboratory workup: PCR, viral culture, Tzanck smear May have keratoconjunctivitis or secondary bacterial infection	Suprainfected eczema
Erythema multiforme	
Symmetrical distribution of target lesions Usually involves palms of the hands and soles of the feet in a symmetrical distribution Maximal involvement of only one mucosal surface	Drug reaction Kawasaki syndrome Other hypersensitivities (SJS) TEN Urticaria Vasculitis Viral syndrome, especially herpes
Henoch-Schönlein purpura	
Patient usually <7 y old Initial maculopapular or urticarial rash Progresses to palpable purpura of lower extremities and buttocks Afebrile May have arthralgia/arthritis, hematuria, and/or abdominal pain May develop ileoileal intussusception	Acute abdomen Drug reaction EM ITP Meningococcemia SLE Juvenile idiopathic arthritis Other vasculitis RMSF
Idiopathic thrombocytopenic purpura	
Patient 2–5 y of age, well appearing History of viral infection or viral immunization 1–6 wk prior Petechiae and ecchymoses (nonpalpable) Bleeding and bruising with minimal or no trauma No generalized lymphadenopathy or hepatosplenomegaly ↓ Platelet count with ↑ MPV; normal WBC and Hgb level	Aplastic anemia Collagen vascular disease Drug reaction Epstein-Barr virus HIV Inflicted trauma Leukemia

Table 12-2. Differential Diagnosis of Serious Rashes, continued

Clinical Features	Differential Diagnosis
Kawasaki disease	
Patient usually <5 y of age Fever >5 d with marked irritability Polymorphic eruption with late desquamation Cracked lips, strawberry tongue, edema of the dorsum of the hands/feet, nonpurulent conjunctivitis with limbic sparing, cervical lymphadenopathy	Adenovirus Drug reaction Juvenile idiopathic arthritis
Meningococcemia	
Fever with rapid progression to toxicity and possible vascular collapse Petechiae and palpable purpura, particularly of the distal extremities	Bacterial sepsis HSP Kawasaki disease RMSF Vasculitis
Necrotizing fasciitis	
Rapidly progressing cellulitis with pain level out of proportion to the visible lesion Becomes edematous, with bullae, areas of hemorrhage, necrosis, and/or erythroderma Fever, marked toxicity, hypotension, altered mental status Severe pain, worsening despite antibiotics	Severe cellulitis Other soft-tissue infection
Rocky Mountain spotted fever	
Erythematous macules beginning on the wrists and ankles Rash spreads centrally, becoming petechial and purpuric Illness may begin with headache, myalgia, malaise, GI complaints Classic triad of fever, severe headache, and rash Patient may have a history of tick bite (60% of cases) Hyponatremia	Enterovirus Kawasaki disease Meningococcemia Mycoplasma Secondary syphilis *Streptococcus* Viral syndrome
Staphylococcal scalded skin syndrome	
Initial erythema progressing to fragile bullae, especially prominent on the flexion creases Fever Fissures around the eyes, nose, and mouth *without mucous membrane involvement* (+) Nikolsky sign	Epidermolysis bullosa Nutritional deficiency Scalding burn TEN
Systemic lupus erythematosus	
Erythema over the nose and cheeks, spreading in a butterfly distribution Fever, myalgia, fatigue, headache, arthralgia, behavioral changes Arthritis, pleuritis, pericarditis (+) ANA, anti–double-stranded DNA, antiphospholipid antibodies, anti-Smith antibodies	Fibromyalgia Lymphoma Malignancies Rheumatologic diseases Viral syndrome

Chapter 12: Rashes Associated With Serious Underlying Disease

Continued

Table 12-2. Differential Diagnosis of Serious Rashes, continued	
Clinical Features	**Differential Diagnosis**
Toxic epidermal necrolysis/Stevens-Johnson syndrome	
New medication started in the past month: antiepileptics, sulfon-amides, β-lactams, macrolides	Bullous disorder
Symmetrical purpuric/erythematous/targetoid macules and bullae that coalesce	Burns
	Epidermolysis bullosa
Rapid progression to detachment of the epidermis, exposing the underlying raw, red skin	EM
	Graft vs host disease
Epidermal detachment <10% in SJS, 10%–30% in SJS/TEN overlap, >30% in TEN	Kawasaki syndrome
	SSSS
Hemorrhage, crusts, and erosions on multiple mucosal surfaces (lips, tongue, buccal mucosa, rectum, genital mucosa)	
Conjunctivitis, keratitis, uveitis	
(+) Nikolsky sign	
↑ Liver transaminase levels, CRP level/ESR; hematuria/proteinuria	
Toxic shock syndrome	
May be staphylococcal or streptococcal	Drug reaction
Prodrome of malaise and myalgia, followed by vomiting, diarrhea, altered mental status	Kawasaki disease
	Leptospirosis
Diffuse macular erythroderma	Meningococcemia
Fever, hypotension, tachycardia, multi-organ failure	RMSF
Mucous membrane involvement	SJS/TEN
Desquamation 1–2 wk later, especially of the palms of the hands and soles of the feet	SSSS
	Viral syndrome
↑ Platelet count and fibrinogen and albumin levels	
↓ Liver transaminase levels, D-dimer levels, CRP levels/ESR, CPK levels, BUN/Cr levels	

Abbreviations: ANA, antinuclear antibodies; BUN, blood urea nitrogen; CPK, creatine phosphokinase; Cr, creatinine; CRP, C-reactive protein; DRESS, drug reaction with eosinophilia and systemic symptoms; EM, erythema multiforme; ESR, erythrocyte sedimentation rate; GI, gastrointestinal; Hgb, hemoglobin; HHV-6, human herpesvirus 6; HSP, Henoch-Schönlein purpura; ITP, idiopathic thrombocytopenic purpura; LFT, liver function test; MPV, mean platelet volume; PCR, polymerase chain reaction; RMSF, Rocky Mountain spotted fever; SJS, Stevens-Johnson syndrome; SLE, systemic lupus erythematosus; SSSS, staphylococcal scalded skin syndrome; TEN, toxic epidermal necrolysis; TFT, thyroid function test; WBC, white blood cell count; +, positive finding.

Drug Reaction With Eosinophilia and Systemic Symptoms Syndrome

For drug reaction with eosinophilia and systemic symptoms (DRESS) syndrome, immediately discontinue any medication that could be a possible etiology and treat the patient with prednisone (1–2 mg/kg/d) for at least a few weeks, followed by a slow taper. Transfer the patient to an intensive care unit (ICU) if there is significant hepatic, renal, or other systemic involvement.

Eczema Herpeticum

For eczema herpeticum, administer acyclovir, 10 mg/kg every 8 hours intravenously, if the renal function is normal. Change to oral medication once no new lesions are erupting.

Idiopathic Thrombocytopenic Purpura

In idiopathic thrombocytopenic purpura (ITP), avoid medications that affect platelet function, such as nonsteroidal anti-inflammatories and salicylates. If the platelet count is less than $20,000/mm^3$ (20×10^9/L), consult a hematologist to discuss treatment options.

Meningococcemia

Immediately obtain a blood culture and treat the patient with intravenous (IV) antibiotics, either ceftriaxone (100 mg/kg/d divided into doses administered every 12 hours, with a maximum of 2 g per dose and 4 g/d) or cefotaxime (200 mg/kg/d divided into doses administered every 6 hours, with a maximum of 12 g/d). Administer antibiotic prophylaxis to the patient's household and nursery or child care contacts, as well as persons who have contact with the patient's secretions. Options include a single dose of oral ciprofloxacin (>1 month of age, 20 mg/kg; maximum, 500 mg), rifampin (<1 month of age, 5 mg/kg taken orally twice a day for 2 days; >1 month of age, 10 mg/kg taken orally twice a day for 2 days; maximum, 600 mg per dose), or a single dose of intra-muscular ceftriaxone (125 mg if <15 years of age, 250 mg if >15 years of age).

Necrotizing Fasciitis

In the event of necrotizing fasciitis, immediately consult a surgeon to perform debridement. Administer broad-spectrum antibiotics to prevent infection with aerobic and anaerobic organisms. Begin treatment with piperacillin/tazobactam, basing the dose on the piperacillin (<2 months of age, 300–400 mg/kg/d divided into doses administered every 6 hours; 2–9 months of age, 240 mg/kg/d divided into doses administered every 8 hours; >9 months of age, 300 mg/kg/d divided into doses administered every 8 hours; maximum dose, 16 g/d) *plus* vancomycin (if normal renal function, 15 mg/kg/d, with a maximum dose of 1,250 mg; <13 years of age, administer a dose every 6 hours; >13 years of age, administer a dose every 8 hours).

Rocky Mountain Spotted Fever

Treat a patient of any age with doxycycline (4 mg/kg/d divided into doses administered twice a day; maximum of 100 mg per dose). Transfer the patient to an ICU if unstable or if close monitoring is required.

Staphylococcal Scalded Skin Syndrome

Obtain a CBC, blood culture, and electrolyte levels and perform a polymerase chain reaction for the toxin. Admit the patient to an ICU or burn unit and treat with clindamycin (40 mg/kg/d divided into doses administered every 6 hours; 4.8-g/d maximum) or vancomycin, as for necrotizing fasciitis.

Systemic Lupus Erythematosus

Defer treatment decisions to a rheumatologist.

Toxic Epidermal Necrolysis

Admit the patient to a burn unit and treat like a severe burn, with meticulous skin care and aggressive fluid resuscitation. Place the patient in reverse isolation if the rash is extensive. Discontinue any medication that could be a possible cause.

Toxic Shock Syndrome

For toxic shock syndrome (TSS), perform a CBC, blood cultures, electrolyte level evaluation, liver function tests, blood urea nitrogen/creatinine level evaluation, and assessment of prothrombin time/partial thromboplastin time. Admit the patient to an ICU and provide fluid resuscitation as needed. Treat with clindamycin (40 mg/kg/d divided into doses administered every 6 hours; 4.8-g/d maximum) *and* vancomycin, as for necrotizing fasciitis. Remove any possible foreign bodies (tampons) and drain any infected wounds.

Indications for Consultation

- **Burn service:** TEN/SJS
- **Cardiology:** Kawasaki disease
- **Dermatology:** DRESS syndrome, eczema herpeticum, systemic lupus erythematosus (SLE), SSSS, TEN/SJS
- **Hematology:** ITP
- **Infectious diseases:** Meningococcemia, necrotizing fasciitis, Rocky Mountain spotted fever (RMSF), TSS
- **Ophthalmology (if the eyes are involved):** Eczema herpeticum, SLE, TEN/SJS
- **Rheumatology:** HSP (severe), SLE
- **Surgery:** Necrotizing fasciitis

Disposition

- **Burn unit:** TEN/SJS
- **Pediatric ICU:** Meningococcemia, TSS, necrotizing fasciitis, RMSF, SSSS
- **Discharge criteria:** Nontoxic appearance, adequate oral hydration, no need for IV medication

Pearls and Pitfalls

- The distribution of the rash and the presence of mucosal involvement are often key features for assigning the correct diagnosis.
- Rapid diagnosis and treatment are important. If the patient appears seriously ill, consult a specialist and treat the patient early.
- Some causes of rashes require notification of the local departments of health.

Bibliography

Blanter M, Vickers J, Russo M, Safai B. Eczema herpeticum: would you know it if you saw it? *Pediatr Emerg Care.* 2015;31(8):586–588

Burkhart CN, Morrell DS, eds. *VisualDx: Essential Pediatric Dermatology*. Philadelphia, PA: Wolters Kluwer Lippincott Williams & Wilkins; 2010:34–35, 186–189, 195–211

Ferrandiz-Pulido C, Garcia-Patos V. A review of causes of Stevens-Johnson syndrome and toxic epidermal necrolysis in children. *Arch Dis Child.* 2013;98:998–1003

Handler MZ, Schwartz RA. Staphylococcal scalded skin syndrome: diagnosis and management in children and adults. *J Eur Acad Dermatol Venereol.* 2014;28(11):1418–1423

Hussain Z, Reddy BY, Schwartz RA. DRESS syndrome: Part I. Clinical perspectives. *J Am Acad Dermatol.* 2013;68(5):693–708

Hussain Z, Reddy BY, Schwartz RA. DRESS syndrome: Part II. Management and therapeutics. *J Am Acad Dermatol.* 2013;68(5):709–720

Jumal N, Teach SJ. Necrotizing fasciitis. *Pediatr Emerg Care.* 2011;27(12):1195–1202

Paller A, Mancini AJ. *Hurwitz Clinical Pediatric Dermatology.* 5th ed. London, United Kingdom: Elsevier; 2016:238, 342–347, 363–364, 400, 476–483, 503–508

Skin and Soft-Tissue Infections

Introduction

Skin and soft-tissue infections (SSTIs) encompass a variety of disease processes that affect the dermis and subcutaneous layer of the skin. Most cases are caused by either *Staphylococcus aureus* or *Streptococcus pyogenes* (group A *Streptococcus*), and most patients admitted to the hospital present with cellulitis or abscess. Recently, there has been an increase in admissions attributable to SSTI, particularly those caused by methicillin-resistant *S aureus* (MRSA). As a result, knowledge of local antibiotic susceptibilities is critical for proper evaluation and management of SSTIs.

Usually, an SSTI can be managed on an outpatient basis. Admitted patients generally have an atypical history, rapidly progressing infection, or extensive area or serious site of involvement; are unable to tolerate oral antibiotics; have not received the appropriate empirical antimicrobial coverage; or have signs of sepsis/systemic infection.

Clinical Presentation

History

Important considerations in SSTIs are immune status, exposure to animals, bite wounds, exposure to marine environments, possible foreign body, penetrating injuries, trauma, surgery, travel history, and current/recent country of residence. Assess the patient for MRSA risk factors, such as prior MRSA infection, MRSA nasal colonization, recent hospitalization, recent antibiotic use, or a family member with previous MRSA infection.

Physical Examination

At presentation, SSTIs appear with a combination of erythema, warmth, induration, and pain/tenderness, and may be accompanied by fever, lymphangitis, or lymphadenitis. Cellulitis is specifically characterized by erythema, warmth, and tenderness, with poorly defined borders. It involves the deeper dermis and subcutaneous fat and lacks the fluctuance of an underlying suppurative focus. However, it may be a sentinel for a deeper or more complicated pyogenic infection, such as an abscess, fasciitis, or bone involvement. Erysipelas is a form of cellulitis with sharply demarcated borders and typically affects the lower limbs and face.

A skin or subcutaneous abscess involves the dermis and deeper tissues. The superficial skin will usually have a warm, erythematous, tender nodule or mass, often with underlying fluctuance; in some cases, a central superficial pustule may be seen.

Laboratory Workup

No laboratory tests are necessary if the patient is well appearing and immunocompetent. If there is a concern about sepsis, perform a complete blood cell count (CBC) and blood culture. Obtain a C-reactive protein level and/or an erythrocyte sedimentation rate if an underlying fasciitis or associated osteoarticular infection is possible. Perform a culture of any abscess drainage. Do not perform a superficial swab for culture from intact skin or perform a needle aspirate for culture when there is no detectable abscess.

Radiology Examinations

In general, imaging is not needed. However, if the patient has a rapidly spreading cellulitis or if there is concern for deeper infection, order ultrasonography (US) to determine whether there is a drainable abscess. If there is concern for foreign body, perform screening US or plain-film radiography; but if the object is deep, the patient will likely need to undergo magnetic resonance (MR) imaging. Also perform MR imaging when there is a concern about fasciitis, pyomyositis, osteomyelitis, or more extensive infection or if the site of involvement is near a vital structure.

Differential Diagnosis

Generally, confirming the diagnosis of a SSTI is straightforward. However, there are a number of conditions with similar appearances that are either more serious or require different therapy (Table 13-1).

Treatment

General principles of management include closely monitoring the extent and progression of the infection by marking the margins of the affected area.

The first-line treatment for a fluctuant abscess is incision and drainage. Depending on the size of the wound and local practice, keep the abscess cavity open with either a drain or packing. Abscesses are more likely to be attributable to S aureus. Treat with clindamycin or alternatives (discussed in the next paragraph) while awaiting culture identification and susceptibility results. Use warm compresses if an underlying abscess has not been drained.

Table 13-1. Differential Diagnosis of Skin and Soft-Tissue Infections

Diagnosis	Differentiating Features
Abscess	Well-demarcated, overlying erythema May be fluctuant or spontaneously draining
Cellulitis	Poorly demarcated macular or raised edges Erythematous and warm
Erysipelas	Well-demarcated or raised edges Extremely painful (St Anthony's fire)
Fungal infection (deep)	Superficial crusted lesion (papule, pustule, plaque) May have a history of foreign body at the same site
Hidradenitis suppurativa	Affects apocrine sweat glands or sebaceous glands Superficial pustules and deep follicular rupture May cause scarring and tract formation
Local allergic reaction (insect bite)	Pruritus Central punctum within the swelling Usually seen in skin not covered by clothing
Necrotizing fasciitis	Superficial progressive destruction of fascia and fat Has a "wooden-hard" feel Painful edges with an anesthetic center
Necrotizing skin and soft-tissue infection	Deeper and more devastating than cellulitis Constant pain, bullae, ecchymosis, systemic signs
Panniculitis	Inflammation of subcutaneous fat tissue Tender skin nodules or papules
Pyoderma gangrenosum	Pustule or lesion with surrounding edema Progresses to ulcerated lesion Associated with systemic disorders (leukemia)
Pyomyositis	Purulent foci within individual muscle groups Severe localized pain
Staphylococcal scalded skin syndrome	Diffuse erythematous rash with wrinkled appearance (+) Nikolsky sign

+, Positive finding.

The microbiology of SSTI is of particular importance in guiding specific antimicrobial management. Because of the increasing prevalence of MRSA, use intravenous (IV) clindamycin (40 mg/kg/d, divided into doses administered every 6–8 hours; maximum, 900 mg per dose or 2.7 g/d) as first-line therapy. However, if there is a significant rate of clindamycin resistance in the community (>20%) or if the patient has a history of frequent hospitalizations or clindamycin-resistant MRSA, administer IV trimethoprim/sulfamethoxazole (10 mg trimethoprim/kg/d, divided into doses administered every 12 hours) *and* a first-generation cephalosporin (cefazolin 100 mg/kg/d divided into doses administered every 6–8 hours; 6-g/d maximum) *or* a semisynthetic penicillin (nafcillin 100–150 mg/kg/d divided into doses administered every 6 hours; 12-g/d maximum) for adequate *S pyogenes* coverage in cellulitis. If the organism identity and sensitivities are known, change to directed monotherapy.

If an apparent focal cellulitis or abscess fails to respond to the above choices for empirical antimicrobial coverage or if the patient is initially seriously ill or toxic, use vancomycin (45–60 mg/kg/d divided into doses administered every 6–8 hours; maximum, 2 g per dose). The goal is to maintain trough values at 10 to 15 µg/mL. In serious staphylococcal infections, add empirical bactericidal coverage for methicillin-susceptible *S aureus* by using nafcillin or a first-generation cephalosporin (as discussed in the previous paragraph), particularly if the involved site is near a vital structure.

For a septic-appearing patient, add ceftriaxone or cefepime (100 mg/kg/d divided into doses administered every 12 hours; 4-g/d maximum) to the staphylococcal coverage if there are concerns for gram-negative rod involvement (eg, environmental contamination or an immunocompromised host).

Another option for MRSA coverage is oral or IV linezolid. The dosing is age dependent (<12 years old, 30 mg/kg/d, divided into doses administered every 8 hours; ≥12 years old, 1,200 mg/d, divided into doses administered every 12 hours; maximum, 600 mg per dose). Linezolid may cause bone marrow suppression as early as the second week of therapy, so monitor the CBC weekly. Oral or IV doxycycline (2–4 mg/kg/d, divided into doses delivered every 12–24 hours; maximum, 100 mg per dose or 200 mg/d) is an alternative in a patient older than 8 years who does not have severe or disseminated staphylococcal disease.

When a patient does not respond appropriately to antibiotics, perform imaging to look for a deeper source of infection, foreign body, or adjacent deep venous thrombosis. Start with US.

Indications for Consultation

- **Infectious disease:** Unusual exposures, immunocompromised patient, failure to respond to therapy, severe illness, institutional approval of certain antimicrobial agents
- **Pediatric surgery or interventional radiology:** Abscess drainage

Disposition

- **Intensive care unit transfer:** Sepsis or a severe disease, such as necrotizing SSTI, necrotizing fasciitis, or staphylococcal scalded skin syndrome
- **Discharge criteria:** Afebrile, stable, or receding margins of involvement, tolerance of oral antibiotics or home IV therapy arranged

Follow-up

Primary care: 2 to 3 days to evaluate the continued response to treatment and removal of packing and/or drain (if placed)

Pearls and Pitfalls

- Streptococcal cellulitis may be caused by a nephritogenic strain, placing the patient at risk for subsequent acute glomerulonephritis.
- Recent or concurrent varicella infection is a risk factor for the development of streptococcal necrotizing fasciitis, as is concurrent ibuprofen use.
- Clindamycin solution has good enteral bioavailability but an unpleasant taste. Ask the pharmacy to flavor it to improve patient adherence. Or, prescribe the capsules and have the parent sprinkle the contents onto a spoon of applesauce or pudding.
- Inducible clindamycin resistance presents as a recrudescence of symptoms after several days of improvement.

Bibliography

Fenster DB, Renny MH, Ng C, Roskind CG. Scratching the surface: a review of skin and soft tissue infections in children. *Curr Opin Pediatr.* 2015;27(3):303–307

Liu C, Bayer A, Cosgrove SE, et al. Clinical practice guidelines by the Infectious Diseases Society of America for the treatment of methicillin-resistant *Staphylococcus aureus* infections in adults and children: executive summary. *Clin Infect Dis.* 2011;52(3):e18–e55

Mistry RD. Skin and soft tissue infections. *Pediatr Clin North Am.* 2013;60(5):1063–1082

Stevens DL, Bisno AL, Chambers HF, et al. Practice guidelines for the diagnosis and management of skin and soft tissue infections: 2014 update by the Infectious Diseases Society of America. *Clin Infect Dis.* 2014;59(2):147–159

Ear, Nose, Throat

Cervical Lymphadenopathy

Introduction

Cervical lymphadenopathy is a common and generally benign finding among many preschool- and school-aged children. There are 3 types of cervical lymphadenopathy.

1. Reactive adenopathy secondary to a viral or bacterial illness
2. Adenitis, an infection of the node itself (most commonly *Staphylococcus aureus* or group A *Streptococcus*, although viral, anaerobic, nontuberculous mycobacteria and *Mycobacterium tuberculosis* can also result in cervical adenitis)
3. Adenopathy secondary to systemic disease (especially Epstein-Barr virus [EBV], cytomegalovirus [CMV], autoimmune diseases, and malignancies)

Clinical Presentation

History

The patient's history is often diagnostic. Determine the duration of the adenopathy. Ask about exposure to sick persons and animals (kittens or puppies, *Bartonella henselae;* rabbits or ticks, tularemia; goats, cattle, or swine, brucellosis), recent travel (tuberculosis or bubonic plague), dental history (caries, abscess), and ingestion of medications (especially antiepileptic drugs), unpasteurized animal products (brucellosis, *Mycobacterium bovis*), or raw or undercooked meat (toxoplasmosis). Assess the patient's immunization status, especially focusing on the mumps vaccination.

With reactive adenopathy, there is usually a history of preceding or concurrent viral or bacterial infection in the head or neck. The onset of adenitis may be insidious in nature, or there may be a history of exposure to such an illness. A patient with a systemic disease may have symptoms such as fever, weight loss, and fatigue. With a malignant process, there may be a history of increasing size of the node, weight loss, weakness, pallor, night sweats, fever, and easy bruising.

Physical Examination

Perform a thorough examination of the head, neck, oral cavity, skin, and respiratory tract to look for infections that may be draining into the affected node(s). Check for generalized lymphadenopathy and hepatosplenomegaly.

Reactive lymph nodes are typically multiple, shotty, discrete, nontender, mobile, nonfluctuant, and smaller than 2 cm in diameter. The overlying skin is intact, with normal texture and color.

At presentation, adenitis appears as a tender, enlarged node, initially firm but becoming more fluctuant with time. The node may be erythematous, with warm, adherent overlying skin. The physical examination is different for a nontuberculous mycobacteria infection, in which the node is often nontender, without warmth, but with a violet or purplish color, while the patient is well-appearing, without fever. A tuberculous node typically has overlying erythema and often suppurates, and the patient usually presents with systemic signs and symptoms (fever, weight loss, fatigue).

A malignant node is fixed, hard, and matted and is most often located in the supraclavicular region.

A systemic disease may have associated diffuse lymphadenopathy and/or hepatosplenomegaly.

Laboratory Workup

No laboratory testing is necessary for adenitis, but obtain a culture if the node is drained. If a systemic disease is a concern (generalized lymphadenopathy, hepatosplenomegaly, weight loss, night sweats, hard or irregular-shaped node), perform a complete blood cell count (CBC), evaluation of erythrocyte sedimentation rate or C-reactive protein level, liver function tests, EBV and CMV serology, blood culture (if febrile and toxic appearing), and, if a malignancy is suspected, evaluate lactate dehydrogenase (LDH) and uric acid levels and obtain a chest radiograph. Test for *Bartonella* bacteria, brucellosis, and HIV if the history and physical examination suggest the possibility. Perform a tuberculin skin test (TST) if the patient has persistent cervical lymphadenopathy, especially if the node is firm, rubbery, or matted. If the patient is at least 5 years old, a blood-based interferon-gamma release assay (such as QuantiFERON-TB Gold In-Tube [Quest Diagnostics] and T-SPOT.TB tests [Oxford Diagnostic Laboratories]) may be used in place of a TST.

In general, imaging studies are not indicated, although ultrasonography (US) can be helpful in assessing whether there is abscess formation and determining when to perform surgical drainage. Order computed tomography of the neck if there are signs of airway compromise.

Differential Diagnosis

Determine whether the node is infected versus reactive to a local infection or secondary to a systemic disease (Table 14-1). See Chapter 17 for the differential diagnosis of neck masses.

Table 14-1. Differential Diagnosis of Cervical Lymphadenitis	
Diagnosis	**Clinical Features**
Adenitis (*Staphylococcus*, *Streptococcus*, anaerobic bacteria)	Node is erythematous, warm, and tender Unilateral
Nontuberculous mycobacteria	Afebrile Node is nonerythematous and nontender Evolves over weeks to months
Bartonella bacteria	Scratch or bite from a kitten or puppy 1–8 wk prior Patient well appearing May have conjunctivitis
Branchial cleft cyst	Recurrent abscesses in the same location, such as the lower border of the sternocleidomastoid Cyst may be draining
Epstein-Barr virus or cytomegalovirus	Fatigue Generalized lymphadenopathy Hepatosplenomegaly
Kawasaki disease	≥5 d of fever Mucous membrane changes Nonpurulent conjunctivitis Edema of the hands and feet Polymorphous rash Lymphadenopathy: acute, nonsuppurative, often unilateral, and with at least one node ≥1.5 cm
Malignancy	Weight loss, fever, fatigue, hepatosplenomegaly Node is firm, fixed, matted, increasing in size
Parotitis	Obscures the angle of the jaw Drainage from the Stensen duct
Tuberculosis	Fever, fatigue, weight loss Overlying erythema Node may drain spontaneously

Chapter 14: Cervical Lymphadenopathy

Treatment

Treat bacterial adenitis parenterally, initially with clindamycin (40 mg/kg/d, divided into doses administered every 6–8 hours; 2.7-g/d maximum) if methicillin-resistant *S aureus* is a concern. Otherwise, use nafcillin or oxacillin (150 mg/kg/d, divided into doses administered every 6 hours; 12-g/d maximum), cefazolin (75 mg/kg/d, divided into doses administered every 8 hours; 6-g/d maximum), or ampicillin/sulbactam (150 mg/kg/d, divided into doses administered every 6 hours; 8-g/d maximum). If the patient's condition deteriorates or if the patient does not respond to therapy after 48 hours, add vancomycin (45 mg/kg/d, divided into doses administered every 8 hours; 4-g/d maximum). Also, order warm compresses every 4 hours. If the node becomes fluctuant, arrange for incision and drainage by a general surgeon or otolaryngologist. Perform US if it is unclear whether the node is ready for drainage. Switch to an equivalent oral antibiotic once the patient responds to treatment.

If bartonellosis (cat scratch disease) is suspected, treat the patient as described previously, with adequate staphylococcal and streptococcal antimicrobial coverage. Although azithromycin, rifampin, trimethoprim/sulfamethoxazole, or gentamicin may offer some advantage, it is not necessary to specifically treat an immunocompetent patient who is not acutely or severely ill.

Surgical excision and culture constitute the treatment of choice if a nontuberculous mycobacterial infection is suspected. Avoid incision and drainage, which can result in a chronic draining fistula. If complete excision is not possible, arrange for curettage and administer antimycobacterial therapy with azithromycin (5 mg/kg administered every day; 500-mg/d maximum) or clarithromycin (15 mg/kg/d, divided into doses administered every 12 hours; 1-g/d maximum) plus rifampin (20 mg/kg/d, divided into doses administered every 12 hours; 600-mg/d maximum) and/or ethambutol (15 mg/kg administered every day; 2.5-g/d maximum).

If a malignancy is suspected, obtain a CBC with reticulocyte count, LDH level, uric acid level, complete metabolic profile, and chest radiograph and consult a hematologist/oncologist. The treatment of Kawasaki disease is discussed in Chapter 67.

The treatment for EBV, CMV, and other mononucleosis-like syndromes is supportive. However, if the patient has significant upper airway obstruction, insert a nasopharyngeal tube (nasal trumpet) and administer methylprednisolone (1 mg/kg every day).

Indications for Consultation

- **General surgery or otolaryngology:** Incision and drainage or surgical excision needed
- **Infectious disease:** Suspected *Mycobacterium* infection
- **Oncology:** Suspected malignancy
- **Rheumatology:** Suspected collagen vascular disease

Disposition

- **Intensive care unit transfer:** Airway compromise or a rapidly progressing infection that is not responsive to parenteral therapy
- **Discharge criteria:** Patient afebrile for more than 24 hours with improvement in adenitis, no respiratory distress, and tolerating adequate oral intake

Follow-up

- **Primary care:** 2 to 3 days
- **Hematology/oncology (malignancy suspected):** Immediate
- **Infectious diseases:** 1 week (suspected *Mycobacterium* infection)

Pearls and Pitfalls

- Adenopathy that persists for more than 3 weeks requires further workup, including tuberculosis testing and possible biopsy for malignancy.
- Incision and drainage of a node suspected to have *Mycobacterium* infection can lead to chronic draining sinus tract or disseminated disease.
- Posterior cervical adenopathy is almost always reactive or viral.
- A well-appearing patient with adenitis can be discharged on oral antibiotics and warm compresses, with follow-up for incision and drainage if the node becomes fluctuant.
- Do not administer steroids if a neoplastic process is a possibility.

Bibliography

Healy CM, Baker CJ. Cervical lymphadenitis. In: Cherry JD, Harrison GJ, Kaplan SL, Steinbach WJ, Hotez PJ, eds. *Feigin and Cherry's Textbook of Pediatric Infectious Diseases.* 7th ed. Philadelphia, PA: Elsevier Saunders; 2014:175–188

Locke R, Comfort R, Kubba H. When does an enlarged cervical lymph node in a child need excision? A systematic review. *Int J Pediatr Otorhinolaryngol.* 2014;78(3):393–401

Neff L, Newland JG, Sykes KJ, Selvarangan R, Wei JL. Microbiology and antimicrobial treatment of pediatric cervical lymphadenitis requiring surgical intervention. *Int J Pediatr Otorhinolaryngol.* 2013;77(5):817–820

Nolder AR. Paediatric cervical lymphadenopathy: when to biopsy? *Curr Opin Otolaryngol Head Neck Surg.* 2013;21(6):567–570

Rosenberg TL, Nolder AR. Pediatric cervical lymphadenopathy. *Otolaryngol Clin North Am.* 2014;47(5):721–731

Infectious Croup

Introduction

Croup is a disease of the upper airway in which the subglottic area becomes inflamed and edematous. The narrowest part of the pediatric airway is within the cricoid cartilage, so 1 mm of edema here can decrease airflow exponentially. Parainfluenza viruses are the most common cause of croup, but many other respiratory viruses, such as rhinovirus, respiratory syncytial virus (RSV), and influenza, cause the same clinical picture.

Viral infectious croup occurs between 3 months and 3 years of age, with a peak incidence at 2 years. There is a slight male predominance, and the disease occurs more frequently in the fall and winter months.

Clinical Presentation

History

Usually, there is a gradual onset of nonspecific upper respiratory symptoms, including coryza, cough, sore throat, and low-grade fever. On day 2 or 3 of illness, patients develop a hoarse voice, barky or seal-like cough, tachypnea, and inspiratory, or in some cases, biphasic stridor. Symptoms are often reported to be worse at night.

Physical Examination

Stridor is primarily inspiratory, but if the narrowing has extended beyond the thoracic inlet, it can be biphasic. Mild disease is characterized by minimal or absent retractions and stridor and normal air entry. Biphasic sounds indicate that narrowing has extended beyond the thoracic inlet. In moderate disease, stridor is present at rest and worsens with agitation. Other findings include mild to moderate retractions and decreased lung aeration. Severe disease and impending respiratory failure are characterized by agitation, decreased mental status, cyanosis, continuous stridor, severe retractions, markedly decreased lung aeration, and/or hypoxemia.

Radiology Examinations

Since croup is a clinical diagnosis, routine imaging is not necessary. If an anteroposterior neck radiograph is obtained, look for subglottic narrowing (steeple sign). However, this finding may be absent.

If a congenital or acquired anatomic airway abnormality is suspected (<3 months of age, recurrent croup, unusually persistent or severe disease), order 2-view chest radiography. Consult an otolaryngologist to discuss additional diagnostic workup, such as laryngoscopy.

Differential Diagnosis

The differential diagnosis of croup is summarized in Table 15-1.

Treatment

Systemic steroids are the mainstay of treatment for infectious croup. Dexamethasone is preferred because of its long half-life, low cost, and ease of administration. Administer a single dose (0.15–0.60 mg/kg; 12-mg maximum) to any patient with croup, including those with mild disease. Use a dose of 0.3–0.6 mg/kg (12-mg maximum) for a patient with moderate to severe disease. Oral, intravenous (IV), and intramuscular (IM) routes are equally effective, so reserve IM or IV administration for a patient who cannot tolerate

Table 15-1. Differential Diagnosis of Croup	
Diagnosis	**Clinical Features**
Angioedema	History of allergies or exposure to an offending substance Swelling of the face/lips/tongue Urticarial rash
Bacterial tracheitis	Abrupt onset of upper airway obstruction in a patient recovering from a viral illness (croup, influenza) Toxic appearance with high fever Copious, purulent secretions at suctioning
Epiglottitis (very rare)	Abrupt onset with fever and toxicity Rapid progression to airway obstruction Patient prefers a "sniffing" posture Patient unimmunized
Foreign body aspiration	History of choking/gagging Sudden onset of cough, stridor, and dyspnea No prodrome of upper respiratory infection or fever
Peritonsillar abscess	Older children and adolescents Severe sore throat, dysphagia, muffled voice, and trismus Exudative tonsillitis with uvula deviation
Retropharyngeal abscess	Fever, toxicity, and dysphagia with drooling Muffled stridor without barking cough Limited neck extension
Spasmodic croup	Recurrent episodes of nighttime barky cough and stridor No upper respiratory infection or fever May have a history of allergies

oral medication or who has severe respiratory distress. The benefit of repeat steroid dosing is unclear. If a hospitalized patient experiences continued respiratory distress and repeated nebulized epinephrine treatments are needed, administer a second dose of dexamethasone 24 to 48 hours after the first dose.

Nebulized epinephrine has rapid onset and alleviates airway obstruction until dexamethasone becomes effective. Administer nebulized racemic epinephrine (0.05 mL/kg, 0.5-mL maximum, diluted in 3 mL of normal saline) to patients with moderate to severe disease. Racemic epinephrine lasts about 2 hours, so repeat the dose every 2 to 4 hours, as needed. Symptom rebound may occur, so monitor patients prior to discharge for 4 to 6 hours. If racemic epinephrine is unavailable, use L-epinephrine (both isomers are equally effective).

If there is severe airway obstruction with signs of impending respiratory failure, intubate the patient and transfer him or her to an intensive care unit (ICU). Because significant subglottic edema exists, use an endotracheal tube that is at least 0.5 mm smaller than the size calculated for the patient's age. Call an anesthesiologist if a difficult intubation is anticipated.

Avoid agitating the patient, since crying increases negative intrathoracic pressure and worsens airway obstruction. Do not administer humidified oxygen unless the patient is hypoxic, because it does not improve symptoms and forcing a mask on an agitated patient only exacerbates respiratory distress. Similarly, attempting to perform a blood gas analysis prior to intubation will only serve to agitate the patient. At this time, routine use of heliox is not recommended, but it may be initially helpful in patients with moderate to severe disease.

Indications for Consultation

- **Anesthesia:** Emergent airway management required
- **Otolaryngology:** Significant airway compromise; age <3 months; long duration of symptoms (>1 week); recurrent croup episodes (>2 episodes per season); concern for epiglottitis, bacterial tracheitis, or foreign-body aspiration; or evaluation for congenital or acquired airway narrowing

Disposition

- **ICU transfer:** Severe respiratory distress and hypoxemia
- **Discharge criteria:** Mild respiratory distress, no nebulized epinephrine treatment in 6 hours, oxygen saturation greater than 94% with room air, adequate oral intake

Follow-up

- **Primary care:** 1 to 3 days
- **Otolaryngology:** 1 to 2 weeks if the patient has an underlying airway anomaly

Pearls and Pitfalls

- Reserve nebulized epinephrine for patients with moderate to severe disease.
- The cricoid cartilage is located in the subglottic area and is the narrowest part of the pediatric upper airway. Only 1 mm of edema in this area can decrease airflow by as much as 80%.
- When intubating a patient with croup, use an endotracheal tube size that is 0.5 mm smaller than the size calculated for the patient's age.

Bibliography

Bjornson CL, Johnson DW. Croup in children. *CMAJ*. 2013;185(15):1317–1323

Joshi V, Malik V, Mirza O, Kumar BN. Fifteen-minute consultation: structured approach to management of a child with recurrent croup. *Arch Dis Child Educ Pract Ed*. 2014;99(3):90–93

Petrocheilou A, Tanou K, Kalampouka E, Malakasioti G, Giannios C, Kaditis AG. Viral croup: diagnosis and a treatment algorithm. *Pediatr Pulmonol*. 2014;49(5):421–429

Zoorob R, Sidani M, Murray J. Croup: an overview. *Am Fam Physician*. 2011;83(9):1067–1073

Mastoiditis

Introduction

Mastoiditis is a bacterial infection of the mastoid bone and air cells. It is the most common suppurative complication of acute otitis media (AOM), secondary to spread of the infection beyond the middle ear via bony erosion or through the emissary vein of the mastoid. Acute mastoiditis can be further categorized into acute mastoiditis with periostitis (purulent material in mastoid cavities) or coalescent mastoiditis (destruction of bony septa between mastoid air cells; may be followed by abscess formation). The most common pathogens are *Streptococcus pneumoniae*, *Streptococcus pyogenes*, and *Staphylococcus aureus* (including methicillin-resistant *S aureus*), although gram-negative bacilli (*Pseudomonas aeruginosa*, nontypable *Haemophilus influenzae*) are also implicated.

Clinical Presentation

History

Usually there is a history of AOM during the preceding 2 weeks. Typical complaints include fever (>38.3°C; >101°F), along with headache, otalgia and/or otorrhea, and pain over the mastoid process. A younger patient may have nonspecific complaints, such as irritability, anorexia, and fatigue.

Chronic mastoiditis may occur and can be subclinical or appear with prolonged otorrhea and otalgia at presentation.

Physical Examination

In mastoiditis, the mastoid process and postauricular area are swollen, erythematous, tender (can be severe), and occasionally fluctuant. The auricle is displaced both anteriorly and inferiorly (or down and outward in a patient <2 years of age), while the ipsilateral tympanic membrane frequently, but not always, shows signs of AOM (erythema, bulging, loss of landmarks). Usually the neurologic examination is nonfocal, although with more severe disease, cranial nerve involvement may occur (most frequently cranial nerves VI and VII or the ophthalmic branch of cranial nerve V). As a result, the patient may have facial palsy, double vision, and/or transient hearing loss.

Radiology Examinations and Laboratory Workup

If mastoiditis is suspected, perform computed tomography (CT) of the temporal bones, because plain mastoid radiographs are unreliable. Typical findings include clouding of the mastoid air cells and loss of the intermastoid cell septa secondary to the osteomyelitic process. Fluid in the middle ear and mastoid, without the loss of bony septa, can be seen with AOM and is nondiagnostic. Other findings may include abscess formation and intracranial extension. Persistent infection in the mastoid cavity can lead to coalescent mastoiditis or empyema of the temporal bone. This is divided into the following 5 stages (increasing in severity):

- Stage 1: Hyperemia to the mucosal lining of the mastoid air cells
- Stage 2: Transudate and/or exudate within the mastoid air cells
- Stage 3: Necrosis of the bone
- Stage 4: Septation loss with abscess formation
- Stage 5: Extension beyond the mastoid area (ie, intracranial abscess, sigmoid sinus thrombosis, meningitis)

Obtain a complete blood cell count, erythrocyte sedimentation rate (ESR) and/or C-reactive protein (CRP) level, and a blood culture. Typically, the patient has a leukocytosis with a left shift, as well as increased CRP level and ESR. The blood culture result will be positive in approximately 5% of cases.

Differential Diagnosis

Usually the diagnosis is clear, based on fever, ipsilateral AOM, and displacement of the pinna with swelling, erythema, and tenderness of the posterior auricular area. Distortion or swelling of the pinna may also be seen with an insect bite reaction or a chondritis. The differential diagnosis of mastoiditis is summarized in Table 16-1.

Treatment

Consult with an otolaryngologist, because surgical drainage is indicated if a subperiosteal or intracranial abscess is seen on CT images or if the patient does not improve clinically after 24 to 48 hours of intravenous (IV) antibiotic administration. Other surgical interventions may include myringotomy and tympanocentesis, as well as simple or radical mastoidectomy.

After CT is performed, a lumbar puncture is indicated if the patient presents with altered mental status or signs of intracranial extension. Consult a neurosurgeon if intracranial extension is confirmed.

Table 16-1. Differential Diagnosis of Mastoiditis

Diagnosis	Clinical Features
Acute otitis media	No erythema, tenderness, or swelling over the mastoid Pinna not displaced
Basilar skull fracture	No fever or ipsilateral AOM Pinna not displaced Ecchymoses over the mastoid, which may be bilateral
Chondritis	Erythema and swelling contiguous with break in the skin No ipsilateral AOM
Insect bite reaction	No fever Punctum may be evident No ipsilateral AOM
Langerhans cell histiocytosis	Recurrent AOM Seborrheic rash
Posterior auricular lymphadenopathy	Mobile, circumscribed Pinna not displaced
Otitis externa	Otorrhea and otalgia No erythema, tenderness, or swelling over the mastoid Pinna not displaced

Abbreviation: AOM, acute otitis media.

Begin treatment with IV ceftriaxone (100 mg/kg/d, divided into doses administered every 12 hours; 4-g/d maximum) or IV cefotaxime (200 mg/kg/d, divided into doses administered every 6–8 hours; 12-g/d maximum), *in addition to* clindamycin (40 mg/kg/d, divided into doses administered every 6–8 hours; 2.7-g/d maximum). For patients with a history of recurrent otitis media or recent antibiotic therapy, use IV ceftazidime (150 mg/kg/d, divided into doses administered every 8 hours; 6-g/d maximum) or IV cefepime (150 mg/kg/d, divided into doses administered every 8 hours; 6-g/d maximum) plus IV vancomycin (60 mg/kg/d, divided into doses administered every 6 hours; 4-g/d maximum). Also add vancomycin if intracranial spread is suspected, if there is no response to therapy within 24 hours, or if there is a high local rate of clindamycin resistance. For disease of stages 3 to 5, a minimum of 6 weeks of IV or parenteral antibiotics is necessary, tailored to the specific organism (if identified). Add a topical antimicrobial agent for chronic mastoiditis (ciprofloxacin optic drops, 0.25 mL, administered twice a day for 7 days).

For stage 1 and 2 disease, administer a shorter IV course (7–10 days), followed by oral therapy (to complete a 2–4 week course), once the patient has been afebrile for 24 hours and there is improvement in the inflammatory markers and physical examination.

Indications for Consultation

- **Neurology and neurosurgery:** Signs of intracranial extension
- **Otolaryngology:** All patients

Disposition

- **Intensive care unit transfer:** Intracranial spread or associated meningitis
- **Discharge criteria:** Patient afebrile for 48 hours, with significant clinical improvement and downward trending of inflammatory markers

Follow-up

- **Primary care:** 1 week
- **Otolaryngology:** 2 weeks

Pearls and Pitfalls

- An infant may not have the classic displacement of the pinna.
- Not every case of mastoiditis is associated with an ipsilateral AOM.
- A patient with mastoiditis is at risk for hearing loss, so audiology follow-up is necessary.

Bibliography

Choi SS, Lander L. Pediatric acute mastoiditis in the post-pneumococcal conjugate vaccine era. *Laryngoscope.* 2011;121(5):1072–1080

Kordeluk S, Kraus M, Leibovitz E. Challenges in the management of acute mastoiditis in children. *Curr Infect Dis Rep.* 2015;17(5):479

Lin HW, Shargorodsky J, Gopen Q. Clinical strategies for the management of acute mastoiditis in the pediatric population. *Clin Pediatr (Phila).* 2010;49(2):110–115

Marom T, Roth Y, Boaz M, et al. Acute mastoiditis in children: necessity and timing of imaging. *Pediatr Infect Dis J.* 2016;35(1):30–34

Psarommatis IM, Voudouris C, Douros K, Giannakopoulos P, Bairamis T, Carabinos C. Algorithmic management of pediatric acute mastoiditis. *Int J Pediatr Otorhinolaryngol.* 2012;76(6):791–796

Tamir SO, Roth Y, Dalal I, Goldfarb A, Marom T. Acute mastoiditis in the pneumococcal conjugate vaccine era. *Clin Vaccine Immunol.* 2014;21(8):1189–1191

CHAPTER 17

Neck Masses

Introduction

The etiologies of pediatric neck masses include inflammatory, congenital, and neoplastic processes. Most involve lymph nodes and are benign and inflammatory in nature (reactive cervical lymphadenopathy or lymphadenitis) (see Chapter 14, Cervical Lymphadenopathy). The most common congenital neck masses are branchial cleft anomalies (BCAs) and thyroglossal duct cysts (TDCs). Malignant processes are rare but must always be considered in the differential diagnosis.

Congenital anomalies may be present at birth or may not become apparent until a rapid phase of growth or infection occurs. TDCs and branchial cleft sinuses and fistulas typically become apparent during infancy and early childhood, while branchial cleft cysts appear later in adolescence or early adulthood. Lymphoma and thyroid carcinomas most often occur in older children and adolescents.

Clinical Presentation

History

Ask the caregiver about the child's rate of growth and associated symptoms. Rapid growth suggests a benign process, with the exception of non-Hodgkin lymphoma. Slow growth associated with systemic symptoms (fever, fatigue, weight loss, night sweats) is more typical of a malignancy. Cysts often fluctuate in size, increasing with upper respiratory tract infections. Chronic, intermittent drainage is consistent with a sinus tract and/or fistula. Ask about prior antibiotic treatment, because a failure of empirical treatment is concerning for either atypical organisms (such as nontuberculous mycobacteria) or malignancy. Also ask about tuberculosis risk factors and exposure to cats (*Bartonella* bacteria).

Physical Examination

Assess the characteristics of the mass, including the location, consistency, mobility, and any signs of infection (redness, warmth, tenderness). The location suggests the most likely diagnoses. Masses located anterior to the sternocleidomastoid muscle are usually benign, except for thyroid malignancies. TDCs are cystic, midline masses that move with tongue protrusion and swallowing. They are found anywhere from the base of the tongue to the thyroid gland. Second branchial cleft cysts, which account for more than 90% of branchial cleft anomalies, are located along the anterior border of the sternocleidomastoid muscle. First branchial cleft cysts can be located anywhere from the external auditory canal to the angle of the mandible. A fluctuant mass is usually an abscess or cyst. An orifice suggests a sinus tract or fistula.

Findings that are suggestive of a malignancy include a firm, painless mass that is matted or fixed to underlying structures, a persistent solitary lymph node larger than 2 cm in diameter, a mass that has not responded to antibiotic treatment, and a supraclavicular mass.

Perform a complete physical examination. Cranial nerve deficits, stridor, and tracheal deviation suggest impingement on surrounding structures. Pay particular attention to generalized lymphadenopathy and hepatosplenomegaly, which can suggest a systemic process, such as certain viral syndromes (Epstein-Barr virus, HIV) or malignancy.

Radiology Examinations

If there is diagnostic uncertainty, order ultrasonography (US) to evaluate the mass. US will also help to determine if fluid is present for drainage or diagnostic sampling. Depending on the results, computed tomography (CT) or magnetic resonance (MR) imaging may be needed to fully visualize the mass, especially if there is a tract or fistula. If malignancy is suspected, discuss the case with the radiologist and consulting surgeon and/or oncologist to determine the best radiologic modality (US with or without CT or MR imaging). For a TDC, perform a thyroid scan to look for thyroid tissue prior to surgical excision.

Laboratory Workup

Order a complete blood cell count with differential if infection or malignancy is suspected. If concerned about malignancy, also obtain a peripheral blood smear, a complete metabolic panel—including phosphorus and lactate dehydrogenase levels—and uric acid level. For cases that are atypical or concerning for malignancy, discuss with the surgeon whether a fine-needle aspiration (FNA) or biopsy is indicated. Certain conditions, such as mycobacterial infection, can be complicated by FNA. If aspiration is performed, order a Gram stain, routine anaerobic and aerobic cultures, histopathology, and cytology. If tuberculosis is suspected, perform a purified protein derivative skin test. If *Bartonella* bacteria is suspected, order *Bartonella henselae* titers.

When a diagnosis of TDC is assigned, check the thyroid studies to assess the patient for hypothyroidism because ectopic thyroid glands are commonly associated with TDCs.

Differential Diagnosis

The priorities are to rule out a neoplasm and address a life-threatening complication, such as airway compression. The differential diagnosis is summarized in Tables 17-1 and 17-2.

Table 17-1. Differential Diagnosis of Congenital Neck Masses	
Diagnosis	**Clinical Features**
Dermoid cyst	Midline painless, doughy, or rubbery mass that moves with the doughy overlying skin Does not move with tongue protrusion or swallowing
Hemangioma	Red to blue soft mass that is present at birth or shortly thereafter Rapid growth phase, followed by slow involution
Lymphovascular malformation	Soft, painless, compressible mass that transilluminates and is located in the posterior triangle
Teratoma	Common cause of neonatal airway obstruction Firm mass with irregular borders Imaging: bulky, heterogeneous mass with solid and cystic components

Table 17-2. Differential Diagnosis of Neoplastic Neck Masses	
Diagnosis	**Clinical Features**
Benign neoplastic masses	
Lipoma	Soft, painless, subcutaneous mass
Neurofibroma	Soft, skin-colored, cutaneous or subcutaneous nodule
Thyroid nodule	Midline nodule that moves with the thyroid gland Consider the nodule to be malignant until proven otherwise
Malignant neoplastic masses	
Hodgkin lymphoma	Slow-growing neck mass Painless, rubbery, or firm lymph node (anterior or posterior cervical, preauricular, supraclavicular) Fever, night sweats, weight loss, hepatosplenomegaly

Neuroblastoma	Metastatic disease (primary abdominal or thoracic tumor)
	  Proptosis, periorbital swelling, and ecchymoses
	  Acute cerebellar ataxia (opsoclonus-myoclonus and nystagmus)
	Primary cervical disease
	  Lateral or retropharyngeal neck mass
	Symptoms of mass impingement on surrounding organs (cranial nerve palsies, Horner syndrome, cough, stridor, dysphagia)

Non-Hodgkin lymphoma	Rapidly enlarging neck mass Painless, firm to hard lymph node (spinal accessory, supraclavicular) Fever, weight loss, bone and joint pain
Rhabdomyosarcoma	Painless, hard mass Anterior and posterior cervical location Symptoms of mass impingement on surrounding organs (hoarseness)
Thyroid carcinoma	Firm mass that feels different from other thyroid tissue Patient has history of irradiation

Treatment

See Chapter 14, Cervical Lymphadenopathy, for the antibiotic treatment of cervical lymphadenitis. If a phlegmon or abscess is present, consult a surgeon to determine whether drainage is indicated (if so, order a Gram stain and routine aerobic and anaerobic cultures). When the patient is clinically improved, change to an equivalent oral antibiotic regimen or a narrow-spectrum antibiotic if culture results are known to complete a 10- to 14-day course of treatment.

For a BCA, TDC, or other congenital neck mass, consult a surgeon (in otolaryngology or general surgery) to discuss the timing of surgery, which can usually be scheduled as an outpatient procedure.

If a malignant mass is suspected, consult an oncologist for recommendations about additional imaging, blood work, and biopsy (FNA vs excisional). Also discuss which surgical service is most appropriate for managing the patient's condition, as well as whether to transfer the patient to an oncology or surgical service.

Indications for Consultation

- **Oncology:** Malignant neck masses
- **Otolaryngology or general surgery:** TDC, BCA, or any other neck mass that requires biopsy or surgical excision

Disposition

- **Tertiary care center transfer:** If malignancy is considered, to expedite obtaining and processing biopsy specimens
- **Intensive care unit transfer:** Airway obstruction
- **Discharge criteria:** Patient clinically improving and tolerating oral intake; appropriate diagnostic and treatment plan is in place (surgical intervention or oncologic consultation if indicated)

Follow-up

- **Primary care:** 3 to 4 days
- **If surgery was performed:** 1 to 3 days with the surgical service

Pearls and Pitfalls

- Consult a surgeon prior to any drainage attempts because some conditions can be complicated by aspiration.
- About 1% of patients with a preoperative diagnosis of TDC will actually have a median ectopic thyroid gland that contains all of the functional thyroid tissue.

Bibliography

Brigger MR, Cunningham MJ. Malignant cervical masses in children. *Otolaryngol Clin North Am.* 2015;48(1):59–77

Geddes G, Butterfly MM, Patel SM, Marra S. Pediatric neck masses. *Pediatr Rev.* 2013; 34(3):115–125

Goins MR, Beasley MS. Pediatric neck masses. *Oral Maxillofac Surg Clin North Am.* 2012;24(3):457–468

LaPlante JK, Pierson NS, Hedlund GL. Common pediatric head and neck congenital/ developmental anomalies. *Radiol Clin North Am.* 2015;53(1):181–196

Meier JD, Grimmer JF. Evaluation and management of neck masses in children. *Am Fam Physician.* 2014;89(5):353–358

Prosser JD, Myer CM. Branchial cleft anomalies and thymic cysts. *Otolaryngol Clin North Am.* 2015;48(1):1–14

CHAPTER 18

Orbital and Periorbital Cellulitis

Introduction

Orbital (postseptal) cellulitis and periorbital (preseptal) cellulitis are major infections of the orbital tissues. There has been a notable increase in cases of both in recent years, possibly as a consequence of the increase in multi–drug-resistant organisms. Periorbital cellulitis is by far more common. However, orbital cellulitis is an ocular emergency because there is significant morbidity and mortality associated with it, including intracranial extension in up to 5% of patients. A rare complication is osteomyelitis of the frontal bone (Pott puffy tumor).

The orbital septum is a fibrous membrane that runs from the periosteum of the orbital bones to the tarsal plates. It functions as a barrier between the skin/subcutaneous tissues of the periorbital space and the intraorbital structures, preventing superficial (ie, periorbital/preseptal) infections from extending inward. It also prevents orbital cellulitis from extending beyond the supraorbital and infraorbital ridges.

Orbital cellulitis is most often secondary to extension of sinusitis (most often chronic ethmoid) through the thin and porous medial orbital wall (lamina papyracea), although it can also occur via hematogenous spread or from direct trauma or surgery. As a consequence of the association with sinusitis, it is most common during the winter months, secondary to group A *Streptococcus*, *Streptococcus pneumoniae*, and *Staphylococcus aureus*. *Pseudomonas*, *Klebsiella*, *Eikenella*, and *Enterococcus* bacteria are less common, while fungal pathogens are a concern in an immunocompromised patient. A polymicrobial infection with both aerobic and anaerobic bacteria can occur in an older adolescent. The venous system of the orbital space is valveless, which can facilitate extension of an infection to intracranial structures.

Periorbital cellulitis is most often secondary to disruption of the skin barrier from trauma, such as insect bites, animal bites, or abrasions to the periorbital region. Common organisms are the same for superficial skin infections, including *S aureus* and group A *Streptococcus*. Less often, sinusitis can extend to the periorbital spaces, so that nasopharyngeal organisms such as *S pneumoniae* and anaerobes may be involved. Rare causes associated with specific exposures include fungi and mycobacteria.

Clinical Presentation

History

Ask about recent sinus infections, facial trauma, insect/animal bites, and dental procedures. In addition, confirm that the patient has normal immune status.

Physical Examination

Orbital Cellulitis

The patient typically presents with fever, malaise, and warm, tender, erythematous eyelid swelling. The cardinal signs are proptosis, conjunctival chemosis, pain with eye movement, and ophthalmoplegia, which may be noted by the patient despite severe lid swelling, preventing direct observation of the extraocular movements. However, all of these signs are not always present. Increased intraocular pressure and a purulent nasal discharge are other possible findings. Decreased visual acuity or presence of visual field defects, which may manifest initially or later in the course of the disease, is an ophthalmologic emergency secondary to involvement of the optic nerve. Unremitting headache and altered mental status suggest intracranial extension, while forehead swelling occurs with Pott puffy tumor.

Periorbital Cellulitis

The patient typically presents with swelling, warmth, and redness of the periorbital region, often in association with an obvious break in the skin integrity (insect bite, scratch, etc). Importantly, there is no proptosis, conjunctival chemosis, pain with eye movement, or ophthalmoplegia. Fever may or may not be present. The orbital septum effectively limits the spread of preseptal cellulitis, so the infection does not spread backward to the orbital space.

Laboratory Workup and Radiology Examinations

If orbital cellulitis is suspected, perform contrast-enhanced computed tomography (CT) of the orbits and sinuses to look for an orbital abscess, subperiosteal abscess, or intracranial extension. Head CT is inadequate because head CT protocols specifically avoid imaging of the orbital space to reduce radiation exposure to the lens of the eye. Also obtain a complete blood cell count, erythrocyte sedimentation rate and/or C-reactive protein level, and blood culture. A lumbar puncture is indicated if there is concern for cerebral or meningeal involvement, provided there is no evidence of increased intracranial pressure. No laboratory testing is necessary for periorbital cellulitis. Specifically, the blood culture result is rarely positive.

A sinus series will not allow differentiation of orbital from periorbital cellulitis, because sinus involvement complicates a significant percentage of cases of periorbital cellulitis. Orbital ultrasonography can be used to identify orbital abscesses, but ultimately, magnetic resonance imaging may be needed for better evaluation of intracranial extension.

Differential Diagnosis

It is essential to distinguish orbital cellulitis from periorbital cellulitis, because more aggressive medical and surgical intervention is required with the former. Passively open the patient's eyelids and examine the eyes for conjunctival injection, discharge, proptosis, chemosis, pain with eye movement, and ophthalmoplegia, and check the patient's visual acuity. Lack of ocular swelling beyond the infraorbital and supraorbital ridges suggests periorbital cellulitis. However, the forehead swelling associated with Pott puffy tumor can be mistaken for a periorbital infection. The differential diagnosis is summarized in Table 18-1.

Treatment

Orbital Cellulitis

If orbital cellulitis is suspected or confirmed, promptly consult both an oto-laryngologist and an ophthalmologist for possible surgical intervention. Treat with one of the following intravenous (IV) antibiotic regimens:

IV or intramuscular (IM) ceftriaxone (50-75 mg/kg/d, divided into doses administered every 12 hours; 2-g/d maximum); use 100 mg/kg/d (4-g/d maximum) if intracranial extension is suspected
or
IV or IM cefotaxime (150–200 mg/kg/d, divided into doses administered every 6–8 hours; 12-g/d maximum)
or
IV or IM ampicillin/sulbactam (300 mg/kg/d, divided into doses administered every 6 hours; 12-g/d ampicillin/sulbactam maximum [8-g/d ampicillin component maximum])
or
IV piperacillin/tazobactam (300–400 mg/kg/d, divided into doses administered every 8 hours; 16-g/d piperacillin component maximum)

Table 18-1. Differential Diagnosis of Periorbital and Orbital Cellulitis

Diagnosis	Clinical Features
Eyelid edema	
Conjunctivitis	May be bilateral No fever or toxicity
Epstein-Barr virus	Dacrocystitis Lacrimal gland/duct inflammation Other signs of Epstein-Barr virus infection
Insect/animal bite	Punctum may be evident Patient may have a history of a bite No fever or toxicity
Allergic reaction	No fever or toxicity Patient may have urticaria or swelling elsewhere Pruritus
Nephrotic syndrome	No fever or toxicity Usually bilateral eye swelling with edema in other dependent areas Proteinuria
Trauma	Patient may have a history or evidence (ecchymoses) of trauma No fever or toxicity
Hordeolum	No fever or toxicity Obstructed gland is often evident
Exophthalmos	
Orbital neoplasm	Slowly progressive swelling May have visual changes No fever or toxicity
Hyperthyroidism	Tachycardia, palpitations, lid lag, heat intolerance Goiter may be palpated
Forehead swelling	
Preseptal cellulitis	Patient may have a history of trauma or a break in the skin No limitation of extraocular movement, proptosis, or chemosis
Pott puffy tumor	Patient is an adolescent History is compatible with frontal sinusitis No or limited orbital swelling

Add IV vancomycin (40–60 mg/kg/d, divided into doses administered 4 times per day; 4-g/d maximum) if local antibiograms suggest that methicillin-resistant *S aureus* (MRSA) is possible or if the patient appears toxic.

Add anaerobic antimicrobial coverage, such as metronidazole, in the event of a brain abscess.

Periorbital Cellulitis

Treatment is as for any other soft-tissue infection (see Chapter 13, Skin and Soft-Tissue Infections). Local resistance patterns determine whether MRSA antimicrobial coverage is necessary. Also treat associated sinusitis (see Chapter 22, Sinusitis). Topical treatment is not effective or indicated.

Indications for Consultation (Suspected or Confirmed Orbital Cellulitis)

- **Ophthalmology:** All patients
- **Otolaryngology:** All patients

Disposition

Orbital Cellulitis

- **Intensive care unit transfer:** Intracranial extension
- **Interinstitutional transfer:** Ophthalmology or otolaryngology service not immediately available
- **Discharge criteria:** Patient afebrile for 48 hours, with significant clinical improvement, including normal visual acuity and extraocular movements, as well as a downward trend of the inflammatory markers; continue oral antibiotics for a minimum of 2 weeks' total treatment

Periorbital Cellulitis

Discharge criteria: Patient afebrile for 48 hours, with significant clinical improvement; continue oral antibiotics for 7 to 14 days' total treatment

Follow-up (Orbital Cellulitis)

Otolaryngology and/or ophthalmology: Weekly during the antibiotic course of treatment

Pearls and Pitfalls

- A subperiosteal abscess may respond to IV antibiotics and may not require drainage.
- There is a 10% risk of residual loss of visual acuity.
- Ninety percent of cases of orbital cellulitis result from the direct spread of sinusitis (most commonly of the ethmoid). Fifteen percent of cases of periorbital cellulitis result from sinusitis.

Bibliography

Bedwell J, Bauman NM. Management of pediatric orbital cellulitis and abscess. *Curr Opin Otolaryngol Head Neck Surg*. 2011;19(6):467–473

Blumfield E, Misra M. Pott's puffy tumor, intracranial, and orbital complications as the initial presentation of sinusitis in healthy adolescents, a case series. *Emerg Radiol*. 2011;18(3):203–210

Mathew AV, Craig E, Al-Mahmoud R, et al. Paediatric post-septal and pre-septal cellulitis: 10 years' experience at a tertiary-level children's hospital. *Br J Radiol*. 2014;87(1033):20130503

Meara DJ. Sinonasal disease and orbital cellulitis in children. *Oral Maxillofac Surg Clin North Am*. 2012;24(3):487–496

CHAPTER 19

Parotitis

Introduction

As a result of the mumps immunization, parotitis is now rare in children. Risk factors include dehydration, poor oral hygiene, medications (antihistamines, anticholinergics), immunosuppression or deficiency, and anatomic abnormalities. Most cases are infectious in nature. Less common are inflammatory etiologies, including juvenile recurrent parotitis (JRP) and Sjögren syndrome.

Viral parotitis occurs in children aged 3 to 10 years, secondary to either mumps paramyxovirus (in both immunized and unimmunized patients) or other viral infections, such as Epstein-Barr virus, human herpesvirus 6, parainfluenza viruses, and HIV. With the exception of HIV parotitis, which is recurrent or chronic, viral parotitis is self-limited over 7 to 10 days.

Bacterial parotitis occurs in infants younger than 2 months and sporadically in children older than 10 years. The most common pathogen is *Staphylococcus aureus*, but streptococci, gram-negative bacilli, and anaerobic bacteria can also be involved. *Bartonella henselae* can cause chronic parotitis.

Clinical Presentation

History

At presentation, viral parotitis involves several days of fever, malaise, and headache before parotid gland swelling develops. The swelling and pain are initially unilateral but eventually become bilateral.

Bacterial parotitis presents with acute, unilateral swelling and intense tenderness of the parotid gland, with erythema and warmth of the overlying skin. High fever and toxicity are common.

Juvenile recurrent parotitis manifests at a mean age of 6 years, with unilateral parotid gland swelling, fever, and pain for days to weeks. These episodes recur every 3 to 4 months. The disease ultimately disappears by the time the child reaches puberty.

Sjögren syndrome is an autoimmune chronic inflammatory disorder that can appear with gradual, bilateral parotid swelling at presentation. It is associated with dry mouth and eyes, secondary to decreased salivary and lacrimal production.

Physical Examination

The patient will have fever and parotid gland pain and swelling that obscure the angle of the jaw. Examine the mass carefully to ensure that the swelling originates from the parotid gland itself and not the surrounding structures, such as lymph nodes. Check for trismus and extension of the infection beyond the parotid gland, as evidenced by swelling, redness, and tenderness beyond the angle of the jaw.

Bacterial, viral, and recurrent parotitis can be differentiated by examining the skin overlying the parotid gland and by applying external pressure to the parotid gland while observing the Stensen duct (located in the buccal mucosa opposite the upper second molar). In bacterial parotitis, the overlying skin is extremely tender, erythematous, and warm. The duct opening is inflamed and prominent, with purulent secretions. In viral parotitis, there is tender swelling without erythema or warmth, and the duct appears erythematous but secretions are clear. In JRP, overlying skin findings are rare. Diagnostic sialendoscopy may be helpful in some cases.

Laboratory Workup

If viral parotitis is suspected, no further workup is required unless HIV is a concern, in which case, perform specific virus polymerase chain reaction (PCR) studies. If bacterial parotitis is suspected and there are increasing rates of local antibiotic resistance, express pus from the Stensen duct and send it for Gram stain and aerobic and anaerobic cultures. Perform fungal and mycobacterial cultures if the patient has an immunodeficiency or a chronic disease. Obtain a blood culture if the patient is severely ill or immunocompromised. *Bartonella* serology or PCR is indicated for chronic cases only.

Radiology Examinations

Do not order imaging at presentation, unless there is clinical suspicion of a focal abscess, extension of the infection into surrounding structures (jaw osteomyelitis, jugular thrombophlebitis), JRP, or an anatomic abnormality (strictures or stones).

Differential Diagnosis

The differential diagnosis is summarized in Table 19-1.

Table 19-1. Differential Diagnosis of Parotitis	
Diagnosis	**Clinical Features**
Bartonella bacterial infection	Tender, swollen lymph node Overlying erythema, can be suppurative Enlarged lymph nodes proximal to the inoculation site
Bulimia	Patients are usually adolescent females Painless, bilateral parotid swelling Dental enamel erosion
Granulomatous parotitis	Painless, enlarging parotid mass without surrounding inflammation Pathogens include *Bartonella*, *Mycobacteria* (*Mycobacterium tuberculosis* and atypical *Mycobacteria*), *Actinomyces*, *Francisella tularensis*, and *Brucella* species Patient may have other signs of sarcoid
HIV	Parotitis can be the first sign of HIV Bilateral tender parotid enlargement
Lymphadenitis	Tender, swollen lymph node Overlying erythema and swelling Angle of the jaw is not obscured
Neoplasm (lymphoma, leukemia, MALT tumor)	Constitutional or systemic symptoms Cervical adenopathy rather than parotid inflammation
Pneumoparotid	Unilateral/bilateral parotid swelling ↑ Intraoral pressure (from playing musical instruments or receiving anesthesia) forces air into the Stensen duct
Sjögren syndrome	History of autoimmune disease Bilateral parotid swelling Xerophthalmia, xerostomia, and conjunctivitis

Abbreviation: MALT, mucosa-associated lymphoid tissue.

Treatment

Manage viral parotitis and JRP conservatively with analgesics, such as acetaminophen (15 mg/kg administered orally every 4–6 hours) or ibuprofen (10 mg/kg administered orally every 6 hours); hydration; gland massage; sialagogues (lemon drops or candy); and good oral hygiene. Prophylactic antibiotics are ineffective in preventing recurrences of JRP. Cold compresses help when acutely inflamed. Warm compresses help between acute inflammations.

Treat bacterial parotitis with intravenous (IV) clindamycin (40 mg/kg/d, divided into doses administered every 8 hours; 2.7-g/d maximum) for antimicrobial coverage of *S aureus* and anaerobes. If there is a high prevalence of clindamycin-resistant methicillin-resistant *S aureus*, treat with IV vancomycin (45 mg/kg/d, divided into doses administered every 8 hours; 4-g/d maximum) plus IV ampicillin/sulbactam (200 mg ampicillin/kg/d, divided into doses administered every 6 hours; 8-g/d maximum for ampicillin) for anaerobic antimicrobial coverage. Clinical improvement typically occurs within the first 48 hours of IV treatment. Switch to oral antibiotics once the patient is afebrile with decreased swelling and pain, and complete a 7- to 14-day course of treatment.

If there is no response to antibiotics, replace clindamycin (if it was the initial antibiotic) with vancomycin (as detailed previously) and add a third-generation cephalosporin, such as IV cefotaxime (50-mg/kg/d, divided into doses administered every 8 hours; 6-g/d maximum) for antimicrobial coverage of gram-negative pathogens. Order ultrasonography to evaluate the patient for abscess formation. Consult an otolaryngologist if there is an abscess or severe, refractory, or recurrent parotitis. If saliva or pus is not expressed from the Stensen duct, cannulation and dilation may be required.

Indications for Consultation
- **Immunology:** JRP, HIV
- **Infectious diseases:** HIV
- **Otolaryngology:** Parotid abscess, anatomic abnormality, JRP
- **Rheumatology:** Sjögren syndrome

Disposition
- **Intensive care unit transfer:** Sepsis, shock, spread of infection to surrounding tissues with airway compromise
- **Discharge criteria:** Patient tolerating oral intake, improvement in parotid gland swelling and pain, pus no longer expressed from the Stensen duct

Follow-up
- **Primary care:** 2 to 3 days
- **Otolaryngology (if involved):** 1 to 2 weeks

Pearls and Pitfalls
- If Stensen duct obstruction occurs, secretions will not be present.
- The keys to diagnosis are the appearance of the skin overlying the parotid gland and duct secretion composition.
- If unilateral, consider bacterial etiology.
- Consider the diagnosis of HIV in patients with parotitis.

Bibliography

Barskey AE, Juieng P, Whitaker BL, et al. Viruses detected among sporadic cases of parotitis, United States, 2009–2011. *J Infect Dis*. 2013;208(12):1979–1986

Campbell JR. Parotitis. In: Cherry JD, Harrison GJ, Kaplan SL, Steinbach WJ, Hotez PJ, eds. *Feigin and Cherry's Textbook of Pediatric Infectious Diseases*. 7th ed. Philadelphia, PA: Elsevier Saunders; 2014:189–193

Ellies M, Laskawi R. Diseases of the salivary glands in infants and adolescents. *Head Face Med*. 2010;6:1

Francis CL, Larsen CG. Pediatric sialadenitis. *Otolaryngol Clin North Am*. 2014;47(5): 763–778

Michaels MG, Nowalk AJ. Infectious disease. In: Zitelli BJ, McIntire SC, Norwalk AJ, eds. *Zitelli and Davis' Atlas of Pediatric Physical Diagnosis*. 6th ed. Philadelphia, PA: Saunders/Elsevier; 2012,469–529

Peritonsillar Abscess

Introduction

Peritonsillar abscess (PTA), or quinsy, is a collection of pus located in the space between the tonsil and the superior pharyngeal constrictor muscle. It is the most frequent deep neck infection in older children and adolescents but is relatively uncommon in young children.

Infections are polymicrobial. The most common pathogens are *Streptococcus pyogenes* (group A *Streptococcus*), *Staphylococcus aureus* (including methicillin-resistant S *aureus* [MRSA] and methicillin-sensitive S *aureus* [MSSA]), and mixed oropharyngeal anaerobes, including *Fusobacterium, Prevotella, Bacteroides, Porphyromonas,* and *Peptostreptococcus* species.

A PTA can extend into or impinge on adjacent structures, causing airway obstruction, ipsilateral vocal cord paralysis, internal jugular vein thrombosis (Lemierre syndrome), and mediastinitis.

Clinical Presentation

History

There is usually a history of a recent infection, such as tonsillitis, streptococcal pharyngitis, or viral respiratory illness (especially mononucleosis). Typical complaints include fever, severe sore throat, drooling, dysphagia, a muffled or "hot potato" voice, and trismus (inability to fully open the mouth secondary to irritation and reflex spasm of the internal pterygoid muscle). Other symptoms include odynophagia, neck pain, and ipsilateral ear pain.

Physical Examination

Classic findings are trismus, a bulging tonsil covered with exudate, and deviation of the uvula away from the affected side. Other findings include halitosis, pooling of saliva in the floor of the mouth, and tender ipsilateral cervical lymphadenopathy.

Laboratory Workup

No laboratory testing is needed. Although empirical antibiotic coverage is often successful, if a drainage procedure is performed, send the specimens for Gram stain and aerobic and anaerobic cultures.

Radiology Examinations

Imaging is not necessary to assign the diagnosis of PTA and is contraindicated in a patient with airway compromise. However, perform computed tomography of the neck with intravenous (IV) contrast material if it is difficult to differentiate PTA from other deep neck space infections or if there is a concern for a serious complication. Intraoral ultrasonography can be used to distinguish PTA from peritonsillar cellulitis and help guide needle aspiration.

Differential Diagnosis

The differential diagnosis is summarized in Table 20-1.

Treatment

Immediate surgical drainage is indicated if there is airway compromise. Otherwise, arrange for either needle aspiration or incision and drainage. The type of initial drainage procedure varies based on the availability of a provider trained in needle aspiration or the otolaryngologist's preference.

A quinsy tonsillectomy (tonsillectomy with simultaneous abscess drainage) is indicated if the initial abscess drainage is inadequate, as evidenced by abscess recurrence or persistence of symptoms. It is also the preferred approach by the otolaryngologist if the patient has a history of severe or recurrent pharyngitis or obstructive sleep apnea.

Medical management includes analgesia (avoid nonsteroidal anti-inflammatory drugs until discussed with the otolaryngologist), hydration, and

Table 20-1. Differential Diagnosis of Peritonsillar Abscess	
Diagnosis	**Clinical Features**
Angioedema	Patient has a history of allergies or exposure to an offending substance Swelling of the lips/tongue, urticarial rash Stridor and respiratory distress
Bacterial tracheitis	Abrupt onset of upper airway obstruction in a patient recovering from a viral illness (croup, influenza) Copious, purulent secretions
Epiglottitis (very rare)	Abrupt onset, with fever and toxic appearance Rapid progression to respiratory obstruction Patient prefers a "sniffing" posture
Retropharyngeal abscess	Occurs in preschool-aged children No peritonsillar swelling or uvula deviation Limited neck extension
Uvulitis	Swelling and erythema of the uvula No peritonsillar swelling

antibiotics. Treat with IV clindamycin (45 mg/kg/d, divided into doses administered every 8 hours; maximum, 900 mg per dose), although IV ampicillin/sulbactam (200 mg/kg/d of ampicillin, divided into doses administered every 6 hours; maximum, 3 g per dose) will suffice if the local prevalence of MRSA is low. However, in communities with high rates of clindamycin-resistant *Staphylococcus* bacteria (MRSA or MSSA), treat with clindamycin *and either* IV vancomycin (15 mg/kg/d, divided into doses administered every 8 hours; 4-g/d maximum) *or* IV linezolid (<12 years of age, 30 mg/kg/d, divided into doses administered every 8 hours; ≥12 years of age, 20 mg/kg/d, divided into doses administered every 12 hours; 1.2-g/d maximum). Continue IV therapy until the patient is afebrile and has clinically improved, at which time treatment should be changed to oral therapy, such as empirical clindamycin (45 mg/kg/d, divided into doses administered every 8 hours; maximum, 600 mg per dose) or a narrow-spectrum antibiotic, based on known sensitivities, to complete a 14-day course of treatment. Once the acute illness is over, the surgeon may schedule a tonsillectomy for 1 to 3 months in the future, particularly if the disease course was complicated or if the patient experiences recurrences.

Do not use corticosteroids in the treatment of PTA.

Indications for Consultation

- **Anesthesia:** Signs of airway compromise, including stridor, increased work of breathing, hypoxemia
- **Otolaryngology:** No response to antibiotics, drainage procedure needed, recurrent abscess formation

Disposition

- **Intensive care unit transfer:** Signs of airway compromise or complications, such as severe aspiration pneumonia, coronary artery erosion, internal jugular vein thrombosis, or mediastinitis
- **Discharge criteria:** Patient febrile, improved range of motion in the neck, adequate pain control achieved with oral medication, adequate oral intake

Follow-up

- **Primary care:** 3 to 5 days
- **Otolaryngology (if surgery was performed):** During the outpatient antibiotic course

Pearls and Pitfalls

- If there are signs of airway compromise, promptly consult both an otolaryngologist and an anesthesiologist and move the patient to a setting where an emergent artificial airway can be secured.
- PTA recurs in 5% to 15% of patients.

Bibliography

Baldassari C, Shah RK. Pediatric peritonsillar abscess: an overview. *Infect Disord Drug Targets*. 2012;12(4):277–280

Goldstein NA, Hammerschlag MR. Peritonsillar, retropharyngeal, and parapharyngeal abscesses. In: Cherry JD, Harrison GJ, Kaplan SL, Steinbach WJ, Hotez PJ, eds. *Feigin and Cherry's Textbook of Pediatric Infectious Diseases*. 7th ed. Philadelphia, PA: Elsevier Saunders; 2014:167–175

Kim DK, Lee JW, Na YS, Kim MJ, Lee JH, Park CH. Clinical factor for successful nonsurgical treatment of pediatric peritonsillar abscess. *Laryngoscope*. 2015;125(11):2608–2611

Nguyen T, Haberland CA, Hernandez-Boussard T. Pediatric patient and hospital characteristics associated with treatment of peritonsillar abscess and peritonsillar cellulitis. *Clin Pediatr (Phila)*. 2015;54(13):1240–1246

Qureshi H, Ference E, Novis S, Pritchett CV, Smith SS, Schroeder JW. Trends in the management of pediatric peritonsillar abscess infections in the U.S., 2000–2009. *Int J Pediatr Otorhinolaryngol*. 2015;79(4):527–531

CHAPTER 21

Retropharyngeal Abscess

Introduction

Retropharyngeal abscess is a suppurative bacterial infection of the retropharyngeal space, which is the area between the pharynx and cervical vertebrae that extends from the skull into the superior mediastinum.

Retropharyngeal lymph nodes drain the nasopharynx, adenoids, posterior paranasal sinuses, and middle ear structures. These nodes are prominent in young children but begin to atrophy before puberty, accounting for the increased incidence in younger children and relatively rare occurrence in adolescents, except after posterior pharyngeal wall trauma. A preceding oropharyngeal infection leads to retropharyngeal cellulitis that organizes into a phlegmon and then into an abscess. While the incidence of retropharyngeal abscesses has increased, the percentage of patients undergoing surgical intervention has decreased, with a trend toward nonsurgical medical management initially.

Infections are polymicrobial. The most common pathogens are *Streptococcus pyogenes* (group A *Streptococcus*), *Staphylococcus aureus* (including methicillin-resistant *S aureus* [MRSA] and methicillin-sensitive *S aureus* [MSSA]) and respiratory anaerobes (*Fusobacterium*, *Prevotella*, *Bacteroides*, *Porphyromonas*, and *Peptostreptococcus* species).

The morbidity and mortality of retropharyngeal abscesses result from extension into adjacent structures. Complications include airway obstruction, abscess rupture and subsequent aspiration, mediastinitis, internal jugular vein thrombosis (Lemierre syndrome), carotid artery aneurysm, and sepsis. These complications are very rare because of early diagnosis and treatment.

Clinical Presentation

History

A young child presents with an antecedent history of ear, nose, throat, or nonspecific upper respiratory tract infection, while an older patient will often have a history of preceding pharyngeal trauma (penetrating foreign body, endoscopy, intubation, dental procedure).

The most common symptoms at presentation are fever, neck pain, neck swelling, sore throat, dysphagia, and odynophagia. Other complaints may include decreased oral intake, muffled voice, trismus, and drooling. Stridor and upper airway obstruction are uncommon symptoms at presentation in children.

Physical Examination

Typical findings of retropharyngeal abscess include neck tenderness, limitation of neck movements (especially neck extension), and torticollis. Cervical lymphadenopathy is common. Inspection of the oropharynx may reveal midline or unilateral posterior pharyngeal swelling, but this is absent in more than 50% of younger children.

Laboratory Workup

No laboratory testing is needed. If the patient is toxic appearing or does not respond to empirical antibiotic therapy, attempt to assign a definitive microbial diagnosis by arranging surgical incision and drainage and sending specimens for Gram stain and aerobic and anaerobic cultures.

Radiology Examinations

If the diagnosis of retropharyngeal infection is equivocal and the patient has no signs of airway obstruction, obtain a screening lateral neck radiograph. This will confirm retropharyngeal swelling but will not allow differentiation between cellulitis, phlegmon, and abscess. Proper radiographic technique is important to avoid an artificially thickened appearance of the retropharyngeal soft tissues. Ensure that the radiographs are acquired during inspiration, with the neck extended and the patient in a true lateral position. Widened prevertebral soft tissues, exceeding the anteroposterior diameter of the adjacent vertebral body, are consistent with retropharyngeal inflammation.

If a retropharyngeal abscess is suspected on the basis of clinical assessment or soft-tissue swelling noted on radiographs, perform neck computed tomography (CT) with intravenous (IV) contrast material. This will allow identification of the location of the infection, as well as any extension into other adjacent neck or chest spaces. Findings suggestive of an abscess include ring enhancement and irregular abscess border (referred to as *scalloping*).

Differential Diagnosis

The differential diagnosis of retropharyngeal abscess is summarized in Table 21-1.

Treatment

Immediate surgical drainage is indicated for any patient with airway compromise. Otherwise, treat medically for 24 to 48 hours and obtain an otolaryngology consult if there is no improvement. Findings associated with drainable fluid at surgery include symptoms for more than 2 days, prior antibiotic

Table 21-1. Differential Diagnosis of Retropharyngeal Abscess

Diagnosis	Clinical Features
Anaphylaxis	Swelling of the lips/tongue Urticarial rash Stridor and respiratory distress
Bacterial tracheitis	Abrupt onset of upper airway obstruction in a patient recovering from croup Patient has a toxic appearance Copious, purulent secretions at suctioning
Croup	Harsh, barky cough; stridor; and drooling No limitations to neck movement No posterior pharyngeal swelling
Epiglottitis (rare)	Abrupt onset, with fever, toxicity, and drooling Rapid progression to respiratory obstruction Patient prefers a "sniffing" posture
Meningitis	Patient is ill appearing and irritable, with photophobia Limited neck flexion and other meningeal signs
Peritonsillar abscess	Older children and adolescents Severe sore throat, muffled voice, and trismus Exudative tonsillitis with uvula deviation
Uvulitis	Swelling and erythema of the uvula

therapy, and a fluid collection with a cross-sectional area larger than 2 cm^2 on CT images.

Treat with IV clindamycin (45 mg/kg/d, divided into doses administered every 8 hours; maximum, 900 mg per dose), although IV ampicillin/sulbactam (200 mg/kg/d of ampicillin, divided into doses administered every 6 hours; maximum, 3 g per dose) will suffice if the local prevalence of MRSA is low. However, in communities with high rates of clindamycin-resistant *Staphylococcus* bacteria (MRSA or MSSA), treat with clindamycin *and either* IV vancomycin (15 mg/kg/d, divided into doses administered every 8 hours; 4-g/d maximum) *or* IV linezolid (<12 years of age, 30 mg/kg/d, divided into doses administered every 8 hours; ≥12 years of age, 20 mg/kg/d, divided into doses administered every 12 hours; 1.2-g/d maximum).

Continue IV therapy until the patient is afebrile and has clinically improved, at which time treatment should be changed to oral therapy with empirical clindamycin (30 mg/kg/d, divided into doses administered every 8 hours) or a narrow-spectrum antibiotic based on known sensitivities to complete a 14-day course of treatment.

If there is no clinical improvement after 24 to 48 hours of antibiotic therapy, perform neck CT with IV contrast material to evaluate the patient for the presence of a drainable fluid collection.

Indications for Consultation
- **Anesthesia:** Signs of airway compromise, including stridor, increased work of breathing, and hypoxemia
- **Otolaryngology:** Surgical drainage needed

Disposition
- **Intensive care unit transfer:** Signs of airway compromise or complications, such as mediastinitis, internal jugular vein thrombosis, or coronary artery aneurysm
- **Discharge criteria:** Patient afebrile with significant clinical improvement, including increased neck range of motion, decreased pain, and good oral intake

Follow-up
- **Primary care:** 2 to 3 days
- **Otolaryngology (if surgery was performed):** During the outpatient antibiotic course

Pearls and Pitfalls
- If there are signs of airway compromise, promptly consult both an otolaryngologist and an anesthesiologist and move the patient to a setting where an emergent artificial airway can be secured.
- Stridor and other signs of airway compromise are uncommon findings at presentation.

Bibliography
Abdel-Haq N, Quezada M, Asmar BI. Retropharyngeal abscess in children: the rising incidence of methicillin-resistant *Staphylococcus aureus*. *Pediatr Infect Dis J*. 2012;31(7):696–699

Elsherif AM, Park AH, Alder SC, Smith ME, Muntz HR, Grimmer F. Indicators of a more complicated clinical course for pediatric patients with retropharyngeal abscess. *Int J Pediatr Otorhinolaryngol*. 2010;74(2):198–201

Goldstein NA, Hammerschlag MR. Peritonsillar, retropharyngeal, and parapharyngeal abscesses. In: Cherry JD, Harrison GJ, Kaplan SL, Steinbach WJ, Hotez PJ, eds. *Feigin and Cherry's Textbook of Pediatric Infectious Diseases*. 7th ed. Philadelphia, PA: Elsevier Saunders; 2014:167–175

Grisaru-Soen G, Komisar O, Aizenstein O, Soudack M, Schwartz D, Paret G. Retropharyngeal and parapharyngeal abscess in children—epidemiology, clinical features and treatment. *Int J Pediatr Otorhinolaryngol*. 2010;74(9):1016–1020

CHAPTER 22

Sinusitis

Introduction

Obstruction of the sinus ostia can be caused by inflammation of the mucosal lining secondary to an upper respiratory infection (URI) or allergic symptoms. This impedes mucous drainage and encourages the overgrowth of bacteria, leading to acute bacterial sinusitis. While acute viral sinusitis is a normal accompaniment of URI, up to 8% of children with a viral URI may subsequently develop acute bacterial sinusitis. Outpatient watchful waiting or antibiotic treatment will suffice for most cases, although a patient may require inpatient therapy if there is evidence of toxicity, failure of outpatient treatment, or an underlying immunodeficiency. Serious complications of bacterial sinusitis can occur secondary to the spread of infection. The most common complications are periorbital and orbital cellulitis or abscess. Less often, intracranial extension can cause a brain abscess, meningitis, or cavernous venous sinus thrombosis. Uncommonly, cranial vault involvement, with osteomyelitis of the frontal bone and subperiosteal abscess (Pott puffy tumor), may result from frontal sinusitis, most commonly in a teenaged male.

A history of recurrent bacterial sinusitis raises the possibility of an underlying chronic allergic condition, immunodeficiency, or defect (anatomic or mechanical), causing poor sinus drainage (cystic fibrosis, immotile cilia syndrome, sinonasal polyps).

The most common causes of acute bacterial sinusitis are *Streptococcus pneumoniae*, nontypable *Haemophilus influenzae*, and *Moraxella catarrhalis*. However, with severe, complicated, and chronic infections, *Staphylococcus aureus* (including methicillin-resistant strains), anaerobic bacteria, and fungi may be involved.

Clinical Presentation

History

At presentation, uncomplicated acute bacterial sinusitis typically appears with persistent or worsening signs and symptoms for 10 or more days, although rarely, it can be rapidly progressive, severe, and even fulminant. Symptoms can include low-grade fever, nasal discharge of any quality, daytime cough (which may be worse at night), headache (which can be severe and positional), or facial pain or pressure. A more severe form of acute bacterial sinusitis occurs with 3 or 4 days of a temperature of at least 39°C (102.2°F) and purulent nasal discharge in an ill-appearing child. There may be other complaints that are related to complications, such as vomiting and severe headache (intracranial spread) or eye pain and visual disturbances (orbital cellulitis).

Physical Examination

Perform a thorough ear, nose, and throat examination and neurologic examination. The patient may appear toxic, with swelling of the forehead, face, or eyelids. There can be pain with eye movements and/or decreased visual acuity. Nasal speculum examination of the nasopharynx might reveal a purulent discharge material from under the middle turbinate. With intracranial spread, there may be painful ophthalmoplegia, as well as bradycardia, hypotension, nuchal rigidity, and palsy in cranial nerve VI secondary to increased intracranial pressure.

Laboratory Workup

No specific laboratory testing is needed, other than aerobic and anaerobic cultures if sinus drainage is performed. Obtain a blood culture if the patient appears toxic. If there is a concern for intracranial extension, perform a lumbar puncture (to evaluate the patient for increased intracranial pressure and pleocytosis) and perform head computed tomography (CT) with contrast material or magnetic resonance (MR) imaging.

Radiology Examinations

The clinical presentation of acute bacterial sinusitis is sufficient to assign the diagnosis, so routine imaging of the sinuses is unnecessary. However, if the patient has a clinical picture consistent with a complication, perform contrast-enhanced head CT or MR imaging or MR venography of the orbits (orbital cellulitis) or head (Pott puffy tumor, venous thrombosis).

Differential Diagnosis

The presentation of the complications of acute bacterial sinusitis is summarized in Table 22-1.

Treatment

Treat acute bacterial sinusitis with either cefotaxime (150 mg/kg/d, divided into doses administered every 6 hours; 6-g/d maximum), ceftriaxone (100 mg/kg/d, divided into doses administered every 12 hours; 4-g/d maximum), or ampicillin/sulbactam (100 mg/kg/d, divided into doses administered every

Table 22-1. Complications of Sinusitis	
Diagnosis	**Clinical Features**
Brain abscess	Headache Altered mental status
Cavernous sinus thrombosis	Toxicity, headache Altered mental status Ophthalmoplegia (cranial nerves III, IV, V1, V2, VI) Signs of ↑ ICP
Meningitis	Headache Photophobia Meningismus
Orbital cellulitis or abscess	Proptosis, chemosis Limited EOMs
Pott puffy tumor	Marked forehead swelling May have signs of ↑ ICP
Preseptal cellulitis	May have a break in the skin integrity No ophthalmoplegia No chemosis No visual changes or EOM limitation

Abbreviations: EOM, extraocular movement; ICP, intracranial pressure.

6 hours; 8-g/d maximum). Add vancomycin (60 mg/kg/d, divided into doses administered every 6 hours; 4-g/d maximum) if there is a serious complication (orbital or periorbital cellulitis, cavernous sinus thrombosis, or Pott puffy tumor) or a failure of appropriate inpatient therapy (as indicated previously). Tailor the antibiotic choices on the basis of clinical response, culture results (if any), and community patterns of antimicrobial resistance. Continue the intravenous antibiotics until the symptoms improve, then change to oral antibiotics to complete at least a 14-day course of treatment. In a more severe or complicated case, the patient may require antibiotic therapy for up to 4 weeks. Consult an otolaryngologist and/or infectious diseases specialist for consideration of sinus drainage if the patient demonstrates clinical deterioration, does not improve after 48 hours of adequate empirical therapy, or presents with signs or symptoms of a complication. In addition, consult a neurosurgeon if the clinical picture suggests intracranial extension.

Do not use adjunctive therapies, such as nasal saline irrigation, antihistamines, mucolytics, or decongestants.

Indications for Consultation

- **Allergy and immunology:** Suspicion of an immunodeficiency or recurrent episodes of sinusitis that may be allergic in nature

- **Infectious disease:** Recurrent sinusitis, isolation of a rare or treatment-resistant pathogen, complication of sinusitis, sinusitis unresponsive to standard antimicrobial therapy
- **Neurosurgery:** Possible intracranial extension
- **Ophthalmology:** Possible orbital or intracranial extension
- **Otolaryngology:** Recurrent or chronic sinusitis, complication of sinusitis, need for sinus aspiration

Disposition

- **Intensive care unit transfer:** Intracranial extension, sepsis
- **Discharge criteria:** Patient afebrile for 24 to 48 hours, clinical improvement, and good oral intake, including the ability to take the appropriate antibiotic

Follow-up

- **Primary care:** 1 week, to assess the need for an extended antibiotic course
- **Otolaryngology (if involved):** 1 week

Pearls and Pitfalls

- If the patient is asymptomatic, do not treat an incidental finding of sinus inflammation seen on CT images.
- If the patient has recurrent bacterial or chronic sinusitis, consider an evaluation for allergic rhinitis, cystic fibrosis, immunodeficiency, Kartagener syndrome and other immotile cilia syndromes, and polypoid disease.
- Plain radiographs, transillumination, and ultrasonographic images of the sinuses are unreliable.

Bibliography

Blumfield E, Misra M. Pott's puffy tumor, intracranial, and orbital complications as the initial presentation of sinusitis in healthy adolescents, a case series. *Emerg Radiol.* 2011;18(3):203–210

Hicks CW, Weber JG, Reid JR, Moodley M. Identifying and managing intracranial complications of sinusitis in children: a retrospective series. *Pediatr Infect Dis J.* 2011; 30(3):222–226

Magit A. Pediatric rhinosinusitis. *Otolaryngol Clin North Am.* 2014;47(5):733–746

Shaikh N, Wald ER. Decongestants, antihistamines and nasal irrigation for acute sinusitis in children. *Cochrane Database Syst Rev.* 2014;10:CD007909

Wald ER. Applegate KE, Bordley C, et al; and American Academy of Pediatrics. Clinical practice guideline for the diagnosis and management of acute bacterial sinusitis in children aged 1 to 18 years. *Pediatrics.* 2013;132(1):e262–e280

Endocrinology

CHAPTER 23

Acute Adrenal Insufficiency

Introduction

Adrenal crisis is a rare but life-threatening emergency with a high mortality rate, unless it is recognized and treated promptly. At presentation, adrenal crisis may be a sign of adrenal insufficiency, or the crisis may occur in a patient with known adrenal insufficiency because of inadequate hormonal replacement. Since the signs and symptoms of adrenal insufficiency are non-specific, the diagnosis may not be suspected until late in the disease course, when the patient presents with a life-threatening cardiovascular collapse. The ultimate cause of adrenal crisis is mineralocorticoid insufficiency.

Primary adrenal insufficiency is secondary to diseases that affect the adrenal gland itself. The most common cause of primary adrenal insufficiency is congenital adrenal hyperplasia (CAH). Other etiologies include damage to the adrenals from infection (commonly tuberculosis, HIV, and fungal infections), hemorrhage, autoimmune diseases, metabolic diseases (adrenoleukodystrophy), and medications (ketoconazole, etomidate). Secondary adrenal insufficiency might be caused by deficient adrenocorticotropic hormone (ACTH) production or by suppression from prolonged pharmacologic doses of glucocorticoids. Such a patient requires additional doses of glucocorticoids when subjected to physiological stress. Inadequate or no replacement may then precipitate an adrenal crisis.

Clinical Presentation

History

The patient will initially present with nausea, abdominal pain, and vomiting, a clinical picture that is frequently misinterpreted as a gastrointestinal (GI) illness. Acute decompensation can occur rapidly and is often precipitated by stress from surgery, trauma, or infection, in which case the patient may be febrile. A patient with undiagnosed adrenal insufficiency may have chronic complaints, such as weakness, fatigue, anorexia, and weight loss. A history of a psychiatric illness (anorexia, depression) or other endocrine problem (diabetes, hypothyroidism) may also be present. Salt craving can occur in a patient with chronic primary adrenal insufficiency.

Physical Examination

The patient will typically appear unwell and have clinical evidence of hypovolemia. Tachycardia, hypotension, shock, and altered mental status are common. Skin hyperpigmentation in areas not exposed to sunlight, such as the axillae and palmar creases, is typically seen in patients with chronic adrenal insufficiency.

Laboratory Workup

If adrenal insufficiency is suspected, order a chemistry panel to look for metabolic acidosis, hyperkalemia, hypoglycemia, and hyponatremia. If the crisis is triggered by infection, inflammatory markers and white blood cell count may be increased. If possible, obtain blood to evaluate cortisol levels, ACTH levels, plasma renin activity, and aldosterone levels before administering exogenous steroids. However, *do not delay definitive treatment* if these test samples cannot be obtained immediately. If CAH is suspected in a neonate, obtain blood for a 17-hydroxyprogesterone test.

Differential Diagnosis

Consider adrenal crisis in any critically ill patient who has a history of previous adrenal insufficiency or is receiving replacement or pharmacologic doses of exogenous corticosteroids. In addition, consider adrenal insufficiency in a patient with shock who is unresponsive to usual fluid resuscitation and inotropic medications.

Treatment

- **Fluids.** If adrenal crisis is suspected, administer 20-mL/kg boluses of dextrose 5% in 0.9% normal saline solution as needed, depending on the patient's clinical condition. Once the patient's blood pressure has been stabilized, continue administration of the same fluid at 1.5 to 2 times the maintenance rate. Monitor the glucose level and change to normal saline solution, if necessary, once the glucose level has been stabilized (see the following).
- **Steroids.** Administer stress doses of steroids simultaneously with the fluid resuscitation. Intravenous (IV) hydrocortisone is the treatment of choice because of its mineralocorticoid activity. The dosing is as follows: 0 to 3 years of age, 25 mg; ≥3 to 12 years of age, 50 mg; and ≥12 years of age, 100 mg. Follow this with the same IV dose per day, either continuously or divided into 4 daily doses. Administer the hydrocortisone intramuscularly if IV access is not readily available. Do not use methylprednisolone or

dexamethasone, because these drugs do not have mineralocorticoid effects.

- **Glucose.** If blood pressure remains low despite the initial bolus with dextrose 5% in normal saline solution, deliver a bolus of 2 mL/kg of 10% dextrose to restore euglycemia. In an adolescent, use 1 mL/kg of 25% dextrose. Ensure proper needle or catheter placement to avoid extravasation, because it may cause tissue damage.

- **Potassium.** If hyperkalemia is present, immediately obtain an electrocardiogram. If findings are consistent with hyperkalemia (peaked T waves, shortening of the QT interval, prolonged PR interval, widened QRS complex) or if the potassium level is higher than 7 mEq/L (7 mmol/L), initiate treatment in an intensive care setting to transiently redistribute potassium: 25% dextrose (2 mL/kg administered over 30 minutes, repeat every 30 minutes), along with regular insulin (1 unit/kg/h) and nebulized albuterol. Also administer 10% calcium gluconate (1 mL/kg = 100 mg/kg per dose delivered every 3–5 minutes) to protect the myocardium. To enhance potassium excretion, use a loop diuretic (IV furosemide 1–2 mg/kg, administered every 6 hours) and rectal polystyrene sulfonate (1 g/kg).

- **Additional treatment.** If an underlying illness precipitated the adrenal crisis, further treatment may be needed (eg, antibiotics for bacterial infections).

- **Stress dosing.** In a patient with known adrenal insufficiency who is hospitalized for fever, vomiting, diarrhea, inadequate oral intake, burn, or surgery, start delivery of stress doses of steroids. Administer hydrocortisone at a dose of 30 to 50 mg/m^2 per day (approximately 3 times the daily dose), divided into 3 or 4 administered per day for 24 to 48 hours. Consult a pediatric endocrinologist if prolonged stress dosing is required or if major surgery or sepsis is the cause.

Indications for Consultation

- **Endocrinology:** Patients with acute adrenal crisis or those with a history of adrenal insufficiency who are admitted to the hospital for major surgery or sepsis or if stress dosing is anticipated for more than 48 hours
- **Intensivist:** All patients in adrenal crisis

Disposition

- **Intensive care unit transfer:** All patients in adrenal crisis
- **Discharge criteria:** The cause of fever, infection, or trauma that precipitated the crisis has been identified and treated; patient is able to tolerate oral medications and hydration

Follow-up
- **Pediatric endocrinologist:** 1 to 2 weeks
- **Primary care:** 2 to 4 weeks

Pearls and Pitfalls
- Adrenal crisis can initially mimic a benign GI illness.
- Do not delay treatment of an adrenal crisis while awaiting confirmatory testing.
- Suspect adrenal crisis if there is hypotension and shock disproportionate to the underlying illness.
- Hydrocortisone is the drug of choice for adrenal crisis because of its glucocorticoid and mineralocorticoid effects.
- At discharge, ensure that the patient has a medical emergency bracelet and carries an emergency medical information card.

Bibliography

Auron M, Raissouni N. Adrenal insufficiency. *Pediatr Rev*. 2015;36(3):92–102; quiz 103, 129

Levy-Shraga Y, Pinhas-Hamiel O. Novel insights into adrenal insufficiency in childhood. *Minerva Pediatr*. 2014;66(6):517–532

Shulman DI, Palmert MR, Kemp SF; and Lawson Wilkins Drug and Therapeutics Committee. Adrenal insufficiency: still a cause of morbidity and death in childhood. *Pediatrics*. 2007;119(2):e484–e494

White PC. Adrenocortical Insufficiency. In Kliegman RM, Stanton B, St Geme JW, Schor NF, eds. *Nelson Textbook of Pediatrics*. 20th ed. Philadelphia, PA: Elsevier; 2016:2703–2714

Zeitler PS, Travers SH, Nadeau K, Barker JM, Kelsey MM, Kappy MS. Endocrine disorders. In: Hay WW Jr, Deterding RR, Levin MJ, Abzug MJ, eds. *Current Diagnosis & Treatment: Pediatrics*. 22nd ed. New York, NY: McGraw-Hill Education; 2014: 1086–1096

CHAPTER 24

Diabetes Insipidus

Introduction

Diabetes insipidus (DI) is classified as either central, which is caused by a deficiency of antidiuretic hormone (ADH), or nephrogenic, which is secondary to insensitivity to ADH in the kidneys. Both causes prevent water reabsorption in the kidneys, leading to hypotonic polyuria. Central DI is caused by genetic defects, congenital abnormalities (septo-optic dysplasia, holoprosencephaly), disruptions in hypothalamic-pituitary ADH production (trauma, neoplasms, infections, autoimmune disorders), or idiopathic causes. Nephrogenic DI may be genetic, idiopathic, or acquired, including kidney disease (chronic renal failure, pyelonephritis, obstructive uropathy, polycystic kidney disease), medications (amphotericin B, gentamicin, lithium), and electrolyte disorders (hypokalemia, hypercalcemia).

Clinical Presentation

History

The patient may present with nonspecific findings, such as irritability, intermittent fever, vomiting, seizures, hypotonia, or failure to thrive. Obtain a detailed history to assess fluid intake, urine output, and voiding pattern. The patient's parents may report polydipsia, polyuria (>2 L/m^2/d), and clear-colored urine. Extreme thirst and nighttime fluid intake can also lead to sleep disturbances and daytime tiredness. However, polydipsia may be absent if the patient does not have an intact thirst mechanism. Enuresis in a previously toilet-trained child is also common. A patient with known DI may present with some other cause for disruption of homeostasis, such as an intercurrent illness.

Physical Examination

The initial priority is to assess the patient for evidence of severe dehydration or shock (dry mucous membranes, delayed capillary refill time, skin tenting, weak peripheral pulse). Also, look for other sequelae of pituitary gland dysfunction (adrenocorticotropic hormone or growth hormone deficiency), visual and central nervous system dysfunction (headache, visual field changes), and craniofacial midline defects (septo-optic dysplasia).

Laboratory Workup

Check serum osmolality and electrolyte levels, as well as urine osmolality, urine specific gravity, and glucose levels. If an intracranial pathologic condition is suspected, perform brain magnetic resonance (MR) imaging with gadolinium-based contrast material, because computed tomography lacks the detail necessary to properly evaluate the hypothalamus and pituitary gland. The characteristic "bright spot" of the posterior pituitary gland seen at T1-weighted MR images, which indicates functional integrity, is often decreased or absent in patients with central DI.

The key laboratory findings in DI are

- Urine output greater than the upper limit of normal (150 mL/kg/d for infants; 110 mL/kg/d for toddlers; 40 mL/kg/d for older children)
- Low urine specific gravity (<1.005)
- Urine osmolality less than serum osmolality
- Urine osmolality <300 mOsm/kg (<300 mmol/kg; often remains <150 mOsm/kg [<150 mmol/kg])
- Serum hyperosmolality (>300 mOsm/kg [>300 mmol/kg])

Consult a pediatric endocrinologist to perform a water deprivation test, followed by a vasopressin test, to differentiate between central and nephrogenic DI. The differential diagnosis of polyuria is summarized in Table 24-1.

Table 24-1. Differential Diagnosis of Polyuria	
Diagnosis	**Clinical Features**

Primary polydipsia
  Psychogenic (compulsive)
  Dipsogenic (abnormal thirst)
	Serum and urine osmolality normal to low normal

Osmotic diuresis (diabetes)	Hyperglycemia ↑ Serum osmolality Serum sodium level normal or ↓
Postobstructive diuresis	Serum sodium level/osmolality normal Urine osmolality normal or ↓
Cushing syndrome	Hyperglycemia Characteristic physical findings: round face, upper-body fat, striae
Fanconi syndrome	Acidosis, hypokalemia, hyperchloremia Rickets, osteomalacia Growth failure
Urinary tract infection	Urinary symptoms: dysuria, urgency
Hypercalcemia	↑ Calcium level (>12.0 mg/dL [>3 mmol/L]) Weakness, altered mental status

Treatment

Fluid Replacement

- **Resuscitation.** The initial priority in diabetes insipidus is fluid resuscitation with 0.9% normal saline if the patient presents with hypovolemic shock (see Chapter 10, Shock). Then, correct the hypernatremia and dehydration after calculation of the fluid deficit by using 0.45% normal saline over 48 hours to prevent a rapid decrease in serum sodium levels and cerebral edema.
- **Free water deficit (in milliliters).** Calculate the free water deficit as follows:

    4 mL/kg × body weight (in kilograms) × (Na$^+$ concentration measured – Na$^+$ concentration desired [145 mEq/L or 145 mmol/L]). Then, administer this volume as dextrose 5% in 0.45% normal saline at a rate of 3 to 6 mL/kg/h.

- **Maintenance and ongoing urine losses.** Calculate maintenance fluids (1,600 mL/m^2/d) and ongoing fluid loss from urine output and replace these amounts with 0.45% normal saline.
- **Monitor.** Monitor the serum sodium level every 1 to 2 hours until it is 145 mEq/L (145 mmol/L), then every 3 to 6 hours until the sodium level is normal. The goal is a rate of correction of <0.5 mEq/L/h (<0.5 mmol/L/h) or <10 mEq/L/d (<10 mmol/L/d) to prevent cerebral edema.

Central DI

Treat central DI with desmopressin, which is available in oral, intranasal, and subcutaneous preparations. Desmopressin decreases urine output by causing increased water reabsorption in the renal collecting ducts. The doses are

- **Oral:** Start with 50 µg administered twice daily, then titrate to the desired response (<12 years of age, 100–800 µg/d; ≥12 years of age, 100–1,200 µg/d; divided into two daily doses)
- **Intranasal:** 3 months to 12 years of age, 5 to 30 µg/d, divided into doses administered twice a day; ≥12 years of age, 5 to 40 µg/d, divided into doses administered 3 times a day
- **Subcutaneous:** 2 to 4 µg/d, divided into doses administered twice a day

Nephrogenic DI

Manage nephrogenic DI with a low-sodium diet (300–500 mg/d) and diuretics.

- Hydrochlorothiazide: <6 months of age, 4 mg/kg/d, divided into doses administered twice a day; ≥6 months of age, 1 to 2 mg/kg/d, divided into doses administered twice a day
- Amiloride: 0.3 mg/kg/d

Indications for Consultation

- **Endocrinology:** All patients
- **Neurology, neurosurgery, and/or oncology:** Abnormal MR imaging findings

Disposition

- **Intensive care unit transfer:** Patient has severe dehydration and hypovolemic shock that requires fluid resuscitation; patient will be undergoing water deprivation and vasopressin tests
- **Discharge criteria:** Clinical improvement, electrolyte abnormalities corrected, pharmacologic regimen in place, comorbid conditions adequately managed, and family educated about measuring urine output and administering doses of desmopressin

Follow-up

- **Primary care:** 1 to 2 weeks
- **Endocrinologist:** 2 to 3 days

Pearls and Pitfalls

- Surgical or accidental trauma may cause central DI in a previously healthy child if the pituitary gland is damaged.
- At presentation, central DI may be the initial sign of a brain tumor (germinoma, craniopharyngioma).
- The current standard of reference for diagnosing DI is the measurement of vasopressin production during graded hyperosmolar stimulation. Simpler tests to better aid in diagnosis (measurement of copeptin) are being developed.

Bibliography

Ball S. Diabetes insipidus. *Medicine.* 2013;41:519–521

Chang Y. Diabetes insipidus. In: Perkin RM, Swift JD, Newton DA, Anas N, eds. *Pediatric Hospital Medicine: Textbook of Inpatient Management.* 2nd ed. Philadelphia, PA: Lippincott Williams & Wilkins; 2008:534–537

Di Iorgi N, Napoli F, Allegri AEM, et al. Diabetes insipidus – diagnosis and management. *Horm Res Paediatr.* 2012;77:69–84

Fenske W, Allolio B. Current state and future perspectives in the diagnosis of diabetes insipidus: a clinical review. *J Clin Endocrinol Metab.* 2012;97(10):3426–3437

Qureshi S, Galiveeti S, Bichet DG, Roth J. Diabetes insipidus: celebrating a century of vasopressin therapy. *Endocrinology.* 2014;155(12):4605–4621

Diabetic Ketoacidosis

Introduction

Diabetic ketoacidosis (DKA) is the leading cause of morbidity and mortality in children with diabetes. DKA occurs when there is a disruption in the balance between insulin and the counterregulatory hormones, either from a lack of circulating insulin (type 1 diabetes mellitus [T1DM]) or increased counterregulatory hormones in response to stress (trauma, acute gastroenteritis, sepsis). This imbalance leads to a catabolic state, which precipitates the hallmarks of DKA: hyperglycemia, hyperosmolality, increased lipolysis, ketonemia, and metabolic acidosis. An osmotic diuresis ensues, causing dehydration and the production of more counterregulatory hormones, which further disrupts the balance.

At presentation, DKA can be the initial sign of T1DM, primarily in children younger than 5 years and those whose families do not have easy access to medical care. In a patient with known T1DM, DKA tends to occur when there is missed insulin dosing or mismanagement of insulin during illness or in the setting of a severe febrile or gastrointestinal (GI) illness. While DKA is a more common presentation in T1DM, as many as 25% of children with diabetes mellitus type 2 initially present with DKA.

A young patient (<5 years old) with severe DKA (severe acidosis, low bicarbonate level, high blood urea nitrogen level) is at increased risk for clinically significant cerebral edema (CE). This potentially fatal complication of DKA, the pathogenesis of which remains unclear, can manifest 4 to 12 hours after treatment is initiated.

Clinical Presentation

History

A patient with DKA often presents with a history of polyuria, polyphagia, polydipsia, and weight loss, sometimes accompanied by nausea, vomiting, or severe abdominal pain. However, nocturia, enuresis, or nonspecific systemic complaints (lethargy or fatigue) can be the initial symptoms. The family or patient may also complain of glucosuria or ketonuria at presentation, because urine dipsticks were used at home.

Physical Examination

The patient presents with signs of dehydration (delayed capillary refill time, dry mucous membranes, tachycardia, skin tenting), Kussmaul breathing (rapid, deep sighing), and possibly a fruity breath odor. In severe cases, there may be evidence of hypovolemic shock (hypotension, oliguria, weak pulse, cool extremities) and weight loss. In addition, the patient may have an altered mental status or be obtunded, which is worrisome for CE. Other signs of CE associated with intracranial hypertension are inappropriate slowing of the heart rate and increasing blood pressure.

Laboratory Workup

Use the following laboratory criteria to confirm the diagnosis of DKA:

- **Diabetic:** Hyperglycemia (blood glucose level >200 mg/dL [>11.1 mmol/L])
- **Ketotic:** Ketonemia (serum β-hydroxybutyrate level >3 mmol/L) and ketonuria
- **Acidotic:** Venous pH level <7.3 or bicarbonate level <15 mEq/L (<15 mmol/L)

For any patient suspected of having DKA, obtain a complete blood cell count, serum comprehensive metabolic panel and osmolality level, and hemoglobin A1c and β-hydroxybutyrate levels, and perform a venous or arterial blood gas analysis and urinalysis to check for ketones. If DKA is the initial sign at presentation in a child with new-onset diabetes, also obtain a C-peptide level, insulin level, insulin autoantibody level, islet cell autoantigen 512 and glutamic acid decarboxylase 65 antibody levels, tissue transglutaminase antibody levels, total immunoglobulin A levels (to evaluate the patient for celiac disease), and thyroid peroxidase antibody and thyroglobulin antibody levels (to evaluate the patient for autoimmune thyroid disease). If infection is suspected, obtain appropriate cultures (urine, blood, throat, wound, etc).

The serum sodium level may be low because of dilutional hyponatremia or pseudohyponatremia. The excess glucose is confined to the extracellular space, which causes the osmotic movement of water into the space, resulting in a relatively lowered sodium concentration. As the hyperglycemia is corrected with treatment and the osmotic movement of water is reversed, the serum sodium level will increase.

$$\text{Corrected sodium level} = \text{serum sodium level} + 1.6 \times$$
$$[(\text{serum glucose level in milligrams per deciliter} - 100)/100]$$

There is a total body depletion of potassium as intracellular stores are lost from transcellular shifts (exchange of K^+ for extracellular H^+; glycogenolysis and proteolysis from insulin deficiency causes potassium efflux from cells); osmotic diuresis, which leads to increased urinary losses; and GI losses from vomiting. However, the serum potassium level may be normal, high, or low. If timely measurement of serum potassium level is not available, obtain an electrocardiogram to look for evidence of hypokalemia (flat T waves, appearance of U waves, widened QT interval) or hyperkalemia (peaked T waves, short QT interval). Once correction of electrolyte abnormalities is started, the serum potassium level will decline. Close monitoring and replacement, as needed, are essential.

Differential Diagnosis

While there are a number of different causes for metabolic acidosis, polyuria, and hyperglycemia, only DKA causes all 3. The differential diagnosis is summarized in Table 25-1.

Table 25-1. Differential Diagnosis of Diabetic Ketoacidosis	
Diagnosis	**Clinical Features**
Metabolic acidosis, ketosis	
Salicylate poisoning	Metabolic acidosis (with or without respiratory alkalosis) No ketosis Serum glucose level ↓ or ↑ (usually <300 mg/dL [<16.65 mmol/L])
Sepsis	Fever, toxic appearance, source of infection Serum glucose level normal or increased No Kussmaul breathing or fruity breath odor
Severe gastroenteritis/ dehydration	May have diarrhea Lactic acidosis can cause metabolic acidosis Serum glucose level mildly increased, decreased, or normal
Starvation	No hyperglycemia or glycosuria Bicarbonate level usually >18 mEq/L (>18 mmol/L)
Polyuria	
Postsurgical/relief of obstructive uropathy	No glucosuria/ketonuria Serum glucose level normal No metabolic acidosis
Urinary tract infection	Urinary symptoms: dysuria, urgency No metabolic acidosis Serum glucose level normal
Hyperglycemia	
Corticosteroid administration	↑ Serum glucose level No metabolic acidosis
Nonketotic hyperosmolar state	↑ Serum glucose level and osmolality No or minimal ketosis; no metabolic acidosis Stupor or coma
Stress	↑ Serum glucose level No ketonuria No metabolic acidosis

Continued

Table 25-1. Differential Diagnosis of Diabetic Ketoacidosis, continued	
Diagnosis	**Clinical Features**
Glycosuria	
Fanconi syndrome	Normal serum glucose level
	Hypophosphatemia, uricosuria, aminoaciduria
	Growth failure
Benign familial glycosuria	Normal serum glucose level

Treatment

Consult with a pediatric endocrinologist and/or pediatric intensivist early in
the course of treatment. Obtain the patient's height and weight (compare to
the premorbid weight) after assessing the severity of dehydration and level
of consciousness. The goals of therapy are restoring the circulating volume,
correcting metabolic derangements, avoiding treatment complications (hypokalemia, CE), and identifying and treating the underlying cause (infection,
insulin pump malfunction, etc).

Initial Management

The total fluid goal is 2,500 mL/m^2/d, which is approximately maintenance
fluids plus about 6% deficit. Administer an initial normal saline or lactated
Ringer fluid bolus of 10 mL/kg, delivered over 1 hour, and subtract this
amount from the total fluid goal. Repeat once if clinically indicated. Exercise
caution when administering initial fluids so as not to potentiate CE. However,
if there is evidence of shock, administer supplemental oxygen and fluid resuscitation as indicated.

If CE is suspected, elevate the head of the bed to 30 degrees, reduce
the intravenous (IV) fluid rate by one-third, and administer IV mannitol
(0.5–1.0 g/kg) or hypertonic (3%) saline (5–10 mL/kg). Consider intubation
if there is impending respiratory failure. After the patient is stabilized, order
computed tomography of the head to confirm the diagnosis and to look for
other intracranial pathologic findings (eg, thrombosis or hemorrhage).

If there is no evidence of shock or severe dehydration, begin a regular
insulin drip after initiating fluid resuscitation (0.1 units/kg/h) to counteract
the ongoing catabolic state. Use the 2-bag system to efficiently correct
metabolic derangements (Box 25-1).

Monitoring

Successful management of DKA requires meticulous monitoring and frequent
adjustments in treatment on the basis of the patient's response. Monitor the
patient's vital signs, neurologic status, and fluid intake and output. Obtain
finger-stick glucose measurements every hour to adjust the fluid infusion

---

Box 25-1. Two-Bag System

Use finger-stick glucose measurements to adjust the IV rate.

Potassium

- K$^+$ ≤5.5 mEq/L (≤5.5 mmol/L)
  — Bag A: LR/NS + 1.5 mEq (1.5 mmol/L) KCl/100 mL + 2 mmol KPO$_4$/100 mL
  — Bag B: D10 LR/NS + 1.5 mEq (1.5 mmol/L) KCl/100 mL + 2 mmol KPO$_4$/100 mL
- K$^+$ ≥5.5 mEq/L (≥5.5 mmol/L)
  — Bag A: LR/NS
  — Bag B: D10 LR/NS

IV rate

Use the blood glucose level to determine the ratio between the Bag A and Bag B IV rates.

Total IV rate (mL/h) = Bag A rate (mL/h) + Bag B rate (mL/h)

Glucose level

- ≥300 mg/dL (≥16.65 mmol/L): Use only Bag A
- 251–300 mg/dL (13.93–16.65 mmol/L): 75% Bag A and 25% Bag B
- 201–250 mg/dL (11.15–13.88 mmol/L): 50% Bag A and 50% Bag B
- 151–200 mg/dL (8.38–11.10 mmol/L): 25% Bag A and 75% Bag B
- ≤150 mg/dL (≤8.32 mmol/L): Use only Bag B

Abbreviations: D10, 10% dextrose; IV, intravenous; LR, lactated Ringer solution; NS, normal saline.

---

to prevent hypoglycemia. Add dextrose to the infusion earlier if the rate of glucose decrease is >90 mg/dL/h (>5.00 mmol/L/h) or if the patient develops hypoglycemia. The goal is a blood glucose level in the range of 150 mg/dL (8.32 mmol/L). Check electrolyte levels and perform a blood gas assessment every 2 hours times 3, then every 6 hours until metabolic derangements have normalized. Test the patient's urine for ketones at every voiding, until the ketones are cleared.

Transition

Clinical improvement occurs as the metabolic derangements are corrected and the signs of DKA resolve. Transition the patient to oral fluids and appropriately reduce IV fluids when there is substantial clinical improvement. The most convenient time to transition the patient to a subcutaneous (SC) insulin regimen is prior to a meal. Administer rapid-acting SC insulin approximately 15 to 30 minutes or regular SC insulin 1 to 2 hours before stopping the insulin infusion. If an intermediate or long-acting SC insulin preparation is used, be sure to allow a longer overlap time with the insulin infusion and taper the infusion. This overlap period prevents rebound hyperglycemia. Continue to monitor finger-stick glucose levels hourly while the patient continues to receive the insulin infusion. Once the infusion is stopped, monitor the blood glucose level every 2 to 4 hours and, if the patient is stable, transition him or her to monitoring the blood glucose level before meals, in the mid-afternoon, at bedtime, and at 2:00 am.

Indications for Consultation

- **Endocrinologist:** All patients with DKA
- **Nutritionist:** For discharge planning, once the DKA is resolved

Disposition

- **Intensive care unit transfer:** Severe DKA (pH level <7), insulin drip, new-onset DKA in a patient younger than 5 years, altered mental status, signs of sepsis
- **Discharge criteria:** Euglycemia maintained on a carbohydrate-consistent diet and an appropriate insulin regimen, family/patient has been instructed on monitoring glucose levels and managing hypo-/hyperglycemia, and necessary follow-up has been arranged

Follow-up

- **Primary care physician:** 1 to 2 weeks
- **Endocrinologist:** 2 to 3 days

Pearls and Pitfalls

- The measured sodium level increases during treatment and does not indicate worsening hypertonicity. Moreover, failure of the corrected sodium level to increase or declining sodium levels are risk factors for CE.
- In DKA, the anion gap is usually 20 to 30 mmol/L. A gap greater than 35 mmol/L suggests concurrent lactic acidosis.
- The serum pH level may initially decrease as hydration mobilizes peripheral lactic acid. However, once renal perfusion improves, the excretion of organic acids increases. If biochemical derangements are not being corrected, reassess the patient, consider other potential causes of impaired insulin response (infection, errors in insulin preparation), and adjust the insulin therapy if warranted.
- The routine use of bicarbonate to correct metabolic acidosis is contraindicated, unless there is profound acidosis and cardiac dysfunction. Routine use is associated with the development of CE.

Bibliography

Kimura D, Raszynski A, Totapally BR. Admission and treatment factors associated with the duration of acidosis in children with diabetic ketoacidosis. *Pediatr Emerg Care*. 2012;28(12):1302–1306

Olivieri L, Chasm R. Diabetic ketoacidosis in the pediatric emergency department. *Emerg Med Clin North Am*. 2013;31(3):755–773

Rosenbloom AL. The management of diabetic ketoacidosis in children. *Diabetes Ther*. 2010;1(2):103–120

Tasker RC, Acerini CL. Cerebral edema in children with diabetic ketoacidosis: vasogenic rather than cellular? *Pediatr Diabetes*. 2014;15(4):261–270

Wolfsdorf JI. The International Society of Pediatric and Adolescent Diabetes guidelines for management of diabetic ketoacidosis: do the guidelines need to be modified? *Pediatr Diabetes*. 2014;15(4):277–286

Hyperthyroidism

Introduction

Hyperthyroidism is rare in children, but if unrecognized, it can have potentially fatal consequences. The most common cause (95%) of hyperthyroidism in pediatrics is Graves disease (autoimmune hyperthyroidism), which primarily affects female subjects. The etiology is not known, but there is a strong genetic predilection. Other causes of hyperthyroidism include pituitary and thyroid adenomas, hashitoxicosis, and drug-induced (amiodarone, iodine) thyrotoxicosis.

Thyroid storm, or thyrotoxic crisis, is a rare, multisystem medical emergency that may be precipitated by acute illness, surgery, or abrupt withdrawal of antithyroid medications in a patient with hyperthyroidism. It can be fatal if untreated.

Clinical Presentation

History and Physical Examination

Hyperthyroidism has widespread systemic effects, so the patient may present with fatigue or hyperactivity, weight loss despite increased appetite, diarrhea, muscular weakness, and psychological and growth disturbances. Physical examination findings include tachycardia, hypertension, widened pulse pressure, proptosis, and thyromegaly.

A patient with thyroid storm will have an acute onset of high fever, vomiting and diarrhea, hyperactivity, hypotension, seizures, acute psychosis, and coma.

Laboratory Workup

Perform thyroid function tests: a low thyroid-stimulating hormone (TSH) level with increased T3 and T4 levels establishes a diagnosis of hyperthyroidism. Thyroid-stimulating antibodies are present in autoimmune thyroiditis. If the free T4 level is normal but the TSH level is suppressed, then measure the free T3 level (T3 toxicity). Also check the glucose level, white cell count, lactate dehydrogenase level, liver transaminase levels, and cortisol level, which may be consistent with a relative adrenal insufficiency.

Differential Diagnosis

Note that hyperthyroidism and thyroid storm may or may not be a continuum, with symptom overlap. Consider acute mania, severe viral gastroenteritis, pheochromocytoma, and diabetic ketoacidosis in the differential diagnosis. A patient with acute mania might demonstrate impaired judgment, euphoria, irritability, hallucinations, and unpredictable, violent behavior. A patient with severe viral gastroenteritis will not demonstrate mental status changes unless there are concurrent metabolic abnormalities. Pheochromocytoma may be confused with a thyroid storm because of anxiety, weight loss, sweating, and tachycardia. However, a patient with thyroid storm is typically hypotensive and febrile, with muscular weakness and possibly stigmata of preceding hyperthyroidism, such as proptosis. A patient with diabetic ketoacidosis will have hyperglycemia with ketosis.

Treatment

Thyroid storm can be life threatening and must be diagnosed presumptively while awaiting laboratory confirmation. Obtain an urgent endocrinology consult and provide hydration with normal saline as a 20-mL/kg bolus, repeated as needed, followed by maintenance fluids. Other supportive care includes use of antipyretics and cooling blankets, restoring electrolyte imbalances, and providing cardiorespiratory support. Under the direction of an endocrinologist, the definitive treatment for hyperthyroidism is antithyroid medications, such as methimazole (0.5–1.0 mg/kg/d, divided into 1 or 2 doses). Use propylthiouracil (5–10 mg/kg/d, divided into 2 doses daily) only as a second-line drug because of the potential for severe hepatotoxicity. β-blockers (such as propranolol or atenolol), corticosteroids, radioactive iodine, and hemodialysis may be needed, with expert consultation.

Disposition

- **Intensive care unit transfer:** Thyroid storm, until the patient's hemodynamic status is normal and body temperature is stabilized
- **Discharge criteria:** Patient is clinically euthyroid and tolerating medications

Follow-up

- **Primary care:** 1 week
- **Endocrinology:** 1 to 2 weeks

Pearls and Pitfalls

Obtain baseline absolute neutrophil count and liver function tests before starting antithyroid medications, because agranulocytosis is a potential side effect.

Bibliography

Bauer AJ. Approach to the pediatric patient with Graves' disease: when is definitive therapy warranted? *J Clin Endocrinol Metab.* 2011;96(3):580–588

Franklyn JA, Boelaert K. Thyrotoxicosis. *Lancet.* 2012;379(9821):1155–1166

Graber MN, Gill R. Pediatric endocrine & metabolic emergencies. In: Stone CK, Humphries RL, Drigalla D, Stephan M, eds. *Current Diagnosis & Treatment: Pediatric Emergency Medicine.* New York, NY: McGraw-Hill Education; 2014:576-588

Srinivasan S, Misra M. Hyperthyroidism in children. *Pediatr Rev.* 2015;36(6):239–248

CHAPTER 27

Hypoglycemia

Introduction

Hypoglycemia may be an incidental finding, or the patient may be symptomatic. Hypoglycemia can also be physiological, but recurrent or severe episodes must be further evaluated.

Outside of the newborn period, hypoglycemia may be defined as any glucose value that produces a neuroendocrine response and associated symptoms, with rapid resolution after return to euglycemia. For diagnostic purposes, hypoglycemia is a blood glucose level less than 55 mg/dL (3.05 mmol/L), but 70 mg/dL (3.88 mmol/L) is the lowest acceptable value during routine monitoring before intervention is initiated.

Most often, hypoglycemia is found in a patient who is a known diabetic, or the hypoglycemia is physiological and associated with acute illness, fasting, sepsis, or inadequate oral intake (in cases of nausea and/or vomiting). In such situations, no specific workup is necessary. Ketotic hypoglycemia is a relatively common disorder of unknown etiology that appears with hypoglycemia at presentation after prolonged (often overnight) fasting in young children.

Uncommon etiologies are potentially serious and include disorders of insulin action or insulin excess (gene/enzyme-related hyperinsulinism, insulinoma, infant of a diabetic mother, Beckwith-Wiedemann syndrome), glycogen storage diseases (glucose 6-phosphatase deficiency), defective counterregulatory/neuroendocrine responses (hypopituitarism), defective glycogenolysis/gluconeogenesis (pyruvate carboxylase deficiency, galactosemia), abnormal fatty acid oxidation (inborn errors of metabolism, medium-chain acyl-CoA dehydrogenase), and defective glucose transporters ("GLUT" deficiency).

Clinical Presentation

History

Common autonomic symptoms include anxiety, nausea and vomiting, diaphoresis, and weakness. There may also be central nervous system symptoms, such as seizures, psychiatric outburst, and altered mental status.

Ask about recent meals and duration of fasting, illnesses, and similar previous episodes, as well as a family history of a disease that predisposes the patient to hypoglycemia. Determine if the patient has access to hypoglycemic medications.

Physical Examination

At examination, the patient may be tachycardic, hypothermic, and diaphoretic, with altered mental status ranging from somnolence to encephalopathy to coma.

Laboratory Workup

For the term infant without risk factors for hypoglycemia, glucose reference ranges are similar among age groups beyond about 48 hours of life.

Indications for performing reference laboratory tests include physical examination findings suggestive of an inborn error of metabolism (hepatosplenomegaly, hypotonia), family history of unexplained infant death or inborn errors, or an episode that cannot be clearly explained despite a detailed history. It is imperative that laboratory testing (the "critical sample") be performed at the time of the hypoglycemic event, because it will have the highest yield. Ideally, this testing would occur with endocrinologist guidance, but do not delay conducting tests while awaiting consultation. The critical sample includes assessing levels of blood electrolytes, lactate, β-hydroxybutyrate, growth hormone, cortisol, insulin/C-peptide, and ammonia; toxicology testing; and evaluating urine ketones, glucose levels, reducing substances, and urine organic acids. Also obtain an alanine level if ketotic hypoglycemia is suspected.

Differential Diagnosis

Because various disorders may cause hypoglycemia, a detailed history and physical examination paired with evaluation of supporting laboratory values is crucial (see Table 27-1).

Treatment

The treatment for hypoglycemia is glucose. If the patient is able to safely swallow, offer oral sugar (fruit juice, glucose tablets, table sugar, etc). Otherwise, administer intravenous (IV) dextrose as a 0.20- to 0.25-g/kg bolus (2.0–2.5 mL/kg of 10% dextrose) with a maximum dose of 25 g. Infuse the dextrose bolus over several minutes to avoid causing rapid glucose swings, then measure the glucose level frequently. After delivery of the bolus(es), start an IV continuous infusion of 10% dextrose at a rate of 6 to 9 mg/kg/min:

$$\text{Rate (mg/kg/min)} = (\% \text{ dextrose in solution}) \times (10) \times (\text{rate of infusion [mL/hr]}) \div (60 \times \text{body weight [kg]})$$

Table 27-1. Differential Diagnosis of Nonphysiological Hypoglycemia

Possible Disorders	Suggestive Features
Adrenal insufficiency Growth hormone deficiency	Severe hypoglycemia with missed meals ↑ Ketones, ↓ insulin level Acidosis
Enzyme deficiencies	Severe constant hypoglycemia ↑ Ketones, ↑ lipid levels, ↓ insulin level
Fatty acid oxidation defect	Severe hypoglycemia with missed meals (-) Ketones, ↑ FFA level, ↓ insulin level, abnormal LFT result, abnormal acylcarnitine profile and urine organic acid levels
Galactosemia	Hypoglycemia after ingesting milk or milk products ↑ Ketones, abnormal LFT result, ↓ insulin level
Glycogen storage disease	Hypoglycemia with growth retardation Hepatomegaly ↑ Ketones and blood lactate, cholesterol, triglyceride, and uric acid levels Acidosis
Hyperinsulinism	Recurrent, severe hypoglycemia shortly after meals History of other family members affected (-) Ketones ↑ Insulin level, ↓ FFA level
Ketotic hypoglycemia	Severe hypoglycemia with missed meals ↓ Alanine level, ↑ ketones

Abbreviations: FFA, free fatty acids; LFT, liver function test; -, negative finding.

Reserve higher dextrose concentrations for patients with central access because of extravasation risk. If IV access cannot be obtained, administer subcutaneous or intramuscular glucagon at a dose of 0.03 mg/kg (maximum, 1 mg per dose).

Indications for Consultation

Endocrinologist, metabolic disorder specialist, geneticist: Suspected hyperinsulinism or inborn error of metabolism

Disposition

- **Intensive care unit transfer:** Hemodynamic instability, high glucose infusion rates that require central line access
- **Discharge criteria:** Euglycemia restored and maintained, patient/family educated about signs/symptoms of hypoglycemia and appropriate interventions

Follow-up

- **Primary care:** 1 week
- **Endocrinology:** 1 month; sooner if workup is still required
- **Genetics:** 1 to 2 weeks, if an underlying abnormality or inborn error of metabolism is suspected or diagnosed

Pearls and Pitfalls

- Hypoglycemia is a medical emergency. Do not withhold treatment of a symptomatic child to perform blood tests.
- Obtain critical laboratory samples during periods of hypoglycemia or diagnostic fasting, ideally with endocrinologist consultation.
- Glucose meters provide rapid assessment of plasma glucose levels and allow for frequent testing, but none of the commercially available meters are as accurate as laboratory testing.

Bibliography

Ghosh A, Banerjee I, Morris AA. Recognition, assessment and management of hypoglycaemia in childhood. *Arch Dis Child.* 2016;101(6):575–580

Kim SY. Endocrine and metabolic emergencies in children: hypocalcemia, hypoglycemia, adrenal insufficiency, and metabolic acidosis including diabetic ketoacidosis. *Ann Pediatr Endocrinol Metab.* 2015;20(4):179–186

Lang TF, Hussain K. Pediatric hypoglycemia. *Adv Clin Chem.* 2014;63:211–245

Lang TF. Update on investigating hypoglycemia in childhood. *Ann Clin Biochem.* 2011;48(Pt 3):200–211

Langdon DR, Stanley CA, Sperling MA. Hypoglycemia in the toddler and child. In: Sperling MA, ed. *Pediatric Endocrinology.* 4th ed. Philadelphia, PA: Saunders; 2014:920–955

Equipment and Procedures

Intravenous Line Placement

Introduction

Peripheral intravenous (IV) catheter placement is a common, but nonetheless challenging, procedure in pediatrics. The small caliber of the blood vessels, the anxious and often uncooperative patient, and the worried parents add to the complexity of this procedure.

Informed Consent and Patient Preparation

Written consent is not needed to place an IV catheter. However, prior to placement, inform the parents of the procedure and its indications. Also explain it to the patient in developmentally appropriate language. It is helpful to show an anxious child the IV catheter beforehand and demonstrate that only a "thin straw" will be placed in the vein. Be sure to explain each step to the patient during the procedure and emphasize that staying still will make the process easier. Avoid using phrases like "This will not hurt" or "You will not feel a thing," because these are misleading to the patient. If possible, perform the procedure in a treatment room or other area and not with the young child in bed.

Supplies and Setup

The following supplies are necessary when preparing for IV placement:

- IV catheters (18 to 24 gauge)
- T-connector set
- 3- to 5-mL normal saline flushes
- 3-mL and/or 5-mL syringes (if concomitant blood sampling is needed)
- Tourniquet (or rubber band)
- Gloves
- Alcohol swabs (iodine swabs if blood cultures will be obtained)
- Gauze
- Tape or waterproof transparent dressing
- Appropriately sized arm board or footboard

Choosing the correct IV catheter size is integral to proper IV catheter placement and depends on the patient's age, caliber of the veins visualized, and indication for IV catheter placement. In emergent situations where fluid resuscitation is necessary, insert a large-bore IV catheter to facilitate the rapid delivery of large volumes. In most other scenarios, use the smallest IV catheter possible (<1 year of age, 22 or 24 gauge; ≥1 to 8 years of age, 20 or 22 gauge;

≥8 years of age, 20 gauge and larger). Note that the smaller the gauge of the catheter, the larger the diameter.

Prior to IV catheter insertion, apply warm packs or blankets to the patient's extremities to assist with vasodilation and make it easier to visualize potential IV sites. It is helpful to work with an assistant who can restrain the extremity at the joints above and below the intended insertion site and reach for supplies as needed. Attach a saline flush to the T-connector and flush normal saline through the tubing prior to connecting the T-connector to the IV catheter. Attach the T-connector to an empty syringe if the plan is to obtain a blood specimen after IV insertion is completed. Cut the tape in advance into the desired sizes for securing the IV catheter site.

Application of a topical anesthetic prior to IV catheter insertion will alleviate pain and mitigate anxiety associated with this procedure. To provide anesthesia, these creams must be placed on a predetermined IV catheter insertion site 30 to 60 minutes prior to the procedure, so they cannot be used in emergent situations. Other distraction techniques, performed by a child life specialist or another care provider, can also help alleviate some of the pain and anxiety of this procedure.

Procedure

The most common sites for IV catheter insertion in an infant or child are the dorsum of the hand or foot and the antecubital fossa. Place a tourniquet proximal to the IV catheter insertion site. Clean the area with an alcohol swab for better visualization and look for the optimal vein for IV catheter insertion. Start with the most distal vessel possible, leaving the more proximal ones for subsequent attempts or for future central catheter insertion, if needed. If possible, avoid inserting an IV catheter into the patient's dominant hand. If finding a vessel proves difficult, use a transilluminating or ultrasonographic device, which may help localize a vein.

When a vein is localized, clean the area thoroughly with alcohol, or with iodine if blood cultures will be obtained. Use your nondominant hand to hold the skin taut distal to the IV catheter insertion site. Hold the IV catheter bevel up at an angle of 10° to 20° from the skin. Slowly advance the needle through the skin and into the vein. Once a flash of blood is noted, lower the angle slightly before advancing the catheter. Then, hold the needle steady and use your index finger to advance just the plastic catheter over the needle into the vein until the hub is abutting the skin. Retract the needle while applying pressure to the vein so that blood will not pour out when the needle is removed.

Quickly attach the T-connector to the hub of the IV catheter. Secure the hub of the IV catheter with a short piece of tape placed perpendicular to the IV hub near the skin insertion site. Use more tape or a piece of waterproof transparent dressing to secure the IV site. If blood samples are needed, connect the T-connector to an empty syringe and aspirate blood. When the desired amount of blood is obtained, attach a sterile saline flush to the T-connector and flush slowly into the vein. The saline should easily flush through the catheter. If it does not, readjust the hub of the IV catheter because it may be positioned near a valve.

While flushing the T-connector, inspect the site for signs of infiltration, such as redness, warmth, induration, pain, and swelling. If an IV infiltration is suspected, remove the catheter immediately. Apply a warm pack to the skin to help with the induration and pain. Blanching of the skin during the saline flush suggests that an artery, rather than a vein, has been cannulized. Remove the catheter and apply pressure to the site.

After flushing the IV site with saline, remove the syringe from the T-connector and lock the catheter. Secure the T-connector tubing to the patient's skin with another piece of tape. Finally, secure the extremity to an arm board or footboard to minimize potential movement and manipulation.

Infiltration and extravasation of caustic substances, such as peripheral parenteral nutrition, chemotherapeutic agents, certain anti-epileptics, and antibiotics, can cause serious damage and necrosis to surrounding tissues. Signs and symptoms of IV infiltration include blanching of the skin, edema, cool skin temperature, pain, tenderness, fluid leakage, and blistering and skin ulceration at the insertion site. If such an event occurs, stop the infusion immediately. Management of infiltration and extravasation is determined by the specific offending agent. Consultation with a surgeon may be indicated if the injury is severe or if a concern for compartment syndrome exists. Preventive measures, such as frequent IV site assessment and parent education, can decrease the incidence of IV infiltration in the inpatient setting.

Difficult IV Access Score

Use the difficult IV access (DIVA) score to identify a patient for whom it may be challenging to obtain IV access. A total score of 4 and higher can be used to predict a greater than 50% failure rate during the first attempt to place an IV catheter. Therefore, if the DIVA score suggests a difficult IV catheter insertion, arrange for the most skilled clinician available to be present.

- Vein not visible: 2 points
- Vein not palpable: 2 points
- Premature birth (<38 weeks' gestation): 3 points
- 1 to 2 years of age: 1 point
- Younger than 1 year of age: 3 points

Pearls and Pitfalls

Rarely, phlebitis, cellulitis of the IV site, or bacteremia can occur with peripheral IV catheter placement. Changing IV sites every 3 to 5 days will help reduce the risks.

Bibliography

Dougherty L. IV therapy: recognizing the differences between infiltration and extravasation. *Br J Nurs*. 2008;17(14):896–901

Goff DA, Larsen P, Brinkley J, et al. Resource utilization and cost of inserting peripheral intravenous catheters in hospitalized children. *Hosp Pediatr*. 2013;3(3):185–191

Park SM, Jeong IS, Kim KL, Park KJ, Jung MJ, Jun SS. The effect of intravenous infiltration management program for hospitalized children. *J Pediatr Nurs*. 2016;31(2):172–178

Rauch D, Dowd D, Eldridge D, Mace S, Shears G, Yen K. Peripheral difficult venous access in children. *Clin Pediatr (Phila)*. 2009;48(9):895–901

Spandorfer PR. Peripheral intravenous access. In: Zaoutis LB, Chiang VW, eds. *Comprehensive Pediatric Hospital Medicine*. Philadelphia, PA: Mosby Elsevier; 2007:1249–1251

Lumbar Puncture

Introduction

A lumbar puncture (LP) is most commonly performed to evaluate potential central nervous system infections. It is also used to measure intracranial pressure and to obtain cerebrospinal fluid (CSF) during the evaluation of other conditions, such as demyelinating diseases, tumors, and other neurologic diseases. Proper patient positioning and maintaining a "good hold" on the patient during the procedure are the keys to a successful LP attempt. Also, involvement of a child life specialist may help the patient prepare for and tolerate the procedure.

When performing an LP, communicate clearly with consulting specialists to ensure that all of the requested samples are obtained and sent for the correct laboratory studies. In addition, make a habit of saving in the laboratory an extra tube with 1 to 2 mL of refrigerated or frozen CSF, in the event that additional tests are needed.

Risks and Contraindications

- Potential airway and cardiovascular difficulties may arise when a patient with cardiorespiratory compromise is positioned for the procedure. If this is a concern, administer intravenous (IV) antibiotics after a blood culture has been obtained (if the LP is being performed to diagnose an infection) and perform the procedure in a controlled, monitored situation after initial resuscitation and stabilization.
- Herniation is possible in a patient with known, increased intracranial pressure or a mass lesion.
- Infected tissue may overlie the entry site of the spinal needle. This might result in iatrogenic introduction of flora into the CSF space.
- There is potential for uncontrolled bleeding. Ensure that the platelet count is more than 50,000/mm³ (50×10^9/L) prior to performing an LP.
- An uncooperative patient may not be able to remain still. Sedation may be required so that the LP can be performed under controlled circumstances. However, the person performing the LP *cannot also provide the sedation*.

Consent

Use simple and reassuring terms to explain the risks of a "spinal tap" to the patient's parents. For example, "There is always a chance of infection and bleeding whenever the skin is broken, but this risk is not much different than when an IV catheter is inserted. Many babies fall asleep during the procedure."

Parents are often worried that somehow their child might become paralyzed from an LP. It is therefore helpful to raise this issue concretely, even if the parents do not ask: "The needle is being inserted only into the outermost portion of the fluid around the spinal cord. I will take out a teaspoon of fluid, which will be replaced within 1 hour. I have never heard of a child being paralyzed after an LP."

An appropriate layperson's description for a written consent form that parents sign is, "Insert a needle into the lower back to remove spinal fluid for analysis." Offer the parents the option of staying in the room for the procedure if their presence does not cause performance anxiety. Position the parents so that they are facing the infant rather than watching the needle.

Procedure

1. Apply lidocaine/prilocaine (EMLA) cream or lidocaine (LMX) cream over the interspaces as soon as an LP is being considered to minimize delays and maximize analgesia.
2. If mandated by the institution, obtain written informed consent and/or documentation of a required time-out.
3. Prepare the equipment and the person holding the patient. Position the equipment so it is convenient to the location of the patient. Include 4 collection tubes, at least 2 spinal needles, oxygen, suction equipment, pulse oximetry equipment, and other monitors as indicated. Use a 22-gauge, 1.5-inch (3.81-cm) spinal needle for an infant or toddler younger than 2 years; a 22-gauge, 2.5-inch (6.35-cm) needle for a child aged 2 to 12 years; and a 20- or 22-gauge, 3.5-inch (8.89-cm) needle for an adolescent.
4. Choose a patient position, and review the restraint and positioning protocol with the person holding the patient. Position the patient in either the lateral decubitus or sitting position, which expands the intervertebral space and may allow easier and more reliable identification of the midline of the vertebral column. With either position, identify the L4-L5 interspace in the midline at the level of the iliac crests.
5. Take a time-out to identify the patient and follow other institution-specific procedural protocols.
6. Sterilize the field. Position the patient and prepare the draping. Ensure that the surface is clean, flat, and relatively firm. Apply sterile gloves.
7. Prepare and drape the patient.

8. Have the person holding the patient restrain him or her in the optimal position. If the patient is in the lateral decubitus position, apply pressure to the patient's shoulders to get him or her into a fetal position with a C-shaped kyphosis, while avoiding compression to the head. If the patient is in the seated position, place a rolled-up towel anterior to the patient's chest/abdomen to facilitate the desired maximal kyphosis of the fetal position.

9. *Do not compromise on positioning.* Identify landmarks and midline structures and give the person holding the patient feedback about the patient's 3-dimensional space. Maximize kyphosis without inducing lateral scoliosis. If the patient is in the lateral decubitus position, to facilitate midline insertion in the sagittal plane, maintain the patient's back perpendicular to the plane of the bed. Also maintain the patient's back parallel or tangential to the edge of the bed at the skin entry to facilitate a consistent cephalad approach toward the umbilicus.

10. If local anesthesia is administered, raise an intradermal wheal over the L4-L5 site either before or immediately after prepping and drying of the skin. Provide oral sucrose for an infant. For a toddler or older child, inject additional local anesthesia gradually and sequentially into the deeper layers of soft tissue and ligaments, taking care not to inject any into the CSF itself.

11. Use the smallest-gauge spinal needle available to reduce potential pressure shifts and minimize the risk of post-LP headache. Insert the spinal needle, with the trocar in place, through the skin, midline at L4-L5, with the bevel pointing cephalad or parallel to the spine. With either position, angle the needle toward the umbilicus. Keep the trocar in the needle until a pop is felt or until a reasonable depth is reached. Then remove the trocar and gently manipulate (advance, withdraw, rotate) the needle. Observe the hub for CSF return. The needle may be held a number of different ways.

    a. One-handed technique: Hold the needle between the index and middle fingers of the dominant hand and advance with the thumb.

    b. Two-handed technique: Advance the needle with both thumbs, guiding the direction with the index fingers braced against the patient's back.

    If a firm surface is felt, it is likely to be bone—often the bottom of the L4 vertebra. Remove the needle to the level of the outermost ligamentous tissues and angle it somewhat more caudally. If a gush of bright red blood is obtained, the needle is probably lateral of the midline in one of the paravertebral veins. Withdraw the needle completely and try again at L3-L4. If there is no fluid return at all, the needle is probably still within ligamentous tissues. Slowly advance and manipulate the needle; for an infant, 1 to 2 cm will suffice. During the initial LP attempt, in the absence of streaming of blood at the needle hub, homogenously red, translucent CSF that does not clear as additional fluid is collected may be evidence of an intracranial bleed.

12. Collect 1 mL (0.5-mL minimum) of CSF into each of the 4 tubes and send it for testing, as indicated herein. If the tap is traumatic, the culture is still valid and is the priority when insufficient CSF is collected for all of the routine, but immediate, studies. Turbid fluid is presumptive evidence of bacterial meningitis; clear fluid is reassuring but not a guarantee of a normal CSF cell count or protein level.

    a. Tube 1: Gram stain, culture, and sensitivity test

    b. Tube 2: Glucose and protein assessment

    c. Tube 3: Additional studies (herpes simplex virus or enterovirus polymerase chain reaction, myelin basic protein level evaluation, serology)

    d. Tube 4: Blood cell count

13. To measure opening pressure, perform the LP with the patient in the lateral decubitus position. Prepare the manometer, stopcock, and flexible tubing in advance. As soon as CSF flows from the hub, attach the male end of the flexible tubing to the hub with the stopcock in the "off" to "drainage" position. Keep the stopcock at the level of the spinal column and gently straighten the patient's legs and back. The opening pressure is equal to the height of the column in centimeters of water once respiratory variation is observed. Open the stopcock to "drainage" position ("off" to the needle) to collect CSF. Turn the stopcock "off" to the manometer to complete CSF collection.

14. After the 4 specimens are obtained, reinsert the trocar and withdraw the needle.

15. Tell the parents the preliminary findings (clear, traumatic, or turbid fluid) and how their child tolerated the procedure.

16. Write a procedure note. For example, "LP performed to rule out meningitis in a febrile 6-week-old infant. After obtaining informed consent, identifying the patient, and performing a time-out, the patient was prepped and draped in the customary sterile fashion, and a 22-gauge, 1.5-inch (3.81-cm) spinal needle was inserted into the L4-L5 interspace in the first attempt. Five milliliters of clear CSF were obtained and sent for the usual studies. The patient tolerated the procedure well, with no complications."

17. While the traditional recommendation is to keep older children and adolescents flat in bed for 4 to 6 hours to avoid a post-LP or spinal headache, there is little evidence to support this practice. Treatment options for a severe spinal headache include narcotic analgesics, IV caffeine (500 mg), or, for persistent symptoms, an epidural blood patch performed by an anesthesiologist.

Pearls and Pitfalls

- Place lidocaine/prilocaine (EMLA) cream or lidocaine (LMX) cream on the lumbar area as soon as an LP is being considered.
- Spend time making sure that patient positioning is optimal, with the patient in the ideal position and the operator comfortably seated.
- If the LP is part of a workup to rule out sepsis in an infant, get the urine sample first, because the patient may urinate while being manipulated and undressed for the LP.

Bibliography

Bonadio W. Pediatric lumbar puncture and cerebrospinal fluid analysis. *J Emerg Med.* 2014;46(1):141–150

Cronan KM, Wiley JF II. Lumbar puncture. In: King C, Henretig FM, eds. *Textbook of Pediatric Emergency Procedures.* 2nd ed. Philadelphia, PA: Lippincott Williams & Wilkins; 2008:505–514

Gibson T. Lumbar puncture. In: Zaoutis LB, Chiang VW, eds. *Comprehensive Pediatric Hospital Medicine.* Philadelphia, PA: Mosby Elsevier; 2007:1240–1242

Schulga P, Grattan R, Napier C, Babiker MO. How to use… lumbar puncture in children. *Arch Dis Child Educ Pract Ed.* 2015;100(5):264–271

Turnbull DK, Shepherd DB. Post-dural puncture headache: pathogenesis, prevention and treatment. *Br J Anaesth.* 2003;91(5):718–729

CHAPTER 30

Noninvasive Monitoring

Introduction

Monitoring objective data, such as vital signs and pulse oximetry, is essential in the clinical assessment of pediatric patients. Noninvasive monitoring techniques provide continuous measurement of physiological parameters, allowing early recognition of clinical deterioration. Caregivers must remain attentive to the monitors, investigate alarm events promptly, recognize significant physiological changes, and intervene appropriately.

Temperature Monitoring

Opinions differ regarding the ideal thermometer and site for temperature measurement in children. Accurate temperature measurement is most important in young infants, since the presence of fever frequently prompts a laboratory evaluation for sepsis. Rectal temperatures are the most accurate, with the least variability, and are therefore considered the standard of care for young infants. However, axillary, oral, tympanic, and temporal artery temperatures are commonly used, because these methods are easier to use and are better tolerated by children. Axillary temperatures are consistently lower than core temperature and are variable, based on environmental factors. Oral temperatures are reliable estimates of core temperature but require patient cooperation and may be inaccurate because of recent oral intake. Tympanic and temporal artery thermometers use infrared thermal detection to provide quick estimation of the core temperature, but studies regarding their accuracy have had variable results. Whichever method is used, document serial temperatures to establish a trend.

Cardiorespiratory Monitors

With cardiorespiratory (CR) monitors, 3 chest electrodes are used to continuously measure heart and respiratory rates. Inaccuracies may occur because of loose leads, patient movement, and poor detection of respiratory movements. Investigate alarm events with a prompt clinical assessment of the child. Document significant events and any interventions.

Use continuous CR monitoring for patients at risk for cardiac or respiratory deterioration. Monitor serial blood pressures with an appropriately sized pediatric blood pressure cuff. CR monitors may be used to detect simple arrhythmias, but obtain a standard 12-lead electrocardiogram for more precise diagnosis of cardiac conditions.

Do not rely on CR monitors to detect apnea or airway obstruction, because they rely on pneumography and can only be used to detect central apnea, characterized by a lack of respiratory effort. Apnea is more commonly caused by airway obstruction, in which chest wall movements persist and continue to be detected with pneumography. Bradycardia is delayed until profound hypoxia occurs.

Pulse Oximetry

Pulse oximetry provides a noninvasive, accurate estimation of arterial oxygen saturation from a sensor placed on a finger, toe, hand, foot, or ear. Pulse oximetry measurements may be inaccurate because of incorrect sensor placement, patient movement, skin abnormalities, fingernail polish interfering with the finger sensor, ambient light interference, distal hypoperfusion, methemoglobinemia, and carbon monoxide or cyanide poisoning. To ensure accuracy, verify the presence of a steady pulse and/or waveform on the pulse oximetry monitor.

Indications for continuous pulse oximetry monitoring include administration of supplemental oxygen, risk of clinical deterioration, and neonatal resuscitation or procedural sedation. However, use *intermittent* pulse oximetry for assessment of patients with stable respiratory illness. Continuous pulse oximetry monitoring may demonstrate transient decreases in oxygen saturation that are not clinically significant and do not indicate a need for supplemental oxygen. This is especially true for mild desaturation that occurs at night, during sleep.

Pulse oximetry does not provide assessment of adequate ventilation. Use capnography or blood gas analysis to assess the patient for hypercarbia and/or respiratory acidosis. Do not rely on pulse oximetry for detection of apnea and/or airway obstruction, because arterial oxygenation decreases gradually during such events.

Capnography

The standard of reference for assessment of ventilation is arterial blood gas analysis. However, blood gas analysis requires a painful procedure and time for laboratory analysis and only provides intermittent data. Capnography is a noninvasive method of assessing ventilation by sampling the end-tidal CO_2 level in children breathing via face mask or nasal cannula. End-tidal CO_2 level allows accurate estimation of partial pressure of CO_2 in children.

Use capnography for monitoring the ventilation of patients during procedural sedation. Other indications include patients with altered mental status or respiratory illness. Capnography has an emerging role in detecting metabolic acidosis. Use colorimetric carbon dioxide detectors for confirmation of endotracheal intubation, as well as for continuously monitoring endotracheal tube placement and patency in critically ill children.

Applications

Sedation

The use of procedural sedation in pediatrics has increased significantly since the early 2000s. Procedural sedation carries significant risks, such as hypoventilation, apnea, airway obstruction, laryngospasm, and hypotension. Continuous observation of the patient and monitoring of vital signs, pulse oximetry, and capnography are essential to ensure that complications are immediately recognized and interventions rapidly instituted. For patients receiving moderate or deep sedation, a caregiver not involved with the procedure must be present to continuously monitor clinical parameters. Use capnography for prompt detection of apnea, airway obstruction, or hypoventilation during sedation and recovery.

Transport

Noninvasive monitoring is critical during the transport of a patient, because assessment becomes more difficult in an ambulance or aircraft. Rely on continuous noninvasive CR, pulse oximetry, and capnography monitoring to detect clinical changes.

Pearls and Pitfalls

- Excessive monitor alarms may result in nurse desensitization and delayed response to subsequent alarms. Set age-appropriate, individualized alarm parameters to minimize false alarms and prevent "alarm fatigue" in the nursing staff.
- Rectal temperatures are only recommended in young infants and are contraindicated in patients with neutropenia, immunodeficiency, or recent rectal surgery.
- Capnography is essential for prompt detection of apnea or respiratory depression during procedural sedation.

Bibliography

American Academy of Pediatrics, American Academy of Pediatric Dentistry, Coté CJ, Wilson S, Work Group on Sedation. Guidelines for monitoring and management of pediatric patients during and after sedation for diagnostic and therapeutic procedures: an update. *Pediatrics*. 2006;118(6):2587–2602

Becker HJ, Langhan M. Capnography in the pediatric emergency department: clinical applications. *Pediatr Emerg Med Practice*. 2013;10(6):1–24

Bonafide CP, Brady PW, Keren R, Conway PH, Marsolo K, Daymont C. Development of heart and respiratory rate percentile curves for hospitalized children. *Pediatrics*. 2013;131(4):e1150–e1157

Fouzas S, Priftis KN, Anthracopoulos MB. Pulse oximetry in pediatric practice. *Pediatrics*. 2011;128(4):740–752

Graham KC, Cvach M. Monitor alarm fatigue: standardizing use of physiological monitors and decreasing nuisance alarms. *Am J Crit Care*. 2010;19(1):28–34

CHAPTER 31

Suprapubic Bladder Aspiration

Introduction

Suprapubic bladder aspiration is the standard procedure for obtaining a urine specimen for culture in a patient younger than 6 months. It is preferable to catheterization in a male patient with a tight foreskin and in a female patient when the urethral meatus cannot be visualized.

Contraindications

Do not perform a suprapubic bladder aspiration if the patient has a coagulopathy, massive organomegaly, or intestinal obstruction or if there is an infection of the overlying skin. Obtain urine via catheterization instead.

Complications

Very rare complications from the procedure include hematuria and intestinal perforation, although the use of ultrasonographic (US) guidance decreases the risk of perforation.

Procedure

It is best to wait at least 1 hour after the patient's last voiding and/or 45 minutes after a feeding before attempting the procedure. Prior to inserting the needle, perform bedside bladder US examination (if readily available) to confirm the presence of urine in the bladder.

1. Explain the procedure to the patient's parents, including the potential complications, and obtain consent if required by institutional policy. Offer the parents the option of staying in the room if they are able to watch comfortably and if their presence does not cause performance anxiety.

2. Gather all necessary equipment, including topical anesthetic, sterile gloves, a 22- or 23-gauge 1.5-inch (3.81-cm) straight needle, antiseptic solution, 3- to 5-mL syringe, gauze, sterile drape, and sterile specimen container.

3. Apply the topical anesthetic to the skin 1 to 2 cm superior to the pubic symphysis and cover with an adhesive bandage for 20 to 30 minutes. Ensure that the available topical anesthetic can be used safely in the patient's age group.

4. Open the package of gloves and use the interior of the package as the sterile field for the needle, syringe, sterile drape, and gauze.

5. Have an assistant restrain the patient in a supine, frog-leg position. Also have an assistant occlude the urethra in a male patient to prevent urination during preparation.

6. Clean the area from the umbilicus to the pubic symphysis with the antiseptic solution. Put on the sterile gloves and drape the area.

7. Palpate the symphysis pubis. Insert the needle 1 to 2 cm above the symphysis, where the abdominal crease and linea alba intersect. Make sure the needle is aligned so it is perpendicular to the lower abdominal wall and aimed at about a 10° to 20° cephalad angle. Exert suction on the syringe while advancing the needle, but do not go deeper than 1 inch. Aspirate the urine into the syringe, although this often occurs while the needle is being withdrawn.

8. Remove the needle once the aspiration is complete. Clean the patient with water and gauze.

9. Transfer the urine in the appropriately labeled sterile specimen containers.

10. If urine is not obtained, withdraw the needle to the edge of the needle tip but do not remove the needle from the skin. Change the angle so that the needle tip is more caudad. If urine is still not obtained, perform a catheterization if not contraindicated or wait 1 to 2 hours and repeat the suprapubic aspiration.

11. Write a postprocedural note in the patient's medical record.

Pearls and Pitfalls

- Perform the procedure at least 1 hour after the last voiding or 45 minutes after a feeding.
- If available, a bladder US examination can be performed to document that the bladder is full.
- The success rate of the procedure may be improved by using US guidance, which allows confirmation of a full bladder and visualization of the puncture.
- Immediately withdraw the needle if anything other than urine is aspirated into the syringe. Occasionally, the small bowel is perforated and stool is aspirated, but the microperforation is not clinically significant and does not require any treatment.

Bibliography

Buntsma D, Stock A, Bevan C, Babl FE. Success rate of BladderScan-assisted suprapubic aspiration. *Emerg Med Australas*. 2012;24(6):647–651

Eliacik K, Kanik A, Yavascan O, et al. A comparison of bladder catheterization and suprapubic aspiration methods for urine sample collection from infants with a suspected urinary tract infection. *Clin Pediatr (Phila)*. 2016;55(9):819–824

Marin, J, Shaikh N, Docimo SG, Hickey RW, Hoberman A. Videos in clinical medicine. Suprapubic bladder aspiration. *New Engl J Med*. 2014;371(10):e13

Ponka D, Baddar F. Top 10 forgotten diagnostic procedures: suprapubic bladder aspiration. *Can Fam Physician*. 2013;59(1):50

Tosif S, Baker A, Oakley E, Donath S, Babl FE. Contamination rates of different urine collection methods for the diagnosis of urinary tract infections in young children: an observational cohort study. *J Paediatr Child Health*. 2012;48(8):659–664

Tracheostomies

Introduction

A child with medical complexity is often dependent on technology, such as a tracheostomy tube (TT). In the immediate postoperative period, any problems associated with such equipment are best managed by the surgical team who performed the insertion procedure. However, once this period has passed, the hospitalist may be expected to manage a number of malfunctions or infections associated with these devices.

A TT is maintained for chronic respiratory insufficiency or inability to protect the airway. The benefit of the tracheostomy is that it allows for assisted airway clearance and access for intermittent or continuous invasive mechanical ventilation without sedating the patient. However, the direct entry into the tracheobronchial tree represents a portal for infection.

Common complications include inappropriate fit (because of patient growth or weight gain), partial or complete obstruction of the tube, mechanical failure (uncommon), and infection (tracheitis, cellulitis, or abscess). Other complications include pressure necrosis, tracheal granuloma, tracheal stenosis, and fistulae to the esophagus or innominate artery.

Clinical Presentation

A patient with a TT may present with local skin breakdown caused by inadequate stoma care, an inappropriately sized tube, or overly tight tracheostomy ties. Partial tube obstruction is common, although a suction catheter can usually still be passed, which gives the misleading impression that the lumen is clear. Secretions may sometimes obstruct virtually the entire lumen, except for the diameter of the suction catheter.

Ask about the routine care of the TT and tracheostomy site, including the frequency and the materials used for stoma care. Typically, this involves half-strength hydrogen peroxide mixed with sterile water. Determine when the TT was last exchanged (usually monthly), whether it was up- or downsized, and when the most recent direct laryngoscopy and bronchoscopy (DL&B) were performed to assess the health of the stoma site. For a cuffed TT, evaluate the integrity of the balloon by using a 5-mL syringe to deflate the balloon, remove it, and refill it outside of the patient's body to check for leaks.

Laboratory Workup

A simple set of anteroposterior and lateral neck radiographs can confirm the position of a TT but cannot be used to assess functionality. If indicated, order a bedside endoscopy or a DL&B, performed by an otorhinolaryngologist, to assess for any tracheal granuloma or stenosis.

If infection is a concern, obtain a Gram stain and cell count of secretions suctioned from the TT. However, these results must be interpreted with care to properly distinguish between colonization and actual infection. The hallmark of infection is an increased number of white blood cells, along with a predominant organism, in the setting of fever and cough. During infections, TT secretions are usually described as thick, green, and foul smelling.

Differential Diagnosis

The diagnosis of common complications is summarized in Table 32-1.

Treatment

If a patient is unable to effectively clear their secretions, use the following formula to choose a flexible suction catheter that is slightly less than half the diameter of the TT (Table 32-2):

Diameter of TT (in millimeters) × 1.5 = French gauge for suction catheter
(Example: 4-mm TT × 1.5 = 6-F suction catheter)

In general, do not insert the suction catheter any deeper than the length of the TT to avoid mucosal injury. It may sometimes be necessary to gently advance the catheter further, until a cough is stimulated or resistance is met. Apply suction only while the catheter is being removed and never during the insertion process. Use the lowest amount of pressure required to effectively

Table 32-1. Common Acute Complications of Tracheostomies	
Diagnosis	**Clinical Features**
Accidental decannulation	Absent TT at stoma site Change in vocalization (often louder)
Infection (vs colonization)	Fever and increased cough Increased need for suctioning Change in color/odor of tracheal aspirate WBCs on Gram stain of aspirate
Minor bleeding	Suctioning depth, frequency, or pressure is excessive Insufficient humidification of airway Infection (hemoptysis)
Obstruction: complete or partial	Respiratory distress or failure ↑ P_{O_2} level, ↑ P_{CO_2} level

Abbreviations: P_{CO_2}, partial pressure of carbon dioxide; P_{O_2}, partial pressure of oxygen; TT, tracheostomy tube; WBC, white blood cell.

Table 32-2. Equivalency of Common Sizes of TTs and Suction Catheters

	Bivona TTs				Shiley TTs				
Size	ID (mm)	OD (mm)	Length (mm)	Suction Catheter (Fr)	Size	ID (mm)	OD (mm)	Length (mm)	Suction Catheter (Fr)
2.5 NEO	2.5	4.0	30	6	3.0 NEO	3.0	4.5	30	6
3.0 NEO	3.0	4.7	32	6 or 8	3.5 NEO	3.5	5.2	32	6 or 8
3.5 NEO	3.5	5.3	34	6 or 8	4.0 NEO	4.0	5.9	34	6 or 8
4.0 NEO	4.0	6.0	36	6 or 8	4.5 NEO	4.5	6.5	36	6 or 8
2.5 PED	2.5	4.0	38	6					
3.0 PED	3.0	4.7	39	6 or 8	3.0 PED	3.0	4.5	39	6
3.5 PED	3.5	5.3	40	6 or 8	3.5 PED	3.5	5.2	40	6 or 8
4.0 PED	4.0	6.0	41	6 or 8	4.0 PED	4.0	5.9	41	6 or 8
4.5 PED	4.5	6.7	42	6 or 8	4.5 PED	4.5	6.5	42	6 or 8
5.0 PED	5.0	7.3	44	8 or 10	5.0 PED	5.0	7.1	44	8 or 10
5.5 PED	5.5	8.0	46	10 or 12	5.5 PED	5.5	7.7	46	10 or 12

Abbreviations: Fr, French; ID, internal diameter; NEO, neonatal; OD, outer diameter; PED, pediatric.

Chapter 32: Tracheostomies

clear the airway (50–100 mm Hg for a child). Individual institutions have policies that require the use of sterile, modified sterile, or clean technique for suctioning TT.

When in doubt, remove the TT and replace it promptly. Always have 2 spare tubes immediately available for emergencies, one of the same size and one of a size smaller than the one currently in use. If no spare TT is available, inspect the current one for any occlusion. In an emergency, use an endotracheal tube of the same diameter and trim the length after insertion.

Many respiratory therapists are knowledgeable about the mechanics of TT exchange, and this skill is easily mastered by hospitalists. To change a TT, the required supplies include gloves, suction, oxygen, bag valve mask, lubricant, and a fresh set of TT ties. Place the patient in the supine position with a neck roll to extend the cervical spine and deflate the cuff if the current TT has one. Gently remove the TT by using an upward and outward movement. Insert the new TT by following the same arc in reverse, inward and downward. Immediately remove the obturator (if one was used) and hold the TT securely in place until new tracheostomy ties are applied. If the procedure proves to be difficult, insert a suction catheter, then advance the new TT over it (similar to a modified Seldinger technique).

If there is an abscess adjacent to the stoma site, arrange for it to be incised and drained, send a specimen for Gram stain and culture, and select antibiotics that treat both skin and respiratory flora, including methicillin-resistant *Staphylococcus aureus* (intravenous clindamycin, 40 mg/kg/d, divided into doses administered every 8 hours; 4.8-g/d maximum).

Indications for Consultation

- **Wound or stoma team:** Difficult wound
- **Pediatric otolaryngology:** Clinical or radiographic evidence of TT malfunction, dislodgment, or inappropriate fit

Disposition

- **Intensive care unit transfer:** Difficult TT replacement
- **Discharge criteria:** Stable tube and clean site

Follow-up

- **Primary care:** 1 to 2 weeks
- **Surgical subspecialist (if involved):** 1 week

Pearls and Pitfalls

- Two spare, new TTs must be available at all times. One must be of the current size (diameter and length) and one a size smaller.
- It is important to note the difference in neonatal- and pediatric-sized tubes when selecting a TT. While the numeric sizes appear the same, there are significant differences in how they fit (Table 32-2).
- When selecting items for home care, a portable suction machine is preferable.
- Teach family members safe techniques for changing a TT.

Bibliography

Flynn AP, Carter B, Bray L, Donne AJ. Parents' experiences and views of caring for a child with a tracheostomy: a literature review. *Intl J Ped Otorhinolaryngol*. 2013;77(10): 1630–1634

Mitchell RB, Hussey HM, Setzen G, et al. Clinical consensus statement: tracheostomy care. *Otolaryngol Head Neck Surg*. 2013;148(1):6–20

Nelson KE, Mahant S. Shared decision-making about assistive technology for the child with severe neurologic impairment. *Pediatr Clin N Am*. 2014;61(4):641–652

Neupane B, McFeeters M, Johnson E, Hickey H, Pandya H. Transitioning children requiring long-term ventilation from hospital to home: a practical guide. *Paediatr Child Health*. 2015;25(4):187–191

Peterson-Carmichael SL, Cheifetz IM. The chronically critically ill patient: pediatric considerations. *Respir Care*. 2012;57(6):993–1003

Porter SM, Page DR, Somppi C. Emergency preparedness in the school setting for the child assisted by medical technology. Tracheostomies, ventilators, and oxygen. *NASN Sch Nurse*. 2013;298–305

Urinary Bladder Catheterization

Introduction

Urinary bladder catheterization is indicated for diagnosis of a urinary tract infection or pyelonephritis in an infant or young child who cannot provide a reliable clean-catch specimen. It is also used for relief of urinary retention and for intermittent catheterization of a neurogenic bladder.

Contraindications

Do not perform bladder catheterization if the patient has a pelvic fracture or suspected trauma to the urethra (blood at the meatus).

Complications

Potential complications of catheterization include urethral trauma, bladder trauma, vaginal catheterization, urinary tract infection, and intravesical knot (rare).

Procedure

Explain the procedure to the patient's parents, including the potential complications. Obtain consent if required by institutional policy. Once the procedure is completed, write a postprocedural note in the patient's medical record.

Male Patients

1. Gather all equipment needed for the procedure, including 2 pairs of sterile gloves, an appropriately sized catheter (8 F in newborns, 10 F in most children, and 12 F in older children), syringe (at least 10 mL), sterile lubricant, antiseptic solution, sterile fenestrated drape, and sterile specimen container.
2. Open the package of gloves. Use the interior of the package as the sterile field and place the catheter, syringe, and lubricant on the field.
3. Have an assistant hold the patient's legs in a frog-leg position.
4. Once all the equipment is arranged, put on gloves, open the diaper, and quickly, but gently, grab the penis mid-shaft and squeeze to prevent spontaneous urination. Use light, persistent pressure to retract the foreskin and expose the meatus. Prepare the urethral meatus and penis by gently cleaning with the antiseptic solution.
5. Place the fenestrated drape over the patient's penis. Remove the gloves.

6. Put on the fresh pair of sterile gloves and lubricate the catheter. Attach the syringe to the catheter. Have an opened urine cup within reach in case the patient urinates during the preparation, in essence providing a true clean catch.

7. Gently grasp and extend the penile shaft to straighten the urethra. Hold the lubricated catheter near the meatus and insert the catheter into the urethra. Slowly advance the catheter and apply continued pressure to get past the resistance that is typically felt at the external sphincter.

8. Once urine is visualized in the tubing, pull back on the syringe. Remove the catheter once the collection is completed. Do not pull back on the syringe while manipulating the catheter.

9. If a Foley catheter is being placed, use the same technique. In addition, test the integrity of the balloon prior to inserting the catheter. Once the catheter is well inserted into the bladder, inflate the balloon with the recommended amount of saline, then gently retract the catheter until slight resistance is met. Attach the catheter to the collection container by using sterile technique.

10. Place the specimen in the appropriate, labeled container (eg, for urinalysis or urine culture). A trace amount of urine (≤1 mL) is adequate for a culture.

11. Clean off the antiseptic solution with water and gauze.

12. If the patient is uncircumcised, ensure that the foreskin is retracted back over the glans to prevent paraphimosis.

13. Rapidly transport the specimen to the laboratory. Place it on ice if there is any potential for delay.

Female Patients

For female subjects, the principles are similar to catheterization in male patients. Have an assistant spread the labia. The urethral orifice is anterior to the vaginal orifice, and the catheter needs to be advanced just a few centimeters to reach the bladder in female subjects.

Pearls and Pitfalls

- Obtain the urine first if the catheterization is part of a sepsis workup in an infant.
- Always have the urine collection cup open while performing the procedure, in case the patient spontaneously voids.
- If urine is not obtained, leave the catheter in, because the patient will eventually produce urine. There is no need to recatheterize.

Bibliography

Beno S, Schwab S. Bladder catheterization. In: King C, Henretig FM, eds. *Textbook of Pediatric Emergency Procedures.* 2nd ed. Philadelphia, PA: Lippincott Williams & Wilkins; 2008:888–894

Karacan C, Erkek N, Senel S, Akin Gunduz S, Catli G, Tavil B. Evaluation of urine collection methods for the diagnosis of urinary tract infection in children. *Med Princ Pract.* 2010;19:188–191

Manzano S, Vunda A, Schneider F. Vandertuin L, Lacroix LE. Videos in clinical medicine. Catheterization of the urethra in girls. *New Engl J Med.* 2014;371(2):e2

Niël-Weise BS, van den Broek PJ, da Silva EM, Silva LA. Urinary catheter policies for long-term bladder drainage. *Cochrane Database Syst Rev.* 2012;15(8):CD004201

Bibliography

Ethics

Do Not Resuscitate/Do Not Intubate

Introduction

Do not resuscitate (DNR)/do not intubate (DNI) orders are a part of advanced directives for patients with life-limiting illnesses when patients (or their surrogates) believe that attempted resuscitation would not be in their best interest. Also known as *do not attempt resuscitation* ("DNAR") or *allow natural death* ("AND") orders, these are to be used not in isolation but as part of an overall discussion with the patient (if appropriate) and the parents/guardians as to the overall goals of treatment. DNR/DNI orders can be instituted should a cardiorespiratory arrest occur while the patient is undergoing other intensive therapies, such as chemotherapy. DNR/DNI orders can be specific for inpatients or outpatients or apply to both settings as a part of a comprehensive end-of-life plan. Laws and regulations that govern their application vary from state to state.

Use DNR orders to help convey the wishes of patients, parents, or guardians in the event of cardiorespiratory arrest. As part of a comprehensive care plan, related orders (eg, advance directives or advance care plans) can also describe the preferred responses to a deteriorating clinical situation before the point of an arrest. These orders and the documented discussions that generated them can also address pain control, symptom management, medically provided fluids and nutrition, and the psychosocial needs of the family.

Most hospitals have DNR/DNI policies or guidelines, as well as forms or order sets. As a child matures into adolescence, there may be guidelines related to obtaining the patient's assent, in addition to the consent of the parents or guardians. In general, always consider the wishes of the adolescent when making decisions about limiting life-sustaining medical treatments.

Process

When a child or adolescent has a terminal illness or condition or is nearing the end of life, arrange for the attending physician, pertinent consultants, patient (if appropriate), and family to discuss the nature and direction of the patient's care. This dialogue is best accomplished when the child or family is *not in a crisis*. A palliative care team or provider may be able to help facilitate the discussion. For a patient cared for by hospitalists or intensivists, it is especially important to include physicians from the child's medical home in the process. If the child is a ward of the state, involve the designated medical decision maker(s).

Once the overall goals are identified, develop and institute the plans to help accomplish them. Resuscitation options are varied and may be as comprehensive as no intervention in the event of an arrest (no intubation, cardiopulmonary resuscitation, cardiac medications, or intravenous medications). In other cases, a "limited DNR/DNI" order can be created by defining which therapies can be initiated. For example, positive-pressure ventilation with bag, mask, and suctioning might be permitted, while chest compressions, intubation, mechanical ventilation, and cardiac medications are not. The more specific the delineation of the plan, the more effectively it can be performed according to the patient's and family's wishes. In addition to the specific details, it is essential to document the discussion that occurred and the goals of care that were identified.

Have an attending physician, not a trainee, write the orders in the paper chart or electronic medical record. Attempt to avoid verbal orders, which are appropriate only in rare situations, such as with a well-known patient whose previous DNR/DNI orders may have lapsed and need to be reinstituted during a repeat hospitalization. Parental "signing" of DNR/DNI orders is not required in most states and should generally be avoided because it can put an undue burden on the parents by suggesting that they approved allowing their child to die.

As soon as the DNR/DNI plan is ordered, discuss and review it with all members of the health care team so that it is clearly understood by everyone responsible for its implementation. If there is a lengthy hospitalization, review the DNR/DNI orders periodically to ensure that the patient and family continue to feel that the DNR/DNI orders support the goals of care. Some hospitals may have policies that define how frequently the orders must be reviewed or rewritten, and some facilities may allow a home DNR/DNI order to remain in effect after the patient is hospitalized, although the order may need prompt renewal. Others may require new orders to be instituted at admission, so it is useful to become familiar with a given hospital's policies in this area. If a well-defined care plan is in place, a brief discussion at the start of each hospitalization can be beneficial to ensure that no changes have occurred. At the same time, the current team can be informed of the patient's and family's wishes.

DNR/DNI orders are typically rescinded and then need to be reinstituted when a patient goes into surgery, since surgery and anesthesia increase the chance that a patient may require some type of "resuscitation." Some institutions are now recommending an approach called "required reconsideration" prior to surgery to help clarify the situation. According to this policy, the anesthesiologist and surgeon will meet with the patient/family and attending physician to discuss the goal(s) of the DNR order and how to incorporate it into the overall surgical plan.

DNR/DNI orders may be used at home and may therefore stay in effect for longer periods (60–90 days). However, this regulation varies among states, so providers should become familiar with their state regulations and forms. In some states, an outpatient form, such as the POLST (Physician Orders for Life-Sustaining Treatment) or MOLST (Medical Orders for Life-Sustaining Treatment), may be helpful to communicate out-of-hospital goals of care. In such a case, provide copies of the orders to the home care agency involved, as well as to local emergency departments, law enforcement, and emergency responders, as appropriate.

Follow-up

- DNR/DNI may be time limited and may require renewal (eg, every 3–5 days for inpatient orders or when the patient changes service). Be aware of various hospital policies and state and local laws and regulations.
- DNR/DNI orders can be rescinded at any time.

Pearls and Pitfalls

- A delay in initiating discussions about the overall goals and possible resuscitation for a patient with a life-limiting condition is the major obstacle to having a clear plan in place. Ideally, this conversation occurs at admission and not during a crisis.
- Clearly and concisely document the plan.

Bibliography

Berlinger N, Jennings B, Wolf SM. *The Hastings Center Guidelines for Decisions on Life-Sustaining Treatment and Care Near the End of Life.* 2nd ed. New York, NY: Oxford University Press; 2013

Clark JD, Dudzinski DM; The culture of dysthanasia: attempting CPR in terminally ill children. *Pediatrics.* 2013;131(3):572–580

Fallat ME, Deshpande JK; American Academy of Pediatrics Section on Surgery, Section on Anesthesia and Pain Medicine, and Committee on Bioethics. Do-not-resuscitate orders for pediatric patients who require anesthesia and surgery. *Pediatrics.* 2004;114(6):1686–1692

National POLST Paradigm. Physicians Orders for Life-Sustaining Treatment. www.polst.org. Accessed January 30, 2017

Sanderson A, Zurakowski D, Wolfe J. Clinician perspectives regarding the do-not-resuscitate order. *JAMA Pediatr.* 2013;167(10):954–958

Informed Consent, Assent, and Confidentiality

Introduction

Obtaining informed consent from a competent patient younger than 18 years of age is the practical application of respect for a patient's autonomy. Informed consent has limited application in pediatrics, because only patients who have appropriate decisional capacity and legal empowerment can give their informed consent to receive medical care. In all other situations, parents or surrogates provide informed permission, not consent. There are exceptions to obtaining consent or permission, including emergencies, specific disease states, and surrogate decision-making when a patient lacks decisional capacity. When developmentally appropriate, also obtain informed assent, an affirmative action of agreement to receive treatment, from an older child or adolescent.

Informed consent represents a voluntary process and not simply a document. Rather than mere disclosure, it involves communicating, in language the patient or surrogate can understand, the various risks and benefits of a course of treatment, including any alternative therapies. While this does not mean discussing every imaginable outcome, it does require conveying the information that a reasonable person would want and need to make a wise decision.

Consent may be obtained verbally, implied from the cooperation of the parent, or documented and signed on a form that must be easily understood by patients and families. Use written consent for invasive procedures or if the patient will be sedated. Employ developmentally appropriate language and concepts to obtain assent from older children. When needed, use professional interpreters trained in health care language. Have the patient or parent "teach back" the information to confirm comprehension.

Disputes

Sometimes there will be disagreements during the informed consent process. The United States Supreme Court, in *Troxel v Granville,* has "recognized the fundamental right of parents to make decisions concerning the care, custody, and control of their children." However, there are limits to this parental authority. Per American Academy of Pediatrics policy, "Although physicians should seek parental permission in most situations, they must focus on the goal of providing appropriate care and be prepared to seek legal intervention when parental refusal places the patient at clear and substantial risk." In addition, to protect the child, the law requires that physicians, nurses, and other medical personnel be mandatory reporters of neglect and abuse.

Harm Threshold

Relying solely on their own judgment about what is in the best interest of the child can lead medical personnel to offer opinions and recommendations that fail to fully consider the family's needs. In addition, there is a threshold of harm below which society generally does not intervene and overrule parents. For example, while it is not in the best interest of a child to be driven through a blizzard so the parent can buy cigarettes, it would be legally imprudent and procedurally impractical for society to intervene. This harm threshold is dependent on the risk of harm (probability), the exposure (severity of the injury), and the immediacy of the danger. This subjective threshold of what constitutes serious harm varies significantly among jurisdictions. Some judges are activists, while others are more deferential to familial authority, setting a threshold that "No reasonable parent would decline treatment." In addition, accommodating cultural and religious diversity is an endorsed virtue, within limits. There will be situations where parents may legally act against medical advice. Thorough and accurate documentation is essential in all such circumstances.

Counseling, mediation, and obtaining a second opinion are the preferred first-line methods for dealing with conflict, rather than embarking on legal intervention. Social workers, ethics committees, and other consultants (eg, child protection and palliative care consultants) are resources in these situations. If those options fail and the medical personnel want to overrule the parent, there are due process requirements that typically involve petitioning a court and alerting the state Child Protective Services agency. The local expert in child abuse, hospital security personnel, hospital attorney, and social workers may have experience with this process. If the child is in imminent danger, which is a combination of probability, timing, and severity of a potential harm, law enforcement agents may take immediate custody of the child.

Custody

Family and guardianship laws vary by state and local jurisdiction. With the usual joint custody, either parent may have the authority to give permission for medical care to be administered. Sometimes after a divorce, the authority to give permission may be specifically granted to just one parent, even if the other continues to have visitation rights. A noncustodial parent may still have a right to disclosure of medical information. Clarify the social situation if possible, particularly before invasive medical procedures. A grandmother may provide most of the day-to-day care of the child, without having legal guardianship. However, if she brings the child to the emergency department for a nonurgent issue, her permission, in the absence of a written proxy from the true guardian, is not enough to permit an examination and administration of simple treatment. Invasive procedures, however, warrant efforts to obtain formal consent from the true legal parent and guardian. When the patient is in imminent danger, the appropriate action is to protect the child's health.

Consent Obtained Directly From a Minor

There are many exceptions that modify the general principles outlined earlier and permit a minor to give consent. These include

- Declaration of emancipation, which is defined by each state. This gives minors the decision-making power and capacity afforded to adults. Examples usually include being married or serving in the military.
- Consent carve-outs, which again vary state by state. The minor is not emancipated, but in specific medical situations, parental consent is not needed. Examples may include treatment for sexually transmitted infections, substance use, and mental health issues.
- Mature minor clause, which exists in a minority of states, with many differences among the definitions. Some permit all adolescents to give consent, some allow this only if the parents are unavailable, and some permit this for all adolescents who are *capable of giving informed consent*.

Since family law, guardianship law, child protection law, mental health law, and the law of medical practice vary among jurisdictions, knowledgeable local lawyers or hospital counsel can provide the necessary guidance.

Exceptions Based on Other Conditions

A minor has the authority to give informed consent for medical care for certain disorders. Diagnosis and treatment of sexually transmitted infections is almost always allowed on the sole basis of the minor's consent, although some states set a minimum age for this. HIV testing is also permitted in many states. Regulations and laws pertaining to contraception, abortion, and prenatal care are more varied. The Guttmacher Institute has an online table that is updated monthly (see the Bibliography at the end of this chapter). In some localities, a minor may give consent for drug and alcohol treatment and for outpatient mental health services.

Confidentiality and Parental Notification

Confidentiality requirements also vary by jurisdiction, status of the minor, and the medical procedure involved. State law determines most of this, but federal law, federal funding rules, and clinic policies may further regulate confidentiality. Therefore, be explicit when making promises of confidentiality. Inform the adolescent that there are situations, such as suicidal or homicidal ideation or abuse, in which the physician is required by law to take action. In addition, billing statements and medical records made available to the parent are potential leaks of information that can compromise any promised confidentiality, but there are many instances in which this may increase the risk of harm to the minor. It is crucial that the pediatrician take these considerations into account when planning care and support for the adolescent.

Bibliography

Coleman DL, Rosoff PM. The legal authority of mature minors to consent to general medical treatment. *Pediatrics*. 2013;131(4):786–793

Groselj U. The concepts of assent and parental permission in pediatrics. *World J Pediatr*. 2014;10(1):89

Guttmacher Institute. An overview of minors' consent law. https://www.guttmacher.org/state-policy/explore/overview-minors-consent-law. Accessed January 31, 2017

Hein IM, De Vries MC, Troost PW, Meynen G, Van Goudoever JB, Lindauer RJL. Informed consent instead of assent is appropriate in children from the age of twelve: policy implications of new findings on children's competence to consent to clinical research. *BMC Med Ethics*. 2015;16(1):76

Katz AL, Webb SA, American Academy of Pediatrics Committee on Bioethics. Technical report: informed consent in decision-making in pediatric practice. *Pediatrics*. 2016;138(2):e20161485

American Academy of Pediatrics Committee on Bioethics. Policy statement: informed consent in decision-making in pediatric practice. *Pediatrics*. 2016;138(2):e20161484

Gastroenterology

Gallbladder Disease

Introduction

Gallbladder disease in children can include cholelithiasis (gallstones), choledocholithiasis (stones in the common bile duct), calculous or acalculous cholecystitis (inflamed gallbladder with or without stones), and hydrops of the gallbladder (acute distention without inflammation). Historically, gallstones occurred in less than 1% of children, but the incidence rate may be increasing because of increasing rates of obesity and the diagnosis of asymptomatic gallstones via ultrasonography (US). Patients with risk factors have a higher incidence of gallbladder disease, with a prevalence of 40% among adolescents with sickle cell disease. In up to 80% of patients, gallstones are asymptomatic, although pancreatitis can occur in 5% to 10%.

Historically, up to 50% of the cases of cholecystitis in children were acalculous and developed from biliary dyskinesia or acquired biliary stasis secondary to compression of the cystic duct by edema, lymph node, or congenital malformation. Recently, more cases have occurred secondary to gallstone disease.

Hydrops of the gallbladder occurs in up to 20% of children with Kawasaki disease, as well as in patients with other infections or inflammatory conditions.

Clinical Presentation

The presentation of biliary tract disease is summarized in Table 36-1.

History

A patient with gallbladder inflammation, distention, or biliary colic from gallstones presents with complaints of nausea, vomiting, anorexia, and abdominal pain. The biliary colic may be described as a constant right upper quadrant pain that radiates to the right shoulder. There may be a history of previous episodes of cholecystitis. An older child or adolescent may describe the pain as postprandial, especially if the meal eaten was fatty. The patient may have light-colored stools and dark urine, which raises a suspicion for obstructive jaundice. The presentation of hydrops is similar to that of cholecystitis.

Inquire about the following predisposing risk factors: hemolytic disease, obesity, family history of gallstones, Native American descent, artificial heart valve, pregnancy, recent delivery, cystic fibrosis, bowel resection, ileal disease, Down syndrome, bronchopulmonary dysplasia, and recent total parenteral nutrition (TPN), as well as ceftriaxone, cyclosporine, or furosemide use.

Table 36-1. Presentation of Biliary Tract Diseases	
Diagnosis	**Clinical Features**
Acalculous cholecystitis	Fever and pain Leukocytosis with normal LFT results US: thickened gallbladder wall with no gallstones
Asymptomatic gallstones	No pain, nausea, or vomiting Incidental finding at US
Calculous cholecystitis	Fever and pain Leukocytosis with normal LFT results US: gallstones in the gallbladder
Cholangitis	Charcot triad: fever, jaundice, right upper quadrant pain May have acholic stools and dark urine (in infants) Leukocytosis
Choledocholithiasis	Jaundice ($\uparrow$ direct bilirubin level) and pain US: no gallstones in the gallbladder, but stones may be present in the common bile duct $\uparrow$ Alkaline phosphatase and gamma-glutamyl transferase levels
Hydrops	Normal gallbladder wall but dilated lumen
Pancreatitis	Pain may radiate to the patient's back $\uparrow$ Amylase and lipase levels

Abbreviations: LFT, liver function test; US, ultrasonography.

Acalculous cholecystitis risk factors include prolonged fasting, infective endocarditis, TPN, opiate use, and infection (streptococcal and gram-negative sepsis, leptospirosis, Rocky Mountain spotted fever, typhoid fever, ascariasis, and *Giardia lamblia* infection). Other parasitic, candidal, and viral infections can cause acalculous cholecystitis in an immunocompromised host.

Symptoms of complications of gallstones may include pain that radiates to the patient's back in pancreatitis, fever and malaise in cholecystitis, or fever and jaundice in cholangitis.

Physical Examination

In calculous or acalculous cholecystitis, there will be right upper quadrant abdominal pain with a positive Murphy sign (pain during inspiration while palpating the right upper quadrant). The gallbladder may be palpable. Hepatomegaly is uncommon in primary gall bladder disease but may be present if there has been longstanding obstructive cholestasis causing cirrhosis. Jaundice and scleral icterus occur when a gallstone is obstructing the common bile duct. With bacterial cholangitis or cholecystitis, the patient has fever, tachycardia, and tachypnea. Perforation of the gallbladder appears with peritoneal signs at presentation, such as abdominal guarding, rebound tenderness, and a firm or distended abdomen.

Laboratory Workup

If gallbladder disease is suspected, obtain a complete blood cell count with differential, liver function panel with alkaline phosphatase level, amylase level, and lipase level, and, if the patient is febrile, a blood culture.

Radiology Examinations

US examination is the preferred initial imaging study for gallbladder disease, with a sensitivity of up to 96% for cholelithiasis and 81% for cholecystitis. Order abdominal US to look for stones, sludge, or a thickened gallbladder. The patient should have no intake by mouth (nil per os, or NPO) for at least 4 hours before the study. The US findings may be normal if the stone is in the common bile duct or if the patient has gallbladder dyskinesia.

Cholescintigraphy is more sensitive for cholecystitis (96%) but is less readily available and exposes the patient to radiation. Order this test when there are no gallstones in the gallbladder at US but there is still concern for extrahepatic biliary disease or obstruction of the common bile duct (good hepatic uptake but delayed or no gallbladder filling). If the findings are equivocal, order computed tomography or magnetic resonance (MR) imaging.

If a patient has signs of cholecystitis or cholangitis but no stones in the gallbladder at US, order MR cholangiopancreatography (MRCP), which can demonstrate stones in the common bile duct and allow assessment of the biliary tree anatomy for congenital malformations. Request endoscopic retrograde cholangiopancreatography (ERCP) for therapeutic removal of an obstructive stone during imaging.

Differential Diagnosis

The differential diagnosis of right upper quadrant pain is presented in Table 36-2.

Treatment

Acute Cholecystitis

The patient should have NPO. Provide maintenance intravenous hydration with 5% dextrose in one-half normal saline + 20 mEq (20 mmol) KCl and correct any additional electrolyte or fluid deficit. Although cholecystitis is typically an inflammatory disease, secondary infection can occur, so empirical antibiotic administration is usually indicated. Administer antibiotic coverage for gram-negative bacilli and anaerobes, with ampicillin/sulbactam (200 mg/kg/d, divided into doses administered every 6 hours; maximum,

Table 36-2. Differential Diagnosis of Right Upper Quadrant Pain

Diagnosis	Clinical Features
Appendicitis	Atypical location of the appendix (especially in pregnancy)
Fitz-Hugh-Curtis syndrome	Sexually active female subject ↑ CRP level/ESR Possible vaginal symptoms or (+) culture findings
Gastroenteritis	Patient may also have diarrhea
Hepatitis	↑ ALT and AST levels (SGPT and SGOT levels)
Musculoskeletal pain	Afebrile May have point tenderness Normal LFT results, ESR, US findings
Peptic ulcer disease	(+) Guaiac stool Pain relieved by eating meals or taking antacids or H_2 blockers
Pleural effusion	↓ Breath sounds (+) Chest radiographic findings
Pneumonia	↓ Breath sounds or rales (+) Chest radiographic findings
Pancreatitis	↑ Amylase and lipase levels

Abbreviations: ALT, alanine transaminase; AST, aspartate transaminase; CRP, C-reactive protein; ESR, erythrocyte sedimentation rate; H_2, histamine 2; LFT, liver function test; SGOT, serum glutamic oxaloacetic transaminase; SGPT, serum glutamic pyruvic transaminase; US, ultrasonography; +, positive finding.

8 g ampicillin/d), piperacillin/tazobactam (300 mg/kg/d, divided into doses administered every 8 hours; maximum, 16 g piperacillin/d), or the combination of ceftriaxone (50–75 mg/kg/d, divided into doses administered every 12–24 hours; 4-g/d maximum) *and* metronidazole (30 mg/kg/d, divided into doses administered every 6 hours; 4-g/d maximum).

Analgesia is a priority. Start with a nonsteroidal anti-inflammatory drug, such as ketorolac (0.5 mg/kg administered every 6 hours for 5 days; 120-mg/d maximum), which may prevent progression of the cholecystitis. However, the patient may require an opiate, such as morphine sulfate (0.05–0.10 mg/kg per dose administered every 2–4 hours; maximum of 2 mg per dose for infants, 4–8 mg per dose for children, and 15 mg per dose for adolescents).

Consult with a surgeon, because acute cholecystectomy may be necessary if supportive care does not relieve the pain or if there are signs of peritonitis, sepsis, or worsening distress. Otherwise, if the patient improves quickly, elective surgery (preferably laparoscopic cholecystectomy) is indicated 6 to 12 weeks after resolution of the symptoms. However, instruct the patient to return to the hospital immediately to undergo an urgent cholecystectomy if the symptoms of cholecystitis recur.

Cholelithiasis

Manage asymptomatic cholelithiasis on an outpatient basis, with a follow-up US study performed in 6 months. However, if the patient has a hemolytic disease, consult with a surgeon to plan a cholecystectomy.

Choledocholithiasis

In addition to supportive care, consult a gastroenterologist and surgeon. Arrange for the patient to undergo MRCP or ERCP. However, if cholecystectomy is planned, cholangiography is usually also performed to confirm the presence or absence of an obstructing stone.

Acalculous Cholecystitis

Treat the underlying condition, such as by discontinuing the implicated medication or administering antibiotics for the inciting infection.

Hydrops of the Gallbladder

This is usually self-limited, so no specific treatment is necessary.

Indications for Consultation

- **Gastroenterology or surgery (depending on the availability of ERCP):** Choledocholithiasis
- **Hematology or other subspecialists:** As needed for underlying disease
- **Surgery (urgent):** Cholecystitis or hydrops of the gallbladder, with perforation, empyema, or necrosis

Disposition

- **Intensive care unit transfer:** Sepsis or peritonitis
- **Discharge criteria:** Patient afebrile and maintaining adequate oral hydration and pain control

Follow-up

- **Primary care:** 1 week
- **Surgery:** 3 to 5 days (if the patient underwent cholecystectomy); 1 to 2 weeks to arrange for elective cholecystectomy in the next 2 to 3 months

Pearls and Pitfalls

- Consider cholangitis and consult a surgeon if fever and jaundice accompany cholecystitis.
- US is recommended as the primary imaging modality for disorders of the gallbladder.
- Always contemplate gallstone disease in an obese child or teen with abdominal pain.
- While nonsteroidal anti-inflammatory drugs are the first-line analgesics, opiates are not contraindicated.

Bibliography

Bennett GL. Evaluating patients with right upper quadrant pain. *Radiol Clin North Am.* 2015;53(6):1093–1130

Broderick A. Gallbladder disease. In: Kleinman RE, Goulet O, Mieli-Vergani G, Sanderson IR, eds. *Walker's Pediatric Gastrointestinal Disease.* 5th ed. Hamilton, Ontario, Canada: BC Decker; 2008:1173–1182

Kurbegov AC. Pediatric biliary disease. In: Zaoutis LB, Chiang VW, eds. *Comprehensive Pediatric Hospital Medicine.* 1st ed. Philadelphia, PA: Mosby Elsevier; 2007:605–611

Murphy PB, Vogt KN, Winick-Ng J, McClure JA, Welk B, Jones SA. The increasing incidence of gallbladder disease in children: a 20 year perspective. *J Pediatr Surg.* May;51(5):748–752

Svensson J, Makin E. Gallstone disease in children. *Semin Pediatr Surg.* 2012;21(3):255–265

Gastroenteritis

Introduction

Gastroenteritis is an intraluminal inflammation of the gastrointestinal (GI) tract that involves any region from the stomach to the colon. Infectious gastroenteritis may be caused by bacteria, viruses, parasites, or preformed toxins produced by bacteria. Viral causes are the most common.

Clinical Presentation

History

Complete a thorough history to help determine the possible etiology, assess the severity of dehydration, and rule out other serious illnesses that can appear with vomiting and/or diarrhea at presentation. Determine the character of the vomiting and/or diarrhea, including the number of episodes and the presence of bile or blood in the vomitus or blood or mucus in the stools. Ask about fever, abdominal pain, other illnesses, rotavirus vaccine status, injuries, medications, recent contact with sick persons, contact with animals (specifically farm animals or reptiles), travel history, and potential exposure to contaminated food or water. In addition, assess the hydration status and severity of the illness and determine recent oral intake, urine output, acute weight loss (if known), and any change in mental status.

Viral Gastroenteritis

Symptoms of viral gastroenteritis typically manifest 2 to 4 days after exposure, usually beginning with vomiting, followed by frequent loose or watery diarrhea. However, diarrhea may be the only symptom. Depending on the virus, fever may or may not be present, and complete resolution of symptoms typically occurs within 7 days. Some viral infections, such as enteric adenovirus, can be more prolonged, lasting up to 7 to 10 days.

Bacterial Gastroenteritis

Signs and symptoms typically overlap with viral gastroenteritis but may cause a more significant colitis associated with diarrhea with gross blood and/or mucus, fever, myalgia, abdominal pain, and tenesmus.

Extraintestinal manifestations may accompany specific bacterial infections, such as *Campylobacter* (erythema nodosum, glomerulonephritis, reactive arthritis), *Escherichia coli* (hemolytic uremic syndrome [HUS]), *Salmonella* (erythema nodosum, reactive arthritis), *Shigella* (encephalopathy, glomerulonephritis, reactive arthritis, Reiter syndrome, seizures), and *Yersinia* (erythema nodosum, glomerulonephritis, hemolytic anemia, reactive arthritis) infections.

Nontyphoidal *Salmonella*–associated gastroenteritis typically causes fever and watery diarrhea and may result in a more severe inflammatory colitis. The illness may also be complicated by bacteremia, especially in a patient who is immunocompromised or younger than 1 year. Ask about exposure to potential sources of *Salmonella* bacteria, including reptiles and contaminated food products, such as eggs and milk products.

Salmonella typhi and *Salmonella paratyphi* are usually acquired outside the United States and cause a systemic infection, with remitting fever that becomes sustained. Other complaints include abdominal pain and constitutional symptoms, such as headache, malaise, anorexia, and lethargy. The patient may progress to having a blanching, macular rash on the trunk and an altered mental status. *S typhi* can also cause intestinal perforation that appears as peritonitis or septic shock at presentation, although this is rare in a child.

Shigella infection causes symptoms that range from mild, watery stools to dysentery. Certain species of the bacteria may also produce the Shiga toxin that causes endothelial damage and HUS, as well as seizures. *Shigella* bacteria are more resistant to acid when compared with other bacteria and can transmit disease through the stomach. Since only 10 to 100 organisms may cause disease, *Shigella* infection is highly contagious.

Gastroenteritis caused by *Yersinia* infection is relatively uncommon in the United States. A known risk factor is eating chitterlings (pig intestines). In a younger child, *Yersinia* infection may present as a mild, self-limited disease, whereas an older patient may have more prominent symptoms, including abdominal pain and tenderness caused by mesenteric adenitis.

Campylobacter-associated infection is characterized by fever, chills, crampy abdominal pain, and bloody, mucoid diarrhea. It can also cause frank rectal bleeding. The source of *Campylobacter* infection is primarily food, such as poultry and eggs.

E coli, which has several identified classes, can cause the full spectrum of diarrheal illness. The enterohemorrhagic *E coli* O157:H7 organism, in particular, produces the Shiga toxin that may cause HUS. Other classes of the bacteria include enterotoxigenic *E coli,* which causes watery diarrhea in developing countries, and enteroinvasive *E coli,* which typically manifests in foodborne outbreaks of dysentery due to undercooked ground beef, raw milk, and, occasionally, raw vegetables. The enteropathogenic form of the bacteria causes acute and chronic diarrhea in infants, and the enteroaggregative form causes acute and chronic watery diarrhea.

Clostridium difficile is found in cases of antibiotic-associated diarrhea, particularly after treatment with β-lactam antibiotics and clindamycin. As with other bacterial sources of diarrhea, symptoms can range from mild diarrhea to life-threatening enterocolitis.

Parasitic Gastroenteritis

Protozoan gastroenteritis may appear as watery diarrhea at presentation but can also cause a protracted diarrhea that lasts 2 to 4 weeks. *Giardia intestinalis (*formerly *Giardia lamblia* and *Giardia duodenalis)* is the leading cause of waterborne disease in the United States. Typical infections are characterized by explosive, foul-smelling, watery diarrhea, with abdominal cramps and bloating.

Physical Examination

The priority at physical examination is accurate assessment of the patient's hydration status. Categorize the dehydration status as minimal (<3% of body weight), moderate (3%–9% of body weight), or severe (>9% of body weight), which will then guide rehydration protocols. The standard of reference for this calculation is based on the patient's acute weight change; however, providers often do not have this information. Clinical scoring systems have been validated that factor in some combination of the patient's general appearance, mental status, subjective thirst level, heart rate, pulse rate and quality, respiratory effort, potentially sunken eyes, tear production, mucous membrane moistness, skin turgor, capillary refill, mottled appearance of extremities, and urine output. Two examples include the Gorelick Dehydration Score (Table 37-1) and the Clinical Dehydration Scale (Table 37-2). As noted earlier, extraintestinal manifestations noted at physical examination may provide clues to the etiology of infection.

Table 37-1: Gorelick Dehydration Score	
Poor overall appearance[a] Capillary refill time >2 s[a] Absent tears[a] Dry mucous membranes[a]	4-Point scale: 2/4 = Moderate dehydration 3/4 = Severe dehydration
Sunken eyes Abnormal respirations Abnormal radial pulse Tachycardia (>150/min for 1 mo to 5 y of age) Decreased skin elasticity Decreased urine output	10-Point scale: <3 = None/mild dehydration 3–6 = Moderate dehydration ≥7 = Severe dehydration

[a] Use these criteria for a 4-point scale; use all of the criteria for a 10-point scale.
Data from Gorelick MH, Shaw KN, Murphy KO. Validity and reliability of clinical signs in the diagnosis of dehydration in children. *Pediatrics*. 1997;99(5):E6.

Table 37-2: Clinical Dehydration Scale[a]

	Score of 0	Score of 1	Score of 2
Appearance	Normal	Patient thirsty, restless, or lethargic but irritable when assessed	Patient drowsy, limp, cold, or sweaty Patient comatose or not
Eyes	Normal	Slightly sunken	Very sunken
Mucous membranes	Moist	Sticky	Dry
Tears	Tears	Decreased tears	No tears

[a] Score interpretation: 0, no dehydration; 1–3, some dehydration; 5–8, moderate dehydration.

From Tam RK, Wong H, Plint A, Lepage N, Filler G. Comparison of clinical and biochemical markers of dehydration with the clinical dehydration scale in children: a case comparison trial. *BMC Pediatr.* 2014;14:149.

Laboratory Workup

According to guidelines from the U.S. Centers for Disease Control and Prevention and the American Academy of Pediatrics, laboratory testing for uncomplicated acute gastroenteritis with mild or moderate dehydration is not needed. Laboratory evaluation is indicated for patients who exhibit severe dehydration and may have electrolyte imbalances. If there is concern for certain extraintestinal manifestations, such as HUS, obtain a complete blood cell count (CBC), peripheral blood smear, electrolyte levels, and blood urea nitrogen (BUN) and creatinine levels. Perform a CBC and blood culture if there is concern for a serious bacterial illness. If there is suspicion for a urinary tract infection in an infant, perform a catheterized urine culture.

If the patient has dysentery (blood, pus, and mucus in the stools), send stool samples for blood analysis, leukocyte evaluation, and culture. Routine stool cultures will typically include testing for *Shigella*, *Salmonella*, *Campylobacter*, and *Yersinia* bacteria, but if the stools are bloody, specifically order testing for *E coli* O157:H7. Evaluation for *C difficile* toxin is indicated if the patient has severe, persistent diarrhea or predisposing conditions, such as receipt of recent or multiple courses of antibiotics; has an underlying GI disorder or immunodeficiency; or has recently been hospitalized. However, do not routinely test a patient younger than 1 year because false-positive *C difficile* results are frequent. Also, there is no need to test for a cure because the toxin can remain after symptoms resolve. Send a stool sample for ova and parasite evaluation if the patient has a pertinent travel history, has had contact with untreated water, or has experienced prolonged GI symptoms.

Differential Diagnosis

While the patient will most often have viral gastroenteritis, the priority is to ensure that there is not a serious or even life-threatening alternative diagnosis (Table 37-3). This is particularly true if the patient presents with unopposed vomiting (no diarrhea), a toxic appearance, or a widened pulse pressure or if the patient required excessive fluid resuscitation. Similarly, if the patient has an altered mental status that does not respond to fluid intake, consider toxic ingestion, encephalitis, intussusception, or increased intracranial pressure as a potential cause.

Table 37-3. Differential Diagnosis of Gastroenteritis	
Diagnosis	**Clinical Features**
Adrenal insufficiency	Unopposed vomiting Weakness, fatigue, anorexia Previous steroid exposure
Appendicitis	Abdominal pain that precedes vomiting Minimal or no diarrhea Signs of acute abdomen (abdominal guarding, rebound)
Diabetic ketoacidosis	History of weight loss/polydipsia/polyuria but no diarrhea Deep (Kussmaul) breathing Mental status change out of proportion to the vomiting frequency
Increased intracranial pressure	History of trauma or hydrocephalus Headache, cranial nerve abnormalities Unopposed vomiting May have Cushing triad ($\downarrow$ pulse with $\uparrow$ blood pressure)
Inflammatory bowel disease	Chronic symptoms and poor overall growth Extraintestinal symptoms: rash, arthritis, uveitis, microcytic anemia
Poisoning, toxic ingestion Inborn errors of metabolism	Acute onset Mental status change out of proportion to the vomiting frequency
Intussusception	Sudden onset of severe, crampy pain and inconsolability Pain associated with drawing up of legs Patient may have altered mental status Guaiac (+) or "currant jelly" stools (late finding)
Malabsorption syndromes (celiac disease)	Chronic diarrhea and weight loss Diet-related onset
Myocarditis	Usually no diarrhea Tachycardia out of proportion to dehydration level Gallop cardiac rhythm
Peritonitis	Fever (may be high) Worsening abdominal pain Rebound and guarding at abdominal examination
Small-bowel obstruction	Persistent, bilious vomiting Abdominal distention History of previous abdominal surgery
Urinary tract infection	Dysuria, urgency, frequency (+) Urinalysis

"+" indicates a positive finding.

Treatment

Oral rehydration therapy (ORT) is the mainstay of management for mild and moderate dehydration. Intravenous (IV) fluids, such as normal saline or lactated Ringer solution, are only indicated for a patient who is severely dehydrated or has an underlying condition that can be exacerbated by dehydration, such as a metabolic disorder. Even patients who are vomiting will tolerate ORT if administered correctly. Deliver ORT by having the patient drink small, frequent amounts of an oral rehydration solution (ORS) to achieve a 3- to 4-hour fluid goal. For example, give the patient 5 to 10 mL every 5 minutes. For an infant or young child, the parents may accomplish this by using a syringe or spoon to administer the liquid, if the child refuses a bottle or cup. If the patient vomits, pause for 10 to 20 minutes and start again. Enteral hydration is as effective as IV hydration and has many advantages, such as reduced cost, fewer complications, and faster recovery. For a patient with mild to moderate dehydration who does not tolerate ORT, continues to refuse it, or does not have a caregiver or staff member available to administer it, fluids can be administered via a nasogastric tube or IV line. Hydration via a nasogastric tube is an effective alternative, with fewer complications than a peripheral IV line. To use this method, calculate the total 4-hour fluid goal and administer the ORS at a tolerated rate over 4 hours.

An ORS is a glucose electrolyte solution that has an appropriate balance of sodium (45–90 mEq [45–90 mmol]) and glucose (2%) to promote water absorption through the sodium-glucose transporter in cells lining the small intestine. Fluids high in glucose content and low in sodium, such as sports drinks, are ineffective rehydration solutions because of the creation of an osmotic load that causes more fluid secretion.

Mild or No Dehydration

For mild dehydration, replace the fluid deficit with 50 mL/kg of an ORS over 3 to 4 hours. Replace ongoing fluid losses on the basis of the patient's weight. For example, give the patient an extra 10 mL/kg of ORS for each stool passed or for each emesis. If the patient is not dehydrated, replace ongoing losses and encourage continued fluid intake and an age-appropriate diet. For a patient who is not dehydrated, an ORS will likely taste too salty.

Moderate Dehydration

If the patient has moderate dehydration, replace the fluid deficit with 75 to 100 mL/kg of an ORS over 3 to 4 hours. Afterward, encourage continued fluid intake to maintain hydration and an age-appropriate diet and continue appropriate replacement of fluid losses, as done for mild dehydration.

Severe Dehydration

Correct severe dehydration with 1 to 3 20-mL/kg IV boluses of an isotonic fluid, either normal saline or lactated Ringer solution, until the patient no longer has orthostatic vital sign changes and/or has adequate urine output (1 mL/kg/h), with improved peripheral perfusion and mental status. Unless the patient has renal disease, sickle cell disease, or diabetes, the urine output is a good gauge as to whether subsequent boluses are needed. Once the patient is stabilized and has appropriate mental status, begin ORT. If the patient does not void after 3 fluid boluses, insert a bladder catheter and obtain electrolyte, BUN, and creatinine levels. Poor perfusion despite multiple boluses occurs with distributive shock secondary to sepsis. Treat with broad-spectrum antibiotics and vasopressors and transfer the patient to an intensive care unit (ICU) setting.

Frequent reassessments, including input and output (stool and urine assessment with specific gravity), vital signs, and physical examination, are crucial for both tracking ongoing fluid losses and diagnosing an underlying illness other than a viral gastroenteritis. Be particularly suspicious of an alternative diagnosis if the patient has an inadequate response to fluid administration, persistent inability to tolerate oral intake, severe abdominal pain, or persistent altered mental status.

Diet

There is no indication for gut rest. As soon as oral intake can be tolerated, resume an unrestricted diet, including complex carbohydrates, lean meat, fruits, vegetables, milk products, or human milk and/or infant formula. If the patient has persistent nausea and/or vomiting that interferes with resuming oral intake, administer a dose of oral (sublingually) or IV ondansetron (0.05–0.10 mg/kg every 6 hours; 4-mg maximum). Do not use ondansetron if there is any concern about a surgical abdomen (acute abdomen that will likely require surgical intervention) or other underlying medical problems, such as long QT syndrome.

Probiotics

Probiotics are a safe adjunctive therapy that can reduce the duration of diarrhea by 1 day, as well as the risk of diarrhea lasting 4 or more days. If the patient has diarrhea, administer probiotics immediately and treat for 5 to 7 days. Use either *Lactobacillus GG* (daily dose of $\geq 10^{10}$ colony-forming units) or *Saccharomyces boulardii* (250 mg to 750 mg per day).

Antibiotics

The antibiotic treatment of bacterial gastroenteritis is summarized in Table 37-4.

Table 37-4. Treatment of Bacterial Gastroenteritis	
Indications	**Antibiotics**
***Salmonella* (nontyphoidal) infection**	

Unproven benefit
Risk factors for an invasive infection include
  Age <3 mo
  Chronic GI disease
  Hemoglobinopathy
  Malignancy
  HIV infection
  Immunosuppressive illnesses or therapies
See the AAP *Red Book* for additional treatment
  issues
	In areas with susceptible strains, treat with
	TMP-SMX (20 mg/kg/d, divided into doses administered every 6–8 h; 640-mg/d maximum) for 3–7 d
	
	In areas of increased resistance, treat with
	Azithromycin (12 mg/kg/d, 500-mg/d maximum) for 3–5 d *or*
	Ciprofloxacin (20–30 mg/kg/d, divided into doses administered every 12 h; 800-mg/d maximum) for 3–5 d
	
	In a patient with localized invasive disease or bacteremia associated with immunosuppression, treat with
	Ceftriaxone (50 mg/kg/d, 4-g/d maximum) for 3–7 d

***Shigella* infection**	

Culture-positive *Shigella* bacteria
High suspicion for *Shigella* bacteria while awaiting
  culture results
Severe disease or dysentery
Underlying immunosuppressive disorder
Treat symptomatic family members and close
  contacts, as well
	For ampicillin and TMP-SMX–resistant or unknown strains (dosing as above), treat with
	Azithromycin (3 d) *or*
	Ciprofloxacin (3 d) *or*
	Ceftriaxone (2–5 d)

***Campylobacter* infection**	

Treatment can shorten the duration of illness and
  prevent relapse when administered early during
  infection
	Treat with
	Azithromycin (10 mg/kg/d, 500-mg/d maximum) for 3 d *or*
	Erythromycin (40 mg/kg/d, divided into doses administered every 6 h; 2-g/d maximum) for 5 d

***Escherichia coli* infection**	

Not indicated for O157:H7 enteritis or a clinical or
  epidemiologic picture strongly suggestive of Shiga
  toxin–producing *E coli* infection
	No antibiotics

***Clostridium difficile* infection**	
Treat if the patient is symptomatic Discontinue the offending antibiotic	*Treat with* Metronidazole (30 mg/kg/d PO, divided into doses administered every 6 h; 2-g/d maximum) for 10 d *or* Vancomycin (40 mg/kg/d PO, divided into doses administered every 6 h; 2-g/d maximum) for 10 d

Abbreviations: AAP, American Academy of Pediatrics; GI, gastrointestinal; PO, per os (oral administration); SMX, sulfamethoxazole; TMP, trimethoprim.

Use metronidazole for *Giardia* infection (15 mg/kg/d, divided into doses administered 3 times a day for 5 days; 750-mg/d maximum).

Indications for Consultation

- **Gastroenterology:** Persistent diarrhea (>14 days), significant GI bleeding, or suspected inflammatory bowel disease
- **Surgery:** Possible acute abdomen

Disposition

- **ICU transfer:** Decompensated shock, patient not responsive to fluid boluses, concern for acute adrenal insufficiency, diabetic ketoacidosis, increased intracranial pressure, or myocarditis
- **Discharge criteria:** Dehydration resolved, oral intake adequate to maintain hydration, oral antibiotics (if indicated) tolerated

Follow-up

Primary Care: 2 to 3 days

Pearls and Pitfalls

- Viral gastroenteritis typically presents with vomiting and diarrhea without blood or mucus.
- Bacterial gastroenteritis may appear as dysentery at presentation, with bloody, mucoid stools.
- Vomiting without diarrhea (unopposed vomiting) may be caused by a non-GI disease.
- The presence of diarrhea does not rule out appendicitis.
- ORT is the mainstay of management for mild to moderate dehydration.
- Enteral hydration is preferred over IV hydration in mild to moderate dehydration, and using a nasogastric tube is an effective hydration route when ORT is unsuccessful.

Bibliography

Bruzzese E, Lo Vecchio A, Guarino A. Hospital management of children with acute gastroenteritis. *Curr Opin Gastroenterol.* 2013;29(1):23–30

Freedman SB, Ali S, Oleszczuk M, Gouin S, Hartling L. Treatment of acute gastroenteritis in children: an overview of systematic reviews of interventions commonly used in developed countries. *Evid Based Child Health.* 2013;8(4):1123–1137

Freedman SB, Vandermeer B, Milne A, Hartling L; and Pediatric Emergency Research Canada Gastroenteritis Study Group. Diagnosing clinically significant dehydration in children with acute gastroenteritis using noninvasive methods: a meta-analysis. *J Pediatr.* 2015;166(4):908–916

Goldman RD, Friedman JN, Parkin PC. Validation of the clinical dehydration scale for children with acute gastroenteritis. *Pediatrics.* 2008; 122(3):545–549

Guarino A, Guandalini S, LoVecchio A. Probiotics for prevention and treatment of diarrhea. *J Clin Gastroenterol.* 2015;49(Suppl 1):S37–S45

Szajewska H, Guarino A, Hojsak I, et al. Use of probiotics for management of acute gastroenteritis: a position paper by the ESPGHAN Working Group for Probiotics and Prebiotics. *J Pediatr Gastroenterol Nutr.* 2014;58(4):531-539

Gastrointestinal Bleeding

Introduction

Gastrointestinal (GI) bleeding is a common complaint that requires prompt evaluation. The presentation and differential diagnosis are broad, with a spectrum that ranges from an occult, self-limited bleed to a severe, rapidly progressive, life-threatening hemorrhage that can originate from either the upper GI (UGI) or lower GI (LGI) tract. A systematic approach is critical, beginning with the confirmation of actual blood that originates from the GI tract, an assessment of the severity of the bleeding, and the initiation of appropriate resuscitation, if necessary. Once the patient is stabilized, the priorities are determining the exact cause and site of the bleeding (UGI vs LGI) and planning for subsequent treatment.

Clinical Presentation

History

Ask about the duration of bleeding or symptoms and the estimated amount of blood loss, measured in terms understandable to nonmedical caregivers, such as teaspoons. Document the presence of fever, lethargy, and weight loss, as well as the location, intensity, and pattern of any abdominal pain. Determine if there have been any prior episodes of bleeding or a family history of disease.

Obtain a thorough history regarding the patient's diet, medications, and possible ingestions, because certain foods and drugs can give the false appearance of blood. Any food with a red skin (beets, tomatoes, apples) or anything that contains red food coloring (candy, drinks, gelatin) can be mistaken for frank blood if vomited. Likewise, medications that contain flavoring syrups (antibiotics, certain preparations of acetaminophen) can resemble hematemesis. Spinach, blueberries, plums, grapes, and medications that contain iron or bismuth can cause melena-like stools. For a breastfeeding infant, ask if the mother's nipples are cracked or bleeding.

Inquire about a choking episode prior to the suspected bleeding. Ingested foreign bodies can lead to GI bleeding if they are sharp or caustic (button batteries) or if they become lodged in the GI tract mucosa.

Aspirin, nonsteroidal anti-inflammatory drugs (NSAIDs), and corticosteroids increase the risk of GI bleeding by directly damaging gastric mucosa. Anticoagulants (heparin, warfarin, aspirin, NSAIDs) can affect coagulation and increase the risk of mucocutaneous bleeding. In addition, some medications (doxycycline, aspirin, NSAIDs) can cause esophagitis.

UGI Bleeding

By definition, UGI bleeding originates proximal to the ligament of Treitz and can manifest hematemesis at presentation, which can be coffee ground or bright red in appearance, depending on the source, severity, and chronicity of the bleed. A slow UGI bleed may also appear with melena at presentation or, if the bleeding is brisk enough, hematochezia (bright red or dark blood that passes through the rectum). Ask about a history of lesions or active disease in the nose, mouth, pharynx, larynx, or lungs, which can lead to swallowed blood and mimic a UGI bleed. Ask about a history of prematurity and possible umbilical artery line insertion. Document symptoms of vomiting and retching (Mallory-Weiss tear) and itching and jaundice (liver disease and portal hypertension). Also inquire about a history of abdominal trauma, which can lead to duodenal injury.

LGI Bleeding

Ask about the quality, consistency, and frequency of the patient's stool. A slow LGI bleed can appear with melena at presentation but more commonly presents with hematochezia. Hard stool that is blood streaked on the outside occurs with bleeding in the rectal vault or anal canal. Bloody diarrhea suggests colitis, most often secondary to an infectious etiology, as does the presence of mucus mixed with the stool, whereas "currant jelly" stool is a classic finding of intussusception. Ask about weight loss, rash, joint pain, atopy in the family or patient, or tenesmus, which, along with a family history of chronic bleeding or GI or autoimmune disorders, can suggest inflammatory bowel disease (IBD).

Physical Examination

The patient can appear well or ill as a result of the underlying condition causing the GI bleed or as a consequence of the bleeding itself. Carefully assess the patient's vital signs (including orthostatic changes), growth parameters, general appearance, perfusion, and mental status to determine if aggressive resuscitation or urgent specialty consultation is needed.

Examine the patient's eyes for scleral icterus (indicative of liver disease) and the oral and nasal mucosa for freckles (associated with polyps) or evidence of bleeding or trauma; and examine the abdomen for distention, bowel sounds, tenderness, ascites, masses, hepatosplenomegaly, or signs of acute abdomen. Epigastric tenderness is nonspecific but may indicate peptic ulcer disease, gastritis, or esophagitis, while hepatosplenomegaly in conjunction with caput medusae is highly suggestive of portal hypertension with esophageal varices. Cutaneous hemangiomas raise the suspicion for other vascular lesions within the GI tract (upper and/or lower). Perform a careful anal and rectal examination to look for fissures, skin tags, fistulas, occult blood, impacted stool, or polyps.

Laboratory Workup

The goals of the diagnostic evaluation are to first confirm the presence of blood and then determine the source and severity of the bleed. Perform a complete blood cell count (CBC), a stool guaiac test for both UGI and LGI bleeds, and a gastric occult blood and pH test for a UGI bleed. If the bleeding is either hemodynamically significant or ongoing, repeat the CBC at least every 6 to 12 hours. If there is evidence of liver dysfunction or coagulopathy (easy bruising or a history of recurrent bleeding, liver disease, or anticoagulant use), obtain a comprehensive chemistry profile, with liver function tests and a prothrombin time (PT)/partial thromboplastin time/international normalized ratio. Also obtain a C-reactive protein level and/or erythrocyte sedimentation rate if the clinical picture suggests an inflammatory process based on findings such as weight loss, fatigue, fever, arthralgia or arthritis, purpura, or a prior history of such symptoms.

If the patient has hematochezia, testing for infectious etiology is not always indicated, but when symptoms are excessive (high fever, prolonged diarrhea, systemic symptoms), obtain stool for bacterial stool culture for common pathogens (*Salmonella*, *Shigella*, *Yersinia enterocolitica*, *Campylobacter jejuni*). If suggested by the clinical presentation, also test for *Escherichia coli* O157:H7 and *Clostridium difficile* toxin A and B. If indicated by a recent travel history to endemic areas, send stool for *Entamoeba histolytica* and *Trichuris trichiura* testing. Perform a urinalysis if the initial test results are consistent with hemolytic uremic syndrome (anemia, thrombocytopenia, evidence of hemolysis on a peripheral smear, and renal impairment). For hemodynamically significant bleeds, order a type and screen in anticipation of obtaining blood products.

Nasogastric or orogastric lavage is not routinely indicated, unless the source of a GI bleed is uncertain or the bleeding is clinically significant. If the lavage returns fresh blood, blood-tinged secretions, or coffee-ground secretions, a UGI or nasopharyngeal source of bleeding is confirmed. The lavage may have falsely negative findings if the bleeding has stopped or if the source is distal to a closed pylorus. A lavage with bilious fluid may indicate an open pylorus and/or a small-bowel obstruction. Use warm saline, because cold solutions may cause hypothermia in an infant or young child, while using water may lead to electrolyte imbalances.

Radiology Examinations

Radiologic tests, such as abdominal imaging with anteroposterior abdominal radiography (commonly referred to as "KUB"), ultrasonography (US), computed tomography (CT), UGI series with or without small-bowel follow-through, or barium enema, may be useful for locating the source of the bleeding and determining the appropriate next step in evaluation (ie, upper vs lower endoscopy) and treatment.

Perform abdominal Doppler US when there is evidence of liver disease that is suggestive of portal hypertension and may be associated with esophageal varices. Abdominal CT with intravenous contrast material, abdominal magnetic resonance imaging, or a UGI series can be used to further evaluate the patient for esophageal varices. If esophagogastroduodenoscopy (EGD) is not readily available, perform a UGI series to identify a radio-opaque foreign body and gastric and duodenal ulcers. However, defer radiographic imaging until the patient is hemodynamically stable.

If further visualization of a potential UGI bleed site is needed, EGD performed by a gastroenterologist is the next best plan of action. An EGD can help identify sites of active bleeding so that therapeutic interventions may be initiated, when indicated. Perform emergency EGD when bleeding is considered to be life-threatening. Otherwise, it is best performed in a controlled setting with anesthesia.

If an infant or younger child has an LGI bleed plus vomiting, perform KUB with either an upright or a cross-table lateral view to look for intestinal obstruction, pneumatosis intestinalis, or findings consistent with an intussusception or volvulus. If intussusception is strongly suspected, perform an air-contrast enema, which will be both diagnostic and therapeutic. A UGI series is indicated for possible volvulus. However, perform abdominal CT or US if an ischemic process is suspected in an older child. When a Meckel diverticulum is suspected, perform a Meckel scan with technetium 99m (^{99m}Tc) to identify ectopic gastric tissue seen in either the diverticulum or intestinal duplications. In select cases, capsule endoscopy, exploratory laparoscopy, or laparotomy is necessary to be able to identify the source. If the diagnosis remains uncertain, a slow bleed may be identified with a "bleeding scan" performed with ^{99m}Tc-labeled red cells, and more active bleeding may be detected with angiography.

Differential Diagnosis

The presence of hematemesis, melena, or hematochezia can help narrow the differential diagnosis when evaluated in the context of the patient's age. Hematemesis reflects bleeding proximal to the ligament of Treitz, and melena is secondary to bleeding proximal to the transverse or descending colon, with a slow intestinal transit time that allows bacteria to denature the hemoglobin. Hematochezia usually (but not always) reflects bleeding distal to the transverse colon. Table 38-1 summarizes the most common causes according to age group and location of the bleed.

Table 38-1. Most Common Causes of GI Bleeding	
UGI Bleed	**LGI Bleed**
Neonate	
Coagulopathy (vitamin K deficiency, thrombocytopenia)	Allergic colitis (allergy to cow's milk protein)
Milk protein sensitivity	Anorectal fissures
Swallowed maternal blood	Coagulopathy (vitamin K deficiency, thrombocytopenia)
Vascular malformations	Necrotizing enterocolitis
	Swallowed maternal blood
	Vascular malformation
Patient 1 mo to 2 y of age	
Esophageal varices	Anorectal fissures
Esophagitis	Infectious colitis
Gastritis	Allergic colitis (allergy to cow's milk protein)
Ingestion (toxin, foreign body)	Intussusception
Stress gastritis or ulcer	Meckel diverticulum
Vascular malformation	Polyps
	Lymphonodular hyperplasia
	Vascular malformations
Patient 2–5 y of age	
Esophageal varices	Anorectal fissure
Esophagitis	Henoch-Schönlein purpura
Gastritis	Infectious colitis
Ingestion (toxin, foreign body)	Inflammatory bowel disease
Mallory-Weiss tear	Intussusception
Reflux esophagitis	Lymphonodular hyperplasia
Stress ulcer	Meckel diverticulum
Vascular malformation	Peptic ulcer disease
	Polyps
	Vascular lesions
Older child or adolescent	
Esophageal varices	Henoch-Schönlein purpura
Gastritis	Infectious colitis
IBD	IBD
Mallory-Weiss tear	Meckel diverticulum
Reflux esophagitis	Peptic ulcer disease
Ulcer	Polyps
Vascular malformation	Vascular lesion

Abbreviations: GI, gastrointestinal; IBD, inflammatory bowel disease; LGI, lower GI; UGI, upper GI.

Treatment

The priority for treatment of a GI bleed is hemodynamic stabilization, including correction of any coagulopathies or blood product deficits. Once stabilization has begun, treat active bleeding with empirical gastric acid–reduction therapy with either a histamine 2 (H_2) blocker or a proton-pump inhibitor until a UGI bleed has been ruled out (Table 38-2). If peptic ulcer disease is suspected, treat the patient with a cytoprotective agent, such as sucralfate. If liver disease or a prolonged PT is discovered or if hemorrhagic disease of the newborn is suspected, treat with vitamin K.

Chapter 38: Gastrointestinal Bleeding

		Table 38-2. Initial Treatment of Active GI Bleeding
Indication	**Drug Name (Class)**	**Dose**
Active bleeding	Cimetidine (H_2 blocker)	PO 20–40 mg/kg/d, divided into doses administered q 6 h (800-mg/d maximum)
	Famotidine (H_2 blocker)	PO or IV, 0.5 mg/kg/d, administered either q hs or divided into doses administered bid (40-mg/d maximum)
	Ranitidine (H_2 blocker)	PO: 1.5–2.5 mg/kg q 12 h (600-mg/d maximum) IM or IV: 0.75–1.5 mg/kg q 6–8 h (400-mg/d maximum)
	Lansoprazole (PPI)	Patient ≤30 kg: 15 mg once daily Patient >30 kg: 30 mg once daily
	Esomeprazole (PPI)	Infants: IV 0.5 mg/kg once daily Patient <55 kg: IV 10 mg once daily Patient >55 kg: IV 20 mg once daily Continuous infusion: bolus of 1 mg/kg (80-mg maximum), followed by infusion of 0.1 mg/kg/h (8-mg/h maximum)
	Pantoprazole (PPI)	Patient <40 kg: IV 0.5–1.0 mg/kg/d q day Patient >40 kg: IV 20–40 mg q day Continuous infusion: bolus of 1 mg/kg (80-mg maximum), followed by infusion of 0.1 mg/kg/h (8-mg/h maximum)
	Octreotide (somatostatin analog, vasoactive agent)	1-µg/kg bolus (50-µg maximum) followed by 1 µg/kg/h May increase every 8 h to 4 µg /kg (maximum, 250 mg q 8 h) Taper by 50% for 1–2 d when bleeding is controlled
	Vasopressin (ADH, vasoactive agent)	0.002-0.005 units/kg/min for 12 h, then taper for 1–2 d (maximum, 0.2 units/min)
Peptic ulcer disease Bleeding ulcer	Sucralfate (mucosal adhesive)	PO 40–80 mg/kg/d, divided into doses administered q 6 h (4-g/d maximum)
Liver disease Prolonged PT Hemorrhagic disease of the newborn	Vitamin K	IM, IV, SC 1–2 mg q day SC administration route preferred Severe reactions resembling anaphylaxis or hypersensitivity have rarely occurred after IV or IM administration

Abbreviations: ADH, antidiuretic hormone; bid, twice a day; GI, gastrointestinal; hs, at bedtime; H_2, histamine 2; IM, intramuscular; IV, intravenous; PO, per os (oral administration); PPI, proton-pump inhibitor; PT, prothrombin time; q, every; SC, subcutaneous.

Consult a gastroenterologist if there is severe bleeding. Therapeutic options may include octreotide or vasopressin, vasoactive agents that are infused to control severe bleeds from varices or bleeding ulcers. Furthermore, treatment for specific lesions found at endoscopy or surgical exploration can be accomplished through electrocoagulation; use of a heater probe, multipolar probe, endoscopic hemoclips, or band ligation; sclerotherapy (injection or laser); or ligation and resection of the lesion. Biological therapies, such as monoclonal antibodies to tumor necrosis factor–α, may be needed for treatment of GI hemorrhage caused by IBD.

Indications for Consultation
- **Gastroenterology:** Severe bleeding, endoscopy needed, suspicion of liver disease, portal hypertension, or IBD
- **Surgery:** Possible surgical abdomen (volvulus, intussusception, perforation), abdominal trauma, suspicion of a duplication cyst or Meckel diverticulum, exploratory laparotomy needed

Disposition
- **Intensive care unit transfer:** Hemodynamic instability
- **Discharge criteria:** The cause of the bleeding has been identified and controlled, anemia adequately treated, and nutrition optimized

Follow-up
- **Primary care:** 1 to 2 weeks
- **Gastroenterology and/or surgery:** Depending on the source and expected chronicity of the bleed

Pearls and Pitfalls
- Swallowed blood (from cracked maternal nipples in a breastfed infant), coughing, tonsillitis, lost teeth, epistaxis, genitourinary bleeding, or menarche may give the false appearance of GI bleeding.
- Medications (bismuth subsalicylate [Pepto-Bismol], iron, liquid acetaminophen [Tylenol]) and foods (red juice, beets) can falsely give the physical and chemical appearance of blood.
- Artificial devices (nasogastric or orogastric tubes; tracheostomy tubes; gastrostomy, gastrojejunal, or jejunal tubes) in which the device tip is causing mucosal irritation can lead to ulceration and bleeding.

Bibliography

Friedlander J, Mamula P. Gastrointestinal hemorrhage. In: Wylie R, Hyams JS, Kay M, eds. *Pediatric Gastrointestinal and Liver Disease*. 4th ed. Philadelphia, PA: Elsevier; 2011:146–153

Gremse DA. Acute gastrointestinal bleeding. In: Perkin RM, Swift JD, Newton DA, Anas N, eds. *Pediatric Hospital Medicine*. 2nd ed. Philadelphia, PA: Lippincott Williams & Wilkins; 2008:304–309

Lirio RA. Management of upper gastrointestinal bleeding in children: variceal and nonvariceal. *Gastrointest Endosc Clin N Am*. 2016;26(1):63–73

Neidich GA, Cole SR. Gastrointestinal bleeding. *Pediatr Rev*. 2014;35(6):243–253

Owensby S, Taylor K, Wilkins T. Diagnosis and management of upper gastrointestinal bleeding in children. *J Am Board Fam Med*. 2015;28(1):134–145

Sahn B, Bitton S. Lower gastrointestinal bleeding in children. *Gastrointest Endosc Clin N Am*. 2016;26(1):75–98

CHAPTER 39

Inflammatory Bowel Disease

Introduction

Inflammatory bowel diseases (IBDs), including ulcerative colitis (UC) and Crohn disease (CD), cause chronic intestinal inflammation characterized by clinical exacerbations and remissions. Specific symptoms are dependent on the extent and location of inflammation, with significant individual variability in disease severity. CD can affect any portion of the gastrointestinal (GI) tract but frequently involves the colon and terminal ileum. UC affects the rectum and colon in a continuous pattern. Pediatric IBD most commonly manifests during adolescence, although it can occur in younger children. Most often, patients with IBD are admitted to the hospital to control a symptomatic flare of their disease, but there are also rare, but serious, complications.

Clinical Presentation

History

A patient with new onset or an exacerbation of IBD classically presents with abdominal pain, bloody diarrhea, weight loss, and increased stool frequency, including nocturnal bowel movements. There may also be fever, fatigue, slowed growth velocity, and delayed puberty. However, the onset of IBD may be subtle, appearing solely with growth delay. At some point, about one-third of patients with IBD have extraintestinal manifestations, including arthralgia or arthritis, skin eruption (erythema nodosum, pyoderma gangrenosum), aphthous stomatitis, and ophthalmologic inflammation. Other extraintestinal manifestations and complications include cholelithiasis, nephrolithiasis, primary sclerosing cholangitis, and osteoporosis. On occasion, these extraintestinal manifestations are the sole presenting signs or symptoms of the disease.

Physical Examination

Perform a complete physical examination, including perianal and digital rectal examinations. Plot the patient's height, weight, and body mass index, and assess the Tanner stage. Common findings include abdominal tenderness, inflamed rectal skin tags, perianal fissures, and drainage from enterocutaneous fistula. A mass is sometimes palpable when there is significant intestinal inflammation or an abscess.

Laboratory Workup

If IBD or an IBD exacerbation is suspected, obtain a complete blood cell count; C-reactive protein (CRP) level and/or erythrocyte sedimentation rate (ESR); a comprehensive metabolic panel; and stool for guaiac, culture, ova and parasite testing, and *Clostridium difficile* testing. Also check the amylase and lipase levels if the patient has mid-epigastric pain. Findings can include anemia and thrombocytosis, increased ESR and CRP level, hypoalbuminemia, and guaiac-positive stools, although all of these results can be normal. These studies, in addition to fecal calprotectin, may be helpful in differentiating relapse from other causes of abdominal pain, but sometimes imaging and/or endoscopy/colonoscopy is required. Given the lack of diagnostic predictive value and high cost, do not use an IBD serology panel as a screening test. Obtain blood cultures if a patient with IBD who is receiving immunosuppressive medications is febrile (>38°C [>100.4°F]).

Radiology Examinations

If the patient presents with severe abdominal pain, order an abdominal radiograph to look for small-bowel obstruction (air-fluid levels) or perforation (free air). In severe acute colitis, toxic megacolon can also be identified on a plain-film radiograph (transverse colon dilatation). If a patient known or suspected to have CD presents with persistent or escalating abdominal pain, persistent fever, bilious emesis, cutaneous fistulae, or persistent rectal bleeding without a source at endoscopy, order an upper GI series with small-bowel follow-through, computed tomographic (CT) enterography, or magnetic resonance (MR) enterography to evaluate the patient for internal disease (stricture, fistula, abscess). If there is concern for extraluminal disease, but both MR and CT enterography are unavailable or the patient is unable to tolerate enteral or rectal contrast material or lying still, perform CT with contrast material or, for perianal disease, MR imaging with contrast material.

Diagnostic Procedures

Endoscopy and colonoscopy with biopsy are needed to assign a diagnosis of IBD, but defer them until the patient is clinically stable. These procedures may be indicated intermittently to evaluate the extent of relapsing disease before changing therapy. Both upper endoscopy and colonoscopy are required because CD may affect any site in the GI tract, from the mouth to the anus. Findings that distinguish CD from UC are patchy inflammation and noncaseating granulomas. In UC, there is continuous chronic inflammation that starts in the rectum and extends proximally. However, in some cases, pediatric CD can also appear with pancolitis at presentation, with or without granulomas.

Differential Diagnosis

Infectious colitis may mimic the acute presentation of IBD. Perform stool cultures and *C difficile* toxin A and B assay or polymerase chain reaction. However, the presence of *C difficile* does not rule out IBD, because a patient with IBD is at increased risk for non–antibiotic-associated *C difficile* infection. The differential diagnosis of IBD is summarized in Table 39-1.

Table 39-1. Differential Diagnosis of IBD	
Diagnosis	**Clinical Features**
Bloody diarrhea	
Allergic colitis	Patient usually <5 y of age No extraintestinal manifestations Peripheral eosinophilia
Infectious colitis (*Campylobacter, Clostridium difficile,* CMV, *Entamoeba histolytica, Escherichia coli, Salmonella, Shigella,* or *Yersinia* infection)	Usually more acute presentation Extraintestinal manifestations are rare, other than fever and arthritis
Henoch-Schönlein purpura	Usually more acute presentation Purpura on legs and buttocks May have hematuria Extraintestinal manifestations are rare, other than arthritis
Abdominal pain, diarrhea, and weight loss	
Celiac disease	Nonbloody diarrhea Positive celiac serologic findings Biopsy: villous blunting and intraepithelial lymphocytes
Constitutional symptoms (weight loss, fever, fatigue, ↑ CRP level/ESR)	
Behçet disease	Patient can have genital ulcers Biopsy does not show chronic inflammation
HIV, other immunodeficiencies	Recurrent infections Leukopenia
Juvenile idiopathic arthritis Other connective tissue disorders	GI symptoms are usually less prominent
Malignancy	Patient may have pancytopenia Patient may have tumor lysis
Tuberculosis	Bloody stools are rare

Abbreviations: CMV, cytomegalovirus; CRP, C-reactive protein; ESR, erythrocyte sedimentation rate; GI, gastrointestinal; IBD, inflammatory bowel disease.

Serious Complications

The most common serious complications of CD are a result of stricturing and penetrating disease, including perforation and peritonitis, abdominal and perirectal abscesses, fistula, and small-bowel obstruction. Patients with refractory UC may develop toxic megacolon, leading to perforation and/or sepsis. Patients with IBD are at increased risk for thrombosis and thromboembolism due to a hypercoagulable state. In addition, many medications used to treat IBD cause immunosuppression, leading to a risk of community-acquired and opportunistic infections. See Table 39-2 for other important potential side effects of IBD treatment.

Treatment

The goals of inpatient treatment are to stabilize the patient, treat complications, and improve symptoms, while ideally inducing a disease remission. IBD therapy is individualized and therefore best guided by a gastroenterologist. Acute management may include fluid resuscitation, packed red blood cells (10–15 mL/kg) for symptomatic or significant anemia in the setting of continued blood loss, and 25% albumin infusion (1 g/kg, 25-g maximum) if the serum albumin level is lower than 2 g/dL (20 g/L). Maximize nutrition intake with oral or tube feedings. If enteral nutrition is not feasible, initiate parenteral nutrition. Try to minimize opioid use because it can lead to side effects such as ileus (leading to nausea, vomiting, and constipation symptoms), toxic megacolon in UC, and narcotic bowel syndrome (a paradoxical increase in abdominal pain). The treatment of IBD complications is summarized in Table 39-3.

Table 39-2. Medication Adverse Effects[a]	
Medication	**Adverse Effects[b]**
6-Mercaptopurine	Hepatotoxicity, lymphoma, pancreatitis
Corticosteroids	Adrenal suppression, glaucoma, hyperglycemia, hypertension, mood disturbance, pseudotumor cerebri, poor wound healing, psychosis, osteopenia, and fractures
Calcineurin inhibitors (cyclosporine)	Hypertension, lymphoma, renal impairment
Anti-TNFα (infliximab, adalimumab)	Anaphylaxis, lymphoma, reactivation of latent diseases (tuberculosis, hepatitis B, histoplasmosis, coccidioidomycosis)
Mesalamine	Myocarditis/pericarditis, nephritis, pancreatitis
Methotrexate	Hepatotoxicity, pneumonitis

Abbreviation: TNF, tumor necrosis factor.

[a] Only severe effects are included here; this is not a comprehensive list.

[b] Except for mesalamine, all medications cause immunosuppression.

Table 39-3. Treatment of IBD Complications

Complication	Treatment
Crohn disease	
Complex fistula	IV antibiotics*: regimen A–D[abcd]
	Surgery consultation
Intra-abdominal abscess	IV antibiotics*: regimen A–D[abcd]
	Surgery consultation
Perianal abscess	IV antibiotics*: regimen E–F[ef]
	Surgery consultation
Small-bowel obstruction	NPO
	Decompression with a nasogastric tube
	Urgent surgical intervention
Complications of both Crohn disease and ulcerative colitis	
Perforation	IV antibiotics*: regimen A–D[abcd]
	Urgent surgery consultation
	NPO
	Treat DIC, electrolyte abnormalities, and hypotension
Toxic megacolon	IV antibiotics*: regimen A–D[abcd]
	Urgent surgery consultation
	NPO
	Correct electrolyte abnormalities
Sepsis	IV antibiotics*: regimen A–D[abcd]
	Hemodynamic support
Thrombosis or thromboembolism	Consult with a hematologist and possibly a vascular surgeon and neurologist
	Possible anticoagulation, thrombolysis, or surgery

Abbreviations: DIC, disseminated intravascular coagulation; IBD, inflammatory bowel disease; IV, intravenous; NPO, nil per os (nothing by mouth).

*Choose empirical antibiotics based on local resistance patterns and likely organism. Use broader coverage for critically ill patients and narrow coverage based on identification and sensitivities, if available. Note: Add clindamycin 30 mg/kg/d, divided into doses administered every 8 hours, or vancomycin 45 mg/kg/d, divided into doses administered every 8 hours, if methicillin-resistant *Staphylococcus aureus* is a concern.

[a] Regimen A: Cefoxitin 100–160 mg/kg/d, divided into doses administered every 4–6 hours, with or without gentamicin 7.5 mg/kg/d, divided into doses administered every 8 hours.

[b] Regimen B: Cefotaxime 100–200 mg/kg/d, divided into doses administered every 6–8 hours and metronidazole 30 mg/kg/d, divided into doses administered every 8 hours.

[c] Regimen C: Piperacillin/tazobactam 300 mg/kg/d, divided into doses administered every 8 hours.

[d] Regimen D: Meropenem 60 mg/kg/d, divided into doses administered every 8 hours.

[e] Regimen E: Metronidazole 30 mg/kg/d, divided into doses administered every 8 hours and/or ciprofloxacin 20–30 mg/kg/d, divided into doses administered every 12 hours.

[f] Regimen F: Cefotaxime 100–200 mg/kg/d, divided into doses administered every 6–8 hours and metronidazole 30 mg/kg/d, divided into doses administered every 8 hours.

Indications for Consultation

- **Gastroenterology:** All patients
- **Hematology:** Suspected complication of hypercoagulable state
- **Infectious diseases:** Immunosuppressed patient with a high fever or not improving with appropriate antibiotic therapy

- **Surgery:** Suspected perforation, small-bowel obstruction, or toxic megacolon; abscess, stricture, or fistula; intractable bleeding; UC that has failed to respond to medical management
- **Nutrition:** Malnutrition, inability to tolerate oral feedings, use of exclusive enteral nutrition as therapy

Disposition
- **Intensive care unit transfer:** Shock, impending respiratory failure, peritonitis, life-threatening electrolyte abnormalities, severe postoperative complications, thrombotic complications
- **Discharge criteria:** Patient tolerating maintenance oral or tube diet, intravenous (IV) medications discontinued, pain well controlled, no or minimal blood in stools, stable hemoglobin level with no symptoms of anemia

Follow-up
- **Gastroenterology:** 1 to 2 weeks
- **Primary care:** 2 to 4 weeks

Pearls and Pitfalls
- IBD affects children of all ages. It is known as *very early-onset IBD* in children younger than 5 years.
- Abdominal distention may be caused by obstruction, ileus, perforation, or toxic megacolon.
- A patient with known IBD may have another etiology for acute abdominal symptoms, such as appendicitis or pancreatitis. Pursue a careful differential diagnosis for each presentation.
- In severe acute UC, IV steroids are the first-line therapy. If there is no response to treatment after 5 to 7 days, escalate therapy to infliximab or cyclosporine and discuss the need for possible colectomy.
- Take caution with repeat imaging, because patients with IBD may be exposed to high levels of ionizing radiation from repeat CT scans.

Bibliography

Dotson JL, Hyams JS, Markowitz J, et al. Extraintestinal manifestations of pediatric inflammatory bowel disease and their relation to disease type and severity. *J Pediatr Gastroenterol Nutr.* 2010;51(2):140–145

Oliva-Hemker M, Hutfless S, Al Kazzi ES, et al. Clinical presentation and five-year therapeutic management of very early-onset inflammatory bowel disease in a large North American cohort. *J Pediatr.* 2015;167(3):527–532

Rosen MJ, Dhawan A, Saeed SA. Inflammatory bowel disease in children and adolescents. *JAMA Pediatr.* 2015;169(11):1053–1060

Srinath A, Young E, Szigethy E. Pain management in patients with inflammatory bowel disease: translational approaches from bench to bedside. *Inflamm Bowel Dis.* 2014;20(12):2433–2449

Turner D, Travis SPL, Griffiths AM, et al. Consensus for managing acute severe ulcerative colitis in children: a systematic review and joint statement from ECCO, ESPGHAN, and the Porto IBD Working Group of ESPGHAN. *Am J Gastroenterol.* 2011;106:574–588

Meckel Diverticulum

Introduction

Meckel diverticulum is often discovered as an incidental finding. However, it will come to medical attention acutely if it is the cause of lower gastrointestinal (GI) bleeding (as a result of ectopic gastric mucosa), intestinal perforation, or intestinal obstruction when it serves as a lead point for an intussusception or a focus for a volvulus.

Clinical Presentation

History

The most common symptom of Meckel diverticulum at presentation is painless rectal bleeding, usually manifesting as the passage of dark red stool, but with massive bleeding it can be bright red. A history of crampy abdominal pain may also be present. Less often, there may be melena and abdominal pain. An intestinal perforation or obstruction is uncommon, manifesting as anorexia, severe abdominal pain, and bilious emesis at presentation.

Intussusception is the second most common occurrence at presentation. The patient may have the typical history of intermittent, colicky abdominal pain, with drawing up of the legs, vomiting, lethargy, and a late finding of bloody, "currant jelly" stools.

Physical Examination

Vital signs are usually within normal limits, but there may be hypotension and tachycardia if significant blood loss has occurred. The typical presentation of Meckel diverticulum can be unremarkable, except for rectal bleeding without tenderness at rectal examination. A patient with severe GI bleeding may have altered mental status. Hypoactive bowel sounds, abdominal distention, rebound, rigidity, and abdominal guarding, if present, suggest acute abdomen from possible perforation or obstruction. A painful, right lower quadrant mass may be noted with intussusception.

Laboratory Workup

There is no specific laboratory test that can confirm Meckel diverticulum (see Chapter 38, Gastrointestinal Bleeding). Perform a stool guaiac test to confirm the presence of blood and obtain a complete blood cell count, coagulation profile, and type and screen. Obtain an abdominal radiograph, which may demonstrate evidence of obstruction, perforation, or a mass suggestive of intussusception.

The standard of reference for diagnosis is the Meckel scan, technetium 99m (^{99m}Tc) pertechnetate scintigraphy. It is indicated for a hemodynamically stable patient with painless lower GI bleeding. The ^{99m}Tc is absorbed by ectopic gastric mucosa (if present), producing an increased area of uptake. To increase the sensitivity in an emergent situation, administer subcutaneous pentagastrin (6 µg/kg) 15 to 20 minutes prior to the scan. Otherwise, administer cimetidine (20 mg/kg/d, divided into doses administered every 6 hours for 2 days before scanning) or IV glucagon (50 µg/kg, one dose administered 10 minutes after ^{99m}Tc injection).

Differential Diagnosis

The differential diagnosis is summarized in Table 40-1.

Table 40-1. Differential Diagnosis of Meckel Diverticulum	
Diagnosis	**Differentiating Features**
Rectal bleeding or melena	
Anal fissure	History of constipation or diarrhea Fissure noted at rectal examination
Bacterial enteritis	Fever, abdominal pain May be associated with vomiting and diarrhea
Coagulopathy	Other bleeding manifestations Petechiae, purpura, ecchymoses
Inflammatory bowel disease	Fever, weight loss, oral ulcers, digital clubbing Perianal skin tags/fissures
Milk protein allergy	Usually occurs in neonates and young infants Patient may have vomiting and/or eczematous rash
Peptic disease	Abdominal pain is relieved by eating or taking antacids
Abdominal pain with bilious vomiting	
Ileoileal intussusception	Intermittent abdominal pain with drawing up of legs "Currant jelly" stools (late finding) suggest ileocolic intussusception
Inflicted trauma	Bruising on the abdomen Other signs of trauma
Midgut volvulus	Ill-appearing, sudden-onset bilious emesis Patient may have abdominal distention
Necrotizing enterocolitis	Feeding intolerance Fever, vomiting, abdominal distention Progressive lethargy

Treatment

The priority is treatment of hypovolemia and/or shock (see Chapter 10, Shock). Insert 2 large-bore intravenous lines and deliver 2 to 3 20-mL/kg normal saline boluses. If the patient remains unstable or the hemoglobin level is less than 7 g/dL (70 g/L), arrange for a packed red blood cell transfusion. Consult a surgeon.

If intestinal obstruction is a concern, the patient should have nothing by mouth. Place a nasogastric tube for continuous wall suction, consult surgery, and order an upper GI series. If the patient has an intussusception, the patient should have nothing by mouth, and the usual reduction strategy should be implemented, recognizing that lead points such as Meckel diverticulum are more likely to require surgical reduction and are more common in older children.

Indications for Consultation

Surgery: Confirmed Meckel diverticulum, rectal bleeding associated with signs of shock, concern about an intestinal perforation or obstruction

Disposition

- **Intensive care unit transfer:** Hypovolemic shock
- **Discharge criteria:** No GI bleeding and patient tolerating maintenance oral fluids

Follow-up

- **Primary care:** 1 week
- **Surgery (if resection is performed):** 2 to 3 days

Pearls and Pitfalls

- An inflamed Meckel diverticulum may appear with right lower quadrant pain and fever at presentation, mimicking appendicitis.
- Consider Meckel diverticulum as a lead point when a patient has recurrent intussusception.
- Bowel obstruction is the most common manifestation in the neonatal period.
- A recent upper GI series or barium enema can cause a false-negative Meckel scan finding, while laxatives can result in false-positive results.

Bibliography

Bertozzi M, Melissa B, Radicioni M, Magrini E, Appignani A. Symptomatic Meckel's diverticulum in newborn: two interesting additional cases and review of literature. *Pediatr Emerg Care*. 2013;29(9):1002–1005

Kotecha M, Bellah R, Pena AH, Jaimes C, Mattei P. Multimodality imaging manifestations of the Meckel diverticulum in children. *Pediatr Radiol*. 2012;42(1):95–103

Liang HH, Wei PL, Hung CS, Wang W, Huang CS. Acute abdomen in infant. Meckel's diverticulum and ileo-ileocolic intussusception. *Ann Emerg Med*. 2011;57(1):24, 28

Spottswood SE, Pfluger T, Bartold SP, et al; Society of Nuclear Medicine and Molecular Imaging; and European Association of Nuclear Medicine. SNMMI and EANM practice guideline for Meckel diverticulum scintigraphy 2.0. *J Nucl Med Technol*. 2014;42(3):163–169

Pancreatitis

Introduction

Pancreatitis is an acute, recurrent, or chronic inflammatory condition of the pancreas. Acute pancreatitis may be secondary to systemic viral or bacterial infections, structural abnormalities, medications or toxins, metabolic disorders, trauma, autoimmune disorders, or cholelithiasis, although 25% of pediatric cases are idiopathic (Table 41-1).

Pancreatitis can lead to abnormal endocrine or exocrine function, which usually resolves completely. Rarely, it can progress to necrotizing pancreatitis, with potential pancreatic insufficiency. Recurrent pancreatitis may cause persistent inflammation, ultimately resulting in chronic pancreatitis and inflammatory changes within the ductal system. Severe cases of chronic or hereditary (autosomal dominant) pancreatitis may cause pancreatic insufficiency or insulin-dependent diabetes.

Clinical Presentation

History

The patient presents with acute abdominal pain, vomiting, fever, and, rarely, shock. The abdominal pain is continuous, typically epigastric or in the upper quadrants, and may radiate to the patient's back or shoulders. Pain is worsened by oral intake and is relieved with bending forward. Nausea and vomiting tend to occur as the inflammation progresses.

Table 41-1. Etiology of Acute Pancreatitis	
Category	Examples
Abdominal trauma	Abdominal injuries from motor vehicle accidents, handlebar injuries
Genetic/metabolic origin	α_1-Antitrypsin deficiency, hypercalcemia, hypertriglyceridemia, cystic fibrosis
Idiopathic origin	
Infectious origin	Mumps, mycoplasma
Medications	Azathioprine, valproic acid
Obstruction	Cholelithiasis Abdominal masses or intestinal strictures obstructing the pancreatic duct
Structural abnormalities	Pancreas divisum
Toxins	Alcohol Scorpion and spider bites

Inquire about predisposing factors, including trauma, exposures to drugs or medications, recent illnesses, and family history of hyperlipidemia, gallstones, or pancreatitis.

Physical Examination

The patient may appear restless, with abdominal pain that most commonly localizes to the epigastrium and radiates to the back. Abdominal rigidity, guarding, and hypoactive or absent bowel sounds because of ileus are common. An epigastric mass secondary to a pseudocyst may be palpable. In severe cases, findings may include diminished breath sounds because of pleural effusions, toxic appearance, periumbilical ecchymoses (Cullen sign), or flank ecchymoses (Grey Turner sign). Mild jaundice can occur with any etiology of pancreatitis, but moderate to severe jaundice is typically associated with common bile duct obstruction from gallstones or edema of the pancreatic head.

Laboratory Workup

If pancreatitis is suspected, obtain serum amylase and lipase levels. The amylase level increases within hours of pain onset (usually >160 U/L [>2.67 μkat/L]) but has low sensitivity (75%). In contrast, lipase level increase typically occurs 72 hours after symptom onset but is more sensitive (90%) and specific (90%) for pancreatic inflammation. However, the degree of amylase or lipase increase does not correlate with disease severity. Also obtain a complete blood cell count (to look for an increased white blood cell count), electrolyte levels (including calcium and magnesium), glucose levels, blood urea nitrogen levels, liver function tests (aspartate transaminase, alanine transaminase, alkaline phosphatase, gamma-glutamyl transpeptidase, albumin, and total bilirubin tests), a fasting lipid panel, and coagulation studies (prothrombin time, partial thromboplastin time, international normalized ratio).

Radiology Examinations

Radiologic studies are not required to diagnose pancreatitis but may be useful for determining the etiology. Order an abdominal ultrasonographic (US) examination to evaluate the patient for the presence of gallstones or ductal dilation, characterize pancreatic anatomy, document the presence of cysts or abscess, and rule out other potential causes of abdominal pain. If US examination is unavailable, obtain abdominal radiographs, which can show bowel distention, pancreatic calcification, ileus, or a pancreatic pseudocyst. If US findings are suboptimal, as in cases of severe pancreatic injury or presence of air in the duodenum, perform abdominal computed tomography or magnetic resonance (MR) imaging.

For a patient with recurrent or chronic pancreatitis because of pancreatic duct obstruction, arrange for evaluation of the biliary system with MR cholangiopancreatography (MRCP) and/or endoscopic retrograde cholangiopancreatography (ERCP). ERCP may be therapeutic for ductal abnormalities if stone removal or stent placement is performed. Contraindications include active inflammation, pseudocyst, and abscess. MRCP is preferable if a therapeutic procedure will not be necessary.

Differential Diagnosis

Increased serum amylase level can occur in many other conditions, including salivary gland inflammation, diabetic ketoacidosis, perforated gastric ulcer, gallbladder disease, ruptured fallopian tube, and renal failure. The differential diagnosis of pancreatitis is summarized in Table 41-2. In these other conditions, pancreatic enzyme levels are generally normal.

Treatment

The patient should have no intake by mouth. Insert a nasogastric tube for suction if the patient has repeated vomiting or significant abdominal distention. Provide aggressive fluid resuscitation with 1.0 to 1.5 times maintenance intravenous fluids with dextrose 5% one-half normal saline (NS) solution or

Table 41-2. Differential Diagnosis of Pancreatitis	
Diagnosis	**Clinical Features**
Acute gastroenteritis	Diarrhea is commonly present Pain is generalized and mild and not associated with eating Pain is not relieved by leaning forward
Appendicitis	Pain is constant Pain classically migrates from the periumbilical area to the right lower quadrant
Cholelithiasis	Right upper quadrant colicky pain Pain may worsen with meals
Intussusception	Pain is cramping and intermittent May be associated with drawing up the legs Hematochezia may be present
Peptic ulcer	Epigastric pain, worse before meals, is not relieved by leaning forward May improve by taking antacids Pancreatic enzyme levels are typically normal, may be ↑ with severe ulcer or perforation
Viral hepatitis	Pain is localized to the right upper quadrant Liver enzyme levels are typically ↑, although they may be normal during the acute phase

dextrose 5% NS solution with 20 mEq/L (20 mmol/L) of KCl. If the patient is dehydrated, replace the volume deficit with an isotonic solution (NS, lactated Ringer). Monitor vital signs every 4 hours and clinical examination findings closely, because the patient is at risk for third-spacing fluid (peritoneal or pleural cavity) and intravascular depletion. Monitor electrolyte levels and urine output until normal and address abnormalities with electrolyte-specific correction and fluid replacement.

Provide adequate nutrition early during hospitalization, ideally within 2 days of admission. Enteral feedings are preferred, particularly once the patient's pain is resolving and bowel sounds are present. Jejunal feeding can be initiated for patients with no signs of bowel obstruction or ileus. Normalization of the pancreatic enzyme levels is not necessary before resuming feedings. If the patient is unable to tolerate enteral feeding, provide total parenteral nutrition, without intra-lipids if hypertriglyceridemia is present.

For analgesia, administer morphine (0.05–0.10 mg/kg every 2–4 hours as needed; maximum, 15 mg per dose) because there is no evidence that opiates interfere with biliary drainage. For severe pain, order patient-controlled analgesia; usually just interval dosing without a basal rate will suffice.

Antibiotics are generally not indicated for acute or chronic pancreatitis, except when it is associated with common bile duct obstruction or for necrotizing pancreatitis. In such a case, treat bacterial superinfection with either piperacillin/tazobactam (patient weight <41 kg, 100 mg/kg of piperacillin every 8 hours with a maximum of 4 g; patient weight ≥41 kg, 3 g of piperacillin every 6 hours) or imipenem (15–25 mg/kg every 6 hours, 2–4-g/d maximum) to cover enteric gram-negative organisms. Consult a pediatric surgeon or gastroenterologist for possible drainage if an enlarging pseudocyst or pancreatic abscess is present. Treat the primary or underlying cause of the pancreatitis when applicable.

Indications for Consultation

- **Gastroenterology:** Recurrent or chronic pancreatitis, pancreatic complications, pancreatic insufficiency, need for ERCP
- **Genetics:** Recurrent pancreatitis, hypertriglyceridemia, hereditary pancreatitis
- **Pain service:** Uncontrolled or prolonged pain
- **Surgery:** Pseudocyst, abscess, or necrotizing pancreatitis

Disposition

- **Intensive care unit transfer:** Shock, suspected sepsis, severe respiratory distress caused by pleural effusions
- **Discharge criteria:** Patient tolerating a low-fat diet, electrolyte abnormalities corrected, pain resolved

Follow-up

- **Primary care:** 2 to 3 days
- **Pediatric gastroenterologist:** 2 to 3 weeks if complicated hospital course or consultation is required

Pearls and Pitfalls

- Bowel rest, early initiation of feedings as tolerated, electrolyte level correction, and pain control are the keys of treatment.
- The degree of amylase and lipase level increase does not indicate the severity of pancreatitis. Therefore, trending of enzyme levels is unnecessary. Also, normalization of the pancreatic enzyme levels is not necessary before resuming feedings.
- Pseudocyst is present in 10% of patients with pancreatitis, although it is more frequent in cases related to abdominal trauma.

Bibliography

Darge K, Anupindi S. Pancreatitis and the role of US, MRCP and ERCP. *Pediatr Radiol*. 2009;39(Suppl 2):S153–S157

Restrepo R, Hagerott HE, Kulkarni S, Yasrebi M, Lee EY. Acute pancreatitis in pediatric patients: demographics, etiology, and diagnostic imaging. *AJR Am J Roentgenol*. 2016;206(3):632–644

Srinath AI, Lowe ME. Pediatric pancreatitis. *Pediatr Rev*. 2013;34(2):79–90

Szabo FK, Fei L, Cruz LA, Abu-El-Haija M. Early enteral nutrition and aggressive fluid resuscitation are associated with improved clinical outcomes in acute pancreatitis. *J Pediatr*. 2015;167(2):397–402

Working Group IAP/APA Acute Pancreatitis Guidelines. IAP/APA evidence-based guidelines for the management of acute pancreatitis. *Pancreatology*. 2013;13(4 Suppl 2):e1–e15

Genetics and Metabolism

CHAPTER 42

Genetics

Introduction

Hospitalists are encountering an increasing number of patients with genetic conditions. Genetics is becoming a greater influence on clinical decision-making, as there is now easier access to a wider range of more complex testing. The hospitalist must be able to identify patients whose clinical presentation or family history warrants immediate, inpatient genetic evaluation and consultation.

Clinical Presentation

History

In assessing a potentially heritable disorder, the family history is the first and most cost-effective "genetic test." Construct a multigenerational pedigree of at least 3 generations, which will provide a visual representation of the family history and aid in identifying patterns of occurrence. Online tools, such as "My Family Health Portrait" (familyhistory.hhs.gov/FHH), can help in the development of a robust pedigree.

Pay attention to conditions or diseases that run in the family, particularly malignancies, cardiac disease, neurodegenerative disorders, epilepsy, developmental disabilities, and dermatologic disorders, as well as sudden death. Other useful information includes difficulties with reproduction, such as infertility, birth defects, or problems with pregnancy; early onset of disease, disability, or death; consanguinity; and ethnicity. A family history that includes "too" or "two" descriptors may indicate a genetic condition; for example, too tall or short, too young, too different, too many, two tumors, two birth defects, or two generations. Sometimes, a pattern of inheritance does not reveal itself in a patient suspected of having a genetic disorder. This may be secondary to a complex multifactorial disease process or a de novo mutation in the patient.

Important findings in the patient's medical history include intrauterine growth restriction or small size for gestational age, abnormal stature, failure to thrive, brain malformation, seizures, vision loss, deafness, developmental delays, autism spectrum disorder, and special health care needs.

Physical Examination

Look for signs of growth abnormalities, such as disproportionate growth, over-growth, short stature, or Marfanoid habitus. Likewise, evidence of congenital abnormalities, including dysmorphic features; limb or skeletal malformations;

and internal malformations, such as tracheoesophageal fistula, diaphragmatic hernias, and renal agenesis, can suggest a genetic disorder—especially in combination. Neurologic abnormalities, such as hyper- or hypotonia, spasticity, or micro- or macrocephaly, encompass the widest category of findings that can point to a genetic basis. There may be dermatologic findings consistent with a neurocutaneous disorder (eg, café au lait macules, ash-leaf spots) or an oncologic process (eg, multiple lipomas). Other important findings include cardiomyopathy without viral cause, clotting abnormalities, and multifocal or bilateral malignancies, such as Wilms tumor or retinoblastoma.

Laboratory Workup

Genetic testing is indicated to confirm a diagnosis in a symptomatic patient, identify carrier status, or identify late-onset disorders in presymptomatic patients. Once the decision for testing has been made, consult a genetic specialist to determine test selection, because the number and variability of commercially available tests are increasingly complex. Additionally, more than 1 test may be required to arrive at a final diagnosis. The general approach to genetic testing is to select the most cost-effective test that will provide results in the timeliest manner. The "correct" test or tests depend on the disease or phenotype and the gene or genes suspected. Genetic tests are summarized in Table 42-1.

In a patient with an unknown diagnosis of suspected genetic etiology, chromosomal microarray (CMA) is the standard, first-line genetic test. CMA is more sensitive than the karyotype and combines two technologies, comparative genomic hybridization and single-nucleotide polymorphism.

DNA methylation studies are useful when assessing patients for one of the approximately 200 known disorders of imprinting, which is an example of epigenetic regulation.

Next-generation sequencing can be used to rapidly, and with high fidelity, perform whole-exome and whole-genome sequencing. These 2 modalities enable the diagnosis of single-gene disorders.

Ethics and Testing

Genetic testing is rapidly expanding, and misuse can have significant ethical, psychological, social, legal, and financial consequences for the patient and family. These tests, although potentially diagnostic for a patient's specific condition, may reveal incidental findings of known or unknown significance. Therefore, base all decisions regarding genetic testing on the best interest of the child. With the guidance of a geneticist or genetic counselor, discuss the risks and benefits with the patient and parents/guardians, and, ideally, obtain

Table 42-1. Specific Genetic Testing		
Test	**When to Use**	**Examples of Disorders**
Chromosomal microarray	Global developmental delay of unknown etiology Intellectual disability of unknown etiology Multiple congenital anomalies	Microdeletion disorders Microduplication disorders
Fluorescence in situ hybridization	Suspected deletion at targeted locus	Williams syndrome Miller-Dieker syndrome Smith-Magenis syndrome
Karyotype	Suspected whole chromosome abnormality, translocations, or large deletions or duplications	Down syndrome Turner syndrome Cri-du-chat syndrome
Methylation analysis		Beckwith-Wiedemann syndrome Angelman syndrome Prader-Willi syndrome
Next-generation sequencing		
"Panels" Selective exome sequencing	To obtain genetic explanation for a specific phenotype Only obtained with geneticist consultation	Cardiomyopathy DNA repair defects Epilepsy Hearing loss X-linked intellectual disability
Whole-exome sequencing	Genetic diagnosis unclear Conducted after performing genetic counseling with family	
Whole-genome sequencing	Only obtained with geneticist consultation	

the minor's assent. Testing for therapeutic purposes is acceptable, as well as predictive testing in asymptomatic children with risk for childhood-onset illness. However, defer predictive testing for adult-onset conditions without childhood-initiated interventions. Likewise, do not perform carrier testing when no medical benefits would arise from the results.

Direct-to-consumer (DTC) genetic testing has become more readily available to the public in the past few years. Consumers receive results that are unaccompanied by interpretation from a qualified medical provider, without the benefit of genetic counseling prior to testing. This can lead to myriad complications, including psychosocial stress and pursuing further inappropriate testing. Medical providers must be prepared to handle questions surrounding DTC testing as this becomes more commonplace. The American Academy of Pediatrics and the American College of Medical Genetics and Genomics strongly discourage the use of DTC testing.

Management

While a genetic diagnosis may be confirmed, often there is no potential curative treatment. However, families often report that a diagnosis provides validation to help guide advocacy for their child, as well as a framework for discussing expectations, goals of care, and even future family planning. Families are also better able to seek out support groups once a diagnosis is assigned. Hospitalists and the primary care physician can help guide families to the appropriate services, whether these are subspecialists, rehabilitation staff, or palliative/supportive care.

In rare cases, a curative treatment may be identified after a genetic diagnosis is determined. For example, children with cystic fibrosis (CF) and a specific CF transmembrane conductance regulator (CFTR) gene mutation are eligible to receive a medication that essentially makes their CFTR protein functional; or, a child with a rare glycogen storage disorder could be cured with a liver transplant. Other examples are the many ongoing gene therapy studies that have led to successfully curing certain patients with immunologic or hematologic disorders. Defer such treatment to the appropriate subspecialist.

Indications for Consultation

- **Genetics and genetic counseling:** Suspected or diagnosed genetic disorder; prior to, during, and after next-generation testing; for family counseling
- **Organ-specific subspecialist:** Organ-specific disorder, when considering specific next-generation panel sequencing
- **Nutrition:** Inborn errors of metabolism
- **Palliative and supportive care:** To establish patient and family goals of care and facilitate discussions of end-of-life care

Pearls and Pitfalls

- Testing costs and insurance coverage are variable across institutions and health management plans. Determine whether the patient's insurance will cover these costs.
- Do not perform whole-exome or whole-genome sequencing without input from a genetics specialist.
- A negative chromosomal microarray result does not rule out a genetic disorder.
- Not every variant is pathologic, and variants of unknown significance are the rule and not the exception.

Online Resources

GeneTests: genetests.org

Genetic Testing Registry: ncbi.nlm.nih.gov/gtr

Genetics in Primary Care Institute: geneticsinprimarycare.aap.org

National Organization for Rare Disorders: rarediseases.org

Online Mendelian Inheritance in Man (OMIM): ncbi.nlm.nih.gov/omim

U.S. Department of Health and Human Services, Surgeon General's Family Health History Initiative: hhs.gov/familyhistory/

Bibliography

American Academy of Pediatrics Committee on Bioethics, Committee on Genetics; American College of Medical Genetics and Genomics Social, Ethical, and Legal Issues Committee. Ethical and policy issues in genetic testing and screening of children. *Pediatrics*. 2013;131(3):620–622

American Academy of Pediatrics Committee on Genetics. *Medical Genetics in Pediatric Practice*. Elk Grove Village, IL: American Academy of Pediatrics; 2013

Moeschler JB, Shevell M; and American Academy of Pediatrics Committee on Genetics. Comprehensive evaluation of the child with intellectual disability or global developmental delays. *Pediatrics*. 2014;134(3):e903–e918

Inborn Errors of Metabolism

Introduction

Inborn errors of metabolism (IEMs) encompass deficiencies of enzymes or cofactors that normally aid in the breakdown of carbohydrates, proteins, fats, and other molecules. These defects can cause a buildup of potentially toxic metabolites and a defect in energy production, most commonly leading to hypoglycemia, hyperammonemia, and/or anion gap metabolic acidosis. State newborn screening programs aid in the early diagnosis and treatment of many, but not all, of these illnesses. A patient with an IEM is at highest risk for morbidity when caloric intake (especially glucose) is poor or when there is an intercurrent illness, such that they are dependent on catabolism of stored sugar (glycogen), protein, or fat for energy. A patient with an IEM is frequently admitted preventively at the first signs of a febrile or vomiting illness or pre-operatively for a surgical procedure.

Urea Cycle Defects

The urea cycle metabolizes ammonia from protein breakdown into urea, which is excreted in the urine. Urea cycle defects (UCDs) are caused by an enzyme deficiency in the pathway, leading to hyperammonemia, vomiting, sometimes chronic liver disease, and neurodevelopmental delay. Triggers for hyperammonemic crises include infections, excessive protein intake, and decreased caloric intake.

Fatty Acid Oxidation Disorders

Fatty acids are shuttled to the inner mitochondria by a molecule called *carnitine,* where they are metabolized, 2 carbons at a time, into acetyl coenzyme A and then into ketone bodies when needed for energy. Different enzymes are responsible for breaking down fatty acids at different stages of the process. An enzyme deficiency in this β-oxidation process or in the carnitine transport process leads to hypoketotic hypoglycemia in a fasted or low–caloric intake state.

Amino Acidemias and Organic Acidemias

Amino acidemias are caused by a proximal defect in an amino acid metabolic pathway (eg, maple syrup urine disease). Organic acidemias are caused by more distal defects in metabolic pathways of many compounds. These disorders include methylmalonic acidemia, propionic acidemia, and isovaleric acidemia. Along with specific enzymes, some organic acid breakdown pathways require vitamin cofactors, such as biotin and vitamin B_{12}. Several organic acidemias may cause an increased ammonia level.

Clinical Presentation

History

If a patient with an established diagnosis of an IEM is acutely ill, he or she will often be referred to the hospital by a metabolic geneticist or primary care pediatrician. The patient may present with normal examination findings or appear ill, with possible neurologic symptoms such as seizures, decreased alertness, or irritability. Ask about prior hospitalizations; obtain a detailed diet history, including prescribed formulas, supplements, and medications; and ask whether the family has a "sick plan," which may involve having the patient take increased doses of current home medications (eg, carnitine in fatty acid oxidation [FAO] disorders). Determine how the diagnosis was assigned and whether appropriate follow-up has been conducted with a metabolic geneticist and a metabolic nutritionist.

A patient with an undiagnosed IEM may present with unexplained poor feeding, failure to thrive, or persistent vomiting, associated with a rapid onset of lethargy or coma. There may be a family history of unexplained infant death, which is highly suspicious for an FAO disorder. Some IEMs, mainly storage diseases, appear late in infancy, with developmental delay, hypotonia, cardiomyopathy, and/or seizures at presentation. The patient may have other physical signs, such as coarse facial features or organomegaly.

Physical Examination

The priority is evaluation of cardiorespiratory and mental status. The patient may be acutely hypotonic, lethargic, or irritable from hyperammonemia or hypoglycemia. With a UCD, hyperammonemia can stimulate the respiratory center and cause central hyperventilation. The neurologic examination findings in an older child with acute hyperammonemia may be significant for word-finding difficulties or combativeness.

Aside from possible failure to thrive or hypotonia, a patient with an undiagnosed IEM may appear normal until stressed by an acute illness. Plot measurements on a growth chart to assess the patient for chronic malnutrition. Listen for murmurs or gallops suggestive of cardiomyopathy and assess the patient for hepatosplenomegaly. Examine the skin for pallor or bruising as possible signs of pancytopenia.

Laboratory Workup

For an established patient, perform routine chemistry tests and a venous blood gas analysis to assess the patient for hypoglycemia and metabolic acidosis, respectively. Beyond this, individualize the laboratory evaluation to the type of disorder or the diagnosis and clinical scenario. See Table 43-1 for the approach in a patient with a suspected but not previously diagnosed IEM. Table 43-2 lists the common laboratory abnormalities in various types of IEMs.

For a patient with a suspected but undiagnosed IEM, the *critical* laboratory tests to perform before introducing dextrose-containing fluids are a complete metabolic panel, venous blood gas analysis, urinalysis for ketones, and ammonia level assessment. Several schema have been suggested for comprehensive evaluation, but the laboratory evaluation can be streamlined depending on the initial abnormality or presenting symptom in Tables 43-1 and 43-2.

Table 43-1. Initial Laboratory Evaluations When an Inborn Error of Metabolism Is Suspected	
Clinical Scenario/Indication	**Initial Laboratory Evaluations**
Comprehensive evaluation	CBC with differential, electrolyte and glucose levels, VBG test, lactate level Ammonia, carnitine, and amino acid levels; acylcarnitine profile If there are neurologic symptoms: homocysteine level Urine: Urinalysis, reducing substances, organic acids test
Anion gap metabolic acidosis	Serum: Lactate to pyruvate ratio Amino acid levels, acylcarnitine profile, total and free carnitine levels Urine: Urinalysis (ketones), organic acids test
Chronic metabolic encephalopathy	Serum: Lactate to pyruvate ratio Ammonia, carnitine, and amino acid levels; acylcarnitine profile Urine: Urinalysis, reducing substances, organic acids test
Hyperammonemia: neonate	Amino acid levels Urine: Organic acids test
Hyperammonemia: infant/child	Amino acid levels, acylcarnitine profile, total and free carnitine levels Urine: Organic acids test
Hypoglycemia	Acylcarnitine profile, total and free carnitine levels Urine: Urinalysis (ketones), organic acids test

Abbreviations: CBC, complete blood cell count; VBG, venous blood gas.

Data from Burton BK. Inborn errors of metabolism in infancy: a guide to diagnosis. *Pediatrics.* 1998;102(6):e69.

Table 43-2. Inborn Errors of Metabolism Laboratory Findings			
Laboratory Finding	Urea Cycle Defects	Fatty Acid Oxidation Disorders	Organic Acidemias
Acidosis	-	+/-	+
Cytopenias	-	-	+/-
↑ Creatine kinase level	-	+	-
Hyperammonemia	++	-	+/-
Hypoglycemia	-	+	+/-
Ketonuria	-	-	+
Lactic acidosis	-	+/-	+/-
Transaminitis	+/-	+	-

"-" indicates a negative finding; "+" indicates a positive finding.
Adapted from Häberle J, Boddaert N, Burlina A, et al. Suggested guidelines for the diagnosis and management of urea cycle disorders. *Orphanet J Rare Dis.* 2012;7:32.

In addition, consider a total plasma homocysteine evaluation in any patient who presents with abnormal neurologic examination findings.

Differential Diagnosis

In a neonate, a new-onset IEM can be confused with sepsis, heart disease (congestive heart failure, cardiomyopathy), chromosomal disorders, or liver disease. In an older infant or child, the differential diagnosis also includes child abuse, pyloric stenosis, allergy to milk protein, acute psychosis, cerebral palsy, and developmental delay.

Treatment

If an IEM is being considered, *immediately stop all feedings,* introduce intravenous (IV) fluids that contain 10% dextrose (D10) and appropriate electrolyte levels at a high glucose infusion rate (GIR), and perform the critical laboratory tests. D10 provides a protein-free, fat-free caloric source and stimulates insulin secretion, which switches the body's metabolism from a catabolic state to an anabolic state. For a patient younger than 12 years who weighs less than 50 kg, start with a GIR of 10. For an older or larger patient, start with 10% dextrose administered at 1.5 times the maintenance rate.

GIR (mg/kg/min) = (% dextrose × fluid rate [mL/h])/(6 × body weight [kg])

Once the laboratory values have normalized and the patient is tolerating a regular diet, de-escalate care by tapering the GIR over 12 to 24 hours or according to the recommendations of the metabolic geneticist.

In addition, individual IEMs require different combinations and doses of medications during a metabolic crisis. Review dosing with the metabolic geneticist before administration, since these treatments can be highly toxic.

Disposition

- **Intensive care unit transfer:** Severe hypoglycemia (<50 mg/dL [<2.78 mmol/L]), hyperammonemia (>200 µg/dL [>142.8 µmol/L]), severe acidosis (pH level <7.2)
- **Discharge criteria:** Able to maintain homeostasis without IV fluid administration

Follow-up

- **Primary care:** 1 to 2 days
- **Metabolic geneticist:** 1 to 2 weeks, but encourage phone follow-up sooner if the patient has not recovered fully

Pearls and Pitfalls

- Ketonuria may clear quickly once the patient receives IV fluids with dextrose.
- A falsely increased ammonia level can be caused by a difficult phlebotomy or delayed blood analysis.
- If the serum ammonia level is over 500 µg/dL (>357 µmol/L), urgently consult a nephrologist because dialysis may be necessary.
- When evaluating a patient for a new diagnosis of an IEM, always check that a newborn screening was performed and that a normal result was verified.
- Galactosemia testing (urine-reducing substances) will only yield a positive result if the patient has recently been receiving galactose in the diet.

Bibliography

Ahrens-Nicklas RC, Slap G, Ficicioglu C. Adolescent presentations of inborn errors of metabolism. *J Adolesc Health*. 2015;56(5):477–482

El-Hattab AW. Inborn errors of metabolism. *Clin Perinatol*. 2015;42(2):413–439

Ibrahim M, Parmar HA, Hoefling N, Srinivasan A. Inborn errors of metabolism: combining clinical and radiologic clues to solve the mystery. *AJR Am J Roentgenol*. 2014;203(3):W315–W327

Mak CM, Lee HC, Chan AY, Lam CW. Inborn errors of metabolism and expanded newborn screening: review and update. *Crit Rev Clin Lab Sci*. 2013;50(6):142–162

Rezvani I. An approach to inborn errors of metabolism. In: Kliegman RM, ed. *Nelson Textbook of Pediatrics*. 20th ed. Philadelphia, PA: Elsevier Health Sciences; 2016

Vernon HJ. Inborn errors of metabolism: advances in diagnosis and therapy. *JAMA Pediatr*. 2015;169(8):778–782

Gynecology

Dysfunctional Uterine Bleeding

Introduction

Dysfunctional uterine bleeding (DUB) is a form of abnormal uterine bleeding that is painless, profuse, irregular, and unrelated to any structural or systemic disease. While anovulation caused by hypothalamic-pituitary-ovarian axis immaturity is the most common cause of DUB, there are many other etiologies.

Heavy (>80-mL) or prolonged (>7-days) vaginal bleeding that occurs at regular cyclic intervals is known as *menorrhagia*. Irregular (acyclic) vaginal bleeding is called *metrorrhagia*. Prolonged or heavy periods that occur at irregular intervals are termed *menometrorrhagia*.

A patient with DUB will be admitted to the hospital for hemodynamic instability, severe anemia (hemoglobin level <7 g/dL [<70 g/L] or <10 g/dL [<100 g/L] with severe ongoing bleeding), or continued bleeding after 24 hours of estrogen-progestin combination therapy or if surgical intervention is needed.

Clinical Presentation

History

Obtain the patient's history with and without the presence of the patient's parent or legal guardian. Ask about the age at menarche and whether or not there was heavy bleeding at the first menses. Determine the menstrual cycle interval (3–6 weeks is normal) and the number of days of bleeding. Menstrual loss that requires pad or tampon changes every 1 to 2 hours, with anything longer resulting in "flooding" or "accidents," is excessive, particularly if the menses lasts 8 days or longer. Ask about the effect of the bleeding on the adolescent's psychosocial well-being (eg, missed days at school and inability to participate in sporting and social activities). Use the "HEADSS" assessment tool (home, education, activities/employment, drug use, suicidality, sex) to screen for health risk behaviors. Focus on recent sexual activity, overall number of partners, recent partners, pregnancy, and possibility of sexual abuse. Determine the method of contraception and whether condoms were used at last intercourse.

Ask about associated symptoms, such as lightheadedness, syncope, abdominal or pelvic pain, nausea, vomiting, fever, vaginal discharge, headaches, and weight change (gain or loss). Inquire about a history or family history of excessive bleeding with surgical or dental procedures, easy bruising or petechiae, frequent nose bleeds, or gingival bleeding. Review and document the patient's current medications and ask specifically about hormones, nonsteroidal anti-inflammatory drugs, anticoagulants, platelet inhibitors, chemotherapy, androgens, antipsychotics, and spironolactone.

Physical Examination

Perform a complete physical examination. Record the patient's weight, height, vital signs, and orthostatic blood pressures. Note the body habitus (low hair line, webbed neck, shield chest, widely spaced nipples) and palpate the thyroid. For a suspected pituitary adenoma, check the optic fundi and perform visual field testing. Determine the sexual maturity rating (SMR) of the breasts and assess the patient for galactorrhea. Examine the skin for pallor, petechiae or hematomas, hypo- or hyperpigmentation, acanthosis nigricans, hirsutism, male pattern baldness, acne, or striae. Palpate the abdomen for a uterine or ovarian mass. Examine the genitalia (clitoromegaly, imperforate hymen) and note the pubertal hair SMR. Look for signs of sexual abuse/trauma (abrasions, contusions, or punctuate tears of the perineum and perianal areas) and sexually transmitted infections (STIs) (malodorous vaginal discharge, vaginal erythema, vesicular lesions or ulcers).

If the patient is sexually active, perform a pelvic examination to obtain samples for STI testing. A pelvic examination performed with anesthesia may be necessary for a virginal adolescent with bleeding that cannot be controlled with hormone therapy, significant anemia, or pelvic and abdominal pain.

Laboratory Workup

Perform a pregnancy test and complete blood cell count with differential, platelet count, and reticulocyte count. If the patient requires a blood transfusion for excessive bleeding and/or hemodynamic instability, obtain a type and screen, prothrombin time, partial thromboplastin time, fibrinogen level, and von Willebrand panel (von Willebrand factor [VWF] antigen, VWF activity) prior to transfusion.

If the patient is sexually active, test for STIs, particularly *Neisseria gonorrhoeae* and chlamydia. STI testing can also be performed on a urine sample.

Arrange for a pelvic ultrasonographic examination if the pregnancy test result is positive (to rule out ectopic pregnancy) or if a mass is palpated during the pelvic examination.

Obtain follicle-stimulating hormone (FSH) and luteinizing hormone (LH) levels in girls in whom diagnosis of anovulatory cycles is considered, if possible on day 3 or 5 of their cycle (when their levels are lowest and therefore the most reproducible).

Other laboratory testing is dictated by the history and findings at physical examination and may include thyroid function tests (goiter, short stature, obesity, skin dryness, and myxedema); evaluation of testosterone, free testosterone, dehydroepiandrosterone sulfate, and androstenedione levels; LH:FSH ratio (obesity, hirsutism, and acne suggestive of polycystic ovary syndrome [PCOS]); prolactin evaluation (galactorrhea, headaches, visual field defects, papilledema); and 17-hydroxyprogesterone evaluation (hirsutism, severe acne, clitoromegaly suggestive of late-onset congenital adrenal hyperplasia).

Differential Diagnosis

Most cases of DUB (90%) during the first 2 years after menarche are secondary to physiological anovulation from delayed maturation of the hypothalamic pituitary axis. However, DUB is a diagnosis of exclusion. The differential diagnosis primarily includes pregnancy (either intrauterine or ectopic) and local infections. Systemic etiologies include bleeding disorders, endocrine disorders, and medications. Local causes include trauma, foreign bodies, and, rarely, benign and malignant tumors (Table 44-1).

Anovulation and vaginal bleeding can also be seen in thyroid disorders, PCOS, Turner syndrome, systemic illnesses (cystic fibrosis, inflammatory bowel disease, diabetes mellitus, renal disease, autoimmune disorders), strenuous exercise, or emotional stress (anorexia nervosa).

Table 44-1. Differential Diagnosis of Dysfunctional Uterine Bleeding

Diagnosis	Clinical Features
Anovulation	Menarche within past 2 y No fever or abdominal/pelvic pain
Ectopic pregnancy	(+) Pregnancy test result Abdominal pain, nausea, vomiting
Endometriosis	Abdominal pain Pain with bowel movements or urination
Missed abortion	Low back or abdominal pain Tissue or clotlike material passing from the vagina
Platelet disorders (idiopathic thrombocytopenic purpura, thrombocytopenia, von Willebrand disease, etc)	Heavy vaginal bleeding at the first menses Epistaxis and gum bleeds Family history of excessive bleeding Malignancy or treatment for malignancy
Sexually transmitted infection/pelvic inflammatory disease	Vaginal discharge Fever, abdominal or pelvic pain, nausea and vomiting Cervical motion and/or adnexal tenderness
Trauma, foreign body	Lacerations and/or abrasions Bruising of the perineum and perianal area

"+" indicates a positive finding.

Treatment

For severe uterine bleeding, when the patient cannot tolerate oral medication, start intravenous (IV) conjugated estrogen (25 mg every 4–6 hours for up to 24 hours) until the bleeding stops. Then change to an oral contraceptive (such as 30 µg ethinylestradiol/0.3 mg norgestrel), 1 pill every 6 hours, until bleeding slows down (usually 24–36 hours), then taper by 1 pill every 3 days.

Start an antiemetic (ondansetron 8 mg, 3 times a day) to minimize nausea and vomiting caused by high-dose estrogen and initiate iron therapy (60 mg elemental iron once or twice per day).

A blood transfusion is indicated for a hemoglobin level less than 7 g/dL (<70 g/L) associated with signs of hemodynamic instability (tachycardia, orthostatic hypotension) or ongoing bleeding. Consult with a gynecologist and hematologist for bleeding that persists beyond 24 hours of hormonal therapy.

Indications for Consultation

Gynecology or adolescent medicine specialist: Severe vaginal bleeding that does not respond within 24 hours to IV conjugated estrogen

Disposition

- **Intensive care unit transfer:** Severe bleeding and signs of shock, with poor peripheral perfusion and/or hypotension
- **Discharge criteria:** Patient hemodynamically stable, bleeding under control, patient tolerating oral hormonal therapy

Follow-up

Primary care physician and/or gynecologist: 1 to 2 days

Pearls and Pitfalls

- DUB remains a diagnosis of exclusion. Exclude pregnancy, STIs, and bleeding disorders.
- High-dose estrogen therapy requires the use of antiemetics.
- Maintain a menstrual calendar to monitor response to therapy (by using paper or smart phone apps).

Bibliography

American College of Obstetricians and Gynecologists. ACOG committee opinion no. 557: management of acute abnormal uterine bleeding in nonpregnant reproductive-aged women. *Obstet Gynecol.* 2013;121(4):891–896

Bennett AR, Gray SH. What to do when she's bleeding through: the recognition, evaluation, and management of abnormal uterine bleeding in adolescents. *Curr Opin Pediatr.* 2014;26(4):413–419

Deligeoroglou E, Karountzos V, Creatsas G. Abnormal uterine bleeding and dysfunctional uterine bleeding in pediatric and adolescent gynecology. *Gynecol Endocrinol.* 2013;29(1):74–78

Gray SH, Emans SJ. Abnormal vaginal bleeding in the adolescent. In: Emans SJ, Laufer MR, eds. *Emans, Laufer, Goldstein's Pediatric & Adolescent Gynecology.* 6th ed. Philadelphia, PA: Lippincott Williams & Wilkins; 2012:159–167

Matteson KA, Rahn DD, Wheeler TL 2nd, et al. Nonsurgical management of heavy menstrual bleeding: a systematic review. *Obstet Gynecol.* 2013; 121(3):632–643

Ovarian Torsion

Introduction

Ovarian torsion is the complete or partial rotation of the ovary on its pedicle, leading to ischemia and potential loss of the ovary. Adnexal torsion refers to a twist of the fallopian tube alone or of the ovary and fallopian tube together. Ovarian torsion is an uncommon cause of acute abdominal pain in girls, accounting for about 3% of all cases. While the incidence peaks during puberty, it can occur at any age. Prompt diagnosis and surgical treatment are critical in maximizing the chances of preserving the ovary, but the nonspecific nature of the presenting signs can make rapid diagnosis challenging.

Clinical Presentation

History

The typical presentation of ovarian torsion is the sudden onset of lower abdominal pain with nausea and/or vomiting. Since torsion causes adnexal ischemia, the pain can be severe and out of proportion to the physical examination findings. The pain is typically unilateral and does not usually migrate or radiate. There may be a history of recent episodes of crampy abdominal pain.

Physical Examination

Lower abdominal tenderness is the most common sign, present in up to 90% of patients. There may be a palpable, tender lower abdominal mass. Do not perform an internal pelvic examination in a prepubertal girl, but both an internal and an external examination are indicated for a patient who is sexually active and at risk for a sexually transmitted infection.

Laboratory Workup

The role of laboratory studies in a patient with possible ovarian torsion is to rule out other causes of acute abdominal pain (see Chapter 118, Acute Abdomen). When the diagnosis is uncertain, obtain a complete blood count and electrolyte, amylase, lipase, and hepatic transaminase levels and perform urinalysis and urine culture. Always perform a urine-based pregnancy test in a girl of reproductive age to exclude the possibility of ectopic pregnancy. Although most ovarian masses in children are benign, if one is noted, evaluate serum tumor markers (α-fetoprotein [endodermal sinus tumor, mixed germ cell tumor] and beta human chorionic gonadotropin [choriocarcinoma, embryonal carcinoma]).

Radiology Examinations

When ovarian torsion is suspected, order Doppler-enhanced pelvic ultrasonography (US), although normal Doppler flow does not exclude the possibility of ovarian torsion. In fact, the absence of arterial blood flow is less predictive than finding heterogeneous ovarian enlargement. Free fluid may also be seen in the cul-de-sac at US.

While an ovarian cyst or mass increases the risk of torsion, nearly half of cases occur in ovaries of normal size. Do not order cross-sectional imaging (computed tomography [CT]) when ovarian torsion is suspected.

Differential Diagnosis

The diagnosis of ovarian torsion can be challenging because it mimics other more common conditions. See Table 45-1 for alternative diagnoses and distinguishing features.

Table 45-1. Differential Diagnosis of Ovarian Torsion	
Diagnosis	Clinical Features
Acute appendicitis	Fever Pain migrates from periumbilical area to right lower quadrant Patient may prefer to stay still for comfort
Acute gastroenteritis	Fever, vomiting, diarrhea Pain is usually abdominal and diffuse
Dysmenorrhea	Timing corresponds with menses Recurs monthly
Ectopic pregnancy	May have vaginal bleeding (+) Pregnancy test result
Endometriosis	Dysmenorrhea, pelvic pain, dyspareunia
Intussusception	Episodic pain with drawing up of the legs May have bloody stool (late finding)
Mesenteric adenitis	Pain in the setting of acute gastroenteritis Can mimic appendicitis
Nephrolithiasis	Episodic pain from flank to groin Microscopic hematuria
Pelvic inflammatory disease	Patient sexually active Vaginal discharge, cervical motion tenderness
Ruptured ovarian cyst	Often occurs mid-cycle May cause vaginal bleeding
Urinary tract infection	Frequency, urgency, dysuria (+) Urinalysis and culture findings

"+" indicates a positive finding.

Treatment

When ovarian torsion is suspected, the patient should have no intake by mouth in anticipation of surgery, and intravenous (IV) maintenance fluids should be administered. Treat pain with either IV morphine (0.05–0.10 mg/kg every 3–4 hours as needed; maximum, 10 mg per dose) and/or ketorolac (0.5 mg/kg every 6–8 hours). Antibiotics are not indicated for a patient with isolated ovarian torsion.

Consult a pediatric surgeon or gynecologist early in the evaluation for any patient with suspicious clinical findings or an ovarian torsion visualized at pelvic US. Prompt laparoscopic detorsion is the immediate surgical objective. Decreasing the time between diagnosis and surgical treatment is critical for maximizing ovarian salvage, because surgical detorsion with ovarian preservation is now the standard of care. Oophorectomy is rarely indicated, given the extremely low rate of malignancy in pediatric ovarian masses.

Disposition

- **Interinstitutional transfer:** Appropriate pediatric surgeon or gynecologist not available
- **Intensive care unit:** Shock, toxic appearance, concern for intra-abdominal sepsis
- **Discharge criteria:** Pain well controlled with oral medication and patient tolerating adequate oral intake

Follow-up

- **Primary care:** 3 to 5 days
- **Surgeon:** 2 to 4 weeks

Pearls and Pitfalls

- Always consider ovarian torsion in the differential diagnosis of a girl with sudden onset of lower abdominal pain.
- Normal ovarian appearance and Doppler flow at US do not exclude the possibility of torsion.
- A normal CT finding does not exclude ovarian torsion.
- Prompt surgical treatment is the key factor that leads to ovarian salvage.
- Most ovarian lesions in children are benign.

Bibliography

Guthrie BD, Adler MD, Powell EC. Incidence and trends in pediatric ovarian torsion hospitalizations in the United States, 2000–2006. *Pediatrics.* 2010;125(3):532–538

Lourenco AP, Swenson D, Tubbs RJ, Lazarus E. Ovarian and tubal torsion: imaging findings on US, CT, and MRI. *Emerg Radiol.* 2014;21(2):179–187

Papic JC, Finnell SM, Slaven JE, Billmire DF, Rescorla FJ, Leys CM. Predictors of ovarian malignancy in children: overcoming clinical barriers to ovarian preservation. *J Pediatr Surg.* 2014;49(1):144–148

Schmitt ER, Ngai SS, Gausche-Hill M, Renslo R. Twist and shout! Pediatric ovarian torsion clinical update and case discussion. *Pediatr Emerg Care.* 2013;29(4):518–523

Spinelli C, Buti I, Pucci V, et al. Adnexal torsion in children and adolescents: new trends to conservative surgical approach — our experience and review of literature. *Gynecol Endocrinol.* 2013;29(1):54–58

CHAPTER 46

Sexually Transmitted Infections

Introduction

Chlamydia and gonorrhea are the most common bacterial causes of sexually transmitted infections (STIs) in adolescents. Other STIs include human papillomavirus, herpes simplex virus (HSV), trichomoniasis, bacterial vaginosis (BV), syphilis, and HIV. Although most cases of STI are managed on an outpatient basis, these infections may coexist with or be included in the differential diagnoses of many conditions in hospitalized adolescents. In addition, pelvic inflammatory disease (PID) can have significant long-term consequences, including infertility, ectopic pregnancy, tubo-ovarian abscess, and chronic pelvic pain.

Clinical Presentation

History

Without a parent or partner present, assure the patient of privacy and confidentiality and ask about the number of sexual partners, the sex of their partners, nature of the sexual activity (eg, oral, anal, and/or vaginal), contraception use, partner history of STIs, and history of sexual assault or abuse. In a female patient, ask about vaginal discharge, lesions, odor, pruritus, irritation, dysuria, heavy bleeding, spotting, abdominal or back pain, nausea or vomiting, fever, and dyspareunia. In a male patient, ask about testicular pain, penile discharge, lesions, dysuria, and pruritus. For all patients, elicit any history of arthralgia, malaise, pharyngitis, conjunctivitis, and generalized or localized rashes. However, keep in mind that many STIs are asymptomatic.

Physical Examination

The priority is the genital examination, with a chaperone present. In a post-pubertal female subject, note any external lesions or excoriations. Perform a bimanual examination for adnexal tenderness, cervical motion tenderness (CMT), or uterine/lower abdominal pain associated with PID. If a speculum examination is performed (for excessive vaginal bleeding, possible retained foreign body, or need to visualize an intrauterine device), examine the cervix for friability, as well as blood or mucopurulent material within the endocervical canal. Note the color, consistency, and malodor of any abnormal discharge.

Collect urine for nucleic acid amplification testing (NAAT) for chlamydia and gonorrhea, as well as pH level, KOH level, and saline preparation to identify inflammation, clue cells, trichomonads, and yeast forms. Also feel for lower abdominal pain, rebound tenderness, and right upper quadrant abdominal pain, which can occur with perihepatitis (Fitz-Hugh-Curtis syndrome). Examine a male subject for lesions, urethral discharge, testicular pain, hydrocele, and swelling of the epididymis.

Perform a careful external examination of the anogenital region for signs of trauma and sexual abuse, such as abrasions, contusions, and punctate tears of the perineum and perianal areas. In a prepubertal or virginal female subject, a speculum examination is not routinely indicated, while a bimanual rectal examination will allow for evaluation of the uterus and cervix. If abuse is suspected, involve a child protection/abuse specialist.

In addition, note any pustules, especially on the extensor surfaces of the extremities, or maculopapular exanthem, including the palms of the hands and soles of the feet. Look for conjunctivitis, oropharyngeal lesions, and lymphadenopathy (generalized, inguinal). The clinical findings of STIs are summarized in Table 46-1.

Laboratory Workup

Screen sexually active adolescents for chlamydia and gonorrhea, conduct rapid plasma reagin (RPR) and Venereal Disease Research Laboratory (VDRL) testing for syphilis, and test for HIV. NAAT for urine, cervical, and vaginal testing is highly sensitive and specific for chlamydia and gonorrhea. The sensitivity of chlamydia and gonorrhea culture is considerably lower, but the specificity is 100%, so for medical-legal reasons it is indicated in cases of suspected sexual abuse. Perform a vaginal/rectal culture in a prepubertal female subject (endocervical samples are not necessary). Anorectal and oropharyngeal cultures are indicated for victims of sexual abuse, men having sex with men, and sex workers. Perform a pregnancy test and, if the result is positive, perform ultrasonography (US) to rule out an ectopic pregnancy if the patient has abdominal pain.

If PID is suspected, obtain a complete blood cell count and a C-reactive protein level and/or erythrocyte sedimentation rate and perform liver function testing if there are symptoms of hepatitis/cholecystitis (these are often normal in Fitz-Hugh-Curtis syndrome). Send any abnormal vaginal discharge for NAAT, Gram stain, and microscopy analysis for white blood cells (WBCs), *Trichomonas* infection, candidiasis, and BV.

For a male patient, send any urethral discharge for microscopy analysis, Gram stain, and NAAT. More than 5 WBCs per high-power field is consistent with urethritis.

Culture the base of any unroofed vesicular lesions for HSV, but do not submit a Tzanck preparation, which lacks sufficient sensitivity and specificity.

Table 46-1. Clinical Presentation of Sexually Transmitted Infections	
Sexually Transmitted Infection	**Clinical Features**
Bacterial vaginosis	Homogenous, gray-white, smooth discharge over the vaginal walls External mild irritation, malodorous discharge
Candidal vulvovaginitis	Thick, cheesy, white discharge Irritation and pruritus
Condyloma accuminatum (human papillomavirus)	Flesh-colored, painless anogenital warts May be pruritic
Epididymitis	Unilateral testicular pain and swelling Dysuria, urgency
Gonorrhea (disseminated)	Petechial/pustular exanthema Asymmetrical arthralgia, tenosynovitis, septic arthritis
Herpes simplex virus	Painful/pruritic vesicles or shallow ulcerations Vaginal/penile discharge, dysuria Tender inguinal lymphadenopathy
Pelvic inflammatory disease	Dysmenorrhea, dyspareunia, spotting off-cycle or with intercourse Fever, nausea, vomiting Lower abdominal pain or chronic abdominal pain ↑ Vaginal discharge/bleeding Cervical motion and/or adnexal tenderness
Reiter syndrome (chlamydia)	Conjunctivitis, urethritis, arthritis
Syphilis (primary)	Single painless ulcer (chancre) Nontender inguinal lymphadenopathy
Syphilis (secondary)	Fever, malaise, myalgia, pharyngitis Salmon-pink macules/copper papules involving the palms of the hands and soles of the feet Condyloma lata (anogenital flesh-colored hypertrophic papules) Generalized painless adenopathy
Trichomonas	Malodorous, frothy, yellow-green discharge External irritation

Perform dark-field examinations or direct fluorescent antibody testing for *Treponema pallidum* from ulcerative lesions. Confirm a positive RPR/VDRL result with treponemal tests (fluorescent treponemal antibody absorption, *T pallidum* particle agglutination, enzyme immunoassays).

Radiology Examinations

US may be helpful for evaluating both gynecologic (ovarian) pathology and suspected appendicitis. Constipation can be ruled out with an abdominal radiograph.

Differential Diagnosis

It can be challenging to assign the correct diagnosis in an adolescent female subject with abdominal pain (Table 46-2).

Treatment

Treatment of STIs is allowed, based solely on the minor's consent, although some states set a minimum age for this. No state requires that physicians notify parents regarding STI evaluation or treatment, although 18 states allow physicians to do so if it is determined to be in the patient's best interest. The Guttmacher Institute has an online table that is updated monthly (www.Guttmacher.org).

Table 46-2. Differential Diagnosis of Abdominal Pain in the Sexually Active Female Subject	
Diagnosis	**Clinical Features**
Appendicitis	Pain migrates from periumbilical area to right lower quadrant Vomiting follows onset of pain, anorexia Rebound, abdominal guarding, leukocytosis
Ectopic pregnancy	(+) Pregnancy test finding Missed or late menstruation Vaginal bleeding Abdominal or pelvic pain
Endometriosis	Chronic abdominopelvic or low back pain, may be associated with the menstrual cycle Dysmenorrhea, dyspareunia
Nephrolithiasis	Colicky pain (may occur in paroxysms), flank pain Nausea, vomiting, dysuria May have hematuria
Ovarian cyst	Pelvic pain Menstrual irregularities Acute pain with rupture
Ovarian torsion	Nausea, vomiting Fever uncommon, except with late presentation Severe, acute lower abdominal pain (with rebound or abdominal guarding)
Pelvic inflammatory disease/ tubo-ovarian abscess	Nausea, vomiting, fever Cervical motion/adnexal tenderness ↑ Vaginal discharge ↑ C-reactive protein level/erythrocyte sedimentation rate/white blood cell count
Pyelonephritis	Dysuria, urgency, frequency Costovertebral angle tenderness (+) Urinalysis and urine culture

"+" indicates a positive finding.

The most common STIs encountered in the hospitalized patient are discussed herein. Please refer to the *Red Book: 2015 Report of the Committee on Infectious Diseases* (redbook.solutions.aap.org) or the U.S. Centers for Disease Control and Prevention (CDC) Sexually Transmitted Diseases Treatment Guidelines for specific treatments of less prevalent infections or infections in special populations. Wait for a negative pregnancy test result before treating the patient with metronidazole or initiating HIV prophylaxis.

Pelvic Inflammatory Disease

Initiate treatment for PID as soon as a presumptive diagnosis is assigned to reduce the chances of long-term sequelae. Indications for inpatient treatment include

- Inability to exclude a surgical emergency as the cause of the symptoms
- Pregnancy
- Outpatient therapy failed or not tolerated
- Tubo-ovarian abscess
- Severe illness with high fever, nausea, and vomiting
- Lack of adequate social or financial support to begin or comply with consistent oral therapy

Treat with intravenous (IV) cefotetan (2 g every 12 hours) or IV cefoxitin (2 g every 6 hours) *plus* oral doxycycline (100 mg per os [PO, by mouth] every 12 hours). Continue the IV therapy until the patient is improving for 24 to 48 hours but complete a 14-day course of doxycycline. If the patient cannot tolerate oral medications, start IV clindamycin (900 mg every 8 hours) *plus* IV gentamicin (2 mg/kg administered once [loading dose], then 1.5 mg/kg every 8 hours [maintenance]), since IV administration of doxycycline can be painful. If a tubo-ovarian abscess is present, add PO/IV metronidazole (500 mg twice a day [bid] for 14 days). Cultures and NAAT results do not change empirical coverage, and patient response does not change the total of 14 days of treatment.

If the response to antibiotics (improvement in pain level, CMT, adnexal tenderness, fever) is not prompt (24–72 hours), repeat the bimanual examination and perform pelvic US to look for a tubo-ovarian abscess or other cause of abdominal pain (appendicitis, ovarian torsion, cysts). If minimal improvement is seen with appropriate antibiotics within 3 to 5 days, consult a gynecologist for further evaluation (laparoscopy) and surgical intervention.

Chlamydia/Gonorrhea (Uncomplicated)

Treat urethritis and cervicitis empirically with 1 dose of azithromycin 1 g PO (*or* doxycycline 100 mg PO bid for 7 days) and 1 dose of intramuscular (IM) ceftriaxone 250 mg (*or* cefixime 400 mg PO). This regimen provides antimicrobial coverage for potential coinfection and may limit the development of resistant gonorrhea.

Treat epididymitis with 1 dose of IM ceftriaxone 250 mg *plus* doxycycline (100 mg PO bid for 10 days) *or* azithromycin (1g PO each week for 2 weeks). Also provide bed rest, scrotal elevation, and analgesia.

Herpes Simplex Virus

Treat with IV acyclovir 5 to 10 mg/kg every 8 hours for 2 to 7 days or until there is clinical improvement. Continue with oral therapy (acyclovir 400 mg PO 3 times a day *or* valacyclovir 1 g PO bid) to complete a minimum of 10 total days of treatment. Adjust the dose for renal impairment.

Syphilis (Primary)

Treat with 1 dose of IM benzathine penicillin G (50,000 million units/kg; maximum, 2.4 million units).

Trichomoniasis

Treat with 1 dose of metronidazole 2 g PO or 1 dose of tinidazole 2 g PO.

Bacterial Vaginosis

Treat with metronidazole 500 mg PO bid for 7 days *or* metronidazole gel (0.75%), 1 applicator (5 g) administered intravaginally daily for 5 days, or clindamycin cream (2%), 1 applicator (5 g) administered intravaginally at bedtime for 7 days.

Postexposure Prophylaxis for HIV

Indications for initiation of postexposure prophylaxis (PEP) include

- Exposure where the risk of transmission is high (exposure to blood, genital secretions, or infected body fluids of a person known to be HIV positive)
- Medical care sought within 72 hours after exposure
- Patient or parent able to strictly adhere to a 28-day regimen

PEP is not generally recommended without the presence of all 3 indications because the effectiveness of prophylaxis is unlikely to outweigh the risks and side effects of antiretroviral regimens. Consult a pediatric HIV specialist or, if one is not locally available, the National Clinicians' Post-Exposure Prophylaxis Hotline (888/448-4911) for recommendations about PEP in specific situations. Additional information regarding pediatric and adolescent antiretroviral regimens can be found at the U.S. Department of Health and Human Services Web site for HIV/AIDS (http://aidsinfo.nih.gov/contentfiles/PediatricGuidelines.pdf).

Indications for Consultation

- **Child abuse:** Suspicion of child abuse
- **Infectious diseases:** HIV-positive adolescents with a coexisting STI, new HIV diagnosis or suspected high-risk exposure, complicated disseminated gonococcal infection, complicated HSV
- **Obstetrics/gynecology:** Possible ectopic pregnancy, pregnant female subject with PID, tubo-ovarian abscess, prolonged symptoms of PID
- **Urology:** Possible testicular torsion or abscess or epididymitis

Disposition

- **Intensive care unit transfer:** Complicated HSV infections (central nervous system or disseminated disease), syphilis with cardiac or neurologic involvement, sepsis
- **Discharge criteria:** Improved symptoms and tolerance of oral medications, social supports available

Follow-up

Primary care: 48 hours, then 1 to 2 weeks and 3 to 6 months for chlamydia and gonorrhea retesting

Pearls and Pitfalls

- Maintain high suspicion for PID in a sexually active female subject and treat accordingly, even if test results for chlamydia and gonorrhea are negative (to avoid possible long-term sequelae).
- Notify and treat the partner(s) of an adolescent infected with chlamydia, gonorrhea, or *Trichomonas*. More information regarding state-specific guidelines for expedited partner therapy may be found at www.cdc.gov/std/ept.
- While all 50 states allow minors to consent to confidential STI screening and treatment, be aware of state-specific differences because reporting and insurance confidentiality measures vary.
- Review contraception options and condom use with the patient. Refer to the American Academy of Pediatrics policy statement on contraception for adolescents or the CDC (http://www.cdc.gov/reproductivehealth/contraception/usspr.htm)

Bibliography

American Academy of Pediatrics. Sexually transmitted infections in adolescents and children. In: Kimberlin DW, Brady MT, Jackson MA, Long SS, eds. *Red Book: 2015 Report of the Committee on Infectious Diseases*. Elk Grove Village, IL: American Academy of Pediatrics; 2015:177–188

Gibson EJ, Bell DL, Powerful SA. Common sexually transmitted infections in adolescents. *Prim Care.* 2014;41(3):631–650

Guttmacher Institute. An overview of minors' consent law. http://www.guttmacher.org/statecenter/spibs/spib_OMCL.pdf. Accessed February 2, 2017

Havens PL; and American Academy of Pediatrics Committee on Pediatric AIDS. Postexposure prophylaxis in children and adolescents for nonoccupational exposure to human immunodeficiency virus. *Pediatrics.* 2003;111(6 Pt 1):1475–1489

Straub DM. Sexually transmitted diseases in adolescents. *Adv Pediatr.* 2009;56:87–106

Workowski KA, Bolan GA; and U.S. Centers for Disease Control and Prevention. Sexually transmitted diseases treatment guidelines, 2015. *MMWR Recomm Rep.* 2015;64(RR-03);1–137

Hematology

HEMATOLOGY

Anemia

Introduction

Anemia is defined as a reduced hemoglobin concentration or red blood cell (RBC) mass below the reference range for the patient's age. Any process that causes increased RBC destruction, failure of RBC production, or blood loss can result in anemia. While mild to moderate anemia will typically be addressed in the outpatient setting, the acute onset of anemia or a chronic anemia that outpaces the body's ability to compensate may require inpatient evaluation and/or treatment. In addition, anemia can occur in the inpatient setting as a comorbidity with many conditions.

Clinical Presentation

History

Symptoms of anemia include pallor, fatigue, weakness, lethargy, decreased energy, headache, and shortness of breath. Palpitations and a sensation of light-headedness may also occur. A very young or preterm infant may present with apnea.

Obtain a thorough history, including the time course of the onset of symptoms, diet (including milk, iron-rich food, and supplement intake), growth and development, recent illnesses, medications (sulfonamides, nitrofurans, quinolones, phenazopyridine, etc), evidence of chronic disease, recent or recurring blood loss, and family history of anemia. Review the newborn screening results, if available. The patient's ethnicity and the presence of pica are also important to elicit. Ask about dark urine or a personal or family history of splenectomy or cholecystectomy, which may suggest an underlying hemolytic anemia.

Physical Examination

The priority is to assess the patient for hemodynamic compromise, which requires immediate intervention. This includes hypotension, persistent tachycardia, orthostatic changes, widened pulse pressure, and bounding pulse. A patient with uncompensated anemia may also present with hypoxia, signs of congestive heart failure, syncope, and altered mental status. A systolic ejection murmur and increased prominence of the cardiac apical impulse may also be noted.

A common physical examination finding is pallor, which is best seen in the nail beds, palmar creases, conjunctivae, and mucosal surfaces. Jaundice, frontal bossing, hepatomegaly, and splenomegaly may be noted with a hemolytic process. Evidence of inflammation or systemic disease may be observed in anemia related to chronic disease.

Laboratory Workup

Obtain a complete blood cell count, reticulocyte count, and peripheral blood smear for any anemic patient. If the patient has a clear source of blood loss, these values will serve as baseline measures. If the blood loss is acute, the hemoglobin level may not reflect the true volume deficit and the reticulocyte count may be normal, because the bone marrow may not have had time to respond. If the cause of anemia is unknown, choose additional studies based on the results of these initial tests. It is important to weigh the value of each diagnostic test in relation to the blood volume needed so as not to exacerbate the patient's degree of anemia. Obtain all blood samples prior to receipt of any transfusions so the patient's blood is evaluated and not that of the blood donor.

High Reticulocyte Count

The physiological response to anemia includes an increased reticulocyte count, which is a normal bone marrow response to blood loss or hemolysis. Since the reticulocyte count represents a percentage of the total RBCs, it is important to correct for the anemia as follows:

$$\text{Corrected reticulocyte count} = (\text{Measured reticulocyte count}) \times (\text{Measured hematocrit level}/\text{Normal hematocrit level})$$

To evaluate the patient for hemolysis, or shortened RBC lifespan, order antiglobulin (Coombs) testing. A direct antiglobulin test is used to detect antibodies bound to the RBC membrane and, in general, indicates autoimmune hemolytic anemia when results are positive. An indirect antiglobulin test is used to assess free anti-erythrocyte antibodies in the serum and may yield a positive result in an autoimmune hemolytic anemia if the antibody titer exceeds the antigen-binding capacity. Be aware that certain conditions, such as neonatal ABO incompatibility, are associated with low RBC antigens and will result in a positive indirect antiglobulin test result. Supportive laboratory findings for a hemolytic process include increased aspartate transaminase (serum glutamic oxaloacetic transaminase), indirect bilirubin, and lactate dehydrogenase levels. A decreased haptoglobin level is also indicative of hemolysis, except in a neonate who may intrinsically have a low haptoglobin level. Request a microscopic evaluation of the peripheral blood smear to look for abnormal RBC morphologies, including sickle cells, spherocytes, spiculated cells, poikilocytes, elliptocytes, target cells, and Heinz bodies. Additionally, check the other cell lines to evaluate platelet morphology and leukocyte abnormalities, especially the presence of malignant-appearing cells. Order a hemoglobin electrophoresis test when there is no clear etiology for a hemolytic process, when newborn screening results are unavailable or abnormal, or when the family history supports a hereditary defect.

To evaluate the patient for chronic blood loss, order a stool guaiac test to rule out a gastrointestinal bleed and perform a urinalysis to look for evidence of renal pathology. Consider other occult sources of blood loss, such as intra-abdominal and intramuscular bleeding. In the very young infant, intracranial bleeds may be associated with anemia.

Low Reticulocyte Count

A low reticulocyte count is consistent with inadequate production of RBCs. The peripheral smear may demonstrate RBC microcytosis or macrocytosis or abnormalities of the other cell lines, including hypersegmented neutrophils or lymphoblasts. Evaluate the C-reactive protein level, iron level and total iron binding capacity, and ferritin level, and perform liver function tests (Table 47-1). Note that ferritin is also an acute-phase reactant and may demonstrate normal levels in a patient with a chronic disease and an iron deficiency. Order parvovirus testing if the patient has anemia, leukopenia, and/or thrombocytopenia, along with a low reticulocyte count. If the mean corpuscular cell volume is increased, assess B_{12} and folate levels.

Table 47-1. Diagnosis of Anemia	
Diagnosis	**Clinical Features**
Blood loss	
Acute blood loss	Overt bleeding Guaiac (+) stool or gastric output May not have reticulocyte level for 1–2 days
Chronic blood loss	May be the presentation of von Willebrand disease in menstruating girls May have guaiac (+) stool ↑ or ↓ Reticulocyte levels May have ↓ serum iron level, TIBC
Decreased RBC production	
Aplastic anemia	Anemia with neutropenia and/or thrombocytopenia ↓ Reticulocyte levels
Chronic inflammation	History of chronic disease ↑ ESR, CRP level, ferritin level ↓ Serum iron level, TIBC

Continued

Table 47-1. Diagnosis of Anemia, continued	
Diagnosis	**Clinical Features**
Chronic renal disease	Uremia ↓ Erythropoietin level
Folate deficiency	Goat milk diet
Iron deficiency	History of inadequate iron in diet ↑ MCV, MCHC, serum iron level, ferritin level, reticulocyte level ↓ RDW
Liver disease	Jaundice, hepatomegaly ↑ LFT values, ↓ albumin level
Red cell aplasia (eg, Diamond-Blackfan anemia)	First year of life Severe presentation Persistence of fetal hemoglobin
Transient erythroblastopenia of childhood	Age: 6 mo to 3 y Neutropenia, normal platelet levels, ↓ reticulocyte levels
Vitamin B_{12} deficiency	Vegan diet or breastfed infant of vegan mother History of terminal ilium resection Hypersegmented neutrophils
RBC destruction	
Autoimmune hemolytic anemia	Acute, severe presentation (+) Coombs test result Hemoglobinuria
Inherited hemolytic anemia	Jaundice, organomegaly ↑ Bilirubin, reticulocyte levels Smear: RBC morphology (sickle cells, spherocytes)
Microangiopathic hemolytic anemia	Associated with HUS/TTP Schistocytes on smear Hemoglobinuria
Thalassemia major	Patient of Mediterranean or African descent Presents during infancy Splenomegaly Severe anemia with ↓ MCV

Abbreviations: CRP, C-reactive protein; ESR, erythrocyte sedimentation rate; HUS, hemolytic uremic syndrome; LFT, liver function test; MCHC, mean corpuscular hemoglobin concentration; MCV, mean corpuscular volume; RBC, red blood cell; RDW, RBC distribution width; TIBC, total iron binding capacity; TTP, thrombotic thrombocytopenic purpura; +, positive finding.

Differential Diagnosis

Use the reticulocyte count to distinguish between anemia caused by a failure in bone marrow production (decreased) versus early RBC destruction or blood loss (increased).

Treatment

The treatment of anemia varies on the basis of the etiology. A significant anemia that has developed slowly can usually be tolerated by the patient and is not necessarily an indication for transfusion. However, in the case of acute blood loss in an unstable patient with hemodynamic compromise, provide urgent volume expansion with packed RBCs. For a critically ill but hemodynamically stable patient, transfuse packed RBCs if the hemoglobin level is below 7 g/dL (70 g/L) or if there are increasing cardiorespiratory symptoms, regardless of the hemoglobin level. The time course for a transfusion varies according to the clinical situation, but in general, provide packed RBCs over a 4-hour period to avoid circulatory overload. A patient with cardiovascular instability may require a slower rate of infusion.

The treatment of a hemolytic anemia depends on the etiology and severity and typically involves consultation with a hematologist. In general, a patient with an inherited hemolytic anemia needs careful monitoring over time and may require occasional transfusions. For life-threatening autoimmune hemolysis, urgently consult with a hematologist, who will determine if treatment with high-dose steroids is indicated. The hematologist may recommend other acute treatment options, such as intravenous (IV) immunoglobulin, plasmapheresis, and exchange transfusion. Long-term management may include splenectomy or immunosuppressant drugs.

Consult with a hematologist if the anemia is associated with abnormalities of other blood cell lines, such as leukopenia, leukocytosis, thrombocytopenia, or pancytopenia. In such cases, bone marrow aspirate and/or biopsy may be necessary to evaluate the patient for bone marrow failure or infiltration.

Treat iron deficiency anemia with oral elemental iron, 3 to 6 mg/kg/d. IV iron sucrose may be a useful alternative if the patient is having difficulty tolerating oral iron. A satisfactory response to treatment is evidenced by an increase in reticulocyte count within 2 to 4 days and an increase in hematocrit level within 2 to 4 weeks. Manage anemia of chronic disease by treating the underlying cause.

Treat postoperative anemia conservatively if the patient is hemodynamically stable. However, a transfusion of packed RBCs may be necessary if the patient is tachycardic, hypotensive, hypoxic, excessively fatigued, or in significant respiratory distress or has ongoing blood loss. Additionally, a transfusion may be indicated to promote postoperative healing of grafts or other injuries, for which the patient may require a higher hematocrit level than what is needed for cardiovascular stability.

Indications for Consultation

Hematology/oncology: Diagnosis unclear, intravascular hemolysis, condition refractory to treatment, concern for bone marrow failure, bone marrow aspirate required, long-term management considerations, suspicion of malignancy

Disposition

- **Intensive care unit transfer:** Hemodynamic instability
- **Discharge criteria:** Hemoglobin level stable, without acute physiological manifestations of anemia

Follow-up

- **Primary care:** 1 to 2 weeks, depending on condition at discharge
- **Hematology:** 1 to 2 weeks, depending on diagnosis and condition at discharge

Pearls and Pitfalls

- If possible, perform blood studies prior to transfusion of blood products.
- Be cautious about the volume of blood drawn in the anemic child, because iatrogenic blood loss may acutely worsen the patient's anemia and cause clinical decline.
- Occult sources of internal blood loss are the abdomen, head (neonate), and thigh and chest (trauma victim). Except for a neonate, it is uncommon for intracranial hemorrhage to cause anemia in the absence of neurologic findings at physical examination.
- Steroid treatment can change the appearance of the bone marrow and alter the subsequent treatment and prognosis of certain malignancies. Therefore, if there is any possibility of a malignancy (generalized lymphadenopathy, hepatosplenomegaly, other cell lines affected, etc), consult with a hematologist before starting steroid therapy in an anemic patient.

Bibliography

Hartung HD, Olson TS, Bessler M. Acquired aplastic anemia in children. *Pediatric Clin North Am*. 2013;60(6):1311–1336

Heeney MM. Anemia. In: Rudolph CD, Rudolph AM, Lister G, First LR, Gershon AA, eds. *Rudolph's Pediatrics*. 22nd ed. New York, NY: McGraw Hill; 2011:1542–1545

Lanzkowsky P. *Manual of Pediatric Hematology and Oncology*. 5th ed. Oxford, United Kingdom: Elsevier; 2011:86

Lerner NB. The anemias. In: Kliegman RM, Stanton BF, St Geme JW III, Schor NF, Behrman RE, eds. *Nelson Textbook of Pediatrics*. 20th ed. Philadelphia, PA: Elsevier; 2016:2309–2311

Powers JM, McCavit TL, Buchanan GR. Management of iron deficiency anemia: a survey of pediatric hematology/oncology specialists. *Pediatr Blood Cancer*. 2015;62(5):842–846

Wang M. Iron deficiency and other types of anemia in infants and children. *Am Fam Physician*. 2016;93(4):270–278

Complications of Cancer Therapy

Introduction

The survival rate for children with malignancies continues to improve but is still associated with significant toxicities and late effects. Chemotherapy, which targets rapidly dividing cells, leads to significant cytotoxic side effects. While the effects of radiation therapy are more localized, there can be profound consequences, including nausea, vomiting, pain, and skin changes. Surgery can lead to issues with wound care, infection, and pain management. Although most pediatric oncology patients are treated at tertiary care centers, the hospitalist will occasionally care for such children.

Clinical Presentation and Diagnosis

Many chemotherapeutic agents share a number of side effects (Table 48-1), which commonly include the following.

Adrenal Insufficiency

Steroids are used in treating pediatric cancers such as acute lymphoblastic leukemia, certain lymphomas, and local edema surrounding brain tumors.

Table 48-1. Side Effects of Chemotherapeutic Agents			
Onset	**Common Side Effects**	**Occasional Side Effects**	**Rare Side Effects**
PEG-asparaginase			
Within 1–2 d	Diarrhea Local allergic reaction	Anaphylaxis Rash	
			Hyperuricemia
Within 2–3 wk	↑ Ammonia level Coagulation abnormalities	Hyperglycemia Pancreatitis	DIC/hemorrhage Thromboses
Bleomycin			
Within 1–2 d	High fever	Rash	Anaphylaxis Hypotension
Within 2–3 wk	Skin hyperpigmentation		Alopecia Onycholysis
~3 mo	Raynaud phenomenon	Interstitial pneumonitis Pulmonary fibrosis	
Carboplatin			
Within 1–2 d	Nausea/vomiting	Anaphylaxis Hypersensitivity reaction	Metallic taste in the mouth
Within 2–3 wk	Myelosuppression	Hepatotoxicity Nephrotoxicity	Mucositis
After 2–3 wk		Ototoxicity	Peripheral neuropathy

Continued

Table 48-1. Side Effects of Chemotherapeutic Agents, continued

Onset	Common Side Effects	Occasional Side Effects	Rare Side Effects
Cisplatin			
Within 1–2 d	Nausea/vomiting	↓ Magnesium level Metallic taste in the mouth	Anaphylaxis
Within 2–3 wk	↓ Magnesium level High-frequency hearing loss Nephrotoxicity	↓ Calcium, ↓ potassium, ↓ sodium levels Peripheral neuropathy	Hepatotoxicity Seizures Vestibular dysfunction
Corticosteroids			
Within 1–2 d		Gastritis	Hyperuricemia
Within 2–3 wk	Hyperphagia Personality changes Pituitary-adrenal axis suppression	Hyperglycemia Hypertension Poor wound healing	Intraocular pressure Pancreatitis
Cytarabine (cytosine arabinoside)			
Within 1–2 d	Conjunctivitis Nausea/vomiting	Fever Flulike symptoms	Acral erythema Anaphylaxis Cerebral/cerebellar dysfunction

Within 2–3 wk	Alopecia
	Myelosuppression
	Stomatitis
		↓ Calcium, ↓ potassium
		  levels
		Diarrhea
		Pulmonary capillary leak
			Hepatotoxicity
			Sinusoidal obstruction
			  syndrome (VOD)

Cyclophosphamide			
Within 1–2 d	Nausea/vomiting	Diarrhea	Anaphylaxis Transient blurred vision SIADH
Within 2–3 wk	Alopecia Myelosuppression	Hemorrhagic cystitis	Cardiac toxicity
Dasatinib/Imatinib			
During use	Diarrhea Nausea	Abdominal pain Chest pain Pericardial effusion Mucositis Myalgia	Severe tumor lysis PRES Cardiac dysfunction GI ulceration/stricture
Dinutuximab (immunotherapy/antibody therapy)			
During infusion	Hives Pain (somatic and neuropathic) Cough Rash	Allergic reaction Dyspnea Blood pressure instability Numbness	Visual changes Anaphylaxis Anemia

Table 48-1. Side Effects of Chemotherapeutic Agents, continued			
Onset	**Common Side Effects**	**Occasional Side Effects**	**Rare Side Effects**
Doxorubicin/Daunorubicin			
Within 1–2 d	Nausea/vomiting Pink/red body fluid discoloration	Hyperuricemia	Diarrhea
Within 2–3 wk	Myelosuppression	Mucositis	
After 2–3 wk		Cardiomyopathy	
Etoposide (VP-16)			
Within 1–2 d	Nausea/vomiting	Urticaria	Anaphylaxis Hypotension during infusion
Within 2–3 wk	Alopecia Myelosuppression	Diarrhea	Mucositis Peripheral neuropathy Stevens-Johnson syndrome
Ifosfamide			
Within 1–2 d	Nausea/vomiting	CNS toxicity	↓ Potassium level Encephalopathy
Within 2–3 wk	Myelosuppression	Cardiac toxicity Hemorrhagic cystitis	Hepatotoxicity
After 2–3 wk			Fanconi-like syndrome Renal failure
Irinotecan			
Within 1–2 d	Cholinergic symptoms (profuse diarrhea) Nausea/vomiting	Headache	Anaphylaxis Dyspnea
Within 2–3 wk	Hepatotoxicity Myelosuppression		Colitis Renal failure
Isotretinoin			
During use	Dry eyes, skin Cheilosis Headache Blisters Hair loss ↑ Sensitivity to the sun	Blurred vision Tinnitus Hepatitis Seizure Mental status changes Anaphylaxis	
Methotrexate			
Within 1–2 d	↑ Transaminase level	Diarrhea Nausea/vomiting	Acral erythema Stevens-Johnson syndrome Toxic epidermal necrolysis
Within 2–3 wk		Mucositis Myelosuppression	CNS toxicity Renal toxicity

Continued

Table 48-1. Side Effects of Chemotherapeutic Agents, continued			
Onset	**Common Side Effects**	**Occasional Side Effects**	**Rare Side Effects**
Mercaptopurine (6-MP)			
Within 1–2 d		Diarrhea Nausea/vomiting	Hyperuricemia Urticaria
Within 2–3 wk	Myelosuppression	Hepatotoxicity Mouth sores	Pancreatitis
Topotecan			
Within 1–2 d	Nausea/vomiting	Hypotension Rash	Anaphylaxis Rigors
Within 2–3 wk	Myelosuppression	Hepatotoxicity Mucositis	Paresthesia
Vinblastine			
Within 1–2 d			Jaw pain Seizure
Within 2–3 wk	Alopecia Myelosuppression	Constipation	Hemorrhagic enterocolitis Peripheral neuropathy Ototoxicity/vestibular dysfunction
Vincristine			
Within 1–2 d	Abdominal pain Extremity pain	Headache Jaw pain	Bronchospasm Fever
Within 2–3 wk	Alopecia Constipation	Ptosis Vocal cord paralysis	Ptosis/diplopia Seizures
After 2–3 wk	Loss of deep tendon reflexes	Peripheral paresthesia	Autonomic neuropathy Sinusoidal obstruction syndrome

Abbreviations: CNS, central nervous system; DIC, disseminated intravascular coagulation; GI, gastrointestinal; PEG, pegylated *Escherichia coli*; PRES, posterior reversible encephalopathy syndrome; SIADH, syndrome of inappropriate antidiuretic hormone hypersecretion; VOD, veno-occlusive disease.

Depending on the duration of treatment, patients may be at risk for adrenal insufficiency (see Chapter 23, Acute Adrenal Insufficiency).

Signs of adrenal suppression can be subtle and hard to differentiate from chemotherapy-related toxicities, including dizziness, weakness, poor appetite, muscle aches, and persistent nausea. More commonly, severe adrenal insufficiency appears with signs of infection, hypotension, shock, or vital sign instability at presentation. Laboratory abnormalities may include hyponatremia, hyperkalemia, and metabolic acidosis with a normal anion gap.

Extravasation

Some chemotherapeutic agents may cause damage if they extravasate into surrounding tissue. Initially, local reactions may include erythema and pain, but they may progress over days to weeks to blistering, ulcerations, and necrosis.

Severe pain and loss of function may result if the necrosis extends to the nerves, ligaments, tendons, and bones.

Fever and Myelosuppression

Bone marrow suppression leads to anemia, thrombocytopenia, and leukopenia. Because granulocytes have the shortest life span and are the first line of defense against bacterial infection, oncology patients are at risk for neutropenia and subsequent infections. A patient with fever and neutropenia (absolute neutrophil count <500/mm^3) requires immediate attention. Fever is defined differently at many centers, but commonly it is a temperature higher than 38.3°C (101°F) or several low-grade fever temperatures (37.8°–38.3°C; 100.1°–100.9°F) in a 24-hour period. However, a patient receiving steroids might not mount a febrile response. It is also critical to assess what type of indwelling catheter the child has (none, peripheral intravenous [IV] catheter, peripherally inserted central catheter, central venous catheter [CVC], tunneled or nontunneled CVC), because these carry differing risks of infection, and antibiotic coverage may differ.

Determine the date of the most recent chemotherapy administration to predict the expected direction of the white blood cell (WBC) trend, because most agents cause suppression 7 to 10 days after infusion. Also note the specific agents and doses administered, recent blood transfusions (a transfusion reaction can cause fever), and a history of other infections, which may help guide antibiotic choices. Perform a thorough physical examination, with focus on the oropharynx and perianal region (looking for mucositis and perianal abscesses) and central venous line insertion sites to assess the patient for erythema, tenderness, or discharge. The patient may not be able to mount a typical inflammatory response to the infection if the WBC count is low or if he/she has recently received steroids. A neutropenic patient is also at risk for neutropenic colitis (typhlitis), a potentially fatal complication, so perform a thorough abdominal examination and consult with a surgeon if there is any concern. Also, except in an emergency, do not permit rectal interventions (taking the patient's temperature or giving medications rectally) in a patient with neutropenia.

Hemorrhagic Cystitis

A patient receiving cyclophosphamide or ifosfamide may present with hematuria secondary to bladder wall irritation. In patients undergoing heavy immunosuppression, such as those who have received a stem cell transplant, BK virus can also be an etiology.

Mucositis

Because chemotherapy affects any rapidly dividing cell, the gastrointestinal mucous membranes are at high risk of becoming inflamed and ulcerated. This can occur anywhere from the mouth to the anus. Signs and symptoms include exquisite pain, drooling, dysphagia, chest pain, abdominal pain, diarrhea, melena, or hematochezia. Mucositis can interfere with adequate oral hydration and also create an entry point for infectious agents. A patient who has received high-dose cytosine arabinoside is at particular risk for a mucositis-related infection, including *Streptococcus mitis*, which can cause life-threatening sepsis.

Nausea and Vomiting

Nausea and vomiting can be caused by chemotherapy and radiation therapy or can occur postoperatively. Chemotherapy-induced nausea and vomiting (CINV) is either acute, occurring within the first 24 hours after receiving chemotherapy, or delayed, occurring more than 24 hours after chemotherapy administration and persisting up to 1 week, or longer, after therapy. The consequences of CINV include dehydration, electrolyte imbalance, anorexia, weight loss, and increased susceptibility to infections.

Skin Manifestations

Both radiation therapy and chemotherapy, such as methotrexate administration, can cause skin changes, such as acrodermatitis in a "stocking-glove" distribution. Abscesses, swelling, and edema at the IV line site can be signs of infection in a neutropenic patient. Skin findings that are especially worrisome include blackened spots or ulcerated/crusted lesions that could be signs of disseminated mold or fungus infection. Radiation therapy can induce skin breakdown and maceration, which can also be a significant nidus for infection. Carefully examine crevices and nonobvious skin folds in or near the radiation field. Chronic, diffuse hyperpigmentation may result from radiation therapy.

Tumor Lysis Syndrome

Tumor lysis refers to metabolic derangements caused by the rapid breakdown of tumor cells with subsequent release of intracellular contents, most often occurring in a patient with leukemia or lymphoma. Tumor lysis syndrome may occur prior to treatment in a patient with a very high WBC count at presentation or in those with rapidly growing tumors (eg, Burkitt lymphoma). Typically, however, it begins 12 to 72 hours after the induction of chemotherapy.

Metabolic derangements include hyperuricemia, hyperkalemia, hyperphosphatemia, and uremia. Because phosphorus precipitates with calcium, the patient can also develop hypocalcemia. Uric acid crystals and calcium phosphorus precipitates can obstruct the renal tubules, producing oliguria and, ultimately, renal failure. Other clinical manifestations include nausea/vomiting, seizures, muscle cramping, tetany, and arrhythmias.

Treatment

Adrenal Insufficiency

Immediately initiate aggressive fluid and steroid replacement (See Chapter 23, Acute Adrenal Insufficiency). If the patient is hypotensive, administer 20 mL/kg 5% dextrose 0.9% normal saline (NS) boluses over 5 to 15 minutes until the blood pressure normalizes. Simultaneously administer a bolus of IV or intramuscular (IM) hydrocortisone (infant, 25 mg; toddler, 50 mg; child or adolescent, 100 mg), followed by 25 mg/m^2 or 1 mg/kg every 6 hours. Treat hypoglycemia (<60 mg/dL [<3.33 mmol/L]) with 2 to 4 mL/kg of 10% dextrose and recheck in 15 minutes. Also treat documented hyperkalemia (see Chapter 23, Acute Adrenal Insufficiency).

Extravasation

If suspected, stop the infusion immediately and institute measures to remove as much of the extravasated drug as possible. Apply warm or cold compresses, depending on the agent (Table 48-2). There are also specific antidotes for some medications.

Table 48-2. Treatment for Specific Agent Extravasation		
Agent	Local Care	Antidote
Actinomycin D	Cold compress	Dimethyl sulfoxide[a]
Cisplatin	Cold compress	Sodium thiosulfate[b]
Daunorubicin	Cold compress	Dexrazoxane[c]
Doxorubicin	Cold compress	Dexrazoxane
Etoposide	Warm compress	Hyaluronidase[d]
Idarubicin	Cold compress	Dexrazoxane[c]
Mechlorethamine	None	Sodium thiosulfate[b]
Mitomycin	None or cold compress	Dimethyl sulfoxide[a]
Paclitaxel	Cold compress	Hyaluronidase[d]
Vinblastine	Warm compress	Hyaluronidase[d]
Vincristine	Warm compress	Hyaluronidase[d]

[a] Dimethyl sulfoxide: Apply 4 drops/10 cm^2 of skin surface area topically to twice the area of the site 3–4 times a day for 7–14 days.

[b] Sodium thiosulfate: Administer 2 mL for each 100 mg of cisplatin extravasation or 2 mL for each 1 mg of mechlorethamine extravasation.

[c] Dexrazoxane: Administer 1,000 mg/m^2 per dose on days 1 and 2 and 500 mg/m^2 per dose on day 3, and administer each dose 24 hours apart.

[d] Hyaluronidase (150 units/mL): Administer 5 injections of 0.2 mL each, infiltrated around the extravasation.

Fever and Myelosuppression

If a neutropenic patient is febrile, obtain a complete blood cell count with differential and blood cultures. Some centers will require culture of all lumens of a central line, as well as a peripheral site. If a child is at risk for urinary tract infections (UTIs) (ie, prior history of UTI, presence of nephrostomy tubes or Foley catheter, <2 years of age), perform a urinalysis and urine culture. Obtain stool cultures and order *Clostridium difficile* toxin testing if abdominal symptoms or significant diarrhea are present. Culture any suspicious lesions on the skin or near surgical or central line sites. Obtain a chest radiograph if there are respiratory symptoms.

Treat with broad-spectrum antibiotics that cover both gram-positive and gram-negative organisms (see Chapter 68, Sepsis), but consult with the oncologist for the preferred regimen. First-line treatment includes any of the following monotherapies:

- IV piperacillin/tazobactam (<2 months of age, 480 mg piperacillin/kg/d, divided into doses administered every 6 hours; ≥2 to 9 months of age, 248 mg piperacillin/kg/d, divided into doses administered every 8 hours; ≥9 months of age, 300 mg piperacillin/kg/d, divided into doses administered every 8 hours; maximum, 16 g piperacillin per day)
- IV cefepime (150 mg/kg/d, divided into doses administered every 8 hours; maximum, 2 g per dose)
- IV meropenem (60 mg/kg/d, divided into doses administered every 8 hours; maximum, 1 g per dose)
- IV imipenem/cilastatin (60–100 mg/kg/d, divided into doses administered every 6 hours; maximum, 4 g/d)

Add a secondary agent, depending on the probable source of infection and local antibiograms. For example, add vancomycin if a central line infection with methicillin-resistant *Staphylococcus aureus* is suspected. Also expand coverage if the likelihood of other resistant organisms is high or if the patient appears septic or is clinically worsening. Add fungal coverage if the fever persists after 72 hours of broad-spectrum antibacterial delivery without an identified source.

Transfusion Guidelines

Consult with an oncologist, because transfusion guidelines vary among treatment centers. Typically, packed red blood cell (RBC) transfusions are indicated if the patient is symptomatic from anemia or if the hemoglobin level is less than 7 to 8 g/dL (70–80 g/L). Prior to procedures and radiation therapy administration, some centers aim for a hemoglobin level closer to 9 to 10 g/dL (90–100 g/L). Ensure that all blood is (a) irradiated to prevent transfusion-associated graft-versus-host disease and *(b)* leukoreduced to prevent transmission of cytomegalovirus, especially before and after a patient receives a bone marrow transplant.

Guidelines for platelet transfusions are also treatment center specific. Generally, a transfusion is indicated if the platelet count falls below 10,000/mm₃ (10×10^9/L). However, maintain a higher count (20,000–30,000/mm³ [$20–30 \times 10^9$/L]) for a patient with residual brain tumor or a patient undergoing bone marrow transplantation or if the child is young or highly active. If a patient will shortly be undergoing a procedure, is at risk for intracranial hemorrhage, or is taking concomitant anticoagulation therapy for a thrombosis, many centers will maintain the platelet count above 50,000/mm³ (50×10^9/L).

Hemorrhagic Cystitis

Treatment consists of vigorous hydration (per the specific chemotherapy protocol), correction of hematologic abnormalities (packed RBC or platelet transfusions, if indicated), and bladder irrigation after placement of a double-lumen Foley catheter by a urologist, if severe. It is also important to rule out viral infections that may cause hemorrhagic cystitis. Prevention involves vigorous hydration to maintain a urine specific gravity below 1.010 or a urinary output of 2 to 3 mL/kg/h and the use of mesna with cyclophosphamide or ifosfamide administration.

Mucositis

Treat mucositis with sponge-tipped applicators soaked in 0.9% sodium chloride for debridement, oral (per os [PO]) nystatin swish and swallow (100,000 units/mL) 5 mL 4 times a day; for analgesia, "magic mouthwash" (2% viscous lidocaine plus liquid diphenhydramine plus liquid aluminum hydroxide with magnesium hydroxide) should be used every 4 to 6 hours. For anal involvement, prescribe stool softeners (docusate sodium, 50–150 mg/d) and "butt paste" (nystatin cream, zinc oxide, and liquid aluminum hydroxide with magnesium hydroxide) for analgesia. The pain associated with mucositis is significant and can often require IV opioid therapy and IV fluid administration or parenteral nutrition while the patient remains nil per os (taking nothing by mouth).

Nausea/Vomiting

Check if the patient already has a specific antiemetic regimen prescribed so that those medications can be instituted or augmented. For acute nausea/vomiting, use PO or IV ondansetron (0.15 mg/kg administered every 8 hours; maximum, 8 mg per dose). Higher doses up to a maximum of 16 mg per dose can be administered once in a 24-hour period, not to exceed a maximum daily allowance of 24 mg. Other 5-HT_3 receptor antagonists are also available, including granisetron and palonosetron. Dexamethasone can be used as an adjunctive antiemetic, but check with the oncologist because it is contraindicated in many cancers. Scopolamine patches are also helpful, as is PO or IV diphenhydramine (1 mg/kg administered every 6 hours; maximum, 50 mg per dose); PO, IV, or IM phenergan (0.25–1.00 mg/kg administered every 4–6 hours; maximum, 25 mg per dose); or PO or IV hydroxyzine (1 mg/kg administered every 6 hours; maximum, 50 mg per dose) when additional relief is needed. If the patient has continued nausea/vomiting, the addition of PO or IV lorazepam (0.04 mg/kg administered every 6 hours; maximum, 2 mg per dose) or PO or IV diazepam (0.2 mg/kg administered every 6–8 hours; 0.6-mg/kg/d maximum) can be effective.

Skin Manifestations

Aspirate or biopsy (as appropriate) any new circumscribed or focal skin lesion. Perform a Tzanck smear and culture of any vesicular lesion that is suspicious for herpes or varicella. Treat radiation-induced skin changes with a lanolin-based ointment. Urgent dermatologic consultation is indicated for blackened spots or ulcerated/crusted lesions that could be signs of disseminated mold or fungus infection.

Tumor Lysis Syndrome

Obtain serum electrolyte, calcium, phosphorus, blood urea nitrogen, creatinine, uric acid, and lactate dehydrogenase levels prior to beginning chemotherapy and every 4 to 6 hours thereafter. Closely monitor the patient's urine output and specific gravity, maintaining a specific gravity below 1.010.

The type of IV fluid used varies among institutions. Prior to starting chemotherapy, many centers prefer to alkalinize the urine with 5% dextrose one-quarter NS with 50 to 100 mEq/L (50–100 mmol/L) $NaHCO_3$ at a 2-times maintenance rate to maintain a pH level of 7.0 to 7.5. Alkalinization is often discontinued once chemotherapy is started to prevent precipitation of calcium phosphorus stones. Administer allopurinol (50 mg/m^2 every 6 hours; 600-mg/d maximum) to decrease the production of uric acid. Add rasburicase (50–100 units/kg administered once but contraindicated in a patient with glucose-6 phosphate dehydrogenase deficiency) if the uric acid or creatinine level remains increased and/or is increasing rapidly despite allopurinol administration and appropriate hydration.

Treat hyperkalemia as described in the Adrenal Insufficiency section of this chapter.

Administer an oral phosphate binder (ie, sevelamer) for hyperphosphate-mia. Calcium replacement for asymptomatic hypocalcemia is not warranted. Dialysis is indicated for the persistence of hyperkalemia or hyperphosphate-mia despite conservative measures and for renal failure with resulting uremia.

Bibliography

Cefalo MG, Ruggiero A, Maurizi P, Attinà G, Arlotta A, Riccardi R. Pharmacological management of chemotherapy-induced nausea and vomiting in children with cancer. *J Chemother.* 2009;21(6):605–610

Koh AY, Pizzo PA. Infectious diseases in pediatric cancer. In: Orkin SH, Fisher DE, Look AT, Lux S IV, Ginsburg D, Nathan DG, eds. *Oncology of Infancy and Childhood*. Philadelphia, PA: Saunders Elsevier; 2009:1099–1120

Schulmeister L. Extravasation management: clinical update. *Semin Oncol Nurs.* 2011; 27(1):82–90

Sparreboom A, Evans WE, Baker SD. Chemotherapy in the pediatric patient. In: Orkin S, Fisher D, Look AT, Lux SE, Ginsburg D, Nathan DG, eds. *Oncology of Infancy and Childhood*. Philadelphia, PA: Saunders Elsevier; 2009:175–207

Ardura MI, Koh AY. Infectious complications in pediatric cancer patients. In: Pizzo PA, Poplack DG, eds. *Principles and Practice of Pediatric Oncology*. 7th ed. Philadelphia, PA: Wolters Kluwer; 2016:1009–1056

Neutropenia

Introduction

Neutropenia may be transient, chronic, isolated, or part of a systemic disorder. It is defined by an absolute neutrophil count (ANC) below the normal reference range for a patient's age and is stratified by clinical significance. In general, an ANC between 1,000 and 1,500 cells/µL is considered mild neutropenia, 500 to 1,000 cells/µL is moderate, and less than 500 cells/µL is severe. Mild and moderate neutropenia are usually managed in the outpatient setting. Severe neutropenia carries a significant risk of infection, although the ANC is only used to measure peripherally circulating neutrophils and does not always reflect the marginated pools or bone marrow reserves. Thus, when determining the clinical significance of a low ANC, take into consideration that neutropenia in the setting of normal reserves does not portend an increased risk of infection because the stored neutrophils may be mobilized when needed.

Clinical Presentation

History

Ask about any previous episodes of neutropenia, as well as any predisposing conditions (drugs, medications, recent illnesses, poor diet). Obtain a thorough infectious history, including the type, frequency, and duration, and note any patterns or periodicity. Specific signs and symptoms to elicit include fever, cough, ear pain, sinus pressure, neck stiffness, headaches, abdominal pain, vomiting, diarrhea, perirectal pain, dysuria, skin infections that include cellulitis or furunculosis, and oral infections that include stomatitis or gingivitis. While in isolation, neutropenia does not increase the risk of viral infections, several viruses can cause neutropenia, which makes viral syndromes relevant, as well.

Determine if there is a family history of hematologic, autoimmune, or other systemic disorders with hematologic findings.

Physical Examination

Assess the patient immediately for evidence of hemodynamic instability that may indicate sepsis. Then, examine the patient for external signs of infection, such as erythema, warmth, tenderness, or swelling. Frank pus or abscesses suggest adequate bone marrow reserve, while a low marrow reserve results in an attenuated inflammatory response, in which case, examination findings may be subtle or absent. Examine the skin, as well as the mucosal surfaces, including the oropharyngeal, perianal, and vulvar areas, for signs of mucositis. Abdominal tenderness may indicate gastrointestinal mucosal involvement that includes typhlitis, also known as neutropenic enterocolitis. Also examine the lungs, ears, and sinuses for evidence of bacterial infection. Look for meningismus. Generalized adenopathy, hepatosplenomegaly, or poor growth may point to an underlying systemic disease associated with neutropenia.

Avoid invasive examinations, such as digital rectal examinations, rectal temperature checks, or speculum examinations, because these may cause bacterial translocation of normal flora and lead to invasive infection.

Laboratory Workup

For patients who are stable with an incidental finding of neutropenia, repeat a complete blood cell count (CBC) with manual differential and peripheral smear to confirm the neutropenia and evaluate other cell lines. If the neutropenia is isolated and the history and examination findings are otherwise benign, arrange for the primary care provider to track the CBC as an outpatient.

If the initial history or physical examination findings have concerning features, consult a hematologist to initiate further workup. Specific tests are dictated by the clinical picture and may include viral studies; antinuclear antibodies to screen for systemic autoimmune diseases; antineutrophil antibodies to screen for an immune-mediated neutropenia; erythrocyte sedimentation rate and C-reactive protein level to assess the patient for a deep-seated infection or systemic inflammatory condition; HIV screening and immunoglobulin levels to look for an underlying immunodeficiency; vitamin B_{12}, folate, and copper levels to look for nutritional deficiencies; genetic testing; and bone marrow biopsy with cytology.

If a neutropenic patient has fever (>38.3°C [>101°F]), collect blood cultures and conduct a clean-catch urinalysis with urine culture prior to antibiotic administration, but do not delay treatment if cultures are not easily obtainable. Never catheterize a neutropenic patient. Order additional cultures and imaging as indicated by the history or physical examination.

Differential Diagnosis

The differential diagnosis of neutropenia is summarized in Table 49-1.

Table 49-1. Most Common Causes of Neutropenia

Diagnosis	Clinical Features
Benign familial neutropenia	African American, Yemenite Jewish, Ethiopian, and certain Arab populations ANC usually ≥800 cells/μL No risk of serious infections
Chronic idiopathic neutropenia	Mild but chronic neutropenia No predisposition to severe infections Diagnosis of exclusion
Acquired/transient neutropenia	
Viral postinfectious neutropenia	Most common cause of transient neutropenia in childhood Can start a few days before viral symptoms and persist up to 1 wk after symptoms resolve Viral etiologies: cytomegalovirus, Epstein-Barr virus, hepatitis A/B virus, HIV, influenza A/B virus, measles, respiratory syncytial virus, parvovirus B19, rubella, varicella, human herpesvirus 6
Bacterial postinfectious neutropenia	Endotoxin-mediated suppression, especially in newborn sepsis Neutropenia improves with treatment of infection Bacterial etiologies: *Staphylococcus aureus*, *Brucella*, *Rickettsia*, tuberculosis

Drug-induced neutropenia	Direct/immune mediated
	    Abrupt onset 1–2 wk after first exposure or immediately with re-exposure
	    Lasts approximately 1 wk
	Toxic suppression
	    Insidious onset, can occur months after drug initiation
	    Lasts days to months
	Common etiologies: penicillins, sulfonamides, dapsone, ibuprofen, indomethacin, hydralazine, phenytoin, carbamazepine, valproate, clozapine, phenothiazines, antithyroid medications

Primary immune disorders	
Autoimmune neutropenia of infancy	5–15 mo of age No risk of infections Spontaneous remission within 7–30 mo
Chronic benign neutropenia Autoimmune neutropenia of childhood (primary)	Most common type of chronic neutropenia in children Appears as early as 6–12 mo of age, generally ≤3 y of age Mild mucocutaneous and upper respiratory infections Usually resolves spontaneously by 5 y of age but may persist into adulthood
Autoimmune neutropenia (secondary)	Patient often has another immune processes (autoimmune lymphoproliferative syndrome, systemic lupus erythematosus, or Evans syndrome) Clinical course varies according to underlying diagnosis
Inherited/syndromic neutropenia	
Severe congenital neutropenia (Kostmann syndrome)	Neurologic abnormalities can occur, such as developmental delay and seizures ANC ≤200 cells/μL (can rarely increase to 500 cells/μL) Autosomal dominant, X-linked, or autosomal recessive (Kostmann disease) Severe infections (primarily skin, mouth, and rectum) in the first month of life High risk of myelodysplastic syndrome and/or AML

Continued

Table 49-1. Most Common Causes of Neutropenia, continued	
Diagnosis	**Clinical Features**
Inherited/syndromic neutropenia, continued	
Cyclic neutropenia	Periodic fever, painful oral ulcers, lymphadenopathy, and recurrent infections Autosomal dominant Low ANC lasting 3–6 d every 21 d

Abbreviations: AML, acute myeloid leukemia; ANC, absolute neutrophil count.

Treatment

In mild to moderate cases of neutropenia, watchful waiting without treatment is appropriate. However, in more severe cases or diagnoses in which the neutropenia is not expected to self-resolve, consult a hematologist to initiate workup and guide management.

A patient with significant neutropenia who presents with fever is at high risk for sepsis and requires broad-spectrum intravenous (IV) antibiotics. Start treatment with one of the following monotherapies:

- IV piperacillin/tazobactam (<2 months of age, 400 mg piperacillin/kg/d, divided into doses administered every 6 hours; 2–9 months of age, 240 mg piperacillin/kg/d, divided into doses administered every 8 hours; ≥9 months of age, 300 mg piperacillin/kg/d, divided into doses administered every 8 hours; maximum, 16 g piperacillin/d)
- IV cefepime (150 mg/kg/d, divided into doses administered every 8 hours; maximum, 2 g per dose)
- IV meropenem (60 mg/kg/d, divided into doses administered every 8 hours; maximum, 1 g per dose)
- IV imipenem/cilastatin (60–100 mg/kg/d, divided into doses administered every 6 hours; maximum, 4 g/d)

Add a secondary agent, depending on the probable source of infection. For example, add vancomycin if the patient has a central line infection. Also expand coverage if the likelihood of resistant organisms is high or if the patient is not improving after at least 24 hours of adequate treatment. Add fungal coverage if the fever persists for more than 5 days of broad-spectrum antibacterial administration, without an identified source.

The organism and site of infection determine the duration of antibiotic use. Transition to oral antibiotics once the patient is clinically well and showing signs of marrow recovery. If no source is identified, continue treatment until the patient is no longer severely neutropenic (ANC >500 cells/μL), culture results are negative for at least 48 hours, and the patient is afebrile for at least 24 hours.

Disposition

- **Intensive care unit transfer:** Hemodynamic instability, septic shock
- **Discharge criteria:** ANC >500 cells/µL, patient afebrile for ≥24 hours, culture results negative for ≥48 hours, antibiotics no longer needed, and patient transitioned to an oral regimen

Follow-up

- **Primary care:** 1 week if benign or if transient cause suspected; check the CBC with differential twice weekly for 6 to 8 weeks to evaluate the patient for resolution and/or patterns of recurrence
- **Hematology/oncology:** 1 to 2 weeks, depending on the final diagnosis

Pearls and Pitfalls

- Infants between the ages of 1 month and 1 year can have ANC values as low as 1,000 cells/µL and be considered normal.
- Standard precautions, including hand hygiene and infection-specific precautions/isolation, are sufficient for hospitalized neutropenic patients. Neither reverse isolation nor strict neutropenic diets are of any benefit.

Bibliography

Boxer LA. How to approach neutropenia. *Hematol Am Soc Hematol Educ Program*. 2012; 2012:174–182

Dinauer MC, Newburger PE, Borregaard N. The phagocyte system and disorders of granulopoiesis and granulocyte function. In: Orkin SH, Fisher DE, Ginsburg D, Look AT, Lux SE, Nathan DG, eds. *Hematology of Infancy and Childhood*. 8th ed. Philadelphia, PA: Elsevier Saunders; 2015:773–848

Freifeld AG, Bow EJ, Sepkowitz KA, et al. Clinical practice guideline for the use of antimicrobial agents in neutropenic patients with cancer: 2010 update by the Infectious Diseases Society of America. *Clin Infect Dis*. 2011;52(4):e56–e93

Lehrnbecher T, Phillips R, Alexander S, et al. Guideline for the management of fever and neutropenia in children with cancer and/or undergoing hematopoietic stem-cell transplantation. *J Clin Oncol*. 2012;30(35):4427–4438

Walkovich KJ, Newburger PE. Leukopenia. In: Kliegman RM, Stanton BF, St Geme JW III, Schor NF, eds. *Nelson Textbook of Pediatrics*. 20th ed. Philadelphia, PA: Elsevier Saunders; 2016:1047–1053

Sickle Cell Disease

Introduction

Sickle cell disease (SCD) is an inherited hematologic disorder characterized by having genes for 2 abnormal hemoglobins that result in the sickling of red cells because of the polymerization of the abnormal deoxyhemoglobin S molecule. The clinical features of the disease then result from chronic hemolysis, as well as end-organ insult secondary to vaso-occlusion and vascular injury. The homozygous hemoglobin SS state is the most common and severe form of SCD, but similar manifestations may occur when the heterozygous hemoglobin S is combined with an alternative hemoglobin abnormality, such as in the conditions of hemoglobin SC (also known as *sickle hemoglobin C disease*) or hemoglobin S β-thalassemia.

The common complications of SCD that lead to hospitalization are infection, including a serious bacterial infection such as sepsis and osteomyelitis, vaso-occlusive crisis (VOC), acute chest syndrome (ACS), stroke, splenic sequestration crisis, aplastic crisis, acute cholecystitis, and, rarely, priapism. A patient with SCD has splenic dysfunction and is therefore at high risk for invasive infection from encapsulated organisms, particularly *Streptococcus pneumoniae*. In addition, there is an increased risk for osteomyelitis from *Salmonella* species and *Staphylococcus aureus*. A patient with SCD is also at increased risk for VOC and ACS after receiving general anesthesia.

Other serious but rare complications include hyperhemolysis, hepatic sequestration, multi-organ failure, orbital compartment syndrome, and subarachnoid hemorrhage.

Clinical Presentation

The presentations of the most common complications of SCD are summarized in Table 50-1, and the serious rare complications are presented in Table 50-2.

History

Ask about the patient's usual blood count levels (hemoglobin, white blood cell count, reticulocyte count), daily medications (penicillin, folate, hydroxyurea), history of ACS, recent surgeries (especially splenectomy), history of asthma, prior transfusions (and the indications), transcranial Doppler ultrasonography (US) results, and the name of the physician (usually a hematologist) managing the SCD. Increased risk factors for ACS include history of asthma, prior

Table 50-1. Common Complications of Sickle Cell Disease	
Diagnosis	**Clinical Features**
Acute chest syndrome	Fever, cough, tachypnea, chest pain Hypoxia New lobar or segmental infiltrate on chest radiographs
Acute cholecystitis Choledocholithiasis	Fever in acute cholecystitis Right upper quadrant abdominal pain (+) Murphy sign
Aplastic crisis	Pallor, fatigue, tachypnea, tachycardia with or without hypotension No ↑ in spleen size ↓ Hemoglobin level (from baseline) with ↓ reticulocyte level (<1%–2%)
Bacteremia/sepsis	Fever Toxicity/patient ill appearing ↑ or ↓ White blood cell count (compared to baseline)
Hepatic sequestration (rare)	Pallor Enlarging liver, right upper quadrant tenderness, ↑ ALT and AST levels ↓ Hemoglobin level (from baseline), normal or ↑ reticulocyte level
Osteomyelitis	Fever Bone pain localized or located at an atypical site
Priapism	Painful erection lasting >4 h
Splenic sequestration	Pallor, fatigue, tachypnea Tachycardia with or without hypotension Left upper quadrant tenderness Increasing palpable splenomegaly from baseline ↓ Hemoglobin level >2 g/dL (>20 g/L) (from baseline), normal or ↑reticulocyte level May also have thrombocytopenia
Stroke	Unilateral weakness or hemiparesis Altered mental status, seizures Slurred speech, aphasia Facial droop
Vaso-occlusive crisis	Acute pain at typical or multiple sites (extremities, chest, back) Occurs with or without fever (usually <38.6°C [<101.5°F])

Abbreviations: ALT, alanine aminotransferase; AST, aspartate aminotransferase; +, positive finding.

history of ACS, and recent surgeries, especially abdominal, which can be associated with poor respiratory effort.

The patient with an established diagnosis of SCD is often admitted for pain and/or fever. Determine the characteristics of the pain, such as location, quality, intensity, radiation, and alleviating and exacerbating factors, and compare these to the patient's typical pattern of sickle cell pain. Common locations for VOC pain are the extremities, abdomen, and back, but specifically note the presence of chest pain or any respiratory complaints. In addition, ask about the response to current and previous pain management strategies, in both

Table 50-2. Rare Serious Complications of Sickle Cell Disease	
Diagnosis	**Clinical Features**
Hyperhemolysis	Causes: RBC transfusion, drugs, infections, G6PD deficiency
	Pallor with worsening scleral icterus and jaundice
	↓ Hemoglobin level (from baseline), normal or reticulocyte level
	Dark, heme (+) urine without RBCs
Multi-organ failure	Confusion (nonfocal encephalopathy)
	Fever
	Rapid decrease in hemoglobin level and platelet count
	↑ AST, ALT, LDH, bilirubin, and creatinine levels
	Failure of lungs, liver, or kidneys
Orbital compartment syndrome (orbital bone infarct)	Eye pain
	Proptosis
Subarachnoid hemorrhage	"Worst headache of my life"
	Altered mental status

Abbreviations: ALT, alanine transaminase; AST, aspartate transaminase; G6PD, glucose-6-phosphate dehydrogenase; LDH, lactate dehydrogenase; RBC, red blood cell; +, positive finding.

inpatient and outpatient settings. Determine if there have been any recent stressors, exposure to cold, or viral illness symptoms, because these are common triggers for a VOC. Note the duration and height of the fever and any measures taken to manage it.

Physical Examination

Priorities at examination are the vital signs, because sepsis is the primary consideration when there is fever higher than 38.5°C (>101.3°F). Tachycardia and tachypnea can occur in ACS, aplastic crisis, and splenic sequestration. Look for other signs of ACS (accessory muscle use, adventitious lung sounds), aplastic crisis (pallor, heart failure), and splenic sequestration (hypovolemic shock). In addition, tachycardia may be secondary to pain, so recheck the vital signs after appropriate analgesia has been administered and reassess the pain level frequently.

Compare the degree of scleral icterus, jaundice, splenomegaly, and location(s) of bone pain to the patient's baseline or typical findings. Palpate areas of pain by paying close attention to the long bones, looking for areas of point tenderness that may suggest a focal inflammatory process. Examine the abdomen for tenderness, distention, organomegaly (spleen and liver), and tenderness over the right upper quadrant (gallbladder). Check the genitourinary area in male subjects if there is a concern for priapism. Perform a complete neurologic examination if there are any neurologic symptoms or a change in mental status.

Laboratory Findings and Radiology Examinations

Obtain a complete blood cell count and reticulocyte count and compare the results to the patient's usual values to look for leukocytosis or leukopenia (compared to the patient's typical baseline values), worsening anemia, thrombocytopenia, or bone marrow suppression. Evaluate electrolyte levels, creatinine level, liver function test results, and C-reactive protein (CRP) level if indicated by clinical findings.

If the patient has a temperature higher than 38.5°C (>101.3°F), also order a blood culture, urinalysis, and urine culture (all female and male patients <12 months of age). Obtain a chest radiograph and blood culture if the patient has lower respiratory symptoms and/or chest pain possibly consistent with ACS. When osteomyelitis is a diagnostic consideration, obtain a blood culture, CRP level and/or erythrocyte sedimentation rate, and magnetic resonance (MR) images of the bone.

If there are concerns for a stroke, order emergent MR imaging/MR angiography (MRA) if the patient is stable enough to tolerate the examination. However, do not delay treatment if a stroke is suspected clinically. Computed tomography of the head is an alternative if MR imaging/MRA is not available.

When there is a concern for hepatobiliary disease (acute cholecystitis, choledocholithiasis), perform US of the right upper abdominal quadrant, as well as MR cholangiopancreatography (if available) or endoscopic retrograde cholangiopancreatography. Also perform abdominal US to visualize the spleen when splenic sequestration is suspected but the spleen is not palpable.

When transfusion might be needed (aplastic crisis, splenic sequestration, ACS, stroke), perform blood typing that includes minor antigens C, D, E, and Kell. Confirm that the blood used for transfusions is sickle negative, leukocyte reduced, matched for the selected minor antigens, and, ideally, irradiated.

Differential Diagnosis

A patient may present with an acute disease that is unrelated to the SCD, such as appendicitis or asthma. Always maintain a broad differential diagnosis and do not assume that the patient's complaints are secondary to SCD.

The most common diagnostic challenge involves the combination of pain and fever. Depending on location of the pain, the differential diagnosis includes infection, VOC, ACS, and osteomyelitis. While both VOC and osteomyelitis appear with pain and swelling in the affected bone(s) at presentation, the pain of osteomyelitis tends to localize to a single site that may represent an atypical location for the patient.

Chest pain associated with fever, cough, wheezing, and tachypnea suggests ACS. A new lobar or segmental infiltrate is required to confirm the diagnosis.

Rule out other potentially life-threatening complications, such as aplastic crisis, hyperhemolysis, and splenic or hepatic sequestration. Pallor, fatigue, tachycardia, and tachypnea occur with aplastic crisis and splenic sequestration. Left upper quadrant abdominal pain can occur with splenic sequestration, while right upper quadrant pain is seen with cholelithiasis, choledocholithiasis, pancreatitis (from gallstones), or hepatic sequestration.

Neurologic signs, such as change in mental status, facial droop, lateralized weakness, aphasia, or slurred speech, may occur with a stroke.

Treatment

Acute Chest Syndrome

Manage pain aggressively (see the Vaso-occlusive Crisis section in this chapter), add orally administered (per os, or PO) azithromycin (10 mg/kg/d, 1,500-mg maximum; 5 mg/kg/d for 4 more days, 250-mg maximum) to the antibiotic regimen described for fever (see the Fever/Presumed Sepsis section in this chapter), and provide oxygen to maintain oxygen saturation at 92% or higher, while encouraging the use of incentive spirometry. If the patient has wheezing or rales, add nebulized albuterol (2.5 mg if the patient weighs <30 kg and 5 mg if the patient weighs >30 kg, every 4–6 hours), methylpred-nisolone 1–2 mg/kg every 12 hours (60-mg/d maximum) or intramuscular (IM), IV, or PO dexamethasone 0.3–0.6 mg/kg once (16-mg maximum) and gastrointestinal prophylaxis with IM/IV ranitidine (2–6 mg/kg/d, divided into doses administered every 6–8 hours; maximum, 50 mg per dose). However, consult with a hematologist before initiating the systemic steroids, as they have been associated with rebound vaso-occlusive episodes and hemorrhagic stroke. Assess the hemoglobin level every 12 hours until it is stable.

If the patient has worsening respiratory symptoms, such as decreased air movement, inspiratory and expiratory wheezing, increasing use of accessory muscles, increasing oxygen requirements, and a hemoglobin concentration more than 1 g/dL (>10 g/L) below baseline, consult with a hematologist to consider a simple transfusion (10 mL/kg packed red blood cells [RBCs]) to a goal hemoglobin level of 9 to 10 g/dL (90–100 g/L) and transfer the patient to an intensive care unit (ICU). Avoid transfusing to a target hemoglobin level higher than 10 g/dL (>100 g/L) to prevent hyperviscosity. Arrange for an exchange transfusion or erythrocytapheresis if there is increasing respiratory distress, persistent oxygen saturation below 90% with supplemental oxygen, worsening pulmonary infiltrates, and continued decrease in hemoglobin concentration after simple transfusion.

Acute Cholecystitis/Cholelithiasis/Hepatic Sequestration

The treatment for biliary disease is the same as for a patient without SCD (see Chapter 36, Gallbladder Disease). Arrange a surgery consult, give the patient nothing by mouth, provide analgesia, and administer antibiotic coverage for gram-negative bacilli and anaerobes. Although urgent surgery may be necessary for worsening pain and fever, cholecystectomy (preferably laparoscopic) is usually performed electively after resolution of the acute episode. For hepatic sequestration, perform a simple or exchange transfusion after consultation with a hematologist.

Aplastic Crisis

The goal of therapy is to prevent cardiovascular compromise secondary to the worsening anemia. If stable, monitor the patient closely and provide IV and PO hydration at maintenance levels until blood is available. If the hemoglobin level is less than 5 g/dL (<50 g/L), transfuse 10 mL/kg of packed RBCs over 4 hours with an expected increase of 2 g/dL (20 g/L) in the hemoglobin level and a goal of achieving a near-baseline hemoglobin level. If the patient is not stable, admit to an ICU and initiate fluid resuscitation while awaiting transfusion. Assume that the patient has a parvoviral infection (pending serologic examination findings) and institute appropriate isolation policies.

Fever/Presumed Sepsis

For the febrile (>38.5°C [>101.3°F]) patient, administer parenteral antibiotics that cover *S pneumoniae* and gram-negative organisms immediately after blood cultures are performed. Do not delay initiating therapy while awaiting laboratory results. Treat with IV cefotaxime (150 mg/kg/d, divided into doses administered every 8 hours; 6-g/d maximum) *or* ceftriaxone (50–100 mg/kg/d, divided into doses administered every 12 hours; 4-g/d maximum) *or* ampicillin/sulbactam (100 mg/kg/d of ampicillin divided into doses administered every 6 hours; 8-g/d maximum) per local antibiotic susceptibilities. If the patient has a known allergy to cephalosporin or penicillin, use IV clindamycin (40 mg/kg/d, divided into doses administered every 6 hours; 4.8-g/d maximum). If the patient is ill appearing or a central nervous system infection is suspected, add IV vancomycin (10–15 mg/kg every 6 hours, 4-g/d maximum).

The treatment of osteomyelitis in a patient with sickle cell disease is the same as for a normal host (see Chapter 97, Osteomyelitis). Administer antimicrobial coverage for both *S aureus* and group A *Streptococcus* with vancomycin and/or clindamycin, depending on the local prevalence of methicillin-resistant, as well as clindamycin-resistant, *Staphylococcus* bacteria. Whichever is prescribed, add ceftriaxone to treat possible *Salmonella* infection.

Priapism

The goals of care in priapism are to control the pain (see the Vaso-occlusive Crisis section in this chapter) and prevent ischemic damage. This requires close consultation with both a urologist and a hematologist. Initiate aggressive PO or IV fluid hydration immediately, along with PO and/or IV analgesia. Corporal aspiration, with or without irrigation, is indicated for persistent priapism that lasts more than 4 hours that is not responsive to fluid hydration and analgesia. If surgical correction is indicated, arrange for a preoperative transfusion.

Splenic Sequestration

The goal of treatment is to prevent the rapid progression of hypovolemic shock while awaiting the release of the blood trapped in the spleen. Transfer the patient to an ICU, consult with a hematologist, initiate IV fluid resuscitation if needed, and order a packed RBC transfusion of 5 to 10 mL/kg, generally over 4 hours, but deliver it more rapidly if the patient is in hypovolemic shock. Aim for a posttransfusion hemoglobin level of less than 9 g/dL (<90 g/L) to prevent hyperviscosity, because once the sequestered blood is returned from the spleen, the hemoglobin level may increase by another 1 to 2 g/dL (10–20 g/L). Obtain a surgical consult to arrange for splenectomy if the patient has had recurrent splenic sequestration episodes or symptomatic hypersplenism.

Stroke

Admit the patient to an ICU and consult with a hematologist to arrange emergent exchange transfusion or erythrocytapheresis. The goal is to increase the hemoglobin level to about 10 g/dL (100 g/L) and decrease the hemoglobin S level to less than 30%. Do not delay transfusion therapy while performing imaging studies and administer oxygen while awaiting the procedure. See Chapter 80, Acute Hemiparesis, for the general management of a stroke.

Vaso-occlusive Crisis

Since a patient admitted for VOC has not responded to home and/or outpatient pain management, use IV opioids via patient-controlled analgesia (PCA), continuous infusion, or scheduled interval dosing, with rescue doses available for breakthrough pain. Titrate the dose to an adequate therapeutic response, which is ideally a minimum of a 50% reduction in pain on the visual scale. Never initiate as-needed dosing alone for a patient with a VOC. A patient with previous opioid exposure may require higher than usual doses of opiates.

The preferred method is PCA, once a child is able to understand that pushing the button decreases pain. For most patients, this occurs by 6 years of age. A typical morphine PCA regimen starts with a total dose of 0.05 to 0.20 mg/kg/h. The usual basal (continuous) rate is one-third to one-half of this total hourly dose. Calculate the PCA dose (demand) by using the remainder of the total hourly dose and dividing it by the number of total potential doses (6–10) available over an hour. For example, using 0.1 mg/kg/h as the hourly dose, start with a basal rate of 0.033 mg/kg/h, with a 0.0067-mg/kg PCA dose permitted every 6 minutes. Therefore, for a 25-kg patient, the continuous rate is 0.8 mg/h with 0.17-mg PCA doses (up to 10 doses in 1 hour). Note that the PCA dose refers to the patient-controlled dose and has many synonyms, including *intermittent dose, interval dose, interval bolus,* and *demand dose.*

Re-evaluate the patient frequently. Additional physician-ordered rescue doses (0.05 mg/kg every 30 minutes) may be needed until the pain is adequately controlled. Readjust the basal and PCA doses every 12 to 24 hours, basing any changes on the total amount of morphine given to control the pain over that period. Increase the basal rate if the patient demands more than 3 PCA doses per hour and decrease the basal rate if the patient appears oversedated. When the pain is well controlled for 24 hours and the patient is using fewer than 3 PCA doses per hour, begin weaning the patient off of the medication by decreasing the basal dose by 10% to 20%, as tolerated.

For a patient unable to use PCA, order scheduled interval dosing of morphine (0.05–0.15 mg/kg every 2–4 hours), although a continuous infusion (0.05–0.10 mg/kg/h) is an acceptable alternative. Treat breakthrough pain with 25% to 50% of the interval dose every 20 to 30 minutes, as needed. Readjust the dose based on the total amount of medication needed to control the pain over time. In some cases, a morphine administration rate greater than 0.1 mg/kg/h may be needed, but this requires careful monitoring for respiratory depression by assessing the respiratory rate, level of sedation, and pulse oximetry. If possible, manage opioid-associated respiratory failure with ventilatory support (bag-valve-mask). The use of naloxone (0.1 mg/kg) may be lifesaving in treating respiratory failure, but it will also reverse pain control. When the pain is well controlled for 24 hours, begin weaning the patient off of the medication by decreasing the infusion or scheduled dosing by 10% to 20%.

Aggressively treat the side effects of opioids. Manage nausea with IV/PO ondansetron (0.05–0.10 mg/kg every 6 hours as needed; maximum, 4 mg per dose) or IV/PO metoclopramide (0.1–0.2 mg/kg every 6–8 hours; maximum, 10 mg per dose). Treat pruritus with either PO diphenhydramine (5 mg/kg/d, divided into doses administered every 6 hours, or 0.5 mg/kg every 2 hours; 300-mg/d maximum) or PO hydroxyzine (2 mg/kg/d, divided into doses administered every 8 hours; 50-mg/d maximum if patient aged <6 years, 100-mg/d maximum if patient aged >6 years, 600-mg/d maximum for adults) or change to IV hydromorphone (0.015–0.020 mg/kg every 3–4 hours). Start a bowel regimen (stool softeners, docusate, polyethylene glycol) if multiple opiate doses are anticipated.

Intravenous (IV) ketorolac (0.5 mg/kg every 6 hours; maximum, 30 mg per dose) is a useful adjunct if there are no contraindications (gastritis, ulcer, coagulopathy, renal impairment). Do not use for more than 5 days.

Begin the transition to oral opioids at an equianalgesic dosing level (see Chapter 115, Pain Management) when the pain is well controlled, the IV morphine dose has been tapered to 0.25 mg/kg/h or less, and the patient has normal gastrointestinal functioning (able to eat and drink without being nauseated). One approach is to first convert the basal rate to the equivalent dose of a long-acting oral opioid, then 24 hours later convert the PCA dose to an equivalent short-acting oral opioid.

To prevent withdrawal symptoms for a patient whose pain has resolved but who has been receiving opioids for 10 days or more, first taper the opioid dose by 10% to 20% per day, as tolerated, with close monitoring, over 5 to 7 days. Then, over the next 3 to 5 days, increase the interval from every 6 hours to every 12 hours to every day.

Supportive therapy includes the correction of any fluid-deficit dehydration, as well as providing (IV and/or PO) maintenance fluid. There is no evidence that increased hydration is helpful, and overhydration can lead to fluid overload; therefore, provide no more than maintenance IV hydration to a euvolemic patient. Provide oxygen as needed to maintain oxygen saturation at 92% or higher. Also order incentive spirometry (10 breaths every 2 hours when awake) and encourage early ambulation to prevent ACS. Other comfort measures include use of heating pads and relaxation techniques.

Rare Complications

Immediately consult with a hematologist if the patient has one of the rare complications listed in Table 50-2. The critical challenge for the hospitalist is to recognize these rare problems as they develop in a patient with SCD who is admitted for another reason.

Patient Requiring General Anesthesia

Order incentive spirometry and perioperative oxygen. Also perform a preoperative transfusion to raise the hemoglobin level to at least 10 g/dL (≥100 g/L) to minimize the risk of VOC or ACS.

Indications for Consultation

- **Hematology:** ACS, splenic sequestration, acute aplastic crisis, hyperhemolysis, priapism, possible cerebral vascular accident, pain difficult to manage
- **Neurology:** Possible cerebral vascular accident
- **Ophthalmology:** Orbital compartment syndrome
- **Surgery:** Consideration of cholecystectomy for gall bladder disease or splenectomy for splenic sequestration
- **Urology:** Priapism lasting more than 4 hours

Disposition

- **ICU transfer:** Septic shock, ACS requiring respiratory support, acute cerebral vascular accident, need for exchange transfusion
- **Discharge criteria:** Septicemia excluded (patient afebrile with negative blood culture results), pain adequately managed with oral medications, ongoing complications (ACS, cerebral vascular accident, etc), patient stable and no longer requiring inpatient interventions

Follow-up

- **Primary care:** 1 to 2 weeks
- **Sickle cell center/pain specialist:** 1 week

Pearls and Pitfalls

- Care coordination between the inpatient and outpatient setting in conjunction with a sickle cell center and pain specialist is essential for the best long-term outcome in a patient with SCD.
- Be careful with fluid administration, because a patient in a chronic high output state secondary to anemia is susceptible to fluid overload and pulmonary edema. This can be difficult to differentiate from ACS.
- As with any immunosuppressed patient, the child's appearance may belie the serious clinical situation.
- If possible, transfuse with minor antigen–matched (C, D, E, Kell), sickle-negative, leukocyte-depleted, packed RBCs.
- A packed RBC transfusion of 10 mL/kg typically increases the hemoglobin level by 2 g/dL (20 g/L).
- Do not transfuse to a hemoglobin level greater than 11 g/dL (>110 g/L), which may then result in hyperviscosity.
- Opioid-induced sedation precedes respiratory depression.

Bibliography

Abbas HA, Kahale M, Hosn MA, Inati A. A review of acute chest syndrome in pediatric sickle cell disease. *Pediatr Ann*. 2013;42(3):115–120

Crabtree EA, Mariscalco MM, Hesselgrave J, et al. Improving care for children with sickle cell disease/acute chest syndrome. *Pediatrics*. 2011;127(2):e480–e488

Kanter J, Kruse-Jarres R. Management of sickle cell disease from childhood through adulthood. *Blood Rev*. 2013;27(6):279–287

Martí-Carvajal AJ, Agreda-Pérez LH. Antibiotics for treating osteomyelitis in people with sickle cell disease. *Cochrane Database Syst Rev*. 2012;12:CD007175

Miller AC, Gladwin MT. Pulmonary complications of sickle cell disease. *Am J Respir Crit Care Med*. 2012;185(11):1154–1165

New England Pediatric Sickle Cell Consortium. Management of acute pain in pediatric patients with sickle cell disease (vaso-occlusive episodes). http://www.nepscc.org/NewFiles/CPG%20Pain%203-09.pdf. Accessed February 6, 2017

Yawn BP, Buchanan GR, Afenyi-Annan AN, et al. Management of sickle cell disease: summary of the 2014 evidence-based report by expert panel members. *JAMA*. 2014;312(10):1033–1048

Hospitalist Practice

Comanagement

Overview

The Society for Hospital Medicine defines *comanagement* as a system of care featuring "shared responsibility, authority, and accountability" for hospitalized patients. Although comanagement originally referred primarily to shared care between hospitalists and surgeons, many programs now involve comanagement between hospitalists and pediatric subspecialists. Because surgical comanagement programs are generally more established, this chapter will focus on those types of programs.

Comanagement programs may refer to a spectrum of care models, from "traditional" consultation to true shared responsibility for care. In traditional consultation, a consulting physician or team sees a patient for a specific clinical reason, documents clinical recommendations, and then has variable ongoing involvement in the case. In comanagement models, the comanaging physician team typically represents a more consistent presence, develops an ongoing relationship with the patient and family, and follows the patient until discharge from the hospital. In some comanagement models, the comanaging physician may make certain medical decisions, write orders, and consult a third service.

Comanagement models offer several potential benefits for patients and hospital systems. Regarding clinical outcomes, comanagement may reduce length of hospital stay, safety incidents, and complication rates, while improving access to clinicians. Patients may also undergo fewer medical interventions, such as parenteral nutrition and laboratory studies. The nursing staff may prefer comanagement because of more consistent access to a pediatric provider who has an ongoing relationship with the patient. Comanagement can also promote patient- and family-centered care through information sharing with patients and families, facilitating active family involvement in the patient's care, and coordinating with the patient's medical home and subspecialists.

Comanagement may also confer benefits to hospital systems. Surgeons and subspecialists may have more time to operate, see outpatients, or perform specialized procedures, since hospitalists, as dedicated inpatient providers, can expediently manage many postoperative issues. Comanaging hospitalists are more likely to identify system issues and engage in quality improvement efforts for surgical or subspecialty patients. As a result of their constant presence, hospitalists can often improve communication, thereby mitigating one of the major factors in malpractice suits and potentially reducing institutional risk.

Structure of Comanagement Programs

Defining and identifying which types of patients are candidates for comanagement remain challenging. The American Academy of Pediatrics suggests that patients younger than 14 years or those weighing less than 40 kg who are being cared for by providers without pediatric training or experience would benefit by having a pediatric-trained provider involved in their care. Thus, in a community hospital, all children undergoing surgery may be appropriate for comanagement. In contrast, in a tertiary care hospital, collaborative agreements may help identify which patients receive comanagement and further delineate the nature of the comanagement relationship. These patients may include those with severe functional limitations or comorbidities, those with technology dependence, or those whose care involves multiple medical subspecialists. These medically complex patients are known to be at high risk for surgical complications, medical errors, readmissions, and increased costs.

Team structure and patient volume may also influence comanagement models. Models that involve a dedicated comanagement hospitalist (surgical or specialist) may offer some advantages over traditional hospitalist–house staff teams in terms of developing competences, rapport, and skills. Two common, but not definitive, examples of comanagement models for orthopedic surgery patients are outlined in Table 51-1.

Keys for Building an Effective Comanagement Relationship

The principles of comanagement are generally not included in a pediatric residency curriculum, although resources do exist. Hospitalists may need to develop new knowledge and skills in specific surgical or subspecialty areas as they enter into a comanagement program. Ongoing professional development in conjunction with primary teams will build knowledge and rapport for both groups.

Initial Goals

- Identify hospitalist, subspecialty, and surgical champions of comanagement
- Articulate program rationale and structure
- Gain hospital leadership support and define resources, including hospitalist salary when overhead is not met by professional billing
- Determine the frequency of reviewing the comanagement arrangement
- Define meaningful metrics

Table 51-1. Comanagement Examples for Surgical Patients in Different Settings		
Type of Care	**Child with <2 Chronic Conditions at a Community Hospital (Surgeon Off-Site)**	**Child with Special Health Care Needs at a Tertiary Care Hospital (Surgical Team With Advanced Practice Nurse, Trainees)**
Primary attending physician	Hospitalist	Surgeon
Team member	Hospitalist and surgeon	Surgeon, trainees, advanced practice providers Hospitalist with or without pediatric house staff
Daily management and rounding	Hospitalist with or without a surgeon	Both teams
Wound care	Surgeon	Surgeon
Drain management	Surgeon	Surgeon
Diet advancement	Hospitalist	Surgeon or hospitalist
Overall nutritional status	Hospitalist	Hospitalist
Fever workup/ management	Shared	Shared
Management of chronic or acute respiratory problems	Hospitalist	Hospitalist
Pain management	Hospitalist	Surgeon or hospitalist
Coordination of care	Hospitalist	Surgeon or hospitalist

Clarify, With the Expectation to Revise

- Clinical care responsibilities, defined as either exclusive or as a shared responsibility between the hospitalist and surgeon/specialist
- Documentation expectations: daily versus as-needed notes
- Legal attending of record: Which is the ultimate primary service?
- Expectations for type of daily patient care communications among surgeon/specialist, hospitalist, and nursing staff: in-person/rounding, verbal, written, text, e-mail (always Health Insurance Portability and Accountability Act compliant)
- Determine appropriate billing approach, which varies according to state insurance regulations: billing independently versus as part of a bundled payment (surgical patients)
- Codify these items in a written service agreement, a document that formalizes the provisions

Communicate Roles

Communicate with nursing, family, and trainees the roles and responsibilities of the hospitalist in the patient's care.

Maintain, Improve, and Measure the Program

- Regularly evaluate comanagement arrangements
- Provide a thorough orientation for new group members
- Track and routinely review program metrics, including quality of care and financial data
- Collaboratively develop and implement clinical pathways
- Jointly review cases

Pearls and Pitfalls

- When establishing a comanagement program, be sure to involve all stakeholders, which may include surgeons, nurses, hospitalists, families, and others.
- Whenever possible, establish joint daily rounding with hospitalists, surgeons, and subspecialists.
- Avoid allowing comanagement to develop "mission creep," whereby hospitalists assume the duties of the surgeons, advance practice providers, and trainees.
- Recognize that the initial costs associated with the program may increase.
- Communication among providers and the patient/family is central to success. Miscommunication and lack of clarity concerning "who is in charge" can cause anxiety, dissatisfaction, and delayed care.
- When developing a comanagement program, consider the needs of learners, such as residents and fellows.
- Recognize possible ethical issues surrounding automatic consults and reimbursement mechanisms.
- A comanagement program may not be able to financially support itself but may represent a "loss leader." Some cost savings, such as surgeons' time and reductions in complications, may not be easily quantifiable.

Bibliography

MedEdPORTAL. Management of postoperative pediatric patients. https://www.mededportal.org/publication/10241. Accessed February 6, 2017

Rappaport DI, Adelizzi-Delany J, Rogers KJ, et al. Outcomes and costs associated with hospitalist comanagement of medically complex children undergoing spinal fusion surgery. *Hosp Pediatr*. 2013;3(3):233–241

Rappaport DI, Rosenberg RE, Shaughnessy EE, et al. Pediatric hospitalist comanagement of surgical patients: structural, quality, and financial considerations. *J Hosp Med*. 2014;9(11):737–742

Rohatgi N, Loftus P, Grujic O, Cullen M, Hopkins J, Ahuja N. Surgical comanagement by hospitalists improves patient outcomes: a propensity score analysis. *Ann Surg*. 2016;264(2):275–282

Schaffzin JK, Simon TD. Pediatric hospital medicine role in the comanagement of the hospitalized surgical patient. *Pediatr Clin North Am*. 2014;61(4):653–661

The Society of Hospital Medicine's (SHM) Co-Management Advisory Panel. A white paper on a guide to hospitalist/orthopedic surgery co-management. http://tools.hospitalmedicine.org/Implementation/Co-ManagementWhitePaper-final_5-10-10.pdf. Accessed February 6, 2017

Cultural Effectiveness

Introduction

The American Academy of Pediatrics (AAP) advocates for care that is accessible, continuous, comprehensive, family centered, coordinated, compassionate, and culturally effective. While these principles are often discussed with respect to pediatric medical homes, they are equally relevant in pediatric hospital medicine, particularly for a population that is increasingly diverse. As such, pediatric hospitalists need to efficiently gather essential information and quickly establish a rapport with patients and their families. Respecting patients' and parents' culture is at the core of this relationship.

Cross-Cultural Health Care Terminology

Culturally effective care is defined as "the delivery of care within the context of appropriate physician knowledge, understanding, and appreciation of all cultural distinctions leading to optimal health outcomes." The practice of culturally effective care is essential to develop the patient- and parent-physician relationships, reduce health care disparities, and promote the health of the patient beyond hospital discharge.

Cultural competency focuses on the acquisition of the knowledge, skills, and attitudes about sociocultural factors to provide high-quality health care. While cultural competence is the foundation of cultural effectiveness, one limitation of competence is that it implies a static outcome. To deliver optimal care to diverse patients, health care providers need to continuously refine their abilities to care for diverse populations.

Key Concepts in Culturally Effective Care

Culture goes beyond race and ethnicity. Religion, sex, age, politics, sexual orientation, socioeconomic status, education, and many other factors (eg, hearing or visual impairment) can shape culture.

Differences *within* races, ethnicities, and cultures can be more pronounced than differences *across* them. For example, low-income, inner-city African American and white families may face comparable barriers to accessing care versus what is experienced by a higher-income African American or white household. Similarly, even amongst people of the same ethnicity, such as Hispanics, there are significant cultural differences across countries of origin. Making inferences about individuals from certain backgrounds based on previous experiences and deductions of the group to which those individuals belong contributes to bias and is a barrier to culturally effective care.

Health care providers must exhibit cultural humility in caring for an increasingly diverse patient population. This is expressed by demonstrating receptiveness and respect in all patient encounters.

Culturally Effective Care in Practice

Provider Education

In addition to practicing the key concepts listed earlier, providers must remain committed to acquiring cross-cultural training and to role-modeling these skills for learners and staff. The AAP *Culturally Effective Care Toolkit* contains resources for providers, many of which are applicable to the inpatient setting.

Linguistic Services

Assess every patient and family for limited English proficiency (LEP) by using the simple two-part U.S. Census screener:

1. Does this person speak a language other than English at home: ☐ Yes ☐ No
   a. If Yes, what is this language:
2. How well does this person speak English?
   ☐ Very well
   ☐ Well
   ☐ Not well
   ☐ Not at all

If a patient is screened as having LEP, always provide a trained professional medical interpreter or bilingual provider, ideally in the patient's and parents' language of choice. Allow additional time for the use of interpretive services, preferably with live personnel. However, in many cases, video remote interpretation services or telephone interpreters may be the only option, depending on the language needed and other hospital issues. Note that it is a Joint Commission standard that pediatric inpatient services have one of these linguistic services available to support effective communication. In addition, have prescriptions and discharge instructions professionally translated.

Patient Interviews

In addition to communicating with patients and parents in their preferred languages, providers can routinely incorporate additional questions and techniques in the medical history to elicit cultural influences. Examples include asking the patient or parent what they believe is causing the illness and what therapies were used at home to treat the illness, while allowing them to fully describe their concerns without interruption. It is important that these be implemented for all patients, not specific patients based on implicit biases. Several models exist to facilitate open dialogue between patients, parents, and their health care providers. One such model is "RESPECT" (Table 52-1).

Table 52-1. RESPECT Model	
Respect	Convey respect for the patient and family
Explain	Use an explanatory model of the illness, where the patient/parents explain their ideas of what is causing the condition and what treatment may entail
Social context	Understand the patient's social context, including strengths, support networks, stressors, and spirituality
Power	Equalize the power in the relationship, including seeking the patient's and parents' input in decision making
Empathy	Convey empathy in the patient encounter
Concerns	Elicit underlying concerns and fears
Trust	Determine and enhance the trust level and come to an agreement on shared goals

Adapted from Mostow C, Crosson J, Gordon S, et al. Treating and precepting with RESPECT: a relational model addressing race, ethnicity, and culture in medical training. *J Gen Intern Med*. 2010;25(Suppl 2):S146–S154, with permission of Springer.

Staff/Health Care Provider Diversity

Staff and providers whose cultural backgrounds are comparable to those of the local patient population can serve as cultural brokers, linking patients and providers with dissimilar backgrounds. There is an increase in trust building when patients are able to engage with medical team members from similar backgrounds. However, this is not always possible, and cultural humility is essential in patient interactions.

Hospital/Community-Based Partnerships

It is often valuable for hospitals to develop relationships with local community-based organizations. These partnerships can provide resources for specific areas of need in providing culturally effective care, such as hiring an interpreter for a particular language or building rapport with certain cultural groups.

In summary, pediatric hospitalists care for an increasingly diverse patient population and must be able to develop rapport with families during a time of a high stress. Delivering culturally effective care is not only a guiding principle but is essential for high-quality patient care. Providers must demonstrate a professional commitment to ongoing cross-cultural training, recognize culture beyond race and ethnicity, remain aware of their own cultural influences in the patient-provider relationship, and approach all patient encounters with cultural humility.

Bibliography

American Academy of Pediatrics. Culturally Effective Care Toolkit. https://www.aap. org/en-us/professional-resources/practice-transformation/managing-patients/Pages/ effective-care.aspx. Accessed February 6, 2017

Kumagai AK, Lypson ML. Beyond cultural competence: critical consciousness, social justice, and multicultural education. *Acad Med*. 2009;84(6):782–787

Mostow C, Crosson J, Gordon S, et al. Treating and precepting with RESPECT: a relational model addressing race, ethnicity, and culture in medical training. *J Gen Intern Med*. 2010;25(Suppl 2):S146–S154

Powell Sears K. Improving cultural competence education: the utility of an intersectional framework. *Med Educ*. 2012;46(6):545–551

Disaster Preparedness

Background

A disaster is an event that destroys property, includes injury and/or loss of life, and affects a large population or area. It is unplanned, sudden, and unpredictable, with enormous effects on the community response system. This necessitates constant preparation for these low-frequency, high-risk events.

All institutions, including those without dedicated pediatric and trauma care, may care for critically ill and injured children in a disaster, because victims will be brought to a local, convenient hospital and not necessarily transported to a pediatric center further away. During a disaster, the emergency triage system has a new focus to optimize the care of the population versus concentrating on the best interests of the individual.

A recent survey found that less than 50% of U.S. hospitals reported having a written disaster plan to address issues specific to the care of children. Hospitals that were more prepared to care for children involved a pediatric emergency care coordinator (PECC). The PECC focuses on the state of the emergency department (ED), with an emphasis on pediatric quality improvement, patient safety, and ensuring supply and equipment availability. Since the pediatric hospitalist may be the only pediatrician in the facility, the hospitalist is an ideal person to fill this role.

Disaster preparedness is a vital role for the hospitalist, who can promote awareness and advise key hospital personnel. The Emergency Medical Services for Children Innovation and Improvement Center (https://emscimprovement. center/) and the National Pediatric Readiness Project (https://emscimprovement. center/projects/pediatricreadiness/) offer essential resources that can assist clinicians in becoming knowledgeable about this issue.

Surge Planning and Alternative Care Sites

Facilities should have about a 30% surge capacity. The pediatric hospitalist may be asked to assist with surge capacity in a variety of ways, including evaluating low-acuity patients in the ED or caring for more inpatients than there are beds available. Identifying, in advance, alternatives within the facility can help to manage the surge. An example of an alternative care site could be the transformation of a postanesthesia care unit into an inpatient unit or a parking garage into a screening facility.

Evacuation Considerations

The TRAIN (Triage by Resource Allocation for IN-patient) matrix, developed by Lucile Packard Children's Hospital, can help in the determination of the transportation needs of pediatric inpatients in the event of an evacuation, as well as the identification of which patients may be safely discharged. Recalculate the patients' scores daily.

Organize a disaster "go bag" with pediatric essentials, in case an evacuation does occur. This might include a bulb suction syringe, intravenous start kits, aerochambers, and appropriately sized respiratory equipment, amongst other items. Be sure to check the expiration dates of the equipment periodically. Attach to the go bag a list of last-minute perishables that can be added before evacuation. Because the hospital may have already organized adult-specific go bags, coordination of disaster evacuation efforts is key.

Since many community hospitals do not have pediatric intensive care services, preemptively establish transfer agreements with facilities that do have such services. Telehealth can virtually bring specialists to the community, serving as an important conduit with the children's hospital. This may be especially vital during a disaster, when resources for transport to children's hospitals are scarce.

Family Reunification

Only about one-third of hospitals have a family reunification plan, which is essential in times of disaster. When a disaster occurs, there will be children who arrive at the hospital with injured family members who are not able to care for them, as well as discharged patients who are awaiting family members. Therefore, define and equip a safe area with adequate supervision and provisions, where children can be cared for until they are reunited with their families. Additionally, these children need identification bands, with a picture and a barcode if possible. Also, when an event occurs in a community, social media coverage may lead family and friends to arrive unexpectedly at a mass casualty event, so there also needs to be a plan for this response.

Drills

To function optimally during a disaster, hospitals and larger communities need to conduct disaster drills at least annually. Include a number of pediatric victims in these drills, proportionate to the number of children in the community (approximately 25%). It is essential to engage community pediatricians, emergency medical services, and other outside resources in these exercises, because they will serve an important role during an actual disaster. Adding family representatives with limited English proficiency or children with special medical needs can augment the realism of the simulation. Adolescents can serve as both mock victims and responders in a drill.

Disaster Preparedness Definitions

Disaster: When needs exceed resources; an event that destroys property, includes injury and/or loss of life, and affects a large population or area

Emergency management: The administrative group charged with creating policies and procedures through which facilities can reduce their vulnerability to hazards and improve their resiliency in disasters

Crisis standards of care: A drastic change in the routine practice of health care operations, including the highest level of care that can be achieved during a disaster

Four Phases of Disaster Management

Prevention: Activities that prevent future emergencies/disasters or minimize their effects; mitigation activities can occur before and after the emergency/disaster

Preparedness: Predisaster activities aimed at strengthening the ability to respond in times of disaster

Response: Emergency operation actions that occur during a disaster to save lives and prevent further damage to property

Recovery: Actions that occur after the disaster has ended to rebuild the community, so its members can function on their own, return to normal life, and protect against future hazards

Pearls and Pitfalls

- Disaster preparedness depends on day-to-day readiness, ideally under the supervision of a pediatric emergency care coordinator
- Family reunification planning must be included in facility disaster drills
- Hospitalists can play a key role in communicating to hospital administrators or emergency care coordinators the need for the facility to develop a pediatric disaster plan

Bibliography

American Academy of Pediatrics. Children & disasters. https://www.aap.org/Disasters. Accessed February 6, 2017

Disaster Information Management Research Center. Health resources on children in disasters and emergencies. https://disasterinfo.nlm.nih.gov/dimrc/children.html. Accessed February 6, 2017

Gausche-Hill M, Ely M, Schmuhl P, et al. A national assessment of pediatric readiness of emergency departments. *JAMA Pediatr.* 2015;169(6):527–534

Han S, Lyons E, Prestidge L. Pediatric disaster preparedness: four phases of disaster management. https://www.aap.org/en-us/advocacy-and-policy/aap-health-initiatives/children-and-disasters/Documents/Han-Article-IL-Newsletter.pdf. Accessed February 6, 2017

Lucile Packard Children's Hospital. Preplanning disaster triage for pediatric hospitals TRAIN toolkit. http://www.acphd.org/media/270195/hospital%20disaster%20triage%20pediatric%20planning%20train%20toolkit%20x.pdf. Accessed February 6, 2017

CHAPTER 54

Family-Centered Rounds

Introduction

Patient-centered care places the patient and family at the focus of medical care by creating a mutually beneficial relationship among the patient, family, and medical providers. Family-centered rounds (FCR) are a manifestation of patient-centered care that incorporates interdisciplinary work rounds *at the bedside,* in which the patient and family *share in the control* of both the management plan and the evaluation of the process itself. The essential component of FCR is the equal relationship between the family and the medical staff, which usually includes the bedside nurse and the physician team. Performing rounds at the bedside allows the family and medical staff to dispense the same information about the patient to everyone.

FCR has become the standard of care in pediatric medicine and offers an ideal setting to role-model professional skills to trainees and conduct case-specific teaching. Medical staff benefits include the opportunity to learn from families, as well as improved communication, coordination of care, and resource use. For patients and families, FCR is empowering because it facilitates participation in rounds and leads to a better understanding of medical issues and the plan of care. Among other benefits, FCR improves patient, family, and staff satisfaction. Potential drawbacks to FCR include an increase in the time it takes to conduct rounds, initial team discomfort with presenting information to families, limitations in discussing emotionally sensitive differential diagnoses, soliciting family participation in case presentations, and crowding in the patient's room. However, with thorough preparation, the benefits outweigh these drawbacks.

How It Works

Who

The medical team consists of the family and the medical staff. The family includes the patient, parent/legal guardian, and other family members, while the physician team, nurses, care coordinators, and other health care providers constitute the medical staff. The physician component is composed of medical students, interns, residents, midlevel providers, fellows, and attending physicians.

Where

FCR occurs at the bedside, in the doorway of the patient's room, or at the nursing station, *with the family*.

Getting Started

Begin by introducing yourself and asking if it is a good time for the family to participate in rounds. Explain the benefits of FCR (as described in the Introduction) to all participants.

Preparing Families

Introduce the family to FCR at admission, either verbally or via brochures or videos. Critical elements are the definition, purpose, and process of FCR and the time at which the family can expect the medical team for rounds. Ask the family if they want to participate in FCR and whom to include; then, confirm before starting the rounds. If they agree, before the rounds begin, ask the family to write down their questions or any observations they want to share. When the case is being presented, have the family correct errors in the history and encourage them to question any unclear medical terminology. Tell the family whether an attending physician will perform a focused physical examination during FCR.

Solicit an adolescent's preferences regarding participating in FCR and determine who should be present. Note that for some topics, like reproductive health, mental health, and substance abuse, adolescent confidentiality laws mandate that the decision regarding parental presence is left to the discretion of the patient. However, be aware of your state's adolescent age definitions and protected health topics, because they can vary considerably. For other health topics, such as asthma and diabetes, the parents have a right to be present. If the teenager does not want a parent present for FCR, then efforts must be made to ensure good rapport with both patient and family.

Preparing the Patient

Help the patient to understand FCR and participate in the process, although this will depend on the child's age, alertness, and developmental level. Explain that a group of people will be in the room to discuss his or her care. Encourage the patient to record and ask questions during FCR. Child life specialists and nurses are a useful resource for facilitating the preparation of the patient for FCR and managing follow-up questions that may arise.

Preparing the Nurse and Other Clinicians

The bedside nurse has the most interaction with the family and patient and is therefore an invaluable resource in FCR. The nurse is uniquely positioned to support the family's participation, assist them in formulating questions for the physician team, and share information about the patient's progress. Other clinicians can also advocate for the family in the same way during FCR.

The Physician Team

Clearly define how the physicians will educate the patient and family about FCR. Meet with the nurse and other team members before entering the room and assign tasks and roles to keep individuals engaged.

- **Introduction:** The team member assigned to the patient introduces the other team members to the patient and family.
- **Presentation:** Sit at the family's level, use lay terminology, and speak in a conversational manner. Talk to the family while the history is being obtained and speak to the family and team during the assessment and plan. Elicit and allow time for questions and observations by the patient, family, nurse, and others present. Clarify the discharge goals.
- **Orders:** Have a physician who is not presenting write/enter any orders and repeat them verbally.
- **Discharge facilitation:** Have one of the nonpresenters begin, update, or complete any discharge paperwork, if appropriate.
- **Resident:** Guide the junior team members in developing their assessments and plans. Ask pertinent questions and introduce the on-call resident to the family, if applicable. Also function as a role model, troubleshooter, and time keeper (the goal is <10 minutes per patient). Arrange consults after exiting the room.
- **Fellow/attending physician:** Be a role model by guiding learners as needed. Take advantage of the opportunity to teach about physical findings, as the family and patient permit. Ensure privacy if a focused physical examination is performed. Confirm with whom the primary care provider is to facilitate comanagement or transition of care at discharge.

Other Medical Staff

Include other staff, such as the care manager/discharge planner, social worker, physical and/or occupational therapist, child life specialist, respiratory and/or speech therapist, dietitian, and pharmacist, if their input is important.

Indications for Consultation

- **Child life specialist:** To help prepare children for rounds or procedures
- **Family advocacy:** To bridge communication gaps when the attending physician or charge nurse has been unable to resolve a conflict; for families to make formal statements about their experience in the hospital; to educate families and staff on the patient's rights and responsibilities
- **Social work:** For resources, including social support

Follow-up

Communicate with the primary caregiver in a timely manner regarding the patient's progress and discharge plan during hospitalization.

Pearls and Pitfalls

- Preparation for FCR includes adapting it to your hospital.
- See Table 54-1 for troubleshooting tips.
- Treat the family as equals on the team. They are the experts on their child.
- In general, families focus on the condition of their child, while medical personnel focus on the plan. Invest time in connecting the diagnosis and patient's condition during the assessment.
- A useful form of communication is a dry-erase board inside the room that includes pertinent information.
- Be selective in the use of handheld electronic devices because they may impair rapport with families. They may be helpful for staying on task, accessing the electronic medical record, and displaying teaching tools for learners and families.

Table 54-1. Troubleshooting FCR Issues	
Potential Solutions Before Rounds	**Potential Solutions During Rounds**
Lack of buy-in	
Staff: Provide a literature review to document benefits of FCR. Family: Clarify expectations for rounds. Presenter: Introduce yourself to the family.	Decrease the number of staff in the room. Identify one person as the team spokesperson. Encourage questions and observations from the family. Involve the primary care provider.
Limited discussion of differential diagnosis and didactic teaching	
Before entering the room, review an expanded differential diagnoses list with the medical team. Make arrangements for a formal didactic session later in the day.	Ask the family if it is okay to teach inside the room. If not, offer teaching points when walking between rooms.

Table 54-1. Troubleshooting FCR Issues, continued

Potential Solutions Before Rounds	Potential Solutions During Rounds
Time constraints	
Review the roles of each individual. Have the presenter practice and review the plan. Before rounds begin, help the family formulate questions and answer the straightforward ones.	Start on time. Be aware of time limitations (<10 min per patient). Politely tell the family that a team member will return later to discuss the less critical issues. Set a time to return.
Family is absent	
Obtain the family's questions and observations and arrange for a different time to talk.	Use a speakerphone to call the family (eg, if the patient's mother is at work).
Use of medical jargon	
Anticipate unavoidable medical terminology and review the definitions with the family.	Provide definitions during the presentation. Encourage the family to ask questions. Give feedback to the presenter after rounds.
Lack of consensus	
Before starting, have a brief planning huddle to quickly review the proposed plan and options.	Ask the family about their major concerns and/or their goals for the hospitalization.
Non–English speakers	
Arrange for a translator to be present (not a family member).	Use an off-site translator via speakerphone or video.
Suspected child abuse	
Clarify with the social worker what information the parents/legal guardians can receive and who makes medical decisions. Practice how to review management decisions in a nonaccusatory way.	Focus on the medical management, safety, and well-being of the patient. Inform the family that the medical staff's role is limited to medical management.

Abbreviation: FCR, family-centered rounds.

Bibliography

Cincinnati Children's Hospital. Patient and Family-centered Rounds. http://www.cincinnatichildrens.org/professional/referrals/patient-family-rounds/default/. Accessed March 21, 2016

Committee on Hospital Care and Institute for Patient- and Family-Centered Care. Patient- and family-centered care and the pediatrician's role. *Pediatrics.* 2012;129(2):394–404

Kuo DZ, Sisterhen LL, Sigrest TE, Biazo JM, Aitken ME, Smith CE. Family experiences and pediatric health services use associated with family-centered rounds. *Pediatrics.* 2012;130(2):299–305

Rosen P, Stenger E, Bochkoris M, Hannon MJ, Kwoh CK. Family-centered multidisciplinary rounds enhance the team approach in pediatrics. *Pediatrics.* 2009;123(4):e603–e608

Videos Explaining FCR for Families

Cincinnati Children's Hospital. Family-centered rounds at Cincinnati Children's Medical Center. http://www.youtube.com/watch?v=XZQ7Yy3gxZU and http://www.cincinnatichildrens.org/professional/referrals/patient-family-rounds/videos/

Texas Children's Hospital. Family-centered care in pediatric hospital medicine. http://www.youtube.com/watch?v=TdgU0VZNfSg

Leading a Team

Introduction

The Pediatric Hospital Medicine competencies call upon pediatric hospitalists to lead various teams within the complex systems of hospitals. These may include clinical, educational, quality improvement, patient safety, and utilization management teams. The requisite leadership skills involve clinical duties (patient- and family-centered care conferences), administration (time management, delegation, and running effective meetings), communication (listening effectively, building consensus, and resolving conflicts), and quality improvement and patient safety. However, most hospitalists have little formal training in leadership, although there are tools available to help them lead effectively. Time spent developing one's leadership skills will pay dividends in job satisfaction and in effectiveness in patient care and systems improvement.

Leading Clinical Teams

Clinical teams are challenged in that there may be fluctuating membership, which requires greater clarity in establishing roles and responsibilities. In addition, the team may include learners, who may have a different set of goals. One common organizing framework is Goals, Roles, Procedures, and Interpersonal Relationships (GRPI). When applied to a clinical team, the four processes are as follows.

Goals

- Quality patient care, including both good clinical care and a good experience of care
- Efficient time management
- Quality educational experience for learners

Roles

- Clear division of responsibilities
- Clear lists of tasks for each role
- Appropriate training, skill, and licensure for the tasks

Procedures

- Clear expectations on how team members interact/communicate with the patient, family, and team members
- Clear delineation of who has decision-making authority for individual tasks and overall team structure and function

- Clear processes for expressing disagreement, especially about potential patient safety issues

Interpersonal Relationships (Interactions)
- Based on trust, mutual support, and collegiality
- State the group culture explicitly
- Group members accomplish their tasks in a timely manner or seek help and apologize for failures
- Leaders address deficiencies promptly, not allowing behavior contrary to the group's culture to continue long enough to be perceived as normal

There is a cascading effect of lack of clarity in each of the domains. Eighty percent of the problems and conflicts on teams are precipitated by unclear goals, with each subsequent domain causing a decreasing percentage of problems.

Teams that reflect on their own performance in real time improve continuously. One method well suited to the inpatient rounding flow is reflection in action—to check in with the team on performance between patient rooms during patient- and family-centered rounds. These pauses for self-reflection also create opportunities for real-time, specific feedback from the leader to improve team performance. Further, explicit role modeling by team leaders at the patient's bedside will affect self-correction and improve team performance.

In settings where there is frequent team member turnover, such as different nurses and/or ancillary providers joining the team based on patient assignment or learners or attending physicians changing teams every 1 to 2 weeks, some centers standardize expectations for team members. Distributing a handout in advance to members joining the team can provide clarity of GRPI expectations, or a chart with GRPI expectations can be posted in teamwork and leisure areas as a reminder. In addition, using a "communication note" in the electronic medical record and/or posting door signs are effective methods of relaying team composition and patient responsibility to staff and families. Simulation exercises are useful to practice team roles for high-stakes events such as code and rapid response.

Leading Other Teams
Leadership of quality improvement (QI) teams, hospital committees, academic medical sections, and other established groups requires skill sets different from those needed for leading clinical teams. With new requirements that residents participate in a QI project, more physicians are learning management tools for this work. (see Chapter 60, Quality Improvement).

Few physicians receive formal training in leading meetings or committees. As a result, many physician-led committees struggle to accomplish their goals efficiently. Applying the GRPI framework can also help when forming new committees, while for standing committees, the leader can partner with members to establish clear ground rules for meetings. The following guiding principles are helpful in establishing ground rules:

- All meetings start on time and end on time.
- Require an agenda for each meeting, including the topic, time allotted, person responsible for the topic discussion, and action needed as a result of the presentation.
- Appoint a facilitator (not necessarily the chairperson) to guide the process and act as timekeeper.
- Adhere strictly to the time allotted. If a person is not finished in the allotted time, a donation of time must be requested from someone later in the agenda. If nobody is willing to give up their time, put the topic on the agenda for the next meeting to finish the discussion. Enforcing the agenda leads to more precise presentations, focused discussions, and realistic agendas.
- Monitor if deliverables are, in fact, delivered and what consequences there are for nondelivery.
- Use a "parking lot" method to record ideas and topics that come up as tangents during the meeting. At the end of the meeting, negotiate which, if any, of the topics that were "parked" are appropriate for being added to the agenda of a future meeting.
- Cancel unnecessary meetings. Some topics are handled more effectively by using a different format.

Pearls and Pitfalls

- Team dynamics can change with the makeup of the team, so a particular management style that worked previously may not fit the next team. Flexibility is key.
- Review team dynamics regularly, in addition to the reflection-in-action, to assess for team function, adherence to stated goals and roles, and any need for change.

Bibliography

Banja J. The normalization of deviance in healthcare delivery. *Bus Horiz.* 2010;53(2):139

Blanchard K, Johnson S. *The New One Minute Manager.* New York, NY: William Morrow; 2015

Chatalalsingh C, Reeves S. Leading team learning: what makes interprofessional teams learn to work well? *J Interprof Care.* 2014;28(6):513–518

Hersey P. *The Situational Leader.* 4th ed. Cary, NC: Center for Leadership Studies; 1992

Jain AK, Thompson JM, Chaudry J, McKenzie S, Schwartz RW. High-performance teams for current and future physician leaders: an introduction. *J Surg Educ.* 2008; 65(2):145–150

Six Sigma. Goal Roles Process and Interpersonal Relations (GRPI). http://www. whatissixsigma.net/grpi/. Accessed February 7, 2017

Stucky ER, Ottolini MC, Maniscalco J. Pediatric hospital medicine core competencies: development and methodology. *J Hosp Med.* 2010;5(6):339–343

Macroeconomics

Introduction

Pediatric hospitalist groups have become collaborative partners with hospitals, especially as external pressures escalate to provide demonstrably efficient, safe, high-quality inpatient care. Most tertiary pediatric institutions and many community hospitals now employ pediatric hospitalists to care for sick children and oversee newborn nurseries. The success and sustainability of these programs depend on revenue primarily generated through patient care that is reimbursed at lower rates than adult medicine services. In pediatrics, unlike many other medical specialties, fees are mostly generated for evaluation and management, rather than procedures.

Hospital Charges Versus Physician Fees

Hospitalists must fully understand the distinction between hospital charges and physician fees. In the United States, a hospitalized patient generally receives one bill from the hospital, which covers the bed space, nursing care, and medicines provided, and then physicians submit their bills separately for intellectual and procedural services. Insurance companies, as well as Medicare and Medicaid, contract with and reimburse hospitals and physicians separately. This piecemeal payment model will change with the evolution of accountable care organizations, in which there will be a single payment for each incident of care.

Pediatric Hospitalist Group Priorities

Most pediatric hospitalist groups use professional fees as the marker of productivity. This can make it difficult for these groups to generate enough revenue to pay their physicians market salaries. Classically, hospitals have supported pediatric hospitalists with value-added payments (see the following section), given the hospitalist's intimate participation in the institution's administrative, quality, and safety initiatives.

There are certain variables that can influence a hospital's payment to pediatric hospitalist groups. These may include

a. **Contracting**. Better contracts with insurers and Medicaid programs, both state run and managed care, can increase revenue. The negotiating leverage here can be quite complex and may require metric demonstration of high-quality and lower-cost care, possibly in comparison with other regional or local services.

b. **Program placement**. Pediatric hospitalist programs employed by or embedded in academic institutions may enjoy some benefits that large, multidisciplinary groups offer, such as protected time and expense sharing. However, the downside is that each dollar collected is shared among more entities. As a result, strictly on the basis of professional fee collection, it may be more difficult to prove that the program breaks even or is profitable.

c. **Scheduling**. Innovative scheduling, in which efficiency opportunities are identified and the ever-evolving balancing act among education, patient safety, and physician overuse is actively considered, can generate financial rewards. One consideration might be prioritizing continuity of care versus considering pediatric hospitalists to be interchangeable and therefore relying on a series of handoffs. The latter approach might provide a more consistent physician presence, while the former might necessitate home call models and periods of lesser resident oversight (in academic institutions).

d. **Services**. Hospitalist groups are often exploring proposals to increase service lines for generating more revenue. This can involve performing a greater number of high-reimbursement procedure-based services, such as sedation or central line placement; building a complex care or medical consulting service; staffing long-term care facilities; marketing services to primary care pediatricians, so the hospitalists assume the care of their inpatients; developing outpatient follow-up clinics; and increasing opportunities for comanagement with surgical specialists.

e. **Billing**. Traditionally, physicians are given very little guidance or education about billing, and they rarely know the charges that are assigned to the *Current Procedural Terminology*® codes they use frequently. Self-auditing is an easy way to ensure proper billing and avoid either overbilling or underbilling. This will be increasingly important as patients continue to shift to high-deductible plans and are thus more responsible for out-of-pocket payments. Informed consumers will then appropriately question the accuracy and veracity of the bills they receive.

Value Added as an Issue

Hospitals are frequently asked to contribute to pediatric hospitalist revenue. A common argument is that hospitalists spend considerable time and contribute significant value to the mission of the hospital and thus deserve to be remunerated for their time expenditure. This includes hours spent streamlining discharge processes, improving communication with primary care pediatricians, facilitating interactions with nursing and ancillary staff, and participating in hospital-wide performance and safety committees. It also includes hours spent on low-revenue overnight shifts (perhaps to teach residents and provide for patient safety) and the care provided to self-pay uninsured patients, which may be a central component of the hospital's community-based service.

Hospitalists must demonstrate their value added to the hospital by developing meaningful quantitative metrics. These may include increased patient and staff satisfaction scores, tracked interactions with students and/or residents, and improved on-site availability for emergencies (such as overnight shifts). Participation in outcome management and performance improvement initiatives, which is always a priority to hospital administrators, will further confirm the nonclinical value added by a hospitalist group and strengthen the hospitalist's position in financial conversations.

Hospital Costs and Revenue as a Variable

In addition to professional fee collection, pediatric hospitalists may contend that they decrease the cost of care and thus increase hospital revenue. This can be measured by metrics such as a decreased length of stay, reduced resource expenditure, fewer insurance denials, fewer readmissions, and improved quality of care (fewer central line placements, nosocomial infections, etc). The validity of this concept is determined either locally or regionally, depending on the contracts hospitals have with payers.

In Medicare-driven adult medicine, the inpatient prospective payment system shifts the financial risk of patient care from the payers to the providers. Specifically, patients are grouped into diagnosis-related groups (DRGs), and a single payment is provided without consideration of resource expenditure. It is understood that some patients will cost more and some less, and with the DRG system, an attempt is made to target the average cost and incentivize the provider to decrease expenditures. This DRG model is less prevalent in pediatric medicine because Medicaid payments are managed at the state level. However, in hospitals with significant DRG contracts, there is certainly validity to the idea that shortening hospital stays or ordering less magnetic resonance imaging is fiscally beneficial. In contrast, if an inpatient pediatric hospitalist program is reimbursed on a per-diem basis, a low-census hospital can potentially lose revenue if length of stay is shortened, since both revenue and costs are decreased. Even in a per-diem environment, hospitals at or near 100% bed occupancy benefit from shortening length of stay and improving throughput.

It is therefore critical for a hospitalist to understand the hospital's types of contracts. DRG-based hospitals may be vested in length-of-stay metrics, while per-diem–based hospitals may be similarly interested in this metric but for the exact opposite reason.

Conclusion

Pediatric hospitalist groups must develop respectful, collaborative partnerships with hospital administrations. In the scope of their everyday practice, they have a clear opportunity to decrease overall costs of care. Since a healthy hospital can provide robust services to a community and a healthy insurance company may be able to provide affordable, broad coverage to more families, this further strengthens the argument for the existence and support of pediatric hospitalist programs.

Bibliography

Frank E, Paul DP, Nersesian R. Hospitalists at an academic medical center, part 1: impact of a voluntary pilot hospitalist program. *Hosp Top*. 2011;89(4):75–81

Greeno R. Funding a hospitalist program: which approach will you take? *Healthc Financ Manage*. 2010;64(8):76–80

Lundberg S, Balingit P, Wali S, Cope D. Cost-effectiveness of a hospitalist service in a public teaching hospital. *Acad Med*. 2010;85(8):1312–1315

Mitchell DM. The critical role of hospitalists in controlling healthcare costs. *J Hosp Med*. 2010;5(3):127–132

Roberts KB. Pediatric hospitalists in community hospitals: hospital-based generalists with expanded roles. *Hosp Pediatr*. 2015;5(5):290–292

Sprague L. The hospitalist: better value in inpatient care? *Issue Brief Natl Health Policy Forum*. 2011;(842):1–17

Microeconomics

Introduction

It is increasingly imperative that pediatric hospitalists understand certain aspects of the business side of medicine. Hospitals depend on physicians not only to care for the patients in a professional and efficient manner but also to provide the necessary documentation that accurately reflects the severity of illness to facilitate proper coding and billing. In addition, in certain states, the hospitalist may be responsible for making the determination, at admission, as to whether a patient will have observation or inpatient status. This may affect the out-of-pocket expenses for the family, since observation status is considered to be the same as outpatient treatment by most insurers and may therefore lead to higher unreimbursed costs for the family. While most clinicians receive little training on the business aspects of medicine, it is crucial to understand what effect the work performed and its documentation has on both the patient/family (out-of-pocket expenses) and the hospital (financial viability).

Documentation

First and foremost in the hospitalist's documentation is a description of the hospitalist's thought processes and clinical assessment, to ensure that others who will be involved in the patient's care have a clear understanding of the clinical picture. This is critical for anyone who will subsequently review the record, including the hospital's coding and billing specialists and the insurers. Depending on the size of the program and the hospital, there may be clinical documentation improvement (CDI) specialists who can help ensure that the documentation is clear and specific enough to allow for accurate coding and billing. As such, during the course of the hospitalization, be as specific as possible in clearly documenting why the patient needs to remain in the hospital. However, avoid copying and pasting your notes, because this can make it difficult to tell what is new each day.

House Staff Documentation

In some settings, the house staff write the history and physical examination notes, daily progress notes, and/or narrative summaries, which are then cosigned by the physician. The hospitalist must then also document that the patient was personally seen, that the findings were discussed with the resident team, and that the hospitalist agrees or disagrees with the assessment and plan of the resident. A correction is mandatory if there is disagreement with any aspect of the resident's notes. On a daily basis, clearly state and substantiate why the patient needs to remain in the hospital. Finally, if a progress note indicates that a patient is expected to be discharged, but instead the patient stays in the hospital, there needs to be clear and specific documentation about what has changed. Add an addendum or another note to explain and justify the ongoing stay.

Billing and Coding

Clinical documentation for the purpose of communicating a patient's status must include all pertinent history and physical examination findings, as well as a detailed plan of treatment. Documentation for the purpose of coding and billing needs to meet additional requirements, such as *ICD-10* (*International Statistical Classification of Diseases and Related Health Problems, 10th Revision*) specificity, although it is not expected for each clinician to know the ins and outs of thousands of *ICD-10* codes. Rather, become familiar with the codes for the most common diagnoses encountered, then start to learn what needs to be documented. CDI specialists can be invaluable in this process. Ask them to organize regular coding in-services for the hospitalist group. The institution may also assign documentation queries to a clinician when clarification is needed on a diagnosis or when further specificity is required to adequately code and bill the patient's hospital stay. Answer such queries in a timely and complete manner.

Admission Status

To determine admission status (inpatient vs observation), some hospitals employ a case management program or a utilization review department to assist in making the determination. Most hospitals and insurers use one of two national guidelines, either Milliman Care Guidelines (MCG) or InterQual Criteria, to also help in determining appropriate admission status. These guidelines provide criteria for when a problem (eg, bronchiolitis) would qualify a child to be admitted as an inpatient (eg, hypoxia that requires supplemental oxygen) and when observation status is sufficient (eg, mild symptoms that need to be monitored for 12–24 hours). Table 57-1 shows examples of MCG inpatient criteria for a few common diagnoses.

Reason for Admission

It is essential that the hospitalists and emergency department (ED) clinicians document clearly why the patient is being admitted (with either observation or inpatient status) rather than being sent home. Status should be determined by the admitting clinician at the time of admission. In some cases,

Table 57-1. MCG Criteria for Admission	
Diagnosis	**Criteria**
Asthma	Oxygen saturation <92% Pao_2 <60 mm Hg Severe or persistent retractions, wheezing, or tachypnea
Bronchiolitis	Apnea Feeding difficulties Oxygen saturation <90% Respiratory rate >60 breaths/min
Gastroenteritis	Bloody diarrhea with fever Severe dehydration (>9%) Severe electrolyte abnormalities
Pneumonia	Oxygen saturation <90% Toxic clinical appearance Respiratory findings that are severe or persistent
Seizures	Altered mental status that is severe or persistent Metabolic disorder (eg, hypoglycemia, hyponatremia) that is severe or persistent New focal neurologic deficit that is severe or persistent

this evaluation may be different than the evaluation conducted by the ED clinicians, especially if some time has passed between evaluations. Avoid using wording such as, "Patient will be admitted as an inpatient to observe how they do," and instead document, "Patient will be admitted as an inpatient for dehydration, acute respiratory distress and hypoxia, and the need for intravenous fluids and supplemental oxygen." This way, both the patient's condition and the plan of treatment are delineated, and the treatment plan and medical necessity of the admission are clearly explained.

Denials

To enhance timely and appropriate payment by payers, it is necessary for claims to accurately reflect the services provided and demonstrate the medical necessity. Payers may deny claims by stating that medical necessity was not met or deny the inpatient admission but approve an observation stay, instead. When a denial occurs, the hospitalist may be contacted to assist the hospital's finance department in developing a plan to convince the insurer that payment for the admission is justified. In some cases, this may involve a peer-to-peer conversation between the hospitalist and the medical director of the insurance plan. Do not take this personally or as an indictment of the care that was provided. To prepare for the telephone call, review the chart in an objective manner and, if possible, review the appropriate MCG (Table 57-1) or InterQual guidelines for the diagnosis. Prepare a clear and concise explanation based on what is documented in the record (not based on assumptions or what was implied) and how it meets a guideline for the type of admission (observation or inpatient), and then present this to the medical director. It is possible that the insurer's medical director does not have certain records in their possession, so that on hearing information directly, the medical director may decide to overturn the denial. If this process is unsuccessful, another option is to write a letter to the insurer on behalf of the hospital, further describing the case, for review by a different medical director.

Bibliography

Charité TL, Kennedy JS. The physician advisor's guide to clinical documentation improvement. https://hcmarketplace.com/aitdownloadablefiles/download/aitfile/aitfile_id/1572.pdf. Accessed February 7, 2017

Lundberg S, Balingit P, Wali S, Cope D. Cost-effectiveness of a hospitalist service in a public teaching hospital. *Acad Med*. 2010;85(8):1312–1315

Michelman MS, Mass S, Ukanowicz D. Optimizing the physician advisor in case management. http://hcmarketplace.com/media/browse/6632_browse.pdf. Accessed February 7, 2017

Mussman GM, Conway PH. Pediatric hospitalist systems versus traditional models of care: effect on quality and cost outcomes. *J Hosp Med*. 2012;7(4):350–357

Palliative Care

Introduction

Pediatric palliative care (PPC) offers physical, psychological, social, and spiritual support to children with life-threatening or life-limiting conditions and their families. The emphasis of PPC is on comfort, quality of life, and goal-directed decision making, with the objective of preventing and relieving suffering through interdisciplinary collaboration. The American Academy of Pediatrics recommends that PPC be instituted from the time of diagnosis of a life-threatening illness and be continued throughout all subsequent phases of therapy, regardless of whether the expected outcome is cure, life extension, or comfort.

PPC is provided by an interdisciplinary team that consists of physicians, nurse practitioners, nurses, social workers, case managers, psychologists, physical and occupational therapists, speech pathologists, child life specialists, music/art therapists, and chaplains. It is essential that hospitalists be able to recognize whom to refer for PPC consultation and when. In addition, it is critical that hospitalists acquire basic proficiencies in treating distressing symptoms and communicating effectively when caring for children with serious illnesses, irrespective of whether their institution has access to a dedicated PPC program.

Indications for PPC

After discussing the case with the medical home team, refer a patient and family for a PPC consultation if there are life-threatening or life-shortening conditions, including (but not limited to) cancer, heart failure, cystic fibrosis and other pulmonary diseases, renal failure, cerebral palsy, advanced HIV/AIDS, and progressive or severe genetic neurologic, metabolic, or immunologic disorders. Other indications include

- Uncertain prognosis and accompanying symptom burden
- Introduction of a new medical technology, such as a feeding tube, tracheostomy tube, or ventilator support for a condition that is not expected to resolve and may preclude living a full, long life
- Disabling or uncontrolled symptoms, such as pain, fatigue, insomnia, depression, anxiety, agitation, spasms, nausea, vomiting, diarrhea, constipation, or dyspnea

- Facilitation of patient-centered and family-centered communication and decision making, both at initial diagnosis and when the goals of care are changing
- Need for psychological, social, or spiritual support, whether for the patient, parents, or siblings
- Multiple admissions for the same diagnosis with undefined goals of care
- Admissions of increasing frequency or severity for the same underlying condition or its complications
- Reliance on full-time medical daycare
- Need for coordination of care across settings (hospital, home, skilled nursing facility, hospice)
- Care and support at the end of life and during bereavement
- Prenatal consultation for a fetus with a life-limiting condition

Statements by Patients and Families That Can Trigger PPC Consultation

- I don't know how much longer we can do this.
- It hurts me to see my child in pain like this.
- We feel like the doctors have given up on us.
- I am so confused. Every new provider tells me something different.
- My child seems to be getting worse, no matter what the doctors are doing.
- My child is so tired of being in the hospital.
- I just want my child to get to be a kid and play.
- We just want to go home.
- There are so many people involved, and no one is really listening.
- I am so worried about my other kids and whether I'll still have my job.

How to Introduce PPC to Patients and Families

The introduction of PPC may be challenging if the family has a pre-existing negative perception about PPC. For example, they may equate PPC with hospice or view PPC as a signal that the medical team is "giving up" on their child. If either of these difficulties arises, consider introducing PPC as an extra layer of support for the family, one that emphasizes doing everything possible to improve the quality of life for the child and family. Also, reassure the family that PPC emphasizes goal-directed care, which will be integrated with curative care. Emphasize that the medical services in your institution often consult the PPC team for a patient with a serious illness when the care plan is complex or when the outcome is uncertain.

PPC Introduction Example

"To best meet the goals of care for your child, we believe it would be helpful to have the PPC service visit with you. The PPC team works with both families and other health care providers. They specialize in improving your child's quality of life by helping to manage symptoms, such as pain, nausea, and fatigue, as well as providing support to your child and family. They can also help you clarify your goals of care and help us think through any decisions as they might arise. Our goal is for all of the teams to work together to provide your child with the best care possible."

Goals of Care

The goals of care are different for each patient and family. To help establish these goals, parents (and if appropriate, the child or any person who plays a vital role in decision making in that family) can be invited for a family meeting with the medical team. It is often useful for the caregivers to meet first, so that all members of the team agree on the diagnosis, prognosis, and recommended treatment plans. To determine the goals of an individual or a family, ask the following key questions:

- What is your understanding of your child's condition?
- What do you expect in the future?
- What are the most important things you desire for your child right now?
- What are you hoping for?
- What are your child's greatest needs right now?
- What are you most worried about, or what keeps you awake at night?

Spiritual Assessment

A spiritual assessment may also be helpful to gain a better understanding of the family's goals. Use the acronym HOPE for assessing the patient's and family's spiritual status and needs.

- **H**ope: What are your sources of hope, strength, comfort, and peace? What do you hold on to during difficult times? What or who sustains you and keeps you going?
- **O**rganized religion: Are you a part of a religious community? How is this helpful to you?
- **P**ersonal spirituality and practices: Do you have other personal spiritual beliefs that are helpful to you? What aspects of your spirituality are most helpful (eg, prayer, meditation, music, nature)?

- **E**ffects on medical care and **e**nd-of-life issues: Has your child's health condition affected your spiritual practices? Are there conflicts between your beliefs and medical situation? Would it be helpful to speak to a chaplain or other spiritual leader?

Continuity of Care

PPC emphasizes interdisciplinary collaboration among the patient's primary medical team, consult services, family, and community-based care providers, with the intention of enhancing communication and improving continuity of care. The process of PPC also includes supporting the family in making difficult decisions. In addition, continuity of care encompasses end-of-life care, whether in the hospital or at home, as well as the provision of bereavement resources for long-term support to the family.

Language Selection

Communication is a key component of successful PPC. Language choices have a meaningful effect on both patients and families, and it is important to choose words carefully (Table 58-1).

Pain Management

Use the World Health Organization pain management 2-step "ladder"

- Step 1: For mild pain, use nonopioids, such as acetaminophen or ibuprofen, with or without adjuvant therapy
- Step 2: For moderate to severe pain, use opioids with or without adjuvant therapy

Table 58-1. Appropriate Language Selection	
Language to Avoid	**Therapeutic Language**
The sickler	The child with sickle cell disease
Your child failed therapy.	Our treatments were not successful in curing your child.
I know how you feel; I know how difficult this situation is for you.	I cannot imagine how difficult this situation is for you.
Do you want us to do everything we can to keep your child alive?	What is your understanding of the decision to attempt life-sustaining interventions?
Are you ready to sign the "do not resuscitate" orders?	Do you agree with the medical recommendation for "do not attempt resuscitation"?
We are going to withdraw support now. We will be pulling the ventilator at this time.	We will stop mechanical ventilation, as it is no longer clinically indicated, but we will continue to provide maximal supportive care.

When discussing medications with patients and parents, use the term "opioid," rather than "narcotic."

Titrate opioids based on clinical response. The "right dose" is the dose that best controls pain with the fewest side effects. The base dosage increases as a percentage of the current dose: 30% increase for mild pain, 50% increase for moderate pain, and 100% increase for severe pain. For chronic, continuous, nonincidental pain, encourage dosing according to a schedule, typically every 4 hours (unless the drug has delayed release or is methadone), to avoid the pain roller coaster that can occur with as-needed (pro re nata, or PRN) dosing.

When using opioids, start a bowel regimen that consists of more than just a stool softener (osmotic agent, with or without a stimulant laxative).

See Chapter 115, Pain Management, for a more complete discussion.

Nonpharmacologic Symptom Management

Use integrative therapies (such as relaxation, meditation, breathing exercises, hypnosis, guided imagery, Reiki, biofeedback, yoga, massage, acupuncture/acupressure, and art/pet/play/music therapy) to help manage pain and other symptoms.

Fatigue: Consider contributing factors, such as anemia, depression, and medication side effects. Sleep, attending to hygiene needs, and gentle exercise may be helpful interventions.

Dyspnea: Try gentle suctioning, repositioning, wearing loose clothing, using fans, minimizing hydration, and doing relaxation exercises. First-line pharmacologic therapy consists of the use of opioids, while sedating medications are second-line line therapy.

Nausea: Try dietary modifications (bland/soft foods, timing/volume of intake), aromatherapy (peppermint or lavender oils), ginger, and acupuncture/acupressure.

Limit painful procedures and address coincident depression and anxiety through counseling and the use of psychopharmacologic agents as needed.

Support for Families

Provide respite care when feasible, such that families may have some time away from caring for the affected child. Child life specialists and volunteers can also provide support for siblings. In addition, enlist the help of the case management and social work teams to explore whether there are appropriate community-based resources available.

Provider Fatigue

Providing PPC to children and families is most often a highly rewarding personal undertaking, but in some instances it can be an overwhelming experience, leading to frustration, stress, hopelessness, or burnout. To avoid or ameliorate these adverse emotional responses, it is critical to maintain open channels of communication with professional colleagues and other health care providers. Establish consistent forums for debriefing, with self-reflection and discussion, to provide a safe place for providers to share and reflect on their experiences.

Disposition and Follow-up

Hospice

The transition into a hospice program can be complex. Prior to hospital discharge, it is important to clarify and clearly document the goals of care. If the child is being enrolled in hospice care, have a representative meet the child, family, and primary care team, ideally prior to discharge from the hospital, to communicate the management plan for symptom control and end-of-life care. Optimize all medications to enhance the patient's quality of life. In addition, be aware that hospice does not necessarily require discontinuation of active therapy. For example, a patient with cancer may continue to receive chemotherapy while under the care of a hospice program.

Home Care

The philosophy of PPC may be successfully implemented in the home, provided that the focus remains on quality of life, physical and psychological comfort, and prevention or alleviation of suffering. A PPC provider may be on call to provide support in the home and can serve as a link among the hospital, specialists, and community caregivers. This PPC provider can help to prevent or facilitate hospital admissions, as well as organize and supervise the provision of respite care and increased home services as needed. The family can benefit from knowing how to obtain help quickly when the clinical condition changes (eg, pain flares, behavior changes, breathing difficulties arise, the patient's color changes).

If the patient is being discharged to go home with goals of care such that resuscitative measures will be limited, complete an out-of-hospital "do not resuscitate" (DNR) form (see Chapter 34, Do Not Resuscitate/Do Not Intubate). These forms are state specific and may be found online through the individual state's Department of Public Health. The DNR protects a patient from aggressive interventions, such as intubation, in the event that emergency medical services are called. Even if the family has signed the form, they may still choose full resuscitative measures at any time.

Pearls and Pitfalls

- If your hospital does not have a dedicated interdisciplinary PPC team, advocate for the creation of one.
- In the absence of a dedicated PPC team, palliative care may still be provided by using the basic skills and competencies required of all physicians and health care professionals.
- The role of the hospitalist may be challenging when PPC concepts have not been addressed with a patient prior to hospital admission at the end of life. However, all hospitalists can readily learn the basic skills and competencies of PPC to provide compassionate care to patients and families at the end of life.

Bibliography

American Academy of Pediatrics Section on Hospice and Palliative Medicine and Committee on Hospital Care. Pediatric palliative care and hospice care commitments, guidelines, and recommendations. *Pediatrics.* 2013;132(5):966–972

Children's Hospice International. http://www.chionline.org/. Accessed February 7, 2017

Downing J, Jassal SS, Mathews L, Brits H, Friedrichsdorf SJ. Pediatric pain management in palliative care. *Pain Manag.* 2015;5(1):23–35

Harvard Medical School Center for Palliative Care. http://www.hms.harvard.edu/pallcare/index.htm. Accessed February 7, 2017

Moore D, Sheetz J. Pediatric palliative care consultation. *Pediatr Clin North Am.* 2014;61(4):735–747

National Hospice and Palliative Care Organization. Pediatric hospice and palliative care. www.nhpco.org/pediatrics. Accessed February 7, 2017

Wolfe J, Hinds P, Sourkes B. *The Textbook of Interdisciplinary Pediatric Palliative Care.* Philadelphia, PA: Elsevier; 2011

World Health Organization. WHO guidelines on the pharmacological treatment of persisting pain in children with medical illnesses. http://apps.who.int/iris/bitstream/10665/44540/1/9789241548120_Guidelines.pdf. Accessed February 7, 2017

Patient Safety

Introduction

Hospitalists are expected to engage in and lead local hospital-based patient safety initiatives and accreditation activities. This requires competence in areas such as causal analysis and sentinel event management, among others. Importantly, hospitalists should adhere to the guiding principle of *primum non nocere* (first do no harm): Patients' well-being is the primary factor that drives intervention decisions. This means that testing and treatments may result in purposeful "not doing" as much as "doing."

Systems improvements and personal accountability are central to developing programs to prevent or respond to medical error or patient harm. The single greatest impediment to error prevention is fear of punishment for making mistakes. It is important to recognize that not all errors may result in harm (eg, administering a double dose of intravenous ampicillin) and that not all harms are preventable (eg, red man syndrome caused by vancomycin). This is best balanced in a system that fosters a "just culture of safety," which encourages the reporting of errors without fear of retribution, supports learning, and focuses on proactive management of system design and behavior choices. A "just culture" distinguishes reckless human actions from at-risk behaviors or human error. Events are addressed in a compassionate, collegial manner, where "second victims"—the team members involved—are supported.

The errors reported most frequently involve medications. However, the most common contributing factors to errors are communication failure, stress, fatigue, and distraction. Errors in patient identification, left/right confusion, and others also exist, but the reporting of these errors is limited. However, diagnostic errors caused by cognitive mistakes are being studied, and there is an emerging body of literature that supports interventions to improve experience (continuing medical education activities, simulation training) and decision making, both retrospective (reflection, case discussion) and concurrent (real-time clinical decision-making support, algorithms). To date, health care systems have not been ranked on the basis of rates of correct treatment or diagnosis, but this is an area of intense interest.

Basic Terms and Tools

Adverse event: Any medical error, regardless of severity or cause.

At-risk behavior: A behavior choice that increases risk, such as not consistently using 2 patient identifiers when indicated. Either the risk is not recognized, or it is mistakenly believed to be justified.

Error: An inadvertent action; a slip, lapse, or mistake. Mistakes are errors due to failure to choose correctly (inexperience). Slips (incorrect action) and lapses (action forgotten) are failures due to inattention.

Failure Mode and Effects Analysis (FMEA): Error analysis conducted either retrospectively or prospectively to determine failures and the relative effects of each failure; allows for prioritization of targets for improvement based on a number (criticality index).

Hard stop: A step in a process that must be completed to continue, such as scanning a patient identification bar code for a medication to be dispensed from a locked cabinet.

Harm: An unintended injury resulting from or exacerbated by medical care.

High-reliability organization (HRO): Any organization that operates under hazardous conditions yet has few adverse events. HROs are preoccupied with failure, resilient when failure occurs, and attentive to operations, and they prioritize a culture of safety.

Just culture: A commitment to safety at all levels in the organization that acknowledges the high-risk, error-prone nature of an organization's activities. This is a blame-free environment with an expectation of collaboration across ranks and a willingness to direct resources to address safety concerns.

Root cause analysis (RCA): A structured method used to identify and evaluate contributing or causal factors associated with adverse events or near misses, implement solutions, and monitor effects of solutions.

Sentinel event: An unexpected occurrence that involves death or serious physical or psychological injury or risk thereof. "Sentinel" means the event requires immediate investigation and response.

Trigger tool: The use of "triggers," or clues, retrospectively (eg, identification of a preceding adverse event by means of the rescue medication given) or prospectively (eg, abrupt discontinuation of a chronically used medication may lead to instability). This is an effective method for measuring the overall level of harm from medical care in a health care organization.

Selected Best Practices

Choosing Wisely: A national campaign initiated by the American Board of Internal Medicine that includes multiple statements from national societies, all focused on preventing harm and overuse by judicious and purposeful avoidance of testing and treatments. Available at http://www.choosingwisely. org/societies/society-of-hospital-medicine-pediatric.

Fatigue recognition training: Education on the effects of fatigue on cognition and motor performance, usually paired with sleep education. The training encourages self-awareness and includes prevention tips.

Safety huddles/daily safety call: Quick team briefings (often 15 minutes long) that focus on key patient safety issues with brainstorming of solutions. In a hospital ward, huddle team members may include nursing and physician leaders and other front-line staff. For a hospital system, participants may include many others from diverse clinical and nonclinical areas; safety huddles may also be performed remotely.

Second victim rapid-response team: A dedicated team with knowledge and experience in supporting practitioners during the acute stages of emotional trauma in the immediate wake of a harmful error. Use of such teams can significantly aid in the recovery of second victims.

Peer review: A clinical review of a case with unintended or complicated outcome and/or unexpected variability compared to similar cases. The review serves to address best practices, diagnostic errors, and systems failures (eg, communication, products, environment); classify the error; and list actions to address these failures.

Postevent debrief (PED): A structured method with a checklist tool used in cases of unexpected complications, unanticipated death or harm, potential sentinel event, or staff request because of potential emotional effects on the staff. Often a first step in a formal RCA, the PED is held within 24 to 48 hours and includes front-line staff (no more than 20).

Safety walk rounds: Typically weekly rounds performed by senior leadership (eg, board members, patient safety officers, chief nursing officers) to connect with front-line staff. Common questions asked are, "Is there anything that might harm your patient today?" and "How can I help?" Focus is on immediately remediable safety issues.

SBAR model: A communication tool that describes the situation, background, assessment, and recommendation related to an acute event.

Stop the line: A policy and procedure that gives all staff, parents, trainees, and visitors the responsibility and authority to immediately intervene to protect the safety of a patient. All staff are expected to immediately stop and respond to the request by reassessing the patient's safety.

Time-out: Per the Joint Commission Universal Protocol, perform a time-out prior to starting a procedure. Ensure that all team members agree on the patient's identity, the anatomic site of the procedure, and the procedure to be performed.

Coding and External Reporting

Insurers may not pay for care that is necessary because of preventable harms. In addition, payment may be affected by proof of adherence to best practices and documenting better outcome. "Pay for performance" is the act of paying a provider for performing at or above a certain standard of quality for a given indicator. Some examples of external reporting include sentinel events (reported to the state), infections (reported to the state public health department), and negligent care delivery (reported to the state medical board). Each can result in mandatory action plans, on-site audits, fines, or other disciplinary or legal actions.

Pearls and Pitfalls

- Lead: Be involved in safety walk rounds or a local initiative. Support just culture and HRO attributes. Integrate safety practices and a 5-minute "safety story" into clinical rounds, conferences, and journal clubs.
- Communicate clearly: Ask clarifying questions, use tools such as SBAR when acute events occur, and use a standardized handoff tool when coming on and off service or transferring patients to other services.
- Seek patient and family input: Anticipate problems by assessing how processes will be completed by patients and families.
- Work with interdisciplinary teams: Engage on hospital committees.
- *Do not* use education and reminders as sole methods to address a problem. These are the least effective methods of error avoidance. Use system-embedded hard stops whenever possible.
- *Do not* fail to report "near misses" or "good catches" in your safety reporting system. These offer great insight into how to do processes well.
- *Do not* fail to perform a thorough RCA when investigating errors, using just culture. Situational, behavioral, and patient-specific issues are often lost if an RCA is not complete. Include "second victim" support.

Information and Training

Agency for Healthcare Research and Quality Patient Safety Tools and Resources: http://www.ahrq.gov/professionals/quality-patient-safety/patient-safety-resources/resources/pstools/index.html

Children's Hospital Association Patient Safety: https://www.childrenshospitals.org/Quality-and-Performance/Patient-Safety

Institute for Healthcare Improvement Open School: http://www.ihi.org/education/IHIOpenSchool/Pages/default.aspx

Children's Hospitals' Solutions for Patient Safety: http://www.solutionsforpatientsafety.org/

The Joint Commission: http://www.jointcommission.org/topics/patient_safety.aspx and http://www.jcrinc.com

Bibliography

Campbell M, Miller K, McNicholas KW. Post event debriefs: a commitment to learning how to better care for patients and staff. *Jt Comm J Qual Patient Saf.* 2016;42:41–49

National Academies of Sciences, Engineering, and Medicine. Improving diagnosis in health care. http://iom.nationalacademies.org/Reports/2015/Improving-Diagnosis-in-Healthcare.aspx. Posted September 22, 2015. Accessed February 7, 2017

Stockwell DC, Bisarya H, Classen DC, et al. A trigger tool to detect harm in pediatric inpatient settings. *Pediatrics.* 2015;135(6):1036–1042

Quality Improvement

Introduction

The increasing shift of the cost of health care to the individual consumer has created a new focus on the delivery of high-value health care, which can be defined as producing the best health care outcomes at the lowest cost. Though seemingly a simple concept, the delivery of the right care for the right reason at the right time and place for the right cost is fraught with complexity and remains the ultimate goal in the transformation of our health care system.

As a result, clinicians must now be trained in the fundamentals of defining, designing, and implementing health care models. The goal is to reduce inappropriate variation, misuse, overuse, and underuse of resources to improve outcomes. Therefore, learning and applying the science of quality improvement (QI) is now a critical skill set for every physician.

The Institute of Medicine (IOM) has defined *quality* as the degree to which health care systems, services, and supplies for individuals and populations increase the likelihood for positive health outcomes and are consistent with current professional knowledge. The IOM has proposed 6 specific aims for improvement. Quality health is

- Safe: Avoid injury from care that is intended to help.
- Effective: Avoid underuse or overuse of services.
- Patient centered: Provide respectful, responsive, individualized care.
- Timely: Reduce wait times and harmful delays in care.
- Efficient: Avoid waste of equipment, supplies, ideas, and energy.
- Equitable: Provide equal care, regardless of personal characteristics, sex, ethnicity, geographic location, and socioeconomic status.

The goal of QI in health care is to provide the right care for every patient, every time.

Right care: Practice evidence-based medicine with judgment, experience, and adaptation to the patient's needs. However, the IOM reported that it may take an average of 17 years for new knowledge generated by randomized controlled trials to be incorporated into practice, so knowing what is right care is not enough. The goal is to translate evidence-based medicine into clinical judgment and patient-centered care.

Every patient: Many reports have demonstrated how care varies for even the most common inpatient pediatric diagnoses, such as gastroenteritis and bronchiolitis. QI methodology is focused on reducing inappropriate variation and improving the delivery of value-based outcomes.

Every time: Most physicians are familiar with the most recent and relevant clinical research (evidence-based medicine) and work to incorporate this knowledge into our daily practice. Unfortunately, it is difficult to do this on a consistent basis.

Every physician should wear this "IOM lens" in evaluating the quality of any health care product. Pediatric hospitalists must be leaders in working toward optimal QI. This requires the knowledge, skills, and attitudes to be successful in leading a system that provides the right care for every patient, every time. The following concepts are critical for hospitalists to recognize as they develop into leaders of QI in their organizations.

System Improvement

Quality improvement is not accomplished by forcing people to work harder, faster, and safer; reusing traditional quality assurance or peer-review methods; or creating order sets or protocols without monitoring their use or effects. To generate meaningful positive outcomes, the hospitalist and other front-line staff must focus on the processes of care, reduce variations in care by shifting entire practices, and change the design of care. Traditional quality assurance focuses on outliers, without changing the process or reducing inappropriate variation, whereas QI focuses on process improvements that lead to more reliable outcomes. Effective QI models that lead to high-value outcomes must also include price transparency, feedback via clinical decision-making support, and dashboards with appropriate process and outcome measures.

Understand How to Measure Quality

Measurement of quality is critical to the QI process. Although measurement systems are inherently imperfect, create local assessment tools to use within the hospital organization. These metrics may further evolve during multiple improvement cycles, allowing individual units (eg, hospital floor units or physician groups) ready access to transparent data that will be meaningful to individuals and will motivate change. Measure relevant information in small samples, over time, and use it for providing feedback to the clinical staff, who can then affect the specific indicators. Provide feedback in a collaborative and nonpunitive manner, so as to build trust, which is essential for further change.

A common framework for addressing QI involves three quality-of-care measures (structure, process, outcome) to benchmark performance against an accepted standard. Structural measures focus on a system's capacity to deliver care and the conditions under which the care is delivered and include information technology, staff, facilities, and policies. Process measures are used to look at how often a recommended health care intervention has been performed within the context of the targeted population—for example, the percentage of patients with asthma who receive a dose of steroids within 1 hour of arrival to the emergency department. Outcome measures reflect the overall result of health care and actual patient outcomes. Examples are the cost and length of stay for a population of inpatients with asthma. Current research documents that alignment and improvement in the structural and process measures almost always lead to positive changes in outcomes. However, it may take multiple rapid improvement cycles to show measurable change in outcomes.

It is important to recognize that government agencies or payers do not initiate the development of quality indicators. Rather, quality indicators often result from the recommendations of professional societies and research studies. Therefore, hospitalists must become involved with national professional bodies and participate in the decision-making process of what are meaningful process and outcome measures.

Build Teams

Traditional medical education focused on training physicians to be autonomous and individualistic, but this model is no longer viable for hospitalists. Today, a quality physician works as part of an effective team, with members representing 3 different components within an organization: system leadership (hospital administrator), technical leadership (physician), and day-to-day leadership (nurses, clerks, housekeepers, respiratory therapists, etc). Front-line staff, such as nurses, clerks, and support personnel, are all important sources of information and potential partners in the improvement process. The principles of family-centered care also apply to QI. Involvement of patients and their families within QI teams is also critical to help break traditional silos.

Implement the Plan-Do-Study-Act Model for Improvement

The plan-do-study-act (PDSA) model for improvement is a powerful and proven tool for accelerating improvement. It provides structure to the improvement process, just as a history and physical examination provide structure to a patient encounter.

- Set aims: "What are we trying to accomplish?" Define an aim that is time specific and measurable and define the population that will be affected.

- Establish measures: "How will we know that a change is an improvement?" Measures help the team determine if a change leads to quantitative improvement.
- Select changes: "What changes can we make that will result in improvement?" Improvement requires change, but not all change leads to improvement. It is the test of change by using rapid cycle methods that will allow QI teams to determine whether meaningful improvement can be measured.
- Test change: "How can we make changes in the real-world setting?" Rapidly initiate a PDSA cycle, with a narrow focus, by using smaller tests of change, before disseminating it across a larger population.
  — Plan: Answer the questions in the first 3 previous steps by setting aims, establishing measures, and selecting changes.
  — Do: Implement the changes. This may range from a "baby step," one small change for a small number of patients, to the widespread use of "bundles," which are packages of evidence-based interventions that help provide consistency of care.
  — Study: Evaluate the pilot change to see if the desired effect occurred and identify any unintended consequences.
  — Act: Adopt, reject, or modify the change plan so that the next cycle can begin.

Sustain the Changes

After several successful PDSA cycles, create a "control" plan to ensure that the "new change" is integrated into a system of care. This control plan is a living document that incorporates a written description of the system for controlling parts and processes, including leadership accountabilities, delineation of standard processes, and educational policies. QI must be sustainable over time, leading to the delivery of reliable outcomes, regardless of changes in team composition.

Spread the Changes

After the hospital or unit has benefited from the improvement, share the process with other organizations to spread best practices. This will also serve as an educational opportunity for the team.

These simple steps have brought profound changes within health care organizations. By developing a system-level approach to improve measurement, building teams, and using the PDSA model of improvement, pediatric hospitalists can be leaders in transforming the culture of an organization, one that is focused on QI. In this way, all members of an organization, from boardroom members to the ward clerks, work together to provide the right care for every patient, every time.

Bibliography

Lannon CM, Levy FH, Moyer VA. The need to build capability and capacity in quality improvement and patient safety. *Pediatrics*. 2015;135(6):e1371–e1373

Pereira-Argenziano L, Levy FH. Patient safety and quality improvement: terminology. *Pediatr Rev*. 2015;36(9):403–411

Santana C, Curry LA, Nembhard IM, Berg DN, Bradley EH. Behaviors of successful interdisciplinary hospital quality improvement teams. *J Hosp Med*. 2011;6(9):501–506

Smith M, Saunders R, Stuckhardt L, McGinnis JM, eds. *Best Care at Lower Cost: The Path to Continuously Learning Health Care in America*. Washington, DC: The National Academies Press; 2013

White HL, Glazier RH. Do hospitalist physicians improve the quality of inpatient care delivery? A systematic review of process, efficiency and outcome measures. *BMC Med*. 2011;9:58

Transition to Adult Care

Introduction

There are an increasing number of children with chronic medical conditions who are surviving into adulthood, and with this evolution, it is imperative that these patients are supported with a continuum of care from childhood into adulthood. The ideal time for this transition is between 18 and 21 years of age, although it is prudent to start preparations several years earlier. This requires a systematic approach that includes policy development and identification of high-complexity conditions, key stakeholders, and barriers to transition, as well as strategies for overcoming those barriers.

Issues of Transition to Adult Care

Adolescents with diagnoses such as type I diabetes, cystic fibrosis, inflammatory bowel disease, and *status post* solid organ transplant are often transitioned to adult care, although for some of these patients, this is done in a haphazard fashion. Children with special health care needs, such as technology dependence or those who underwent major surgical procedures to correct or ameliorate congenital anomalies, are now surviving into adult years and require an organized and well-coordinated transition from pediatric to adult health care.

While patients with congenital heart disease are living into their 30s and beyond, adult-based cardiologists are less familiar with the anatomy, physiology, and clinical effects of repaired congenital heart lesions. Similarly, patients with other congenital malformations that require surgery (eg, esophageal atresia and anorectal malformations) and medical diseases acquired from surgery (eg, short bowel syndrome) are surviving into adulthood, and adult-based general surgeons are less familiar with the anatomy of these lesions.

Technologic advances, such as tracheostomies, home ventilators, gastrostomy tubes, ventriculoperitoneal shunts, and ostomies, now allow patients with severe cerebral palsy, hypoxic-ischemic injury, genetic conditions, and other severe medical conditions to survive into adulthood. Adult-based primary care providers are often unfamiliar with the medical equipment used by these patients, the insurance approval process for replacement of equipment, and the multitude of other services and programs available to support these patients and their families. Also, as these patients age, they may remain small for their age but become at-risk for adult-acquired conditions that require monitoring by physicians familiar with these diseases. Finally, many patients with complex medical care needs often require full and continuous care from aging family members. This poses an additional challenge to address in the transition process.

Stakeholder Identification

Key stakeholders must be identified, including the patients, their families, referring pediatric medical teams and institutions, and adult-based medical teams that will be accepting the patient. While not intimately involved in the transition, other issues that enter the discussion include insurance implications and identification of appropriate adult emergency rooms, hospitals, and long-term care facilities.

Identification of Barriers to Successful Health Care Transition

Barriers to successful transition include inadequate institutional guidelines and policies, lack of perceived and actual patient readiness for transition into adult care, deficient training and comfort level of adult-based clinicians, and inadequate relationships with the adult-based team that will be accepting the patient. To be successful, each institution must identify the common and unique barriers to transition that exist within their individual facilities. Surveys of patients, families, clinicians, and ancillary staff members are a proven method of barrier identification.

Institutional Policy on Transition

Many organizations lack a formal policy on transition of pediatric patients to adult care. Without a written policy that can be used as a guide and a reference, providers and/or patients may be unprepared for the transition and uncertain as to what, exactly, will occur.

Transition Readiness

Transition readiness includes ongoing assessments up until the time of transition. The American Academy of Pediatrics "Got Transition" statement encourages starting the process in the patient's early teens. The American College of Cardiology recommends initiation of the transition process for patients with congenital heart disease in the preteen years, with the goal of completing transition during the college years. A similar approach can be used for other congenital and acquired conditions, but this requires dedicated staffing to create and expand programs to provide uninterrupted transitions of care. Many providers overestimate the readiness and comprehension of their patients, because much of the communication has been with parents or guardians.

Provider Training/Provider Discomfort

Most training in general internal medicine and its subspecialties focuses on the recognition, diagnosis, management, and complications of health conditions acquired in adulthood. As a result, many adult-based hospitalists feel uncomfortable caring for the pediatric patient population, often citing lack of familiarity with the literature and insufficient training in chronic diseases of childhood. Similarly, pediatric physicians are not familiar with the standard monitoring practices for adult-acquired diseases, such as colon cancer, cervical cancer, heart disease, and others.

Relationships With Adult-Based Care Providers and Institutions

Particularly at freestanding children's hospitals, logistics of transfer can be difficult when the institution is not aligned with adult care providers and institutions. In shared pediatric and adult care systems, the logistical barriers are less complex, but the provider-based barriers remain the same. To be successful, the pediatric team must identify the appropriate adult-based ambulatory and inpatient medical homes for the transitioning patient.

Overcoming Barriers

Once established barriers have been identified, action plans can be developed to overcome them.

Institutional policy. A key early step for every organization (ambulatory and/or inpatient) is the development of a written policy that is displayed in a public domain and discussed with patients and families. Important components include expectations of the organization and the process of transition of adolescent patients to adult-based medical teams.

Transition readiness. An early step in accomplishing patient transition can include an ongoing needs assessment, highlighting medical knowledge, independent medical decision-making, self-advocacy, and emotional separation from current pediatric providers. Devote time at each encounter to addressing these needs and encourage teenagers to be actively involved in these discussions. Case management professionals, psychologists, and social workers are key contributors to a successful transition readiness program.

Provider training/provider discomfort. Internal medicine/pediatrics and family medicine–trained physicians have undergone unique training that equips them to serve this population. However, few internal medicine–trained hospitalists have received adequate education about caring for patients with chronic diseases of childhood. Many institutions are establishing adult medicine consult services led by medicine/pediatrics hospitalists to improve the quality of care delivered to this population.

Relationships with adult-based care providers and institutions. Pediatric institutions may establish formal agreements with partnering adult facilities. This may include dual appointments for specific pediatric medical subspecialists and pediatric surgeons and/or formalized institutional agreements. This is especially important for patients who may experience technical complications (eg, malfunction of grafted tissue in patients with congenital heart disease) that necessitate the expertise of physicians (eg, pediatric cardiologists and pediatric cardiothoracic surgeons) who are more familiar with anatomic variations not frequently encountered in adult populations.

There are now a small number of "lifetime specialty clinics" for patients with congenital or acquired childhood disease who require transition to adult care. These specialty clinics employ both pediatric and adult-based physicians who collaborate to provide the optimal care for this specific population. As the number of patients surviving into adulthood with congenital and complex medical diseases grows, an increasing number of "lifetime clinics" will be able to serve as medical homes for these adults.

Bibliography

American Academy of Pediatrics, American Academy of Family Physicians, American College of Physicians, and Transitions Clinical Report Authoring Group. Supporting the health care transition from adolescence to adulthood in the medical home. *Pediatrics.* 2011;128(1):182–200

Fernandes SM, O'Sullivan-Oliveira J, Landzberg MJ, et al. Transition and transfer of adolescents and young adults with pediatric onset chronic disease: the patient and parent perspective. *J Pediatr Rehabil Med.* 2014;7(1):43–51

Hunt S, Sharma N. Pediatric to adult-care transitions in childhood-onset chronic disease: hospitalist perspectives. *J Hosp Med.* 2013;8(11): 627–630

Kovacs AH, McCrindle BW. So hard to say goodbye: transition from paediatric to adult cardiology care. *Nat Rev Cardiol.* 2014;11(1):51–62

Transport

Introduction

Hospitalist involvement in pediatric interfacility transport is evolving. Pediatric hospitalists may find themselves as either the referring physician looking for a higher level of care or the physician accepting the patient at the higher-level institution.

Communication

Securing the correct care team and appropriate transport vehicle depends on complete, accurate, and timely communication Transport programs differ in the method of access for referring physicians. Some have communication centers, which can vary in model, while others have hospital-based personnel who answer the calls and organize all aspects of the transport. Either way, having one telephone number, with 24-hour coverage, that personnel at referring sites can call is the safest and most efficient means to conduct transports.

On both ends, log and save all communications for later review. This transport information then becomes part of the medical record. Triage decisions will depend on the patient's diagnosis and whether the proposed receiving hospital has the higher-level capabilities desired. Personnel answering the telephone must know to whom to triage the call (hospitalist, emergency department [ED], or pediatric intensive care unit [PICU] attending physician) and where to refer the intake call if desired services are unavailable. See the American Academy of Pediatrics (AAP) Guidelines for Developing Admission and Discharge Policies for the Pediatric Intensive Care Unit and Admission and Discharge Guidelines for the Pediatric Patient Requiring Intermediate Care (see the Bibliography) for decisions regarding when to refer a child to a PICU or an intermediate level of care. Sample referring and intake forms are shown in Figures 62-1 and 62-2.

Transport Team Composition

Transport teams vary among institutions, with several different possible combinations that include physicians, nurse practitioners (NPs), registered nurses (RNs), physician assistants, respiratory therapists, emergency medical technicians (EMTs), and paramedics. The medical control physician (MCP), along with the referring physician, assesses the patient's needs and determines the team composition accordingly.

Figure 62-1. Hospitalist Transport Activation—Guidance Card (Referring)

1. Discuss patient with accepting physician
2. Location recommendation: ED, ward, PICU, NICU
3. Time-out: (provide information)

   Today's date and time _____

   Referring physician _____

   Referring hospital _____

   Hospital address (if needed) _____

   Referring hospital phone number _____

   Where is patient located in hospital? _____

   Patient name _____

   Patient date of birth _____

   Patient telephone _____

   Chief concern _____

   Medical history _____

   Vital signs _____

   Pertinent labs and x-rays _____

   Get medical advice until transport arrives _____
4. Ask for anticipated arrival time
5. Ask for call-back number in case patient status changes

There are three levels of transport: basic life support (BLS), advanced life support (ALS), and critical care transport. Individual state pediatric guidelines vary, with some more stringent than others. BLS transports involve only EMTs, usually no medications or intravenous (IV) fluids, and minimal oxygen administration. EMTs are trained in basic cardiopulmonary resuscitation, and just a small percentage of their training and encounters involve children. ALS transport teams involve paramedics and/or RNs and can administer various medications, infuse IV fluids, provide oxygen, and maintain temperature control. Critical care transport teams include specialized RNs, NPs, and/or physicians and can provide higher-level, critical care needs, often for patients with one or more failing organ systems.

Specialized teams have been shown to improve patient outcomes, although this does not necessarily mean that a physician must be present. However, if response time is crucial (ie, the patient requires an emergent procedure

Figure 62-2. Hospitalist Transport Activation—Guidance Card (Intake)

1. Discuss patient with referring physician
2. Consider bed situation
3. Time-out: (collect information)

   Today's date and time _____

   Referring physician _____

   Referring hospital _____

   Hospital address (if needed) _____

   Referring hospital telephone number _____

   Where is patient located in hospital? _____

   Patient name _____

   Patient date of birth _____

   Patient telephone _____

   Chief concern _____

   Medical history _____

   Vital signs _____

   Pertinent labs/x-ray _____

   Give medical advice until transport arrives _____
4. Give referring site anticipated arrival time
5. Activate transport (phone no.):
6. Call admitting resident
7. Await notification of transport arrival at referral site

that can only be performed at the accepting institution), then it may be more beneficial to send a BLS team, which can be mobilized in much less time than an entire critical care team. In addition, sending a critical care team for a patient with simple medical needs can be an inefficient use of resources. It is always helpful to speak with the referring physicians and understand their preferences.

When accepting a patient from a private practitioner's office or clinic, specify that the child will not be exposed to a lower level of care during transit to the hospital. The MCP may decide that the safest approach would be using local emergency medical services to transport the patient to a nearby ED. Referral hospitals must abide by the federal Emergency Medical Treatment and Labor Act, which requires hospital personnel to evaluate all patients who arrive with emergent conditions and to stabilize them before transfer. The MCP must review the case with the referring physician when deciding about the proper composition of the transport team, personnel, and mode. Medicolegal responsibility is shared once a receiving hospital accepts a patient. Therefore, the MCP must work in conjunction with the referring physician to help make these decisions.

Role of the MCP

The MCP starts caring for the patient when the transport team arrives and can provide advice to the referring physician about the continuing evaluation and management of the child. At this point, the MCP may also need to consult with subspecialists. It is important for the MCP to have easy communication with the transport team (via radio or cell phone), especially when difficult decisions arise. Therefore, the MCP should have knowledge of the transport environment and equipment.

Of note, state regulations may dictate who can act in the role of MCP. In many cases, it can be any pediatrician, but in some states, it needs to be a critical care or ED physician. The role of an MCP is evolving, though, and with the increased presence of pediatric hospitalists who are familiar with transport program protocols and the transport environment, a program can rely on the hospitalist to act as the primary MCP.

Equipment

Do not assume that the referring hospital can provide all of the equipment required for transport. Rather, develop and maintain a supply of dedicated specialized storage packs designed to cover pediatric critical care needs for all age and weight ranges. The fourth edition of the AAP *Guidelines for Air and Ground Transport of Neonatal and Pediatric Patients* has sample supply lists (in Tables 6.1, 6.2, and 6.3). Know what supplies accompany every transport and which additional supplies you may need to request for a given service. Check the equipment daily to ensure that oxygen and battery supplies are sufficient for the expected duration of any potential transport.

Vehicle Selection

The three different types of vehicles are ambulance, fixed-wing plane, and helicopter. The MCP makes the decision about which vehicle to use in coordination with the referring hospital. Selection criteria include severity of the illness or injury, distance to the referring hospital, travel time required, weather conditions, vehicle availability, equipment needs, and expense.

Factors to keep in mind when considering whether or not to fly are that fixed-wing planes require several ambulance transfers, flying at certain altitudes can affect partial pressure in body cavities and increase the volume of entrapped air, and space is a constraint in air transport, so equipment and personnel may be limited.

Safety

Safety is a priority with each transport. Air transport may be faster but carries inherent risks, including weather, mechanical failure, and collisions. Weather plays a significant role in all modes of transport. The Commission on Accreditation of Medical Transport Systems offers guidelines for minimal safe weather conditions. If a transport is delayed because of weather, the MCP must continue to guide the management of the patient until a transport can take place. In addition, advise ambulances to never use lights and sirens, because the data indicate that this has no positive effect on patient outcome.

Bibliography

American Academy of Pediatrics Committee on Hospital Care and Section on Critical Care; and Society of Critical Care Medicine Pediatric Section Admission Criteria Task Force. Guidelines for developing admission and discharge policies for the pediatric intensive care unit. *Pediatrics*. 1999;103(4):840–842

American Academy of Pediatrics Section on Transport Medicine. *Guidelines for Air and Ground Transport of Neonatal and Pediatric Patients*. 4th ed. Elk Grove Village, IL: American Academy of Pediatrics; 2016

Edgerton EA, Klein BL. Interfacility transport of the seriously ill or injured pediatric patient. In: Kliegman RM, Stanton BF, St Geme JW III, Schor NF, Behrman RE, eds. *Nelson Textbook of Pediatrics*. 20th ed. Philadelphia, PA: Elsevier; 2016:481–483

Felmet K, Orr RA, Han YY, Roth KR. Pediatric transport: shifting the paradigm to improve patient outcome. In: Fuhrman BP, Zimmerman J, eds. *Pediatric Critical Care*. 4th ed. Philadelphia, PA: Mosby; 2011:132–138

Jaimovich DG; American Academy of Pediatrics Committee on Hospital Care and Section on Critical Care. Admission and discharge guidelines for the pediatric patient requiring intermediate care. *Pediatrics*. 2004;113(5):1430–1433

Orr RA, Felmet KA, Han Y, et al. Pediatric specialized transport teams are associated with improved outcomes. *Pediatrics*. 2009;124(1):40–48

Stroud MH, Trautman MS, Meyer K, et al. Pediatric and neonatal interfacility transport: results from a national consensus conference. *Pediatrics*. 2013;132(2):359–366

Immunology

Immunodeficiency

Introduction

Primary immunodeficiencies (PIs) are inherited disorders of the immune system that predispose patients to recurrent infections, malignancies, and autoimmune diseases. Unusually severe, long-lasting, atypical, or repeated infections are indications for an immune system evaluation. In addition to the 10 classic warning signs of PI (Box 63-1), other clues for immunodeficiency include chronic diarrhea; atypical infections; complications from live vaccines; autoimmune disease, such as idiopathic thrombocytopenic purpura; and malignancies, such as lymphoma.

There are some typical patterns of age of onset, infectious organism(s), and site(s) of infection for each type of PI (Table 63-1). In addition to the classic categories of humoral, cellular, combined, phagocytic, and complement-mediated PI, newly discovered PIs and molecular techniques have caused the classification to be revised to include diseases of immune dysregulation, innate immunity, and autoinflammation.

Clinical Presentation

History

Obtain a thorough history, including age of onset and locations of infections, types of organisms, and need for intravenous (IV) antibiotic therapy. Defects in antibody production typically appear with sinopulmonary infections, once transplacental maternal antibody levels decline after 6 months, in a patient

Box 63-1. Ten Warning Signs of a Primary Immunodeficiency
≥4 New ear infections within 1 year
≥2 Serious sinus infections within 1 year
≥2 Months on antibiotics with little effect
≥2 Pneumonias within 1 year
Failure of an infant to gain weight or grow normally
Recurrent deep skin or organ abscesses
Persistent thrush in the mouth or fungal infection on the skin
Need for intravenous antibiotics to clear infections
≥2 Deep-seated infections, including septicemia
Family history of primary immunodeficiency

These warning signs were developed by the Jeffrey Modell Foundation Medical Advisory Board. Consultation with primary immunodeficiency experts is strongly suggested. © 2016 Jeffrey Modell Foundation.

Chapter 63: Immunodeficiency

Table 63-1. Primary Immunodeficiencies

Presentation	Defects	Examples	Organisms	Onset	Initial Laboratory Workup
Recurrent sinopulmonary infections (sinusitis, otitis media, pneumonia), diarrhea	Antibody deficiencies	XLA, IgA deficiency, CVID	Encapsulated bacteria, *Giardia lamblia*	After 6–9 mo of age	Ig levels (IgA, IgG, IgM)
FTT, rash, thrush, pneumonia, opportunistic infections	Combined defects	SCID, DiGeorge syndrome, Wiskott-Aldrich syndrome, hyper-IgM due to CD40 or CD40 ligand mutations	Adenovirus, *Candida*, CMV, EBV, *Pneumocystis jirovecii*, parainfluenza, varicella	Infancy	Ig levels T, B, NK cells Chest radiography Flow cytometry or mitogen stimulation
Skin or solid organ abscesses, pneumonia, dental infections	Phagocytic defects	CGD, LAD, hyper-IgE syndrome	*Burkholderia cepacia*, *Aspergillus*, *Nocardia*, *Serratia*, *Staphylococcus*	Infancy to young adult	CBC, IgE, CGD assay
Sinopulmonary infections, glomerulonephritis, meningitis	Complement defects	C3, membrane attack complex, regulatory components	Encapsulated bacteria, especially *Streptococcus pneumoniae* and *Neisseria*	Infancy to young adult	CH50
Mucocutaneous fungal infections, mycobacterial multifocal osteomyelitis, MAC	Cellular deficiencies	Chronic mucocutaneous candidiasis, IFN-g/IL-12 receptor deficiency	*Candida*, *Mycobacterium*, *Salmonella*	Young child to adolescent	IFN-g level, DTH or lymphocyte proliferation for *Candida*

Abbreviations: CBC, complete blood cell count; CD40, cluster of differentiation 40; CGD, chronic granulomatous disease; CH50, total complement activity; CMV, cytomegalovirus; CVID, common variable immune deficiency; C3, complement component 3; DTH, delayed type hypersensitivity; EBV, Epstein-Barr virus; FTT, failure to thrive; IFN, interferon; Ig, immunoglobulin; IL-12, interleukin-12; LAD, leukocyte adhesion defect; MAC, *Mycobacterium avium* complex; NK, natural killer; SCID, severe combined immune deficiency; XLA, X-linked agammaglobulinemia.

who is otherwise thriving. Combined T and B cell defects appear early in infancy, with failure to thrive (FTT), diarrhea, rash, opportunistic infections, and pneumonia. Phagocytic defects typically appear in infancy to early adulthood as skin, lymph node, and organ abscesses and pneumonia. Complement component 3, or C3, deficiencies may appear early in life, similar to antibody defects, while late component deficiencies (C5–C9) predispose older children and young adults to recurrent *Neisseria* infections.

Assess the patient's growth pattern and document the vaccine status, as well as whether there have been any severe or unusual adverse reactions to live vaccines. Check the family history for any recurrent infections or known immunodeficiency. Finally, document all previous culture and serologic results.

A PI can also appear with autoimmune disease or malignancy at presentation. Some patients with common variable immune deficiency (CVID) develop immune thrombocytopenic purpura prior to any infections. Some PIs, such as autoimmune lymphoproliferative syndrome and X-linked lymphoproliferative syndrome, are predominantly immune dysregulation that appears with fever, adenopathy, and hepatosplenomegaly at presentation.

Physical Examination

Perform a complete physical examination (Table 63-2), paying special attention to any rash (including in the diaper area); evidence of previous or current skin infections or abscess; thrush; the lack of tonsils or palpable lymph nodes (especially in the neck and groin); and signs of otitis media, sinusitis, or pneumonia. Digital clubbing can be seen with recurrent pneumonias and subsequent bronchiectasis and respiratory failure. Plot the child's growth curves and review them for signs of FTT.

Laboratory Workup

The types of infection(s) guide the initial laboratory testing (Table 63-1). For any patient with suspected PI, perform a complete blood cell count (CBC) with differential and urinalysis and obtain the erythrocyte sedimentation rate or C-reactive protein level, comprehensive metabolic panel, HIV screen, and quantitative immunoglobulin (Ig) levels (IgA, IgG, IgM, and IgE) *prior* to consulting an immunologist. If a patient has any chest symptoms, obtain a chest radiograph. Order a sweat chloride test if the patient has had frequent sinopulmonary infections, especially if the newborn cystic fibrosis screening results are not available. Lymphopenia can be a clue for severe combined immunodeficiency (SCID), so an absolute lymphocyte count less than $2,500/mm^3$ in a newborn must be investigated (see the guidelines herein). Several states now perform standard newborn screening for SCIDs, but this

Table 63-2. Physical Examination Findings and Associated Immune Deficiencies

Physical Examination Findings	Associated Immune Deficiency
Aphthous ulcers	CGD
Ataxia or telangiectasia	Ataxia-telangiectasia
Digital clubbing	Any immune deficiency leading to recurrent pneumonia or bronchiectasis
Delayed separation of the umbilical cord Severe gingivitis	Leukocyte adhesion defect
Failure to thrive	T cell defects (SCID)
Granuloma formation Lymphoid hyperplasia	CGD CVID
Hypertelorism, heart murmur, low-set ears, microcephaly, cleft lip and/or palate	DiGeorge syndrome
Lack of tonsils and palpable lymph nodes (especially in the neck and groin)	XLA SCID
Nonspecific rash	SCID
Otitis media/sinusitis findings (perforated or scarred TMs, purulent nasal discharge)	B cell defects (XLA, IgA deficiency, CVID)
Petechiae	Wiskott-Aldrich syndrome
Severe diaper dermatitis Persistent or recurrent thrush	T cell defects (SCID, chronic mucocutaneous candidiasis)
Severe eczema	Hyper-IgE syndrome Wiskott-Aldrich syndrome
Skin abscess or adenitis (unusual organisms or severe/recurrent infection with *Staphylococcus aureus*)	Phagocytic defect (CGD)

Abbreviations: CGD, chronic granulomatous disease; CVID, common variable immune deficiency; Ig, immunoglobulin; SCID, severe combined immune deficiency; TM, tympanic membrane; XLA, X-linked agammaglobulinemia.

will not allow PIs with normal lymphocyte counts to be identified. A low globulin fraction on a metabolic panel suggests decreased Ig levels.

Obtain an immunology consult if there is a high index of suspicion or abnormal initial laboratory values. However, if immunology services are not available, pursue further workup as described herein.

For recurrent sinopulmonary infections with encapsulated organisms consistent with a B cell defect, obtain IgA, IgM, and IgG levels, although IgG subclasses are typically not helpful. If the Ig levels are less than 2 SDs below normal or if a humoral defect is a concern, order antibody titers (tetanus, diphtheria, *Candida*). After infancy, an IgG level <200 mg/dL (2 g/L) or a total Ig level (IgG, IgA, and IgM) less than 400 mg/dL suggests a severe humoral defect and warrants urgent consult with an immunologist. Most laboratories can determine Ig levels, but confirm that appropriate age-based normal levels are used when interpreting the results.

Suspect a phagocyte deficiency if there are skin, lymph node, or solid organ abscesses, especially with unusual organisms such as *Klebsiella* or *Serratia;* delayed wound healing; cavitary pneumonias; or infections with *Staphylococcus aureus, Burkholderia cepacia, Serratia, Nocardia,* or *Aspergillus.* Obtain a CBC, peripheral smear for neutrophils, total IgE level, and chronic granulomatous disease assay. The dihydrorhodamine oxidative burst assay is preferred over the classic nitro blue tetrazolium test. If there is delayed separation of the umbilical cord (after 4–6 weeks of age) and an increased white blood cell count, order flow cytometry for CD11/CD18, which will be absent in leukocyte adhesion deficiency type 1. Any of these abnormal test results requires prompt consultation.

If an infant has a lymphocyte count less than 2,500 mm^3, an abnormal SCID newborn screening result, or a history of opportunistic infections, check the Ig levels and flow cytometry for T, B, and natural killer cell enumeration. If these tests are not available locally, send the specimens to a referral laboratory accredited for flow cytometry assessments. Low age-based lymphocyte levels warrant urgent immunology consultation. In an infant with hypocalcemia and heart defects, order fluorescence in situ hybridization for chromosome 22q11.2 microdeletions for DiGeorge syndrome.

In a patient with recurrent pyogenic infections (especially if associated with glomerulonephritis) or recurrent *Neisseria* infections, order a CH50 test. A normal CH50 result excludes most serious complement deficiencies. If the CH50 finding is low or if complement deficiency is still suspected, an immunologist can assist with testing specific complement components, such as a mannose-binding lectin assay or an alternate pathway AH50 assay.

A patient with a PI can be predisposed to infectious or inflammatory diarrhea. Obtain stool samples for culture and test for *Clostridium difficile, Giardia,* and other ova and parasites for any patient with PI and diarrhea.

Differential Diagnosis

About 10% of children with recurrent serious infections will end up having a PI. Secondary, or acquired, immune deficiencies (Table 63-3) are more common than primary disorders and must also be considered in a patient with frequent infections. Atopic diseases, such as eczema and asthma; underlying anatomic defects; and chronic diseases, such as cystic fibrosis and diabetes, all predispose children to frequent infections. Because of the success of protocols to prevent vertical transmission, perinatal HIV cases have dramatically decreased in developed countries, but they can still occur,

Table 63-3. Secondary Causes of Immune Deficiency	
Cause	**Examples**
Autoimmune diseases	JIA SLE
Infections	HIV CMV
Immune suppressants	Corticosteroids Chemotherapy Monoclonal antibodies
Malignancies	Leukemia Lymphoma
Immunoglobulin loss	Nephrotic syndrome Protein-losing enteropathy
Asplenia	Sickle cell disease Postsurgical disease
Malnutrition	Protein deficiency Vitamins A and D deficiency Zinc deficiency
Other	Cirrhosis Cystic fibrosis Diabetes mellitus Inborn errors of metabolism Primary ciliary dyskinesia Uremia

Abbreviations: CMV, cytomegalovirus; JIA, juvenile idiopathic arthritis; SLE, systemic lupus erythematosus.

especially in children born in developing countries. Order an HIV screening prior to initiating a complex workup. HIV can appear in a manner similar to SCID at presentation, with FTT, rashes, thrush, pneumonia, and opportunistic infections. However, it will generally manifest later in life, because it may take several years for CD4 counts to decrease to levels associated with AIDS.

Numerous medications, especially chemotherapy and immune suppressants, are common causes of secondary immunodeficiency. Long-term or frequent short-term courses of systemic corticosteroids and rituximab are frequent iatrogenic causes of reduced Ig levels.

Over 50% of recurrent infections occur in normal, healthy children. Preschoolers can get 10 viral infections per year, each lasting up to 7 to 14 days, which means they could be sick frequently throughout the year. Recurrent benign viral infections are rarely a manifestation of an immune deficiency and do not warrant specialized testing. FTT without associated infections (especially opportunistic infections or pneumonia) is rarely the result of a PI.

Treatment

A patient with a phagocytic defect, combined T/B cell immunodeficiency, or severe hypogammaglobulinemia (X-linked agammaglobulinemia, hyper-IgM syndrome, CVID) will typically require hospital admission and aggressive IV antibiotic therapy for a prolonged course (≥2–4 weeks). See Table 63-4 for appropriate antibiotic choices, but use doses that are on the high end of the typical regimens. If possible, try to get a definitive diagnosis (via cultures, bronchoscopy, etc) to guide therapy. The patient will often need a central line catheter for several weeks, but avoid permanent indwelling access devices because they significantly increase the long-term infection risk.

Suspected SCID is an emergency. Immediately consult with an immunologist if lymphocyte studies are low (see the Laboratory Workup section). Patients with SCID are at risk for graft versus host disease and must be given irradiated, cytomegalovirus-negative blood products. For a patient with suspected SCID or complete lack of Ig, administer IVIg (400–500 mg/kg) and repeat in 1 to 3 days and then monthly. If possible, perform the appropriate antibody studies before starting IgG therapy. Also, SCID is a contraindication to breastfeeding to reduce the risk of transmitting cytomegalovirus.

A patient with PI is at increased risk for malignancies and autoimmune diseases. Autoimmune hemolytic anemia, thrombocytopenia, and neutropenia are frequently seen with CVID, hyper-IgM syndrome, and other PIs.

Table 63-4. Antibiotic Therapy for Immunodeficient Patients[a]

Defects	Organisms	Typical Antibiotics[b]
Antibody deficiencies	Encapsulated bacteria	Ceftriaxone or levofloxacin
Cellular deficiencies	*Candida, Mycobacterium, Salmonella*	Ceftriaxone Fluconazole Triple therapy for *Mycobacterium*
Combined defects	Adenovirus, *Candida*, EBV, CMV, parainfluenza virus, *Pneumocystis jirovecii*, varicella	TMP/SMX *plus* extended β-lactam (meropenem, piperacillin/tazobactam, cefepime, etc) If patient appears septic: Add vancomycin Significant thrush or a diaper rash: If MRSA is prevalent, add vancomycin Consider fluconazole Interstitial pneumonia: Add macrolide
Complement defects	Encapsulated bacteria, *Neisseria*	Same as antibody defects
Phagocytic defects	*Aspergillus, Burkholderia cepacia, Nocardia, Serratia, Staphylococcus*	Voriconazole *plus* (TMP/SMX, fluoroquinolone, or meropenem) Add vancomycin if *Staphylococcus* is likely

Abbreviations: CMV, cytomegalovirus; EBV, Epstein-Barr virus; MRSA, methicillin-resistant *Staphylococcus aureus*; SMX, sulfamethoxazole; TMP, trimethoprim.
[a] See specific chapters on infectious diseases for dosing guidelines.
[b] See *Nelson's Pediatric Antimicrobial Therapy* (www.aap.org/nelsonsabx) for dosing.

Consult both an immunologist and a hematologist because the patient may need steroids, high-dose IVIg, or rituximab.

A patient with complete IgA deficiency may have anti-IgA antibodies, which can rarely lead to anaphylactic reactions to IVIg and other blood products. Order washed red blood cells and consider IVIg preparations with low IgA levels, but testing for anti-IgA antibodies is not helpful.

Indications for Consultation
- **Immunology:** Abnormal immune laboratory test results or opportunistic infection
- **Infectious diseases:** Complex or opportunistic infection
- **Pulmonologist:** Chronic pulmonary infections, bronchiectasis

Disposition
- **Intensive care unit transfer:** Septic shock, respiratory failure
- **Discharge criteria:** Afebrile for 24 to 48 hours or longer with appropriate treatment of acute infection underway

Follow-up
- **Primary care:** 1 week
- **Immunology or infectious diseases (if involved):** 2 to 4 weeks

Pearls and Pitfalls
- Admit a patient with severe immune deficiency and temperature of 38.3°C (101°F) or obvious infection and promptly initiate IV antibiotics. A prolonged course of IV antibiotics may be necessary.
- Obtain appropriate cultures as quickly as possible.
- Complete the laboratory evaluation (Ig levels, vaccine and isohemagglutinin titers) prior to treatment with Ig.
- Initiate proper isolation precautions, especially for a patient with suspected SCID.
- While rare, if a patient with complete IgA deficiency is given Ig, monitor closely for anaphylaxis.
- Suspect SCID in an infant with a lymphocyte count lower than 2,500/mm^3.

Bibliography

Bonilla FA, Khan DA, Ballas ZK, et al. Practice parameter for the diagnosis and management of primary immunodeficiency. *J Allergy Clin Immunol*. 2015;136(5):1186–1205

Chinen J, Paul ME, Shearer WT. Approach to the evaluation of the immunodeficient patient. In: Rich RR, Fleisher TA, Shearer WT, Schroeder HW Jr, Frew AJ, Weyand CM, eds. *Clinical Immunology: Principles and Practice*. 4th ed. London, United Kingdom: Elsevier; 2013:381–390

Modell V, Knaus M, Modell F, Roifman C, Orange J, Notarangelo LD. Global overview of primary immunodeficiencies: a report from Jeffrey Modell Centers worldwide focused on diagnosis, treatment, and discovery. *Immunol Res*. 2014;60(1):132–144

Subbarayan A, Colarusso G, Hughes SM, et al. Clinical features that identify children with primary immunodeficiency diseases. *Pediatrics*. 2011;127(5):810–816

Bibliography

Infectious Diseases

Fever in Infants Younger Than 60 Days

Introduction

In an infant younger than 60 days of age, fever is defined as a rectal temperature of 38°C (100.4°F) or higher. In this age group, fever may be the only sign of meningitis, bacteremia, and/or a urinary tract infection (UTI). Other bacterial infections, such as pneumonia, bacterial gastroenteritis, and skin and soft-tissue infections can also cause fever in this age group but generally appear with additional signs or symptoms at presentation. UTI is the most prevalent bacterial infection (7%–10% of cases) in febrile but otherwise well-appearing infants, while bacteremia (2% of cases) and meningitis (<1% of cases) are rare. Risk stratification criteria (eg, Rochester Criteria) can be used to identify infants who are at low overall risk (<2%) of serious bacterial infection (SBI).

The common bacterial organisms encountered in the first 60 days of life include *Escherichia coli,* group B *Streptococcus* (GBS) and *Streptococcus pneumoniae,* and, less commonly, *Staphylococcus aureus, Klebsiella, Salmonella, Enterococcus,* and *Listeria monocytogenes.* Of note, neonates are at higher risk of bacterial infection than older infants.

Clinical Presentation

History

Ask about the infant's temperature at home and how it was obtained; birth history; maternal infection risks (including herpes simplex virus [HSV] and GBS); underlying medical conditions; level of fussiness or irritability; feeding habits; lethargy; change in respiratory status; vomiting and bowel habits; urine output; rashes; immunization history; exposure to ill persons; use of antipyretics; and history of recent travel, immigration, or homelessness.

Of note, axillary and tympanic membrane temperatures are unreliable. However, consider a patient who reportedly had a documented rectal fever at home but is afebrile at presentation to be febrile to the degree reported in the history.

Physical Examination

The physical examination findings may be unremarkable, but always evaluate the patient's vital signs and overall appearance. Concerning findings include irritability, lethargy, hypotonia, grunting, bulging fontanelle, tachypnea, apnea, seizures, mottled skin, cyanosis, poor capillary refill, jaundice, soft-tissue swelling, and difficulty moving an extremity. Meningeal signs may be absent in an infant younger than 2 months. Vesicular lesions involving the skin, eye, or mouth can occur with an HSV infection.

Laboratory Workup

The extent of laboratory workup is age based and somewhat controversial. Several sets of well-validated risk stratification criteria (Boston, Philadelphia, and Rochester Criteria) have been developed to attempt to identify febrile but otherwise well-appearing infants who are at particularly low risk for SBI (Table 64-1). Choose the guideline to follow before performing the laboratory tests and not after the results are obtained. For example, the Boston and Philadelphia Criteria require cerebrospinal fluid (CSF) studies, so if the lumbar puncture is unsuccessful, the patient must be classified as high risk.

In general, for any febrile, well-appearing infant, order a complete blood cell count, urinalysis, and urine culture. Also perform a blood culture if the patient is 28 days or younger, because there is a higher risk of bacterial infection. For any infant who does not meet low-risk criteria, perform blood cultures and CSF studies, if not done previously.

If the patient has respiratory signs or symptoms, obtain a chest radiograph. If a viral respiratory tract infection is a concern for an infant older than 28 days, a respiratory viral panel may help to decrease the length of hospitalization and limit the unnecessary use of antibiotics. If the respiratory panel findings are positive, then an infant who meets low-risk criteria is eligible for discharge at 24 hours. However, a rhinovirus-positive finding is the exception, since it is not significantly predictive of a decreased risk of concurrent SBI. Order an enterovirus polymerase chain reaction (PCR) test between June and

Table 64-1. Summary of Low-Risk Criteria

	Rochester	Philadelphia	Boston
Age	≤60 d	29–60 d	28–89 d
Appearance	Well	Well	Well
WBC count	5–15,000/mm^3	<15,000/mm^3	<20,000/mm^3
CSF	NA	<8 WBC/hpf	<10 WBC/hpf
Urine	≤10 WBC/hpf	<10 WBC/hpf (-) Urine Gram stain	<10 WBC/hpf
Stool	≤5 WBC/hpf (if diarrhea)	No blood or few/no WBCs (if indicated)	NA
Chest radiography	NA	(-) (If obtained)	(-) (If obtained)
Other		Band-to–total neutrophil ratio <0.2	

Abbreviations: CSF, cerebrospinal fluid; hpf, high-power field; NA, not applicable; WBC, white blood cell; -, negative finding.

November if there is CSF pleocytosis. Persistent watery, mucoid, or bloody stools is an indication for a stool for culture.

Disseminated or central nervous system (CNS) HSV is a concern in neonates with sepsis syndrome or seizures with or without a vesicular rash. If disseminated or CNS HSV is a possibility, obtain liver transaminase levels, as well as CSF and blood for PCR assay. Perform oral, nasopharyngeal, conjunctival, and rectal swabs for HSV culture and PCR when there is a possibility of HSV skin, eye(s), and/or mouth (SEM) disease.

Differential Diagnosis

Most patients will have an infectious etiology for the fever. Viral, bacterial, and fungal infections may be acquired vertically or horizontally, so assume that a neonate 7 days of age or younger has a perinatal infection until proven otherwise. The most common viral etiologies include enteroviruses, rhinoviruses, and respiratory syncytial virus. Although bacterial infections are less likely, they can be much more serious, and they must therefore be ruled out. *Listeria monocytogenes* is a rare cause of fever in an otherwise well-appearing infant, because the patient most often appears ill.

Of note, approximately three-quarters of infants who contract HSV were born to women who had no history or clinical findings suggestive of genital HSV infection during or preceding pregnancy. Initial signs of HSV can occur any time between birth and 6 weeks, although almost all infected infants with disseminated, CNS, or SEM disease develop clinical symptoms within the first month of life. Although fever is unusual, consider disseminated or CNS HSV in a neonate with sepsis syndrome, negative bacterial culture findings, seizures, liver dysfunction, coagulopathy, and/or CSF pleocytosis.

Other possible etiologies for fever include a focal abscess, cellulitis, omphalitis, GBS lymphadenitis, osteomyelitis, pertussis, malignancy, and nonaccidental trauma.

Treatment

A full workup—including blood, urine, and CSF cultures—and empirical antibiotics (as detailed herein) are indicated for an ill-appearing infant, regardless of age. Refer to Tables 64-2 and 64-3 for dosing recommendations.

0 to 28 Days of Life

Treat with empirical intravenous (IV) antibiotics, since low-risk assignment may be less reliable. Target therapy for *E coli*, GBS, and *S pneumoniae*. *L monocytogenes* is rare, but treat a patient for *L monocytogenes* in the first month of life or if the CSF results suggest meningitis.

Table 64-2. Antimicrobial Dosing for Patients ≤28 Days Old			
Medication	**Route**	**Dosing for Patients Weighing <2 kg**	**Dosing for Patients Weighing >2 kg**
Ampicillin	IV IM	≤7 d: 100 mg/kg/d, divided into doses administered every 12 h 8–28 d: 150 mg/kg/d, divided into doses administered every 8 h	≤7 d: 150 mg/kg/d, divided into doses administered every 8 h 8–28 d: 200 mg/kg/d, divided into doses administered every 6 h
Gentamicin	IV IM	≤7 d: 5 mg/kg every 48 h 8–28 d: 5 mg/kg every 36 h	≤7 d: 4 mg/kg every 24 h 8–28 d: 4–5mg/kg every 24 h
Cefotaxime	IV IM	≤7 d: 100 mg/kg/d, divided into doses administered every 12 h 8–28 d: 100–150 mg/d, divided into doses administered every 8-12 h	≤7 d: 100 mg/kg/d, divided into doses administered every 12 h 8–28 d: 150 mg/d, divided into doses administered every 8 h
Ceftriaxone	IV IM	50 mg/kg every 24 h	50 mg/kg every 24 h
Vancomycin	IV	Dosing based on creatinine concentration; refer to the AAP *Red Book* for dosing recommendations	Creatinine concentration will not reflect neonatal renal function until about day 5 of life

Abbreviations: AAP, American Academy of Pediatrics; IM, intramuscular; IV, intravenous.

Table 64-3. Antimicrobial Dosing for Patients >28 Days Old			
Medication	**Route**	**Dosing**	**Comments**
Ampicillin	IV IM	200–400 mg/kg/d, divided into doses administered every 6 h (12-g/d adult maximum)	Reserve highest dosing for presumed CNS infections
Gentamicin	IV IM	6.0–7.5 mg/kg/d, divided into doses administered every 8 h May be given in one dose	Use serum concentrations to guide ongoing therapy
Cefotaxime	IV IM	200–225 mg/kg/d, divided into doses administered every 4–6 h (up to 300 mg/kg/d for meningitis)	
Ceftriaxone	IV IM	100 mg/kg/d, divided into doses administered every 12–24 h (2-4-g/d adult maximum)	
Vancomycin	IV	45–60 mg/kg/d, divided into doses administered every 6–8 h	Use serum concentrations to guide ongoing therapy
Acyclovir	IV	60 mg/kg/d, divided into doses administered every 8 h × 14 d for SEM and 21 d for CNS or disseminated disease	

Abbreviations: CNS: central nervous system; IM, intramuscular; IV, intravenous; SEM, skin, eye(s), and/or mouth.

A combination of IV ampicillin *and either* IV gentamicin *or* a third-generation cephalosporin (cefotaxime or ceftriaxone) provides appropriate empirical coverage for the most common bacteria. Ceftriaxone is contraindicated if the patient has hyperbilirubinemia or is receiving an IV calcium-containing solution.

If the patient has evidence of a soft-tissue infection in a community with a significant prevalence of methicillin-resistant *S aureus* (MRSA) and is well appearing with no clinical suspicion of meningitis, administer clindamycin *and* a third-generation cephalosporin, pending culture results. For an infant who is ill appearing or if there is a clinical suspicion for meningitis, use vancomycin instead of clindamycin. In the absence of new or concerning findings during hospitalization, most often an infant younger than 28 days of age can be discharged 36 hours after receiving negative culture findings.

If the clinical presentation is concerning for HSV infection (mucocutaneous vesicles, focal neurologic symptoms, apnea, seizures, CSF pleocytosis, and/or increased liver transaminase levels), treat empirically with IV acyclovir, pending diagnostic studies. However, if HSV testing can be performed rapidly (within a few hours) and the clinical suspicion for HSV infection is low, treatment can be deferred until the test results are available.

29 to 60 Days of Life

An infant that meets low-risk criteria does not necessarily require empirical antibiotics, unless the clinical situation worsens or microbiological cultures suggest a pathologic organism. Treat a non–low-risk infant with a third-generation cephalosporin, pending culture results. Add IV ampicillin if there is a concern for meningitis or if the patient has findings suggestive of an *Enterococcus* infection (eg, if either gram-positive cocci are seen on a urine Gram stain or if *Enterococcus* is locally prevalent).

As with a younger, well-appearing infant, use clindamycin *and* a third-generation cephalosporin if there is evidence of a soft-tissue infection in a community with a significant prevalence of MRSA. Reserve vancomycin for a patient who is ill appearing or if there is a clinical suspicion for meningitis. Once again, in the absence of new or concerning findings during hospitalization, a patient 29 to 60 days of age can be discharged 36 hours after receiving negative culture findings.

Indications for Consultation

Infectious diseases: Atypical presentation and/or clinical course

Disposition

- **Intensive care unit transfer:** Hemodynamic instability despite administration of IV fluids and antibiotics or significant respiratory distress, apnea, or seizures
- **Discharge criteria:** Patient well appearing, good oral intake, and negative culture findings for at least 36 hours

Follow-up

Primary care: 2 to 3 days

Pearls and Pitfalls

- Birth via cesarean section does not eliminate the risk of neonatal HSV.
- HSV CSF PCR findings may be negative during the first few days of the illness. Treat empirically and perform serial CSF testing if there is a high degree of clinical suspicion for HSV.
- Consider enterovirus testing if the patient has a CSF pleocytosis during the warmer months.
- The presence of blood in the CSF is not significantly associated with the rate of HSV meningoencephalitis.
- Persistent fever despite standard empirical antibiotic coverage is most likely secondary to a viral infection and not an atypical bacterial disease.
- Nonaccidental trauma can be a cause of fever.
- *Neisseria meningitidis* is a rare cause of bacterial infection in this age group and may signal an underlying complement deficiency or asplenia.

Bibliography

Kimberlin DW, Brady MT, Jackson MA, Long SS, eds. *Red Book: 2015 Report of the Committee on Infectious Diseases*. 30th ed. Elk Grove Village, IL: American Academy of Pediatrics; 2015

Biondi EA, Byington CL. Evaluation and management of febrile, well-appearing young infants. *Infect Dis Clin North Am.* 2015;29(3):575–585

Biondi E, Evans R, Mischler M, et al. Epidemiology of bacteremia in febrile infants in the United States. *Pediatrics.* 2013;132(6):990–996

Biondi EA, Mischler M, Jerardi KE, et al. Blood culture time to positivity in febrile infants with bacteremia. *JAMA Pediatr.* 2014;168(9):844–849

Byington CL, Reynolds CC, Korgenski K, et al. Costs and infant outcomes after implantation of a care process model for febrile infants. *Pediatrics.* 2012;130(1):e16–e24

Hui C, Neto G, Tsertsvadze A, et al. Diagnosis and management of febrile infants (0–3 months). *Evid Rep Technol Assess (Full Rep).* 2012;205:1–297

Huppler AR, Eickhoff JC, Wald ER. Performance of low-risk criteria in the evaluation of young infants with fever: review of the literature. *Pediatrics.* 2010;125(2):228–233

CHAPTER 65

Fever in the International Traveler

Introduction

With the increasing popularity of and access to overseas travel, there is increasing potential of exposure to pathogens not endemic to the United States, and the pediatric hospitalist may be among the first providers to encounter and manage them. Maintaining a high index of suspicion, timely recognition, management, and containment of these infections are essential for the health of the individual and the community. Recognize that common infections like upper respiratory infections, urinary tract infections, pneumonia, viral gastroenteritis, and infectious mononucleosis will still account for most infections in children with a recent travel history. Therefore, the most important aspect of care of the recent traveler is a careful history and examination. Seek signs of common infections, but be aware of the most important life-threatening infections related to travel and treat these empirically on the basis of initial findings while the evaluation proceeds.

Malaria

Malaria is caused by 1 of 5 species of intraerythrocytic parasites of the genus *Plasmodium* (*Plasmodium falciparum, Plasmodium vivax, Plasmodium ovale, Plasmodium malariae,* and *Plasmodium knowlesi*) and is spread by female mosquitoes of the *Anopheles* genus. Malaria is endemic throughout the tropics, and it is estimated that one-half of the world's population lives in areas where transmission occurs. In the World Health Organization 2015 World Malaria Report, 214 million cases and 438,000 deaths were estimated in 2015.

In the United States in 2012, almost 1,700 cases were reported, resulting in 6 deaths; all of these were acquired through foreign travel. In general, a child is at higher risk for serious disease, and this is further increased if prophylaxis was not received prior to and during travel. Malaria must always be considered as a possible diagnosis for unexplained fever in an international returnee.

Dengue

Dengue (also known as "breakbone fever") is an acute febrile illness caused by infection with one of four dengue virus (DENV) serotypes. Transmission most commonly occurs through the bite of Aedes mosquitoes (*Aedes aegypti* and *Aedes albopictus*). Since dengue viremia can last about 7 days, transmission can also occur through exposure to infected blood, organs, or other tissues. Neonates can contract the virus through perinatal transmission from infected mothers, as well as possibly through human milk.

Dengue is endemic throughout the tropics and subtropics and is a leading cause of febrile illness among travelers from Latin America, the Caribbean, and Southeast Asia. Outbreaks have occurred in North America, as well, including Florida, Hawaii, and along the Texas-Mexico border.

Typhoid Fever

Typhoid fever is caused by *Salmonella* enterica serotype typhi (*Salmonella typhi*). It is prevalent in resource-limited areas of the world with poor sanitation and overcrowding, including the Indian subcontinent, southcentral and southeast Asia, and southern Africa. It is limited to humans and acquired by ingestion of contaminated food or drink. Administration of the typhoid vaccine, available in oral and parenteral forms, is recommended at least 1 to 2 weeks prior to travel but is generally only about 50% to 80% effective.

Paratyphoid fever is caused by *S enterica* serotype paratyphi A, B, or C. However, typhoid and paratyphoid are clinically indistinguishable and are collectively termed *enteric fever.*

Clinical Presentation

History

Malaria

Ask about prophylaxis, high fevers, chills, rigors, sweats, and headache in a patient with a history of travel to a malaria-endemic area. The symptoms may begin as early as 7 days after initial exposure but may also occur as late as several months later. Patients may report cyclic fever (every 2 or 3 days), but absence of this pattern does not rule out malaria. Ask also about nausea, vomiting, cough, tachypnea, arthralgia, myalgia, abdominal pain, and back pain, because these may be present later in the course of illness. Less commonly, patients can present with intravascular hemolysis that leads to anemia, hemoglobinuria, and renal failure ("Blackwater fever").

Dengue

Dengue appears with the abrupt onset of fever at presentation, anywhere from 3 to 14 days after a potential exposure. Fever can be biphasic and lasts up to 1 week. The patient may also have severe headache, retro-orbital pain, myalgia, arthralgia, and bone pain.

The course of disease typically has 3 phases: febrile, critical, and convalescent. The critical phase begins at defervescence and lasts up to 48 hours. While most patients show clinical improvement during this phase, up to 5% develop severe dengue, with complaints consistent with substantial plasma leakage. These include generalized swelling and shortness of breath. Severe bleeding, including hematemesis, hematochezia, melena, or menorrhagia, may also be present. Severe disease is more likely in those who have been infected previously and are now experiencing a repeat infection rather than after an initial exposure.

Typhoid Fever

Typhoid/enteric fever presents with fever and abdominal pain or a true fever without a source after an incubation period of 1 to 4 weeks. The fever tends to be intermittent initially and shows a stepwise pattern and may then become continuous. Early on, the presentation may often be just fever without other localizing signs or symptoms. There may be a history of chills, anorexia, headache, abdominal pain, rash, diarrhea (possibly bloody), or conversely, constipation. Severe manifestations, such as intestinal hemorrhage or perforation, can occur in the second or third week of the illness.

Physical Examination

Malaria

The patient is typically ill appearing but not toxic, although there may be pallor or jaundice in severe cases. Hepatosplenomegaly is a common finding. Signs of severe disease include shock (hypotension, poor perfusion), altered sensorium, seizures, and organ system failure (eg, renal, respiratory, and hepatic).

Dengue

Oropharyngeal and facial erythema may be noted in the first 48 hours of symptoms. A macular or maculopapular rash may be present, and the patient may have petechiae, ecchymoses, purpura, or mild mucosal bleeding. Physical findings of severe dengue include edema (central or peripheral), decreased breath sounds because of pleural effusions, and signs of shock, such as narrowing pulse pressure, hypotension, or signs of end-organ hypoperfusion.

Typhoid Fever

The classic, but uncommon, rash is rose spots, which are macular, salmon-colored lesions over the chest and abdomen. Other findings include hepatosplenomegaly, signs of intestinal bleeding and perforation, altered mental status, and possibly shock.

Laboratory Workup

If any of these 3 diseases is being considered, obtain a complete blood cell count (CBC) with white blood cell differential and platelet count, erythrocyte sedimentation rate (ESR) and/or C-reactive protein (CRP) level, liver transaminase level, and, if the patient appears toxic, blood culture.

Malaria

The standard of reference for diagnosis is a peripheral blood smear to look for parasites. Obtain both thick and thin smears to identify and quantify the parasitemia. Parasite load is important to determine malaria severity and risk of complications. If the pretest probability of malaria is high, 3 negative test sets are necessary to rule out the diagnosis. A rapid antigen-based test is now available and can be used to screen quickly and guide evaluation of the smear, although the test has poor sensitivity for low-density *P vivax* infections. If the result is positive, the diagnosis of malaria is likely, and empirical therapy can be started. If the test results are negative but the clinical concern is high, repeat the smears and CBC (to look for anemia or thrombocytopenia) over the course of the next day to completely exclude the diagnosis.

Some state laboratories will perform polymerase chain reaction (PCR) assays, which can be used to detect low levels of parasitemia (0.5–5.0 parasites/μL). There is also a U.S. Food and Drug Administration rapid antigen-based test available (described earlier), but this must still be confirmed with blood smears.

Other laboratory findings can be suggestive of the diagnosis, including anemia, thrombocytopenia, and transaminitis.

Dengue

Findings may include leukopenia, thrombocytopenia, hyponatremia, and increased transaminase levels. ESR and CRP level are typically normal. Signs of end-organ damage, such as transaminase levels greater than 1,000 IU/L (>16.7 μkat/L), raise the concern for severe disease.

In the United States, reverse-transcription PCR for DENV genomic sequences obtained within 5 days of symptom onset is diagnostic in a patient with compatible clinical and travel history. Immunoglobulin M (IgM) anti-DENV can be detected with enzyme-linked immunosorbent assay (ELISA) after 5 days of illness and is the appropriate test for a patient who presents more than 1 week after fever onset. However, consider potentially cross-reactive flaviviruses (West Nile, yellow fever, Japanese encephalitis viruses, Zika) in a patient with positive IgM findings from a single sample (rather than acute- and convalescent-phase samples) and a compatible history.

Molecular and immunoassay testing is available from commercial reference laboratories, state public health laboratories, and the Centers for Disease Control and Prevention (CDC). Consult with the CDC on dengue diagnostic testing by calling 787/706-2399 or by visiting www.cdc.gov/Dengue/clinicalLab/index.html.

Typhoid Fever

There is no standard of reference for diagnosis, which is often assigned on clinical grounds, with treatment initiated empirically. Nonspecific findings include leukocytosis or leukopenia, anemia, and mild increase of transaminase levels. Cultures of blood (more likely to have positive findings with multiple samples), stool, urine, cerebrospinal fluid (CSF), rose spots, duodenal aspirate, and bone marrow may be performed with varying success, even after several days of incubation. Serologic testing (Widal test) and ELISA are not useful in the acute setting.

Differential Diagnosis

There is much overlap among malaria, dengue, and typhoid fever. However, always consider common local infections, such as influenza, adenovirus, pneumonia, and bacteremia with sepsis. In children with the appropriate travel history, also consider chikungunya virus, meningitis, leptospirosis, and Zika virus.

Treatment

Malaria

For the most up-to-date treatment recommendations, see the current edition of the American Academy of Pediatrics *Red Book* or the CDC malaria guidelines (http://www.cdc.gov/malaria/diagnosis_treatment/treatment.html). It is necessary to know where the disease was transmitted to guide therapy, and the CDC has up-to-date information about worldwide resistance patterns. Consult with an infectious diseases expert, because treatment recommendations change quickly in relation to resistance, and conditions in specific locations can affect treatment choices. If an infectious diseases expert is not immediately available, assistance with management is available 24 hours a day through the CDC Malaria Hotline (770/488-7788 or 855/856-4713, Monday to Friday, 9 am to 5 pm EST; and 770/488-7100 after hours and on weekends and holidays).

Dengue

No specific treatment exists for dengue. Maintain the patient's hydration level and avoid nonsteroidal anti-inflammatory drugs because of the risk for hemorrhagic disease. Treat the fever with acetaminophen. Febrile patients should avoid mosquito bites because they increase the risk of further transmission.

Typhoid Fever

The goal of treatment is to shorten the duration of the illness. Administer 14 days of parenteral therapy with ceftriaxone (80 mg/kg once daily for 14 days, for a maximum dose of 2g/d) or ciprofloxacin (20–30 mg/kg/d, divided into doses administered every 12 hours; maximum, 1.2 g/d). Azithromycin administered orally at 10 mg/kg/d for 1 to 2 weeks is a satisfactory alternative. If a diagnosis is established early in the course of uncomplicated typhoid, oral therapy may be sufficient. Culture results and knowledge of regional resistance patterns, if available, can be used to guide antibiotic choices. For more information, visit www.cdc.gov/typhoid-fever/ or call the CDC public response hotline at 888/246-2675 (English).

Indications for Consultation

Infectious diseases: All patients with malaria, dengue, and typhoid

Disposition

- **Intensive care unit transfer:** Coma, encephalopathy, signs of severe end-organ (liver, kidney) involvement, shock, intestinal perforation or severe bleeding, severe malaria (parasitemia greater than 5% of red blood cells, cerebral malaria)
- **Discharge criteria**
  - **Malaria:** Patients should remain admitted until *Plasmodium* species is identified. If nonfalciparum species, discharge once the patient is tolerating oral intake and maintaining hydration. For *Plasmodium falciparum* malaria, the patient may be discharged once the parasite load is less than 1% and the patient is clinically stable.
  - **Dengue:** Supportive care in the outpatient setting is reasonable for mild dengue, even in the febrile phase, if the patient can maintain adequate hydration and good follow-up. Once admitted, patients should remain inpatients until they are afebrile and until warning signs of severe dengue have resolved and they are clinically stable.
  - **Typhoid fever:** Patients may be discharged after completion of parenteral therapy. In uncomplicated cases with good clinical response, the last 4 of the 14 days may be completed at home.

Follow-up

- **Primary care:** Within a few days of discharge to assess clinical status and look for complications
- **Infectious diseases:** As indicated by local providers; especially important in areas where providers are less familiar with these diseases and future complications

Pearls and Pitfalls

- Treat the patient for malaria empirically if a patient with a negative smear result has a recent possible exposure and no other plausible diagnosis.
- Remember to rule out serious causes of infections, such as meningococcemia or pneumococcal sepsis acquired in this country.
- Dengue, malaria, and typhoid are notifiable diseases.
- Initiate empirical treatment for typhoid while awaiting culture results.
- Cultures of blood, bile, or bone marrow are most likely to yield *Salmonella* bacteria, while stool cultures frequently have negative findings.

Bibliography

Centers for Disease Control and Prevention. Dengue. http://wwwnc.cdc.gov/travel/yellowbook/2016/infectious-diseases-related-to-travel/dengue. Accessed February 13, 2017

Centers for Disease Control and Prevention. Malaria. http://wwwnc.cdc.gov/travel/yellowbook/2016/infectious-diseases-related-to-travel/malaria. Accessed February 13, 2017

Centers for Disease Control and Prevention. Typhoid & paratyphoid fever. http://wwwnc.cdc.gov/travel/yellowbook/2016/infectious-diseases-related-to-travel/typhoid-paratyphoid-fever. Accessed February 13, 2017

Committee on Infectious Diseases, American Academy of Pediatrics. *Red Book: 2015 Report of the Committee on Infectious Diseases*. 30th ed. Elk Grove Village, IL: American Academy of Pediatrics; 2015: 528–535, 322–325, 695–702

Kundu R, Ganguly N, Ghosh TK, Choudhury P, Shah RC. Diagnosis and management of malaria in children: recommendations and IAP plan of action. *Indian Pediatr.* 2005;42(11):1101–1114

Wain J, Hendriksen RS, Mikoleit ML, Keddy KH, Ochiai RL. Typhoid fever. *Lancet.* 2015;385:1136–1145

World Health Organization. Dengue: guidelines for diagnosis, treatment, prevention and control. http://www.who.int/tdr/publications/documents/dengue-diagnosis.pdf. Accessed February 13, 2017

CHAPTER 66

Fever of Unknown Origin

Introduction

Fever of unknown origin (FUO) is defined as a temperature higher than 38.3°C (101.0°F) for at least 2 weeks, during which a cause has not been identified despite a thorough clinical evaluation being conducted. There are a vast number of causes of FUO, with infections (especially in a patient <6 years old) and rheumatologic diseases (in older children) accounting for up to 60% of diagnoses. FUO most often represents a common disease process that appears in an uncommon fashion at presentation, such as an occult viral (Epstein-Barr virus [EBV], cytomegalovirus [CMV]) or bacterial (osteomyelitis, urinary tract infection, missed appendicitis with abdominal abscess) infection. Although rare etiologies may sometimes be considered and diagnosed, initially evaluate the patient for the more conventional illnesses. In approximately one-third of patients, a definitive diagnosis is never confirmed.

Clinical Presentation

History

The diagnosis of the etiology of FUO relies on an exhaustive and repeated history being obtained from the patient (if verbal), as well as all caregivers. Focus on associated symptoms (cough, vomiting, diarrhea, pain, arthralgia, etc), contact with sick persons, and new and chronic medications (including over-the-counter medications and herbal supplements). Specifically ask about exposure to animals (kittens [bartonellosis], reptiles, amphibians [salmonellosis], and farm animals [brucellosis, Q fever, leptospirosis]), consumption of unusual foods (unpasteurized milk or cheese [*Mycobacterium bovis*], squirrel or rabbit meat [tularemia], pica [*Toxocara* infection, toxoplasmosis]), camping (Lyme disease, ehrlichiosis, anaplasmosis), and travel, both internationally (malaria, tuberculosis) and within the United States (Lyme disease, histoplasmosis, coccidioidomycosis, blastomycosis).

Likewise, inquire about HIV risk factors, poor growth or abdominal symptoms (inflammatory bowel disease [IBD]), frequent or unusual infections (immunodeficiency), and genetic background (periodic fever syndromes, familial dysautonomia). A detailed pattern, height, and duration of fevers may provide clues, as in juvenile idiopathic arthritis (JIA) or periodic fever syndromes, but otherwise rarely lead to a diagnosis.

Physical Examination

Perform a thorough and extensive physical examination and, most importantly, repeat it regularly for new clues to aid in the diagnosis. A consistent approach to the examination allows for recognition of salient and evolving changes. Discuss each examined organ system with the family. They may fear a particular diagnosis, such as cancer or HIV, or equate a detailed, prolonged examination of certain organs with pathology.

Evaluate the child in both the febrile and nonfebrile state, because physical examination findings may be different (the evanescent rash of JIA often occurs only with fever, and the heart murmurs of acute rheumatic fever [ARF] or endocarditis will often be accentuated). The absence of sweating during fever occurs with dehydration, familial dysautonomia, or atropine exposure.

Assess the child's growth parameters, including height, weight, and, when appropriate, head circumference. Growth retardation may be a nonspecific finding of any chronic disease, but its presence may suggest an inflammatory process, such as IBD or immunodeficiency. Perform a thorough examination of the head, eyes, ears, nose, and throat to look for signs of sinusitis or rheumatologic/autoimmune disease, such as mucosal ulcerations. At ophthalmologic examination, note red, weeping eyes (connective tissue disease, especially polyarteritis nodosa); icterus (liver dysfunction, hemolytic anemia); palpebral conjunctivitis (measles, coxsackievirus, tuberculosis, EBV, bartonellosis, lymphogranuloma venereum); bulbar conjunctivitis (often purulent with infection; nonpurulent with Kawasaki disease and leptospirosis); uveitis (sarcoidosis, systemic lupus erythematosus [SLE], Kawasaki disease, Behçet disease, JIA); chorioretinitis (CMV, toxoplasmosis, syphilis); or proptosis (tumor, infection, thyrotoxicosis, Wegener granulomatosis). At oral examination, inspect and palpate all teeth for caries.

Ensure that the child is relaxed while a reliable abdominal examination is performed to palpate for masses (neuroblastoma, abscess) and hepatosplenomegaly. Auscultate for new heart murmurs (ARF, endocarditis), rales (pneumonia), or rubs (pleuritis, pericarditis). Other examination priorities include the skin (malar or discoid rash [SLE], petechiae, Janeway lesions, and splinter hemorrhages [endocarditis]) and the presence of lymphadenopathy (EBV, CMV, bartonellosis, lymphoma).

Examine each joint for evidence of arthritis and tenderness (osteomyelitis, JIA, or malignancy). Severe pain that involves multiple joints out of proportion to the swelling may represent leukemia rather than JIA. An abnormal gait may represent infection or malignancy of the lower extremities or a problem with the spine (diskitis, vertebral osteomyelitis, or tumor). Generalized muscle tenderness suggests dermatomyositis, trichinosis, or arboviral infection.

Thoroughly examine the neurologic system for clues, such as failure of pupillary constriction (hypothalamic dysfunction), hyperactive reflexes (thyrotoxicosis), and absence of fungiform papillae (familial dysautonomia).

Laboratory Workup

Base laboratory investigation on the history and physical examination findings. Personally review all findings from laboratory and radiologic evaluations undertaken in other settings and use appropriate consultants for interpretation of biopsy findings, radiographs, or other data. Obtain a complete blood cell count (CBC) with manual differential, C-reactive protein (CRP) level and/or erythrocyte sedimentation rate (ESR), comprehensive metabolic panel, EBV and CMV titers, blood cultures, and urinalysis and urine culture. Perform other tests in tier 1 from Box 66-1 if indicated (*Bartonella* titers if there is contact with a kitten; immunoglobulins if there is a history of frequent infections). Use the ESR to stratify the likely etiologies: An ESR greater than 30 mm/h often indicates infectious, autoimmune, or malignant disease; an ESR greater than 100 mm/h suggests tuberculosis, Kawasaki disease, malignancy, or autoimmune disease. In contrast, CRP levels tend to be markedly increased during infectious processes and less so with malignancies and autoimmune diseases. If fever persists without a diagnosis despite tier 1 evaluation and observation for several days, repeat the CBC with differential, CRP level/ESR evaluation, and any tests from tier 1 that yielded abnormal results; also perform tier 2 tests where indicated.

Box 66-1. Laboratory Tiers for Fever of Unknown Origin

Tier 1 Tests

CBC with manual differential, CRP level, ESR, CMP, serologic tests (EBV, CMV, *Bartonella* infection), quantitative serum immunoglobulin levels, blood cultures, urinalysis and urine culture, stool for analysis of blood/leukocytes and culture[a], upper and/or lower GI endoscopy[a], chest radiography, and TST (INF-γ release assay for a patient >6 y old)

Tier 2 Tests

Repeat selected tier 1 tests; syphilis[b], toxoplasma[b], hepatitis viruses, *Brucella*[b], Lyme[b], and tularemia titers[b]; multiple blood cultures; CT of the sinuses; abdominal US; lumbar puncture[c]; echocardiography; and bone marrow biopsy[d]

Abbreviations: CBC, complete blood cell count; CMP, comprehensive metabolic panel; CMV, cytomegalovirus; CRP, C-reactive protein; CT, computed tomography; EBV, Epstein-Barr virus; ESR, erythrocyte sedimentation rate; GI, gastrointestinal; INF, interferon; TST, tuberculin skin test; US, ultrasonography.

[a] Perform if the patient has suspicious symptoms, such as loose stools or mucus or blood in the stools and abdominal pain.

[b] Perform in patients exposed to endemic areas or those with a history of exposure.

[c] Perform in an infant or toddler with significant headache, abnormal neurologic examination findings, or bulging fontanel.

[d] Perform for unexplained hematologic abnormalities, such as bicytopenia or pancytopenia, blast cells or other abnormal cells on a peripheral smear, or underlying conditions that predispose the patient to malignancy, such as Down syndrome.

Differential Diagnosis

First, differentiate FUO from fever without source, pseudo-FUO, factitious fever, and deconditioning. Fever without source is an acute (<3–5 days) febrile illness, in which the origin of the fever is not initially apparent after obtaining a careful history and performing a physical examination. In pseudo-FUO, there are serial infections in which the fevers abate and recur, but vague symptoms persist. Have the caregiver use a calendar or diary to record symptoms, maximum temperature, and route and method of obtaining the temperature. True fevers that are measured with a thermometer and persistent are more likely to represent FUO, while the pattern for pseudo-FUO is high fevers for several days, followed by low fevers or reporting that the child "felt warm" and had mild, persistent symptoms (slight congestion, improving cough) for several days. The pattern then repeats. Deconditioning is often seen in the adolescent. After a well-defined, self-limited acute illness, the patient develops low-grade or subjective fevers, becomes inactive, and generates increasing concern from extended family members. Vitality and stamina decrease, but true fevers do not persist. Next, assess the patient for life-threatening or severe diseases. The severity of the disease, and not the anxiety of the family or the referring physician, dictates the appropriate pace of the evaluation.

The differential diagnosis is summarized in Table 66-1.

Treatment

Most often, hospitalization is indicated to expedite the evaluation, but reserve empirical antibiotic therapy for a patient who is toxic or has a compromising underlying condition and/or a deteriorating clinical course. Up to 80% of patients will have received 1 dose of antibiotics prior to admission, making the diagnosis more challenging. Avoid prescribing medications such as nonsteroidal anti-inflammatory drugs, because they may mask clues to diagnosis. Reserve their use for symptomatic care, on an as-needed basis, as well as for rheumatologic disease.

Specific treatment depends on the final diagnosis: antibiotics for bacterial disease; steroids, anti-inflammatory agents, and biological agents for rheumatologic disease/IBD; drug discontinuation for drug fever; and education and psychological or psychiatric referral for factitious fever.

If the etiology is not determined or is a virus other than a treatable cause (such as HIV), construct a detailed follow-up plan for the family. This must include symptomatic treatments, both pharmacologic and nonpharmacologic, such as the appropriate use of antipyretic medications, the application of cool cloths/bathing, and the avoidance of potentially harmful cultural techniques

Table 66-1. Differential Diagnosis of Fever of Unknown Origin	
Diagnosis	**Clinical Features**
Bacterial infections	
Bartonella infection	Exposure to kittens Lymphadenopathy Cranial nerve palsy Macular star
Lyme disease	Erythema migrans rash Oligoarticular arthritis (especially the knee) Cranial nerve palsy (cranial nerve VII)
Occult abscess	History of antibiotic use Daily fever spike Pain Poor dentition (dental abscess)
Osteomyelitis	Refusal to bear weight Bone point tenderness ↑ CRP level/ESR
Salmonellosis	Relative bradycardia (pulse doesn't increase with fever) Vomiting and diarrhea (may be bloody) Rose spots and cough (typhoid)
Sinusitis	Cough and postnasal drip Facial erythema or tenderness Swollen, erythematous nasal turbinates
Fungal infections (all can cause influenza-like illness, hilar adenopathy, pulmonary infiltrates, and dermatologic and CNS involvement, usually in an immunocompromised patient)	
Blastomycosis	Travel to Southeast and Central United States
Coccidioidomycosis	Travel to Southwest United States
Histoplasmosis	Travel to Mississippi, Ohio, and Missouri River valley Hepatosplenomegaly in toddlers Erythema nodosum in adolescents
Parasitic infections	
Malaria	Travel to endemic areas Rigors, hepatosplenomegaly Hemolytic anemia
Toxoplasmosis	Lymphadenopathy (especially cervical) Pharyngitis, myalgia
Tick-borne infections (all can cause headache, myalgia, thrombocytopenia)	
Babesiosis	Hemolytic anemia
Ehrlichiosis/ anaplasmosis	Nausea, variable rash (or no rash) in a truncal distribution, leukopenia, ↑ liver transaminase levels
Viral infections	
Epstein-Barr virus, CMV	Pharyngitis, generalized lymphadenopathy, hepatomegaly, atypical lymphocytosis
Hepatitis viruses	Possible travel history Blood/body fluid exposure ↑ LFT and bilirubin levels

Continued

Table 66-1. Differential Diagnosis of Fever of Unknown Origin, continued

Diagnosis	Clinical Features
Collagen vascular diseases	
Acute rheumatic fever	History of streptococcal infection Migratory polyarthritis Carditis (new murmur)
Juvenile idiopathic arthritis	Quotidian fever spikes alternating with subnormal temperatures Lymphadenopathy, evanescent rash Arthritis (may not be present initially)
Systemic lupus erythematosus	Alopecia, arthritis, malar rash Cytopenia Hematuria
Hereditary diseases	
Anhidrotic ectodermal dysplasia	Lack of sweating with fever Dental defects, abnormal facies, sparse hair
Fabry disease	Angiokeratomas (flat or raised red-black telangiectasias) Burning pain and paresthesia of the feet and legs
Familial Mediterranean fever	Serositis (especially peritonitis) Arthritis or arthralgia
Malignancy	
Leukemia	Bruising, pallor Bone pain ↑ LDH and uric acid levels
Neuroblastoma	Proptosis, abdominal mass Opsoclonus-myoclonus (dancing eyes, dancing feet) ↑ Urine catecholamine levels
Other	
Drug fever	Consider all medications, even eye drops Lack of other symptoms CRP level/ESR not increased
Factitious fever	Thermometer manipulation or injection of pyrogens May need video surveillance
Hemophagocytic lymphohistiocytosis	Splenomegaly Cytopenia ↓ Fibrinogen, ↑ ferritin and triglyceride levels
Inflammatory bowel disease	Growth retardation Abdominal pain Arthritis, erythema nodosum, uveitis
Typical Kawasaki disease	Nonpurulent bulbar conjunctivitis Erythematous polymorphic rash Swollen hands and feet Oral changes

Abbreviations: CMV, cytomegalovirus; CNS, central nervous system; CRP, C-reactive protein; ESR, erythrocyte sedimentation rate; LDH, lactate dehydrogenase; LFT, liver transaminase.

to reduce fever (cupping); imposing activity restrictions (taking heat-related illness precautions while fever persists, avoidance of abdominal trauma with splenomegaly); conducting routine follow-up with the primary care pediatrician shortly after discharge; and reviewing indications for emergent visits (severe abdominal pain with EBV that could represent splenic rupture or new signs or symptoms). Communication with the primary care physician regarding evaluation findings and ongoing care can help to decrease parental and physician anxiety and prevent unnecessary readmission.

Indications for Consultation

- **Infectious diseases:** Uncertain diagnosis in a patient who appears toxic or has been exposed to suspicious foods, animals, places, or activities that are associated with infections; immunocompromised patient
- **Ophthalmology:** Difficult eye examination or concern for a diagnosis with potential eye involvement (endocarditis, uveitis, IBD, chorioretinitis, JIA).
- **Various subspecialists:** Based on "most likely diagnosis" information obtained from repeated history and physical examination findings

Disposition

- **Intensive care unit transfer:** Clinical deterioration, respiratory distress, hypotension, monitoring of parents to rule out factitious fever
- **Discharge criteria:** Patient afebrile for ≥48 hours with nontoxic appearance; either the diagnosis is confirmed and continued fever is expected or there is no specific diagnosis after critical inpatient testing has been performed and appropriate consultation obtained, with close outpatient follow-up arranged

Follow-up

- **Primary care:** Within 2 to 3 days
- **Various subspecialists:** Based on the ultimate diagnosis

Pearls and Pitfalls

- The key to the ultimate diagnosis of FUO lies in repeated assessment of both the history and the physical examination findings, not in increasing the extent of the laboratory workup.
- More often than not, FUO represents a common disease process that appears in an uncommon fashion at presentation.

Bibliography

Antoon JW, Potisek NM, Lohr JA. Pediatric fever of unknown origin. *Pediatr Rev*. 2015;36(9):380–390

Arora R, Mahajan P. Evaluation of child with fever without source: review of literature and update. *Pediatr Clin North Am*. 2013;60(5):1049–1062

Kimberlin DW, Brady MT, Jackson MA, Long SS, eds. *Red Book: 2015 Report of the Committee on Infectious Diseases. 30th ed*. Elk Grove Village, IL: American Academy of Pediatrics; 2015

Marshall GS. Prolonged and recurrent fevers in children. *J Infect*. 2014;68 (Suppl 1): S83–S93

Nield LS, Kamat D. Fever without a focus. In: Kleigman RM, Behrman RE, St Geme JW III, Schor NF, Stanton BF, eds. *Nelson Textbook of Pediatrics*. 20th ed. Philadelphia, PA: Elsevier; 2016: 1280–1287

Kawasaki Disease

Introduction

Kawasaki disease (KD) is an acute, self-limited, multi-organ vasculitis of small and medium-sized arteries. Eighty percent of patients are younger than 5 years of age, with a peak incidence at 13 to 24 months, although it can occur in infants younger than 6 months. In the developing world, KD has replaced rheumatic fever as the most common cause of acquired heart disease in children. The etiology of KD is unknown, although epidemics are most common in the winter and spring.

The most significant complication of KD is vasculitis of the coronary arteries, leading to aneurysm formation. This occurs in about 20% of untreated patients but is seen in about 4% if treated appropriately with intravenous immunoglobulin (IVIg) early in the disease course. Risk factors for the development of coronary artery aneurysms include age younger than 12 months or older than 8 years, male sex, duration of fever more than 10 days prior to treatment, and lack of response to initial IVIg dose. Certain laboratory value abnormalities also indicate a higher risk: low hematocrit level, low albumin level, hyponatremia, and increased alanine transaminase level.

Clinical Presentation

History

There are 3 distinct stages of illness in KD. Most patients will present during the acute stage (first 10–14 days), which is characterized by the abrupt onset of high fever (38.9°C–40.0°C [102°F–104°F]) for at least 5 days that is associated with irritability. Within 2 to 5 days of the onset of fever, the patient develops other characteristic features of the illness, including a polymorphous erythematous rash in 90% of cases (often in the diaper area; may involve the palms of the hands and soles of the feet), nonpurulent conjunctivitis (80%–90% of cases), erythema and cracking of the lips or strawberry tongue (75%–90% of cases), cervical lymphadenopathy with a single lymph node larger than 1.5 cm in diameter, and erythema and swelling of the dorsum of the hands and feet. However, some of the classic features, such as conjunctivitis or rash, may have already resolved by the time the patient presents to the hospital. Less common complaints are abdominal pain, vomiting, and arthralgia.

The subacute phase of KD (approximately 2–6 weeks) is characterized by resolution of the classic symptoms (fever, lymphadenopathy, rash, mucositis, extremity changes, conjunctivitis). Periungual desquamation may occur during the second to third week of the illness. Cardiac complications, including coronary artery aneurysms, coronary obstruction and thrombosis, and myocardial and endocardial inflammation, can develop during this time, if not already present. The risk of sudden death is greatest during this phase.

In the final stage, physical findings are no longer apparent. Coronary artery ectasia may resolve, progress to myocardial ischemia or infarction, or remain unchanged.

Physical Examination

Perform a thorough examination of the head, eyes, ears, nose, and throat. Typical findings in the acute stage include conjunctival injection with perilimbic sparing, without exudate; erythema of the mouth and pharynx; strawberry tongue; dry, cracked lips; and a unilateral cervical lymph node larger than 1.5 cm in diameter. Other findings include erythema and swelling of the dorsum of the hands and feet and a polymorphic, erythematous rash that may involve the palms and soles. In many cases, within a few days of the appearance of the rash, desquamation of the perineal/diaper region occurs.

Findings with cardiac involvement may include tachycardia, a flow murmur, muffled heart sounds, or a gallop rhythm.

A less common feature is arthritis that involves the small joints during the acute phase and, later, the large, weight-bearing joints. Myringitis, urethritis with sterile pyuria, aseptic meningitis (nuchal rigidity) and, rarely, hydrops of the gallbladder (right upper quadrant abdominal mass) may also occur.

During the subacute phase, there can be desquamation of the hands and feet. Cardiac manifestations during this stage, if present, are more severe and may reveal signs and symptoms of congestive heart failure, valvular regurgitation, ventricular arrhythmias (premature ventricular contractions, ventricular tachycardia), or myocardial ischemia. Young children with myocardial infarction rarely present with chest pain but rather with shock, vomiting, abdominal pain, and excessive crying.

Laboratory Workup

If KD is suspected, obtain a complete blood cell count with differential; erythrocyte sedimentation rate (ESR) and/or C-reactive protein (CRP) level; serum chemistry values with liver function tests, including γ-glutamyltransferase and alkaline phosphatase levels; and urinalysis findings. Leukocytosis with neutrophil predominance, normocytic normochromic anemia, increase of liver enzyme levels and alkaline phosphatase levels (seen in hydrops of the gallbladder), decreased albumin and serum sodium levels, and sterile pyuria are suggestive of KD. The ESR and CRP level are increased early in the clinical course, whereas thrombocytosis (platelet count >500,000/mm³ [>500 × 10^9/L]) may not occur until the second or third week of illness. Thrombocytosis and increased ESR may persist for 6 to 8 weeks, and normalization of these values coincides with resolution of the disease, although a steady decline in the CRP level promptly occurs after successful treatment with IVIg.

If KD is strongly suspected, obtain an echocardiogram to evaluate the patient for cardiac involvement. However, the absence of cardiac abnormalities does not rule out KD. Obtain an electrocardiogram, which may demonstrate changes such as tachycardia, prolongation of the PR interval, abnormal Q waves, and nonspecific ST wave changes.

Blood, throat, and viral cultures may be helpful in differentiating KD from other infectious causes with prolonged fever. An increased brain natriuretic peptide level may aid in the diagnosis of KD when the etiology of the febrile illness is unclear.

Differential Diagnosis

Strongly suspect KD if a patient between 6 weeks and 12 years of age has a fever for more than 5 days in association with 4 of the following 5 major manifestations:

- Conjunctival injection without exudate
- Erythema of the mouth and pharynx; strawberry tongue; and cracked, red lips
- Erythematous rash of almost any pattern
- Edema and induration of the hands and feet with erythematous palms and soles
- Isolated, unilateral cervical lymphadenopathy larger than 1.5 cm

An atypical presentation, often termed *incomplete KD,* is increasingly common, especially among infants younger than 12 months of age. The patient who is at the highest risk of coronary artery abnormalities has prolonged fever and fewer than 4 of the principal diagnostic features. However, while the physical examination may not be clearly diagnostic, the laboratory value abnormalities follow a pattern similar to what is seen in classic disease. Given that infants and patients with delayed diagnosis of KD are at increased risk for cardiac disease, it is critical to diagnose KD when the clinical picture is "incomplete" but the abnormal laboratory values and echocardiogram findings are consistent with the diagnosis.

There is a broad differential diagnosis for KD, including a wide variety of infectious diseases (toxic shock syndrome, rheumatic fever, scarlet fever, staphylococcal scalded skin syndrome, Rocky Mountain spotted fever, leptospirosis, adenovirus, Epstein-Barr virus, influenza, measles) and noninfectious etiologies (Stevens-Johnson syndrome, drug reaction, juvenile idiopathic arthritis, mercury toxicity) that may have similar symptoms at presentation (Table 67-1).

Treatment

Management in the acute phase is aimed at reducing inflammation in the myocardium and coronary artery wall, as well as preventing thrombosis. The mainstay of inpatient therapy is high-dose IVIg (2 g/kg IVIg administered over 10–12 hours). During the IVIg infusion, many patients will become afebrile, with dramatic improvement in symptoms. However, fever can persist after IVIg administration, so do not consider a patient to be IVIg nonresponsive until there is a documented fever more than 36 hours after the end of the infusion.

Approximately 10% to 20% of patients with KD will ultimately be IVIg nonresponsive and remain febrile beyond 36 hours. These patients are at increased risk for coronary artery abnormalities. Consult with a KD expert to determine whether KD remains the most likely diagnosis and what is the best course of action. Options include a second course of IVIg (2 g/kg) alone or in conjunction with pulse methylprednisolone therapy (30 mg/kg/d) for 3 days or infliximab (5 mg/kg), a tumor necrosis factor inhibitor. Cyclosporine and

Table 67-1. Differential Diagnosis of Kawasaki Disease	
Diagnosis	**Clinical Features**
Acute rheumatic fever	History of strep infection No conjunctivitis Migratory polyarthritis and/or carditis (regurgitation)
Adenovirus	Exudative pharyngitis Purulent conjunctivitis Mild ↑ of inflammatory markers
Juvenile idiopathic arthritis	May have (+) antinuclear antibodies or rheumatoid factor Lack of conjunctival and oral findings Lymphadenopathy more generalized
Measles	Exanthem progresses in a cephalocaudad pattern Purulent conjunctivitis Lack of swelling of the hands and feet
Stevens-Johnson syndrome	Purulent conjunctivitis More severe desquamation of mucosal surfaces Sudden onset with progression to shock if untreated
Toxic shock syndrome	Presence of inciting bacterial agent Signs of shock, including hypotension Renal involvement with ↑ blood urea nitrogen/creatinine level

"+" indicates a positive finding.

methotrexate are additional treatment options, but reserve them for a patient who fails to respond to multiple treatment courses.

During the first 7 to 10 days of the illness, also administer high-dose aspirin (80–100 mg/kg/d, divided into doses administered every 3 days), but switch to low-dose aspirin (3–5 mg/kg/d as a single daily dose) after the patient has been afebrile for 48 hours. Continue the low-dose aspirin until the inflammatory markers (CRP level, ESR) normalize and the patient has completed a follow-up appointment with a cardiologist to confirm that no coronary artery abnormalities have developed. If coronary artery aneurysms are identified, long-term antiplatelet therapy is indicated.

Indications for Consultation

- **Cardiology:** All patients
- **Infectious diseases:** The diagnosis of KD is unclear or there is concern for other infectious etiologies
- **KD expert, if available (may be a cardiologist, rheumatologist, or infectious diseases specialist):** Fever persists for more than 36 hours after first immunoglobulin dose

Disposition

- **Intensive care unit transfer:** Cardiac involvement with compromised function
- **Discharge criteria:** Patient afebrile with improvement of clinical symptoms and decreased inflammatory markers (≥36 hours after completion of IVIg treatment)

Follow-up

- **Primary care:** 1 to 3 days
- **Cardiology:** 1 to 2 weeks

Pearls and Pitfalls

- Incomplete KD may be more common than a classic presentation, especially at the extremes of the age spectrum.
- Siblings of patients with KD are at increased risk for developing the disease.
- KD can appear with an acute abdomen at presentation, resulting in admission to a surgical service, or with "cervical lymphadenitis," resulting in admission to the ear, nose, and throat service.
- Cough, congestion, and petechial, purpuric, and vesicular rashes are not features of KD.
- Defer live virus vaccines for 11 months after administration of IVIg for KD.

Bibliography

Forsey J, Mertens L. Atypical Kawasaki disease—a clinical challenge. *Eur J Pediatr*. 2012; 171(4):609–611

Newburger JW, Takahashi M, Burns JC. Kawasaki disease. *J Am Coll Cardiol*. 2016; 67(14):1738–1749

Patel RM, Shulman ST. Kawasaki disease: a comprehensive review of treatment options. *J Clin Pharm Ther*. 2015;40(6):620–625

Saneeymehri S, Baker K, So TY. Overview of pharmacological treatment options for pediatric patients with refractory Kawasaki Disease. *J Pediatr Pharmacol Ther*. 2015; 20(3):163–177

Shulman ST, Rowley AH. Kawasaki disease: insights into pathogenesis and approaches to treatment. *Nat Rev Rheumatol*. 2015;11(8):475–482

Yang X, Liu G, Huang Y, Chen S, Du J, Jin H. A meta-analysis of re-treatment for intravenous immunoglobulin-resistant Kawasaki disease. *Cardiol Young*. 2015;25(6):1182–1190

Ye Q, Shao WX, Shang SQ, Zhou MM. Value of the N-terminal of prohormone brain natriuretic peptide in diagnosis of Kawasaki disease. *Int J Cardiol*. 2015;178:5–7

Sepsis

Introduction

Sepsis is defined as the presence of a known or suspected infection *and* at least *two of four* qualifying systemic inflammatory response syndrome (SIRS) criteria, including at least one temperature or leukocyte abnormality:

- Abnormal leukocyte count: more or less than the normal range for age *or* bandemia greater than 10%
- Abnormal core temperature: lower than 36.0°C (<96.8°F) *or* higher than 38.5°C (>101.3°F)
- Abnormal heart rate: More than 2 SDs above *or* below the mean for the patient's age
- Tachypnea (age specific): respiratory rate more than 2 SDs above the mean for the patient's age

Since up to 20% of patients in the emergency department qualify for the diagnosis of sepsis (eg, pneumonia with fever and leukocyte increase), there is also a category of *severe sepsis*, defined by sepsis *and* end-organ system dysfunction (either cardiac instability *or* respiratory dysfunction *or* dysfunction of two other end-organs, such as hepatic and renal). *Septic shock* is defined as sepsis with persistent cardiovascular dysfunction despite initial fluid resuscitation (40 mL/kg administered in <1 hour). Note that in its septic shock diagnosis algorithm, the American College of Critical Care Medicine focuses on mental status and perfusion rather than on the SIRS criteria. Severe sepsis and septic shock therefore encompass the continuum of the body's response to infection.

While the etiology of sepsis varies on the basis of patient age, immune status, and geographic location, most cases in children in the developed world are caused by bacterial infections, although viruses and fungi are also implicated. Excluding neonatal sepsis (see Chapter 64, Fever in Infants Younger Than 60 Days), the most common cause of pediatric severe sepsis is pneumonia, followed by bacteremia. Other illnesses (pyelonephritis, osteomyelitis, appendicitis, meningitis) can progress to sepsis, and the pathogenic organism can thus range from being gram positive (*Steptococcus pneumoniae, Staphylococcus aureus*) to gram negative (*Escherichia coli, Neisseria meningitidis*) or anaerobic (*Bacteroides* species), as well as respiratory syncytial virus, influenza, and herpes virus. An immunocompromised patient may have a fungal (particularly *Candida* species) or other viral (cytomegalovirus, herpes zoster) infection.

Clinical Presentation

History

Perform a careful review of the symptoms. Fever pattern, cough, dyspnea, emesis, diarrhea, abdominal pain, dysuria, headache, rash, and focal pain or swelling will yield clues to the type of underlying infection. Recent urine output or mental status may help determine where the patient is on the spectrum of sepsis, severe sepsis, and septic shock. Frequent recurrent infections, chronic diarrhea, and failure to thrive may suggest an immunodeficiency and the possibility of unusual organisms.

Travel to the developing world suggests the possibility of infections such as *Salmonella typhi*, malaria, dengue, and yellow fever. Travel within the United States can raise the concern for exposure to leptospirosis (Hawaii), Rocky Mountain spotted fever (Southeast United States), and Chikungunya virus (Florida, Puerto Rico, U.S. Virgin Islands).

Physical Examination

Carefully assess and frequently reassess vital signs, with special attention to

- Fever or hypothermia (temperature <36.0°C [<96.8°F] or >38.5°C [>101.3°F])
- Tachycardia or bradycardia (see the Introduction)
- Tachypnea: adjust the heart rate for fever: for each 1.0°C (1.8°F) above 38.5°C (101.3°F), subtract 10 beats/min from the heart rate

Capillary refill time longer than 2 seconds, weak pulse, hypotension, and altered mental status for the patient's age are sensitive indicators for abnormal end-organ perfusion with shock. Bradycardia and hypothermia are ominous signs. Focus the remainder of the rapid first physical examination on identifying sources for sepsis to direct the initial antimicrobial choice.

Laboratory Workup

The two goals of laboratory studies are to identify the etiology of infection and to assess the severity of organ dysfunction. Some evaluations, such as C-reactive protein (CRP) level, may be most helpful when repeated to trend the severity of the infection or response to interventions. Indicated basic studies, similar to those for the patient in shock (see Chapter 10, Shock), include

- Complete blood cell count with differential (note bandemia, toxic granulocytes, thrombocytopenia, anemia; smear for hemolysis or abnormal cells)
- Blood culture (aerobic and anaerobic)
- Urinalysis and urine culture
- Basic metabolic panel with liver enzyme evaluation

- Lactate level (≥4 mmol/L is consistent with high risk for sepsis)
- Venous blood gas panel (often includes ionized calcium, sodium, glucose, hemoglobin, and potassium level assessment)
- CRP level
- Chest radiograph
- Electrocardiogram (when pericarditis/myocarditis is suspected)
- Coagulation panel (when disseminated intravascular coagulation is suspected)
- Cerebrospinal fluid studies, viral polymerase chain reaction test, and bacterial culture (if meningitis/encephalitis is suspected; also consider reserving extra fluid for possible specialty viral/fungal/parasitic testing)

Differential Diagnosis

The differential diagnoses of sepsis are summarized in Table 68-1.

Treatment

Initiate treatment within the first hour of symptom recognition. Stabilize the patient by using Pediatric Advanced Life Support pathways to address circulation, airway, and breathing. Immediately provide oxygen to all patients.

A standard of reference in the therapy for all forms of sepsis is fluid resuscitation to the point of hemodynamic stability. Obtain immediate intravenous access, preferably at 2 sites, but if that is not possible, place an intraosseous line. Push boluses of 20 mL/kg of isotonic crystalloid (normal saline or lactated Ringer solution) over 15 to 20 minutes. Repeat boluses as necessary until there is clinical improvement, including normalization of the blood pressure, capillary refill, pulse, and urine output. However, clinical outcome may be negatively affected by fluid overload, especially in a patient with underlying cardiac disease or certain infectious diseases (dengue, malaria, and other illnesses of the developing world). If any signs of fluid overload (new hepatomegaly or pulmonary rales) are noted, start the administration of inotropes instead of continuing fluid resuscitation.

Start antibiotics within the first hour of recognition of symptoms, based on the most likely underlying infection. Do not stop fluid resuscitation for antibiotic administration and do not withhold antibiotics pending culture results, especially the cerebrospinal fluid culture findings, if the patient is not stable enough for a lumbar puncture to be performed. Consequently, empirical antibiotic choices are broad, but narrow the spectrum once an organism and/or source is identified. See Table 68-2 for antibiotic recommendations based on the common etiologies of sepsis. For infants less than 60 days old, see Chapter 64, Fever in Infants Younger Than 60 Days.

Table 68-1. Differential Diagnosis of Sepsis	
Diagnosis	**Clinical Features**
Hemodynamic instability	
Anaphylaxis	Urticaria and/or angioedema
	Wheezing and/or acute respiratory distress
	Emesis, abdominal pain
	Hypotension
Adrenal crisis	History of previous steroid use or underlying primary deficiency
	Nausea/emesis
	Shock unresponsive to IV fluids
	Patient may have hyponatremia with hyperkalemia
Congestive heart failure	Tachypnea/diaphoresis during feeds (infant)
	Cardiomegaly
	Hepatomegaly or pulmonary congestion (rales)
Fever and systemic signs	
Kawasaki disease	Nonpurulent conjunctivitis
	Mucosal changes (strawberry tongue, cracked lips)
	Polymorphous rash
	Cervical adenopathy
	Hand/foot swelling
Inborn errors of metabolism	Symptoms may present at birth, with concurrent illness, or when infant starts fasting through the night
	Emesis, lethargy, altered mental status
	May have ↓ glucose level, ↑ ammonia level, and/or metabolic acidosis
Periodic fever syndromes	Often other family members are affected
	Child is well between episodes that occur at regular intervals
	Abdominal pain, rash, and joint pain are all common
Sympathomimetic ingestion	Psychosis/irritability in a young child
	Hypertension, mydriasis, diaphoresis
Dysautonomia/neurologic storming	History of underlying CNS disease
	Increased dystonia
	Hypertension, tachycardia
Narcotic or baclofen withdrawal	Hypertension, tachycardia
	Diarrhea
	Irritability

Abbreviations: CNS, central nervous system; IV, intravenous.

Disposition

- **Intensive care unit (ICU) transfer:** Hemodynamic instability despite administration of antibiotics and fluid resuscitation (typically after 40–60 mL/kg isotonic fluids in 1 hour) or pressor support required, respiratory failure, evidence of multi-organ dysfunction
- **Institutional transfer:** Need for ICU or specialist consultation not available locally

- **Discharge criteria:** Patient hemodynamically stable with infection identified and therapy demonstrating consistent clinical improvement

Follow-up
- **Primary Care:** 2 to 3 days
- **Infectious Disease:** 1 to 2 weeks if long-term antibiotic therapy is prescribed

Table 68-2. Initial Empirical Antibiotic Choices	
Type of Infection	**Antibiotic(s) of Choice**

Previously healthy patient
  Community-acquired pneumonia
  Pyelonephritis
  Bacterial meningitis
	IV ceftriaxone 50 mg/kg every 24 h
	  Use 100 mg/kg/d if meningitis is suspected
	  (4-g/d maximum)
	and
	Vancomycin 15 mg/kg per dose every 8 h
	(4-g/d maximum; follow up serum levels)

Medically complex patient with risk of aspiration/anaerobic infections	IV ampicillin/sulbactam 50 mg/kg per dose every 6 h (maximum, 3 g per dose) *or* IV clindamycin 13 mg/kg per dose every 8 h (4.8-g/d maximum) *or* IV meropenem 20 mg/kg per dose every 8 h (3-g/d maximum, except for meningitis [6-g/d maximum]) *and if MRSA infection is suspected,* Vancomycin (dosing as above)
Intra-abdominal infection	IV meropenem 20 mg/kg per dose every 8 h (3-g/d maximum) *or* IV piperacillin/tazobactam, 100 mg piperacillin/kg per dose every 8 h (maximum, 3.375 g per dose)

Immunocompromised patient
  Neutropenic (due to chemotherapy
    or underlying immunodeficiency)
  Cystic fibrosis
	Ensure pseudomonal coverage with:
	  IV cefepime 50 mg/kg per dose every 8 h
	  (maximum, 2 g per dose)
	or
	Carbapenems (ie, meropenem, dosing as above)
	and if clinically indicated,
	MRSA coverage with vancomycin (dosing as above)
	Fungal coverage (consult with an infectious diseases specialist)

Abbreviations: IV, intravenous; MRSA, methicillin-resistant *Staphylococcus aureus*.

Chapter 68: Sepsis

Pearls and Pitfalls

- Hypotension is a *late finding* of sepsis and uncompensated shock. Diagnose and treat shock when it is compensated, by using heart rate, perfusion, and core temperature.
- Carefully review the patient's vaccination status.
- Perform fluid resuscitation with the goal of normalizing blood pressure, perfusion, and possibly heart rate, while being alert for signs of fluid overload (new rales, hepatomegaly).
- Narrow the antimicrobial therapy as soon as possible to avoid development of organism resistance.

Bibliography

Dellinger RP, Levy MM, Rhodes A, et al; and Surviving Sepsis Campaign Guidelines Committee including the Pediatric Subgroup. Surviving sepsis campaign: international guidelines for management of severe sepsis and septic shock: 2012. *Crit Care Med.* 2013;41(2):580–637

Randolph AG, McCulloh RJ. Pediatric sepsis: important considerations for diagnosing and managing severe infections in infants, children, and adolescents. *Virulence.* 2014;5(1):179–189

Scott HF, Deakyne SJ, Woods JM, Bajaj L. The prevalence and diagnostic utility of systemic inflammatory response syndrome vital signs in a pediatric emergency department. *Acad Emerg Med.* 2015;22(4):381–389

Singer M, Deutschman CS, Seymour CW, et al. The third international consensus definitions for sepsis and septic shock (sepsis-3). *JAMA.* 2016;315(8):801–810

Standage SW, Wong HR. Biomarkers for pediatric sepsis and septic shock. *Expert Rev Anti Infect Ther.* 2011;9(1):71–79

Ingestions

Esophageal Foreign Body

Introduction

Coins are the most common foreign bodies ingested by children in the United States. Foreign bodies that remain in the esophagus tend to lodge in 3 areas of anatomic narrowing: 60% to 70% are at the thoracic inlet at the upper esophageal sphincter, 10% to 20% are in the mid-esophagus at the level of the aortic notch, and about 20% are just above the lower esophageal sphincter.

Other less common objects include toys or toy parts, needles and pins, chicken or fish bones, and other food. Batteries and sharp, long objects require special consideration because of the higher risk for complications. Button batteries can conduct electricity in the esophagus, causing liquefaction necrosis and perforation that can develop within hours. There is a high risk for perforation with sharp objects, which can get trapped anywhere in the esophagus. If there is an esophageal abnormality, a foreign body can lodge in an atypical location.

Clinical Presentation

History

The presenting symptoms depend on the type and size of the foreign body, as well as the location and duration of impaction. The most common symptoms are drooling, dysphagia, substernal discomfort or a sensation of a foreign body, retching, vomiting, coughing, and difficulty breathing. The presence of fever is concerning because it suggests deep ulceration or perforation. There may be a history of a choking episode, the caregiver may have witnessed the ingestion, or the patient may self-report it. However, up to one-third of patients are asymptomatic, and in as many as 40% of cases there is no history of ingestion. If possible, determine the time since the ingestion, because a longer duration (>24 hours) is associated with greater risk for complications.

Physical Examination

The physical examination findings may be normal, or there may be a range of findings, from drooling to respiratory distress secondary to tracheal compression. Neck swelling, erythema, or crepitus is concerning for esophageal perforation. Rarely, a patient presents with massive gastrointestinal bleeding as a result of a foreign body that causes an aortoesophageal fistula.

Laboratory Workup

Obtain anteroposterior and lateral radiographs of the neck and chest to visualize coins or other radio-opaque foreign bodies. Coins appear as a circle on frontal views and as a line on lateral views. This is in contrast to coins in the trachea, which would have the opposite findings. A radiolucent object will not be visualized on plain radiographs, but its presence may be suggested by compression or displacement of adjacent structures. If the history and physical examination findings are consistent with an esophageal foreign body but the radiograph findings are normal, obtain a contrast-enhanced esophagram to rule out a radiolucent foreign body. Order chest computed tomography if the patient has significant respiratory distress that may be secondary to erosion or extraluminal extension. A handheld metal detector is another option for identifying and localizing coins and other metallic objects.

Differential Diagnosis

The differential diagnosis of an esophageal foreign body is summarized in Table 69-1.

Table 69-1. Differential Diagnosis of an Esophageal Foreign Body	
Diagnosis	**Clinical Features**
Drooling/dysphagia	
Epiglottitis	Fever, toxicity "Sniffing dog" position
Mediastinal mass	Difficulty breathing Recurrent lung infections
Peritonsillar abscess	Trismus, "hot potato" voice Uvula deviated to the contralateral side
Retropharyngeal abscess	Fever, drooling Anterior bulging of the posterior pharyngeal wall Limited neck hyperextension
Cough/choking/cyanosis	
Bronchiolitis	Upper respiratory infection prodrome Respiratory distress and wheezing follows
Gastroesophageal reflux	Intermittent regurgitation Sandifer syndrome
Pneumonia	Fever, cough, tachypnea Infiltrate on chest radiograph
Stridor/wheezing	
Croup	Hoarseness, barking cough Stridor
Laryngotracheomalacia	Positional inspiratory stridor Presentation occurs early in life

Treatment

Management of esophageal foreign bodies depends on the type, location, and size of the object, as well as the patient's size and symptoms. In up to 80% to 90% of cases, the object will pass spontaneously, whereas in 10% to 20% of cases, the object must be removed endoscopically; less than 1% of cases will require a surgical procedure.

If the patient is asymptomatic and has no history of esophageal or tracheal abnormality and if less than 24 hours has elapsed since the ingestion, permit a period of observation (up to 24 hours). Give the patient nothing by mouth, provide continuous cardiac monitoring with pulse oximetry, and administer maintenance intravenous fluids. If the patient remains asymptomatic, repeat the radiography in 12 to 24 hours. Discharge the patient if the object spontaneously passes into the stomach. However, if drooling, substernal chest pain, vomiting, difficulty swallowing, or respiratory distress develop, or if the object does not progress after 24 hours, consult with an otolaryngologist, gastroenterologist, or surgeon to coordinate a removal procedure.

Arrange for immediate removal of a button battery that has lodged in the esophagus. The same is true for large, long, and/or sharp objects. Arrange for emergent endoscopic removal for any patient who has symptoms and cannot manage secretions or who exhibits acute respiratory symptoms. Do not prescribe motility agents, such as glucagon.

Depending on institutional skills and preferences, removal options include rigid esophagoscopy or flexible endoscopy (especially for sharp objects and batteries lodged in the esophagus). Regardless of the technique used, the success rate for removal of an esophageal foreign body is 95% to 100%. If several hours have passed to coordinate the removal procedure, repeat the radiography just prior to the procedure to confirm the position of the foreign body.

During the postremoval period, observe the patient for risk signs from the procedures, such as bleeding, vomiting, stridor, respiratory distress, or hypoxia. If there are no signs of drooling or difficulty breathing, start a trial of clear liquids to ensure that the patient can tolerate liquids.

Indications for Consultation

Gastroenterology, otorhinolaryngology, surgery, or radiology: Depending on who performs the procedure at a given institution

Disposition

- **Intensive care unit transfer:** Impending respiratory failure or signs of shock
- **Discharge criteria:** Normal respiratory status, no oxygen requirement, no drooling, adequate oral intake

Follow-up

If object required removal: 1 to 2 weeks with the physician that performed the procedure

Pearls and Pitfalls

- If the foreign body passes into the stomach, instruct the caregivers to watch for signs of abdominal pain, bleeding, or vomiting.
- The patient may continue to complain of a foreign body sensation for several days after removal.
- Food impaction in an older child or adolescent can be caused by eosinophilic esophagitis.

Bibliography

Green SS. Ingested and aspirated foreign bodies. *Pediatr Rev.* 2015;36(10):430–436

Leinwand K, Brumbaugh DE, Kramer RE. Button battery ingestion in children: a paradigm for management of severe pediatric foreign body ingestions. *Gastrointest Endosc Clin N Am.* 2016;26(1):99–118

Popel J, El-Hakim H, El-Matary W. Esophageal foreign body extraction in children: flexible versus rigid endoscopy. *Surg Endosc.* 2011;25(3):919–922

Sahn B, Mamula P, Ford CA. Review of foreign body ingestion and esophageal food impaction management in adolescents. *J Adolesc Health.* 2014;55(2):260–266

CHAPTER 70

Toxic Exposures

Introduction

Toxic exposures are common among children. In 2013, 61% of calls to poison centers and 7.5% of toxin-related fatalities involved patients younger than 20 years of age. Younger patients (<6 years) have better outcomes because they usually present promptly to a health care facility, have fewer comorbid conditions, are exposed to a single substance, and are not trying to harm themselves. However, some substances are potentially fatal in small doses (Box 70-1).

Box 70-1. Toxins That Are Potentially Fatal With Small Doses	
Antidysrhythmics Antimalarials (chloroquine, hydroxychloroquine, quinine) β-antagonists Botulinum toxin Bupropion Calcium channel antagonists Camphor Clonidine Clozapine	Diphenoxylate-atropine Ethylene glycol Methanol Methyl salicylate Opioids Organophosphates (parathion) Phenothiazines Sulfonylureas Theophylline Tricyclic antidepressants

Clinical Presentation

History

Ask about the timing and onset of concerning symptoms, timing and amount of a known exposure, and available sources of exposure in the house, including prescription and over-the-counter medications, household/cosmetic products, illicit drugs, pesticides, and herbal/alternative and traditional/cultural medications. Determine recent occupational exposures, encounters with venomous/poisonous animals, or exposures to plants. Use historical data and available pharmacy information to determine maximum exposures. Assess intent regarding exposure. Ask about underlying medical conditions (renal or liver disease) that may affect drug metabolism.

Physical Examination

Be aware that some toxic effects have delayed onset (Table 70-1). Physical examination findings are summarized in Table 70-2.

Table 70-1. Toxins With Potential for Delayed Toxicity

Toxin	Toxicity
Acetaminophen	Hepatic and renal failure
Amanita species mushrooms	Hepatic failure
Brodifacoum	Bleeding
Buprenorphine-suboxone	Respiratory failure
Bupropion	Seizures
Colchicine	Gastrointestinal toxicity, multi-organ failure
Diphenoxylate-atropine	Respiratory failure
Diquat	Renal failure, multi-organ failure
Iron	Hepatic, multi-organ failure
Lead	Encephalopathy, seizures, anemia
Paraquat	Pulmonary fibrosis, multi-organ failure
Salicylates	Encephalopathy, seizures, arrhythmias, renal failure, multi-organ failure
Sulfonylureas	Hypoglycemia
Sustained-release β-antagonists	Hypotension, bradycardia
Sustained-release calcium channel antagonists	Hypotension, bradycardia

Table 70-2. Physical Examination Findings for Toxic Exposures

Symptom	Substance/Syndrome
Vital signs	
Hyperthermia	Anticholinergics, sympathomimetics, serotonin syndrome, malignant hyperthermia, neuroleptic malignant syndrome, GABA agonist withdrawal (ethanol, benzodiazepines, barbiturates, baclofen, gamma-hydroxybutyrate)
Hypothermia	Opioids, hypoglycemic agents, carbon monoxide, β-blockers
Tachycardia	Sympathomimetics, anticholinergics, serotonin syndrome, GABA agonist withdrawal, tricyclic antidepressants
Bradycardia	Cholinergics (organophosphates, carbamates), β-blockers, calcium channel blockers, digoxin, opioids, sedatives, clonidine
Hypertension	Sympathomimetics, elemental mercury, serotonin syndrome, GABA agonist withdrawal
Hypotension	Calcium channel blockers, β-blockers, digoxin, clonidine, opioids, TCAs
Tachypnea	Sympathomimetics, anticholinergics, salicylates, hydrocarbons
Bradypnea	Opioids, sedatives, clonidine, cholinergics
Neurologic/mental status	
Agitation	Sympathomimetics, anticholinergics, serotonin syndrome
Hallucinations/ delusions	Sympathomimetics, anticholinergics, dextromethorphan, LSD, cannabinoids, PCP, psilocybin, *Salvia divinorum*
Sedation	Opioids, sedatives, carbon monoxide, hydrocarbon inhalants

Table 70-2. Physical Examination Findings for Toxic Exposures, continued

Symptom	Substance/Syndrome
Neurologic/mental status, continued	
Seizures	Sympathomimetics, anticholinergics, TCAs, antipsychotics, caffeine, isoniazid, propoxyphene, tramadol, theophylline
Head, eyes, ears, nose, throat	
Dry mucosal membrane	Anticholinergics
Miosis	**C:** carbamates, clonidine; **O:** opioids, organophosphates, olanzapine; **P:** phenothiazines; **S:** sedatives
Mydriasis	Sympathomimetics, anticholinergics
Sialorrhea/drooling	Cholinergics, caustics
Visual loss	Methanol
Cardiopulmonary	
Myocarditis	Ipecac (chronic exposure)
Pulmonary edema (noncardiogenic)	Salicylates, opioids, organophosphates, carbamates
Torsades de pointes (prolonged QT interval)	TCAs, methadone, antipsychotics, erythromycin, cisapride, diphenhydramine (see list at crediblemeds.org)
Ventricular tachycardia (prolonged QRS)	Cocaine, TCAs, anticholinergics, halogenated hydrocarbons, propranolol, propoxyphene
Wheezing/dyspnea	Hydrocarbons, organophosphates, carbamates
Gastrointestinal	
Constipation	Anticholinergics, opioids
Diarrhea	Caustics, cholinergics, ipecac, iron, cathartics
Emesis	Caustics, cholinergics, ipecac, ethanol, plants, mushrooms, iron
Hepatotoxicity	Acetaminophen, *Amanita* species mushrooms, phenytoin, ethanol, iron, valproic acid, *Mentha pulegium* (pennyroyal)
Pancreatitis	Ethanol, salicylates, valproic acid
Hematologic and renal	
Bleeding/bruising	Coumadin, brodifacoum (found in certain rat poisons)
Nephrotoxicity	Ethylene glycol, nonsteroidal anti-inflammatory drugs, aminoglycosides

Abbreviations: GABA, γ-aminobutyric acid; LSD, lysergic acid diethylamide; PCP, phencyclidine; TCA, tricyclic antidepressant.

Laboratory Workup

If a toxic exposure is suspected, order a blood glucose level, basic metabolic panel (Table 70-3), 12-lead electrocardiogram, and continuous pulse oximetry. Obtain acetaminophen and salicylate concentrations if there is an unknown exposure or suicidal intent. Order neuroimaging, chest radiography, creatine phosphokinase level, liver enzyme levels, and liver function tests if there is a

Table 70-3. Metabolic Findings Associated With Certain Toxins	
Electrolyte Abnormality	**Possible Toxins**
Hypernatremia	Sodium salts, baking soda, sodium phosphate, drug-induced diabetes insipidus
Hyponatremia	Lithium, diuretics, drug-induced syndrome of inappropriate antidiuretic hormone
Hyperkalemia	Digoxin
Hypokalemia	Sympathomimetics, toluene, insulin, albuterol
Hyperchloremia	Sodium chloride, bromide (spurious)
Metabolic alkalosis	Baking soda
Anion gap metabolic acidosis	Methanol, metformin, iron, isoniazid, ethylene glycol, salicylates, carbon monoxide, cyanide, toluene
Normal anion gap metabolic acidosis	Topiramate, toluene
Hyperglycemia	Sympathomimetics, calcium channel blockers
Hypoglycemia	Insulin, sulfonylureas, β-blockers, ethanol

suspicion of hypoxic injury, such as a patient who is found unconscious. Base other testing on suspected toxin, history, physical examination, and initial laboratory findings. Order a pregnancy test for postpubertal female adolescents.

Confirm urine drug screen results that are indicated for medical, social, or psychiatric management with gas chromatography/mass spectrometry. Send urine and blood samples to the laboratory for storage in patients with suspected malicious poisoning with an unknown substance. Use these samples for future testing with the guidance of subsequent clinical course, history, and consultant expertise.

Differential Diagnosis

At presentation, some toxic exposures can appear the same as common pediatric illnesses. Seizures from sympathomimetics or bupropion are indistinguishable from generalized seizures. Sympathomimetics, anticholinergics, lead encephalopathy, and serotonin syndrome can mimic infectious meningitis. Consider carbon monoxide poisoning in the evaluation of new-onset migraine or tension headaches. Hydrocarbon ingestion can be confused with an asthma exacerbation. Ipecac administration, early acetaminophen or iron poisoning, and viral gastroenteritis will appear with comparable symptoms at presentation. Liver injury from viral hepatitis and acetaminophen toxicity are also similar. Dehydration and sodium chloride toxicity can appear with similar symptoms and laboratory findings. Some poisons appear with constellations of symptoms called *toxidromes* (Table 70-4).

Table 70-4. Common Toxidromes				
	Sympathomimetic	**Opioid**	**Anticholinergic**	**Cholinergic**
Toxins	Cocaine, amphetamines, pseudoephedrine, methylenedioxypyrovalerone	Heroin, morphine, codeine, fentanyl methadone	Diphenhydramine, TCA, atypical antipsychotics, carbamazepine, *Datura* species	Organophosphates, carbamates
Temperature	Hyperthermia	Hypothermia	Hyperthermia	
Pulse	Tachycardia	Bradycardia	Tachycardia	Bradycardia
Blood pressure	Hypertension	Hypotension		
Respiratory rate	Tachypnea	Bradypnea, apnea		Dyspnea (pulmonary edema), tachypnea
Skin	Diaphoresis		Dry	Diaphoresis
Neurologic symptoms	Agitation, seizures	Sedation, coma	Agitation, seizures, coma	
Ocular symptoms	Mydriasis	Miosis	Mydriasis	Miosis
Gastrointestinal symptoms		Constipation	Constipation	Emesis, diarrhea
Genitourinary symptoms	Urinary retention		Urinary retention	Enuresis
Mnemonic symptoms	Mimics "fight-or-flight" response		"Mad as a hatter, hot as a hare, blind as a bat, red as a beet, dry as a bone"	**S**alivation **L**acrimation **U**rination **D**efecation **G**astrointestinal upset **E**mesis

Abbreviation: TCA, tricyclic antidepressant.

Treatment

The initiation of Pediatric Advanced Life Support and supportive care are mainstays of treatment. Discuss treatment and antidote (Table 70-5) administration with a poison center (800/222-1222). Reserve gastrointestinal decontamination (activated charcoal, gastric lavage, whole-bowel irrigation) for the following select cases:

- Activated charcoal (1–2 g/kg; maximum, 50 g): potentially fatal toxin (calcium channel blocker, tricyclic antidepressant), presentation within 1 hour of ingestion, and no aspiration risk

Table 70-5. Select Antidotes

Toxin	Antidote
Carbon monoxide	Oxygen
Cyanide	Hydroxocobalamin
Digoxin	Digoxin-specific Fab
Ethylene glycol, methanol	Fomepizole
Heparin	Protamine
Iron	Deferoxamine
Isoniazid	Pyridoxine
Lead	Succimer, CaNa2EDTA (edetate), dimercaprol
Local anesthetics (cardiotoxicity)	IV lipid emulsion (info at lipidrescue.org)
Organophosphates and carbamates	Atropine and pralidoxime
Toxin-induced methemoglobinemia	Methylene blue
Sulfonylureas	Octreotide
Warfarin, brodifacoum	Vitamin K, fresh frozen plasma

Abbreviations: CaNa2EDTA, calcium disodium versenate; IV, intravenous.

- Gastric lavage: potentially life-threatening toxin that can be withdrawn through a gastric tube (liquid such as organophosphates, ethylene glycol, methanol), presentation within 1 hour of ingestion, and no aspiration risk
- Whole-bowel irrigation (polyethylene glycol 3350 and electrolyte lavage solution, 25 mL/kg/h, 2-L/h maximum, until desired effect is achieved): potentially life-threatening toxin (iron, lead, arsenic) and no aspiration risk

Treat toxin-induced agitation or seizures with intravenous (IV) lorazepam (0.05–0.10 mg/kg per dose, 2–4-mg maximum). Treat seizures refractory to lorazepam with IV phenobarbital (10–20 mg/kg per dose, 1-g maximum).

Treat ventricular tachycardia or a QRS duration greater than 100 msec with an IV sodium bicarbonate bolus (1–2 mEq/kg [1–2 mmol/kg] per dose). For torsades de pointes or a corrected QT interval greater than 500 msec, administer IV magnesium sulfate (25–50 mg/kg per dose, 2-g maximum) and correct hypokalemia, if present.

Naloxone (0.1 mg/kg, repeat every 2 minutes as needed; maximum, 2 mg per dose) can be used for respiratory failure from opioids and for opioid-induced hypotension, particularly when the hypotension is refractory to standard therapies. Do not use flumazenil for non–life-threatening benzodiazepine ingestion because it can cause seizures or benzodiazepine withdrawal. Reserve flumazenil (0.01 mg/kg per dose; 0.2-mg maximum) for confirmed benzodiazepine ingestion with respiratory failure, without co-ingestion of substances that will lower seizure threshold or a history of chronic benzodiazepine use.

Administer IV N-acetylcysteine (NAC) (150 mg/kg/h for 1 hour, then 12.5 mg/kg/h for 4 hours, then 6.25 mg/kg/h for a minimum of 16 hours) for an acute acetaminophen (APAP) ingestion with a serum concentration above the APAP toxicity nomogram treatment line (Figure 70-1), a chronic APAP ingestion with a detectable APAP concentration or with evidence of liver

Figure 70-1. The Rumack-Matthew nomogram

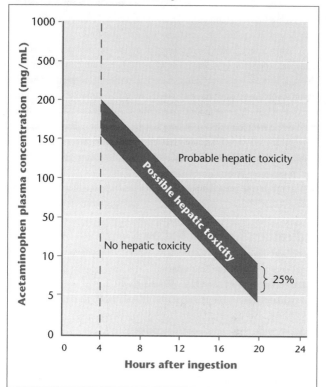

The Rumack-Matthew nomogram for acetaminophen poisoning is a semilogarithmic plot of plasma acetaminophen concentrations versus time. Cautions for the use of this chart: The time coordinates refer to time after ingestion, the serum concentrations obtained before 4 hours are not interpretable, and the graph should be used only in relation to a single acute ingestion with a known time of ingestion. The nomogram is not useful for chronic exposures or unknown time of ingestion and should be used with caution in the setting of coingestants that slow gastrointestinal motility. The lower solid line is typically used in the United States to define toxicity and direct treatment; the upper line is generally used in Europe. (Reprinted from Kostic MA. Poisoning. In: Kliegman RM, Stanton BF, St. Geme III JW, Schor NF, eds. *Nelson Textbook of Pediatrics.* 20th ed. Philadelphia, PA: Elsevier; 2016:447–467.e1. © 2016, with permission from Elsevier.)

injury/decreased function, or hepatotoxicity in a patient with an unknown ingestion (until the etiology is determined). Discontinue the NAC after the 21-hour infusion if the APAP concentration is less than 10 µg/mL and if aspartate transaminase (AST) and alanine transaminase (ALT) levels are within normal limits. If the AST or ALT levels remain abnormal, continue IV NAC at 6.25 mg/kg/h until there is clinical improvement, the ALT is at 50% of its peak or declining and below 1,000 U/L, international normalized ratio (INR) is less than 2, creatinine level is declining or stable, any encephalopathy has resolved, and APAP concentration is less than 10 µg/mL.

To enhance the elimination of salicylates, initiate serum alkalinization for a salicylate concentration greater than 40 mg/dL (2,896 µmol/L) or a detectable salicylate concentration with metabolic acidosis, altered mental status, seizures, vomiting, and/or tinnitus. Put 150 mEq (150 mmol) of sodium bicarbonate in 1 L 5% dextrose in water and administer the IV fluids at 1 to 2 times maintenance requirements. Goals are a serum pH level of 7.40 to 7.45 and a urine pH level of 7.5 to 8.0, but monitor the patient carefully for hypokalemia. Elimination of salicylates, ethylene glycol, methanol, caffeine, and theophylline are enhanced by hemodialysis.

Institute suicide precautions and consult a psychiatrist if there is suicidal or unclear intent.

Indications for Consultation

- **Medical toxicology (if available):** All patients with symptoms that require antidotes or enhanced elimination
- **Poison center (800/222-1222):** All patients
- **Psychiatry:** Suicidal or unclear intent, drug abuse, Munchausen syndrome by proxy
- **Social work:** Home or self-safety concerns

Disposition

- **Intensive care unit transfer:** Seizure, cardiac arrhythmia, hypotension, agitation, respiratory failure
- **Discharge criteria:** Patient is asymptomatic, and any toxin-induced organ injury has resolved; psychiatric and social disposition is established; observation period is met for toxins with delayed toxicity

Follow-up

- **Primary care:** 1 week
- **Psychiatry:** If needed, 1 to 2 weeks

Pearls and Pitfalls

- Fosphenytoin is ineffective for most toxin-induced seizures.
- Avoid premature disposition for a patient who has ingested a substance with delayed toxicity (salicylates, acetaminophen, bupropion, sulfonylureas, ethylene glycol, methanol, sustained-release [SR] β-blockers, SR calcium channel blockers).
- APAP toxicity nomogram is only for acute ingestion of the regular product, not the extended-release product.
- Do not discontinue NAC in APAP toxicity when the APAP concentration is undetectable but hepatotoxicity is worsening.
- IV NAC can increase the prothrombin time and increase the INR as high as 1.9.
- Establish trends by obtaining serial serum concentrations with salicylate or iron ingestion.
- Salicylate concentrations are often reported in units of milligram percent or milligrams per deciliter, rather than milligrams per liter.
- Know which drugs are included in serum or urine drug screenings and use caution when relying on screening tests to prove toxicity, predict prognosis, or rule exposures in or out.
- Always assume that an adolescent has taken more than one drug.

Recommended Additional Resource

Micromedex: Online toxin and toxicant database, acetaminophen toxicity nomogram (www.micromedex.com)

Bibliography

Barrueto F Jr, Gattu R, Mazer-Amirshahi M. Updates in the general approach to the pediatric poisoned patient. *Pediatr Clin North Am.* 2013;60(5):1203–1220

Calello DP, Henretig FM. Pediatric toxicology: specialized approach to the poisoned child. *Emerg Med Clin North Am.* 2014;32(1):29–52

Fine JS. Pediatric principles. In: Hoffman RS, Howland MA, Lewin NA, Nelson LS, Goldfrank LR, eds. *Goldfrank's Toxicologic Emergencies.* 10th ed. New York, NY: McGraw-Hill; 2015:415–427

Lopez AM, Hendrickson RG. Toxin-induced hepatic injury. *Emerg Med Clin North Am.* 2014;32(1):103–125

Mowry JB, Spyker DA, Cantilena LR Jr, McMillan N, Ford M. 2013 annual report of the American Association of Poison Control Centers' National Poison Data System (NPDS): 31st annual report. *Clin Toxicol (Phila).* 2014;52:1032–1283

Nelson ME, Bryant SM, Aks SE. Emerging drugs of abuse. *Dis Mon.* 2014;60(3):110–132

Liver Diseases

Acute Liver Failure

Introduction

Pediatric acute liver failure (PALF) is defined as biochemical evidence of acute liver injury in a patient with no previous history of chronic liver disease and a coagulopathy, which is characterized by either

1. A severe liver-based coagulopathy (prothrombin time [PT] >20 seconds or an international normalized ratio [INR] >2) without hepatic encephalopathy (HE) *or*
2. A mild coagulopathy (PT >15 seconds or INR >1.5) with encephalopathy

The etiology of PALF varies according to age (see Table 71-1). Overall, when a cause can be identified, a viral etiology is the most common known cause, typically hepatitis A. Neonates most commonly have metabolic disease, hemochromatosis, and unknown (indeterminate) causes. Over 1 year of age, viral hepatitis, drugs, and indeterminate causes are the most common etiologies, followed by autoimmune and Wilson disease. Acetaminophen overdose

Table 71-1. Etiologies of Acute Liver Failure	
Etiology	**Examples**
Infants	
Metabolic	Galactosemia, hereditary fructose intolerance, mitochondrial disorders, Niemann-Pick disease type C, tyrosinemia, urea cycle disorder, Wilson disease
Viral	Adenovirus, cytomegalovirus, enterovirus, coxsackievirus, hepatitis B and C, herpes simplex, human herpesvirus 6
Other	Hemophagocytic syndrome
Children	
Indeterminate	Up to 50% of cases
Viral	Cytomegalovirus, Epstein-Barr virus, herpes simplex, varicella, viral hepatitides (A, B, C, D coinfection, and E)
Other	Autoimmune, drug induced, or infiltrative ischemic etiology (leukemia, hemophagocytic lymphohistiocytosis); *Salmonella;* sepsis; tuberculosis; vascular; Wilson disease
Adolescents	
Indeterminate	Up to 50% of cases
Viral	Hepatitis A and B, hepatitis non-A and non-B, cytomegalovirus, Epstein-Barr virus, herpes simplex
Drug induced	Acetaminophen (most common), anticonvulsants
Other	Autoimmune, ischemic, or infiltrative etiology (leukemia, hemophagocytic lymphohistiocytosis); *Salmonella;* sepsis tuberculosis; vascular Wilson disease

is an important cause in adolescents. However, a specific etiology cannot be identified in approximately 50% of PALF cases.

Clinical Presentation

History

The typical presentation is a flulike illness with symptoms that include anorexia, vomiting, abdominal pain, malaise, and lethargy with or without fever. This will be followed by progressive jaundice over days to weeks. Encephalopathy may occur hours to weeks later and will manifest as confusion, somnolence, or altered consciousness, although encephalopathy may not be detected in infants and young children until it is severe.

Ask about exposure to sick persons with infectious hepatitis, a history of blood transfusion, and what medications (both prescribed and over the counter) are in the home that the child has or might have taken. A history of developmental delay, failure to thrive, or seizures raises the concern for a metabolic disease. There may be a family history of liver disease, autoimmune conditions, infant death, α1-antitrypsin deficiency, or Wilson disease. An adolescent making a suicide attempt or gesture will often take an overdose of acetaminophen, with or without other drugs. In addition, it is important to specifically ask about acetaminophen use, because toxicity can occur from dosing errors during a prolonged therapeutic course.

Physical Examination

Priorities include the growth parameters and skin evaluation for jaundice, bruises, and petechiae. Perform an abdominal examination for hepatomegaly, splenomegaly, and ascites, and look for peripheral edema. A thorough neurologic examination is also essential. Assess mental status, which may range from mild confusion (excessive crying in infants) to coma with hyperreflexia and decorticate/decerebrate rigidity (late stages). The patient may also have signs of hypoglycemia (pallor, diaphoresis), cerebral edema, and/or signs of increased intracranial pressure (ICP). In contrast, findings not usually present in a child with PALF are Kayser-Fleischer rings of Wilson disease, asterixis, and fetor hepaticus.

Complications

A severe coagulopathy is the major complication and an independent risk factor for death or the need for liver transplant. Cerebral edema with increased ICP is another serious complication of PALF. Other complications include sepsis (most often caused by *Staphylococcus aureus*), hypotension, ascites, gastrointestinal bleeding, seizures, and hypoglycemia secondary to depletion of hepatic glycogen storage and impaired gluconeogenesis. Renal failure may develop in the later stages.

Laboratory Workup

In general, the consulting gastroenterologist or liver specialist will guide the workup of PALF. Not all laboratory studies need to be performed immediately, and a tiered workup is usually appropriate. There may be limitations on blood volume that can be drawn because of the small size of the patient; therefore, testing needs to be prioritized. At initial evaluation, obtain a complete blood cell count (CBC) and electrolyte, glucose, calcium, and phosphorous levels and perform liver function tests, including alanine transaminase (ALT), aspartate transaminase (AST), γ-glutamyltransferase, albumin, and total and direct bilirubin levels. Assess the degree of coagulopathy with PT and INR, as well as factor V and VII assays. Other initial tests include fibrinogen, ammonia, lipase, and amylase levels. Base further workup on the most likely suspected etiologies; however, the early identification of conditions that are amenable to treatment is the priority for early diagnosis.

If a viral etiology is suspected, send serologic samples for hepatitis A (anti–hepatitis A virus immunoglobulin [Ig] M), B (surface antigen of the hepatitis B virus, antibody to the hepatitis B core antigen), C (anti–hepatitis C virus), and D (anti–hepatitis D virus RNA).

Obtain a serum acetaminophen level for every patient with PALF. If the time of ingestion is unknown, the acetaminophen level may be very low, despite markedly increased ALT and AST levels (>3,500 IU/L [58.4 μkat/L]).

See Chapter 43, Inborn Errors of Metabolism, for the laboratory evaluation of a suspected metabolic disorder.

If an autoimmune disease is a possibility, obtain immunoglobulin (IgG, IgA, IgM), antinuclear antibody, anti–smooth muscle antigen, and liver-kidney microsomal antibody levels, and perform complement component tests (C3 and C4).

Radiology Examinations

Abdominal and Doppler Ultrasonography

Ultrasonography is useful to assess liver size, identify ascites and a liver mass, and establish the patency and flow in the hepatic vein (allowing exclusion of Budd-Chiari syndrome), hepatic artery, and portal vein.

Head Computed Tomography

Computed tomography (CT) findings are usually normal in HE, while early cerebral edema may not be evident. Head CT is also useful for ruling out intracranial bleed or structural causes of encephalopathy.

Magnetic Resonance Imaging

Use of a T1-weighted sequence confirms the presence of abnormal water accumulation, even in patients with minimal grades of encephalopathy, and documents its resolution after hepatic transplantation or successful treatment of hepatic failure. However, magnetic resonance imaging may be impractical for a critically ill patient.

Differential Diagnosis

Generally, the diagnosis of PALF is clear, based on the definition noted earlier. However, an abnormal PT or INR may also be caused by factor VII or vitamin K deficiency, warfarin ingestion, and sepsis. Liver failure may be the present-ing manifestation of a systemic condition such as leukemia. Severe hypoten-sion caused by trauma, hemorrhage, cardiomyopathy, or heart failure can lead to liver failure. Increases of liver transaminase levels (ALT and/or AST) may be a consequence of hemolysis, infectious mononucleosis, muscle injury or myositis, pancreatitis, myocardial injury, and hepatotoxic drugs.

Treatment

The treatment of PALF requires an intensive care unit (ICU) setting with a multidisciplinary team that includes a hepatologist, critical care special-ist, neurologist, neurosurgeon, nephrologist, metabolic specialist, and liver transplant surgeon. If this is not available locally, immediately consult with a pediatric gastroenterologist to guide initial treatment and arrange for transfer. Care is mostly supportive and involves managing increased ICP and multi-organ failure while awaiting recovery of liver function or liver transplant.

General treatment includes admission to an ICU with continuous cardio-respiratory and oxygen monitoring, as well as frequent assessments of neuro-logic status. Closely monitor input and output and measure the blood glucose level every 6 hours, electrolyte levels and PT/INR every 12 hours, and the CBC daily. If fluid resuscitation is not required, restrict intravenous fluids to 85% to 90% maintenance levels to avoid overhydration while continuing to provide sufficient glucose and phosphorus. More specific management guidelines are summarized in Table 71-2.

Table 71-2. Management of Acute Liver Failure	
Complication	**Management**
Ascites	*If the ascites is causing respiratory symptoms* Fluid restriction Diuresis Spironolactone 1–3 mg/kg/d, divided into doses administered 2 or 3 times a day *or* Furosemide 1 mg/kg per dose every 6–8 hours
Cerebral edema	Elevate head of bed to 30° Fluids: 2/3 maintenance levels, if no sign of dehydration or hypovolemia Consult a neurosurgeon for possible intracranial pressure monitoring Maintain oxygen saturation >95% and diastolic pressure >40 mm Hg
Coagulopathy	If there is active bleeding, INR >7, or an invasive procedure required Fresh frozen plasma (10 mL/kg) or recombinant factor VII (90 µg/kg) Platelet transfusion: Platelets <50,000/mm³ (50 × 10⁹/L)
Encephalopathy	Minimize stimulation and sedation Reduce protein intake Analgesia: short-acting opiates (fentanyl)
Hypoglycemia	10% Dextrose in water at 6–8 mg/kg/min (3.6–4.8 mL/kg/h)

Liver transplant is a consideration, but decision making can be challenging. Many patients with PALF will have spontaneous recovery. The goal is to let spontaneous recovery occur but transplant when recovery does not occur. The prognosis can be extremely challenging to predict.

Pearls and Pitfalls

- Early identification of conditions that are amenable to treatment is a critical priority.
- Always consider acetaminophen poisoning, especially in an adolescent. There may be marked increase of liver function test (LFT) values, with a normal or mildly increased total bilirubin level.
- Coagulopathy is an excellent tool for monitoring the patient's status and assessing the prognosis. In contrast, LFT values do not correlate with severity of disease. They will increase terminally and are markedly increased in metabolic diseases.
- Alkaline phosphatase to bilirubin ratio less than 2 differentiates fulminant Wilson disease from other causes of acute liver failure (ALF).
- For ammonia testing, samples must be obtained from a free-flowing catheter, placed on ice, and rapidly transported to the laboratory.
- Sedation is contraindicated in a nonintubated patient with ALF.

Bibliography

D'Agostino D, Diaz S, Sanchez MC, Boldrini G. Management and prognosis of acute liver failure in children. *Curr Gastroenterol Rep.* 2012;14(3):262–269

Devictor D, Tissieres P, Durand P, Chevret L, Debray D. Acute liver failure in neonates, infants and children. *Expert Rev Gastroenterol Hepatol.* 2011;5(6):717–729

Dhawan A. Acute liver failure in children and adolescents. *Clin Res Hepatol Gastroenterol.* 2012;36(3):278–283

Squires RH, Alonso EM. Acute liver failure in children. In: Suchy FJ, Sokol RJ, Balistreri WF, eds. *Liver Disease in Children.* 4th ed. New York, NY: Cambridge University Press; 2014

Sundaram V, Shneider BL, Dhawan A, et al. King's College Hospital Criteria for non-acetaminophen induced acute liver failure in an international cohort of children. *J Pediatr.* 2013;162(2):319–323

CHAPTER 72

Neonatal Hyperbilirubinemia

Introduction

While jaundice is a common and benign finding in the neonatal period, the potential for neurotoxicity makes early detection of dangerous levels imperative. The most common scenarios involve unconjugated (indirect) hyperbilirubinemia, resulting from physiological jaundice, breast milk jaundice, or ongoing hemolysis from ABO incompatibility, glucose-6-phosphatase dehydrogenase (G6PD) deficiency, and other hereditary hemolytic disorders. However, timely identification of conjugated (direct) hyperbilirubinemia and its underlying pathology is critical, because early intervention reduces long-term morbidity for biliary atresia and may be lifesaving. Jaundice that persists at 3 weeks of age or later raises the concern for biliary atresia and neonatal hepatitis. The Kasai procedure for biliary atresia, if performed under 30 to 45 days of life, improves outcomes and significantly delays the need for future liver transplantation.

Clinical Presentation

History

Ask about jaundice that occurs in the first 24 hours of life, because this is almost never normal and is usually a result of hemolysis. Determine if the infant has symptoms of acute bilirubin encephalopathy, including lethargy, high-pitched cry, vomiting, poor feeding, and poor weight gain. Opisthotonus and seizures occur with extremely high bilirubin levels.

Obtain feeding and bowel histories, including frequency, amount, source of nutrition, and composition of any formula, and ask about dark urine or clay-colored stools. Review the maternal and birth history (including fetal ultrasonography [US] results), look for evidence of a congenital viral infection, and determine percentage of weight loss, if any. Ask about a family history of jaundice or consanguinity.

Physical Examination

Obtain vital signs and growth parameters and assess the patient for signs of dehydration. Measure the size and note the consistency of the liver and spleen. Palpate for abdominal masses and ascites. Document the level of jaundice and the presence of bruising or cephalohematomas. Note dysmorphic features that can be associated with syndromes, such as triangular facies in Alagille syndrome, macroglossia in hypothyroidism, and microcephaly in congenital cytomegalovirus (CMV).

Laboratory Workup

Obtain total serum bilirubin (TSB) and direct bilirubin levels, complete blood cell count (CBC) with differential and smear, reticulocyte count, and blood type and perform a direct antibody test (Coombs test) if previous results are unavailable. If the TSB level is 25 mg/dL or greater (≥427.6 µmol/L) (or ≥20 mg/dL [≥342.08 µmol/L] in a sick or preterm infant), send blood for type and crossmatch and an albumin level evaluation. Calculate the ratio of TSB to albumin, which is an additional criterion for determining the need for an exchange transfusion. Bilirubin that is unbound to albumin more readily crosses the blood-brain barrier and is associated with increased risk of kernicterus in sick and preterm newborns. Check the results of the newborn screen (galactosemia, G6PD level, thyroid).

If the history and physical examination findings suggest sepsis, obtain blood, urine, and cerebrospinal samples for culture and full analysis. Also, new-onset jaundice after 2 weeks of age can be the presenting sign of a urinary tract infection (UTI), especially in a patient with galactosemia.

Obtain a quantitative G6PD level if suggested by ethnic or geographic origin (African, Mediterranean, Middle Eastern, Southeast Asian) or if there is a poor response to phototherapy in a patient with evidence of hemolysis (decreasing hematocrit level associated with increased serum glutamic oxaloacetic transaminase [SGOT] and lactate dehydrogenase levels). G6PD screening can have falsely negative findings during acute hemolytic episodes, so perform a quantitative G6PD assay.

If the infant has conjugated or direct hyperbilirubinemia, consult a gastroenterologist to determine the appropriate testing, which may include obtaining blood for culture and CBC; albumin, SGOT, serum glutamic pyruvic transaminase, alkaline phosphatase, and glucose levels; prothrombin time, partial thromboplastin time, and hepatitis serologies; as well as urine for bacterial and CMV culture, urinalysis, and reducing substances. If clinically suspected, repeat testing for galactosemia and hypothyroidism, because these require urgent management to prevent serious sequelae. If the results are negative for sepsis, UTI, or other specific disease, perform abdominal US and obtain α1-antitrypsin levels.

Differential Diagnosis

The differential diagnosis of unconjugated hyperbilirubinemia is summarized in Table 72-1, and the differential diagnosis of conjugated hyperbilirubinemia is presented in Table 72-2.

Table 72-1. Differential Diagnosis of Unconjugated Hyperbilirubinemia	
Diagnosis	**Clinical Features**
Common diagnoses	
Breast milk jaundice	Presents after 7 d and may last for weeks ↑ Total bilirubin level <0.5 mg/dL/h (<8.55 µmol/L/h), and total level usually does not reach phototherapy levels
Dehydration/breastfeeding jaundice	Often due to poor feeding Poor weight gain <3–4 stools/d and <6–7 wet diapers/d
Physiological origin	Presents at 24–72 h and resolves by 10 d (-) Coombs test
Less common diagnoses	
ABO/Rh incompatibility	Can present in first 24 h of life (+) Coombs test ↓ Hemoglobin level compared to level measured in the newborn nursery
G6PD deficiency	African, Mediterranean, Middle Eastern, or Southeast Asian ethnicity Poor response to phototherapy Abnormal G6PD enzyme assay
Hypothyroidism	Delayed stool production after birth Macroglossia, large fontanelles May be conjugated
Infection/sepsis	Vomiting, lethargy, temperature instability Suspect urinary tract infection if onset after 2 wk May be conjugated
Rare diagnoses	
Crigler-Najjar syndrome	Presents at 1–3 d of life Total bilirubin level >15 mg/dL (>256.56 µmol/L) Type I responds to phenobarbital treatment
Other hemolytic disorders	Can present in first 24 h of life (-) Coombs test Peripheral smear: abnormally shaped red blood cells
Polycythemia	Plethora, lethargy/irritability, jitteriness Hematocrit level >65%
Sequestered blood	Cephalohematoma, bruising, central nervous system hemorrhage

Abbreviations: G6PD, glucose-6-phosphate dehydrogenase; -, negative finding; +, positive finding.

Table 72-2. Differential Diagnosis of Conjugated Hyperbilirubinemia

Diagnosis	Clinical Features
Common diagnoses	
Biliary atresia	Presents in the first 2 mo of life Usually a full-term female subject Hepatosplenomegaly
Idiopathic neonatal hepatitis	Recovery without intervention (most cases) Diagnosis usually requires liver biopsy
TPN cholestasis	Usually after 2 wk of TPN Reverses when TPN stops
UTI/sepsis	Vomiting, lethargy, temperature instability May be unconjugated
Less common diagnoses	
α1-Antitrypsin deficiency	(+) Family history Liver biopsy: (+) PAS granules
Alagille syndrome	Facies: broad forehead, deep-set eyes, pointed chin Congenital heart disease, butterfly vertebrae Liver biopsy: paucity of small bile ducts
Choledochal cyst	May have a palpable RUQ mass Can present at this age or later
Congenital infection	CMV, other TORCH, HIV, parvovirus B19, HBV, HCV IUGR, hepatosplenomegaly, thrombocytopenia, rash Abnormal funduscopic or slit-lamp exam findings
Cystic fibrosis	May have (+) family history Delayed stool production, meconium ileus Abnormal newborn screen results, (+) sweat test
Galactosemia	Poor growth, hypotonia, cataracts, liver dysfunction *Escherichia coli* sepsis or UTI Abnormal newborn screen results, quantitative GALT test (+) Urine reducing substances
Gallstones/biliary sludge	May have history of TPN, hemolysis, or fasting (+) Ultrasonography
Hypothyroidism	Delayed stool production after birth, lethargy, hoarse cry Macroglossia, large fontanelles, poor growth May be unconjugated
Panhypopituitarism	Normal growth parameters, micropenis Lethargy, hypotension, temperature instability Hypoglycemia, electrolyte disturbances
Tyrosinemia	FTT, vomiting, diarrhea, bleeding, hepatomegaly Cabbage-like odor Abnormal newborn screen results and/or plasma amino acid and urine organic acid analysis findings

Abbreviations: CMV, cytomegalovirus; FTT, failure to thrive; GALT, gut-associated lymphoid tissue; HBV, hepatitis B virus; HCV, hepatitis C virus; IUGR, intrauterine growth restriction; PAS, periodic acid–Schiff stain; RUQ, right upper quadrant; TORCH, toxoplasmosis, other agents, rubella, cytomegalovirus, herpes simplex; TPN, total parenteral nutrition; UTI, urinary tract infection; +, positive finding.

Treatment

Unconjugated Hyperbilirubinemia

For an infant 35 weeks or older, check the Bilitool Web site, which is consistent with the American Academy of Pediatrics guidelines, for treatment recommendations with intensive phototherapy (www.bilitool.org). Have the following information available when entering the site: date and time of birth, date and time of blood sampling (or the infant's age in hours), and total bilirubin level. Recommendations for intensive phototherapy will depend on TSB level, gestational age, and risk factors for hyperbilirubinemia and neurotoxicity. The latest-generation biliblankets are equivalent to single- or double-bank phototherapy and can allow for continuous treatment while the caregiver holds and feeds the baby.

Monitor the therapeutic effect by retesting the TSB level in 2 to 12 hours, depending on the infant's age and prior levels. Transcutaneous bilirubin (TcB) measurements on exposed (uncovered) skin are unreliable once treatment is initiated, since phototherapy bleaches the skin. Risk factors for severe hyperbilirubinemia are summarized in Box 72-1. The criteria for exchange transfusion are TSB level above exchange transfusion thresholds, the bilirubin rate of increase is >0.5 mg/dL/h (>8.55 µmol/L/h) despite intensive phototherapy, or the patient has clinical symptoms of acute bilirubin encephalopathy, regardless of bilirubin level. Intravenous (IV) gamma globulin (0.5–1.0 g/kg) is a safe and effective adjunctive therapy.

Encourage more frequent feeding (every 2–3 hours) with either milk-based formula or expressed breast milk. Do not administer IV hydration unless the infant is severely dehydrated or unable to tolerate oral feedings.

If jaundice is caused by an acute illness (UTI, sepsis, hypothyroidism), treat the underlying cause.

Box 72-1. Important Risk Factors for Severe Hyperbilirubinemia	
Predischarge TSB or TcB measurement in the high-risk zone	Exclusive breastfeeding, especially with poor latch and/or excessive weight loss
Younger gestational age	Previous sibling with jaundice
Cephalohematoma/bruising	Isoimmune or other hemolytic disease
Jaundice in the first 24 h of life	East Asian race

Abbreviations: TcB, transcutaneous bilirubin; TSB, total serum bilirubin.

Adapted from the American Academy of Pediatrics Subcommittee on Hyperbilirubinemia. Management of hyperbilirubinemia in the newborn infant 35 or more weeks of gestation. *Pediatrics*. 2004;114(1):297-316.

Conjugated Hyperbilirubinemia

If there is evidence of biliary obstruction, consult with a gastroenterologist and/or a pediatric surgeon. Urgent workup and management are necessary to avoid morbidity and mortality from conditions such as inborn errors and surgical conditions such as biliary atresia. Treatment options include the Kasai procedure (biliary atresia), liver transplantation (tyrosinemia, late biliary atresia), choledochal cyst excision, cholecystectomy, and bile duct resection.

Ensure adequate nutritional support and medical management of underlying disorders. Consult with a geneticist and an experienced nutritionist for dietary guidelines for liver and metabolic diseases.

Discharge Management (Unconjugated Hyperbilirubinemia)

Discontinue phototherapy and discharge the patient to go home when the TSB level decreases to less than 13 to 14 mg/dL (<222.4–239.5 μmol/L). In general, observing the patient for rebound is not necessary if it delays hospital discharge, since significant rebound that results in a readmission is rare. However, obtain a follow-up level 6 to 12 hours after discontinuation of phototherapy for an infant with a positive Coombs test finding, who is at increased risk for a clinically significant rebound that may require the reinstitution of phototherapy.

Indications for Consultation

- **Gastroenterology:** Conjugated hyperbilirubinemia
- **Geneticist:** Suspected metabolic disease
- **Pediatric surgery:** Suspected extrinsic/biliary obstruction

Disposition

- **Intensive care unit transfer:** Need for exchange transfusion
- **Discharge criteria (unconjugated hyperbilirubinemia):** TSB level less than 13 to 14 mg/dL (<222.4–239.5 μmol/L), good oral intake with adequate urine output and stool production patterns

Follow-up

Primary care: Within 24 hours for a follow-up bilirubin level evaluation

Pearls and Pitfalls

- Some infants with cholestatic jaundice exposed to phototherapy may develop a dark, grayish-brown discoloration of the skin, serum, and urine (bronze infant syndrome). This is not a contraindication to continued phototherapy.
- Chronic bilirubin encephalopathy (kernicterus) is characterized by severe athetoid cerebral palsy, paralysis of upward gaze, hearing loss, and intellectual impairment.
- Universal predischarge bilirubin screening may be performed by using TSB or TcB measurements; however, obtain a TSB level if the TcB value is at least 70% of the level recommended for use of phototherapy, because TcB values tend to lead to underestimation of TSB values at higher levels. In addition, TcB values are not useful after phototherapy.
- Clinical assessment of TSB, as well as TcB measurements, are particularly inaccurate in darker-skinned infants.
- Blue LED lights are most effective at lowering TSB level. At these wavelengths (450–475 nm), light penetrates the skin and is maximally absorbed by bilirubin.
- Breastfeeding jaundice and breast milk jaundice are *not* contraindications to continuing breastfeeding, even if other fluid supplementation is needed.

Bibliography

Kaplan M, Bromiker R, Hammerman C. Hyperbilirubinemia, hemolysis, and increased bilirubin neurotoxicity. *Semin Perinatol.* 2014;38(7):429–437

Maisels MJ. Managing the jaundiced newborn: a persistent challenge. *CMAJ.* 2015; 187(5):335–343

Muchowski KE. Evaluation and treatment of neonatal hyperbilirubinemia. *Am Fam Physician.* 2014;89(11):873–878

Soldi A, Tonetto P, Chiale F, et al. Hyperbilirubinemia and management of breastfeeding. *J Biol Regul Homeost Agents.* 2012;26(3 Suppl):25–29

Taylor J, Burgos AE, Flaherman V, et al. Discrepancies between transcutaneous and serum bilirubin measurements. *Pediatrics.* 2015;135(2):224–231

Nephrology

Hemolytic Uremic Syndrome

Introduction

Hemolytic uremic syndrome (HUS) is a disorder characterized by the triad of microangiopathic hemolytic anemia, thrombocytopenia, and acute renal injury that classically follows the prodrome of a diarrheal illness. While most patients (73%) will recover completely, 3% to 5% will progress to renal failure. HUS affects boys and girls equally, and most cases occur in children younger than 5 years old. HUS occurs most frequently during the summer and fall.

Cases of HUS are now classified as either primary (formerly atypical or diarrhea negative) or secondary (formerly typical or diarrhea positive). Approximately 10% of cases of HUS are classified as primary, which include genetic or acquired disorders of regulatory components of the complement system. This form of HUS is less common but has a poorer prognosis, with higher rates of both relapse and progression to end-stage renal disease. Most cases of HUS are classified as secondary and are primarily associated with infections, most commonly Shiga toxin–producing *Escherichia coli* serotypes or other bacteria, such as *Shigella*, *Salmonella dysenteriae*, and *Streptococcus pneumoniae*, and HIV. Other associated, but rare, triggers for secondary HUS include drug toxicities, autoimmune disorders, and pregnancy.

Clinical Presentation

History

Secondary HUS is preceded by a nonspecific diarrheal illness (often bloody) that appears with nausea, vomiting, abdominal pain, tenderness, and low-grade fever at presentation. A patient with HUS will then develop the sudden onset of pallor, irritability, weakness, and oliguria or anuria. These symptoms occur several days (often 5–7 days) after the onset of the diarrheal illness, typically when the colitis is improving. Approximately one-third of patients may experience neurologic changes at the onset of symptoms, ranging from mild irritability and lethargy to seizures, stroke, or coma.

Physical Examination

Perform a thorough physical examination, because abnormal findings reflect the severity of the cascade of hematologic and renal dysfunction. The patient is often ill appearing, with significant pallor and possibly mild jaundice. Hypertension and tachycardia are common. There may be petechiae, but purpura is rare. Generalized edema is often present and is more prominent in dependent areas. Nonspecific neurologic findings are common and include irritability and generalized weakness or fatigue. However, more severe neurologic changes, such as seizures, encephalopathy, coma, or focal neurologic deficits consistent with stroke, may be seen secondary to metabolic derangements or thrombotic events.

Generalized abdominal pain and tenderness are common and are typically related to the inciting infectious colitis. More focal abdominal pain and tenderness can be seen with complications such as hepatitis (right upper quadrant tenderness, hepatomegaly), pancreatitis (epigastric pain and tenderness radiating to the back, severe emesis), intestinal obstruction, intussusception, or perforation (distention, severe emesis, decreased bowel sounds). Cardiovascular complications include severe tachycardia, hypertension, or signs of heart failure (dyspnea, tachypnea, rales, hepatomegaly, cool extremities, delayed capillary refill). These physical findings are secondary to severe anemia, fluid overload, electrolyte abnormalities, and acute renal insufficiency. Myocarditis is a rare complication.

Laboratory Workup

Initially repeat the complete blood cell count every 8 to 12 hours, because HUS causes microangiopathic hemolytic anemia. The hemoglobin level is typically less than 8 g/dL (80 g/L) and may decrease rapidly as a result of intense, ongoing hemolysis. The cells are normochromic and normocytic, with schistocytes/helmet cells seen on a peripheral smear. Assess the patient for other markers of nonimmune-mediated hemolysis, including increased reticulocyte count, indirect bilirubin level, and lactate dehydrogenase level, with decreased haptoglobin level and a negative Coombs test result. The patient may have thrombocytopenia, with a platelet count less than 73,000/mm³ (73×10^9/L) megakaryocytes on a peripheral smear and an increased D-dimer level, but the coagulation factors (prothrombin/partial thromboplastin time, D-dimer and fibrinogen levels) are otherwise normal. Mild leukocytosis is seen, but it is rarely greater than 20,000/mm³. A low complement component 3, or C3, level may be noted in some cases of primary HUS.

During the acute phase, monitor the electrolyte levels every 12 hours to look for hyperkalemia, hyper- or hyponatremia, metabolic acidosis, hyperphosphatemia, and hypocalcemia. The blood urea nitrogen and creatinine levels might be markedly increased, although there is no correlation between the degree of anemia and the severity of the renal disease. The patient may also have increased liver transaminase and hypoalbuminemia levels from enteric protein losses. If the pancreas is involved, amylase and lipase levels will be increased, and the patient may be hyperglycemic. Also perform urinalysis to assess the patient for hematuria, proteinuria, and possible red blood cell casts.

Perform a stool Shiga-toxin assay, as well as a stool culture for enterohemorrhagic *E coli*. Stool cultures performed more than 6 days into the diarrheal illness may have a low yield, and blood cultures typically have negative results.

Radiology Examinations

While imaging is not routinely indicated, perform abdominal imaging (anteroposterior abdominal radiography, computed tomography [CT], ultrasonography [US]) if there is a concern for obstruction, perforation, or intussusception. Renal US can be used to exclude renal vein thrombosis and assess the patient for cortical necrosis. Perform magnetic resonance imaging or non–contrast-enhanced head CT if the patient experiences seizures, coma, or signs of a stroke. Order an electrocardiogram if the patient has severe hyperkalemia and order an echocardiogram, troponin level, and/or brain natriuretic peptide level if there are signs of congestive heart failure, pericardial effusion, or myocarditis.

Differential Diagnosis

The differential diagnosis of HUS is summarized in Table 73-1.

Treatment

The management of secondary HUS is mostly supportive and includes meticulous attention to fluid and electrolyte balance, based on the intravascular fluid status and renal function of the patient. Thus, rehydrate a hypovolemic patient, but restrict fluids in a patient with increased intravascular volume and diminished urine output (provide insensible losses only: 400–730 mL/m^2). Early volume expansion targeted to increase body weight by 10% can improve the outcome, with a decreased rate of renal replacement therapy, shorter duration of intensive care, shorter length of stay, and a trend toward decreased central nervous system (CNS) involvement.

Correct electrolyte abnormalities and follow the patient's daily weight. Administer furosemide (1 mg/kg per dose every 6–24 hours) to help maintain some urine output and prevent progression from oliguria to anuria. Antimotility agents and antibiotics are contraindicated and may worsen the disease course. Optimization of nutritional support is essential, preferably by the enteral route, if the clinical status permits.

Table 73-1. Differential Diagnosis of Hemolytic Uremic Syndrome

Diagnosis	Clinical Features
Gastrointestinal etiology: No microangiopathic hemolytic anemia or thrombocytopenia	
Appendicitis	Acute onset of periumbilical pain that migrates to the right lower quadrant Diarrhea uncommon Normal blood urea nitrogen/creatinine levels and liver function test results
Infectious colitis	Fever, severe abdominal pain, tenesmus (+) Fecal leukocytes
Inflammatory bowel disease	Diarrhea or constipation Weight loss and/or growth failure Oral ulcers and perianal skin tags/fissures
Henoch-Schönlein purpura	Arthralgia/arthritis Palpable purpura of extensor surfaces of the lower extremities Patient may have severe abdominal pain, which can be due to intussusception Heme (+) stools
Hematologic etiology	
Bilateral renal vein thrombosis	Flank pain No gastrointestinal symptoms
Disseminated intravascular coagulation	Prolonged prothrombin time/partial thromboplastin time ↓ Fibrinogen level, fibrin split products, D-dimer level
Sepsis	Absence of microangiopathic hemolytic anemia Signs/symptoms of infection/systemic inflammatory response system May be associated with DIC
Thrombotic thrombocytopenia	Usually occurs in adults Unlikely if platelet count is <30,000/mm^3 (<30 x 10^9/L) or if ↑ creatinine level More central nervous system involvement
Renal etiology	
Acute glomerulonephritis	Absence of hemolysis No gastrointestinal symptoms
Severe dehydration	Return of renal function with fluid resuscitation No hematologic findings
Vasculitis	Rash, arthralgia/arthritis Gastrointestinal symptoms may occur with gut involvement Persistent systemic symptoms

Abbreviations: DIC, disseminated intravascular coagulation; +, positive finding.

Despite rigorous management of fluid and electrolyte status, dialysis may eventually be required. Indications for dialysis include refractory hyperkalemia (>6.0–6.5 mEq/L [>6.0–6.5 mmol/L]), severe metabolic acidosis, symptomatic uremia, calcium/phosphate imbalance, or volume overload with persistent anuria that is not responsive to diuretic therapy. In addition, management of nutritional support and transfusions for severe anemia may require administration of large volumes of fluid, necessitating dialysis.

Emergent antihypertensive treatment may be required. Administer a bolus of intravenous hydralazine (0.2–0.6 mg/kg; maximum, 20 mg per dose) or labetalol (0.2–1.0 mg/kg; maximum, 40 mg per dose), followed by a continuous infusion of either nicardipine (start with 0.5–1.0 g/kg/min and titrate to a maximum of 4–5 g/kg/min) or labetalol (0.25–3.00 mg/kg/h). In the setting of hypertensive urgency in a patient who can tolerate oral medications, administer isradipine (0.05–0.10 mg/kg; maximum, 5 mg per dose) or clonidine in an older child or adolescent (0.05–0.10 mg per dose every 1 hour; maximum, 0.8 mg per dose). In the acute phase of renal injury, avoid nephrotoxic drugs, such as angiotensin-converting enzyme inhibitors and nonsteroidal anti-inflammatory medications, because they alter glomerular perfusion.

Transfuse packed red blood cells (5–10 mL/kg) if the hemoglobin level is less than 6 to 7 g/dL (60–70 g/L) or if there are signs of cardiovascular compromise. Transfuse slowly with a posttransfusion goal of a hemoglobin level of 8 to 9 g/dL (80–90 g/L). Monitor the patient closely for signs of fluid overload and treat with furosemide (1 mg/kg per dose), if necessary, before and/or during the transfusion. Avoid a platelet transfusion unless there is a significant hemorrhage or an invasive procedure is necessary. A patient with significant CNS involvement or primary HUS may require eculizumab or plasmapheresis.

Indications for Consultation

- **Cardiology:** Carditis or heart failure
- **Gastroenterology/surgery:** Complications from colitis or acute abdomen
- **Hematology:** Complications from anemia or thrombocytopenia
- **Nephrology:** Suspected or diagnosed HUS
- **Neurology:** Coma, stroke, or seizure

Disposition

- **Intensive care unit transfer:** Severe electrolyte abnormalities, refractory hypertension requiring antihypertensive infusions, status epilepticus, coma, stroke, or heart failure
- **Discharge criteria:** Improving renal function, anemia, and thrombocytopenia, with stable electrolyte levels; adequate oral intake and nutrition; hypertension resolved or stable with oral medication

Follow-up

- **Primary care:** 2 to 3 days
- **Nephrologist:** 1 week; however, long-term follow-up is needed for persistent or recurrent hypertension and proteinuria

Pearls and Pitfalls

- Maintain a high index of suspicion for a patient with a recent diarrheal illness and abrupt onset of pallor or change in urine output or activity.
- Avoid using antibiotics or antimotility agents in a patient with a diarrheal illness.
- Consider obtaining central access early to facilitate management and monitoring of fluid and electrolyte status, nutritional support, hematologic derangements, transfusions, and possible dialysis, through a right internal central venous catheter and not a peripherally inserted central catheter.
- There is no correlation between the severity of the hematologic findings and that of the renal disease.
- Avoid platelet transfusions.

Bibliography

Ardissino G, Tel F, Possenti I, et al. Early volume expansion and outcomes of hemolytic uremic syndrome. *Pediatrics.* 2016;137(1):e20152153

Bitzan M, Schaefer F, Reymond D. Treatment of typical (enteropathic) hemolytic uremic syndrome. *Semin Thromb Hemost.* 2010;36(6):594–610

Delmas Y, Vendrely B, Clouzeau B, et al. Outbreak of *Escherichia coli* O104:H4 haemolytic uraemic syndrome in France: outcome with eculizumab. *Nephrol Dial Transplant.* 2014;29(3):565–572

Lapeyraque AL, Malina M, Fremeaux-Bacchi V, et al. Eculizumab in severe Shiga-toxin-associated HUS. *N Engl J Med.* 2011;364(26):2561–2563

Pape L, Hartmann H, Bange FC, Suerbaum S, Bueltmann E, Ahlenstiel-Grunow T. Eculizumab in typical hemolytic uremic syndrome (HUS) with neurological involvement. *Medicine (Baltimore).* 2015;94(24):e1000

Scheiring J, Rosales A, Zimmerhackl LB. Clinical practice. Today's understanding of the haemolytic uraemic syndrome. *Eur J Pediatr.* 2010;169(1):7–13

CHAPTER 74

Henoch-Schönlein Purpura

Introduction

Henoch-Schönlein purpura (HSP), also known as *anaphylactoid purpura,* is a systemic, predominantly immunoglobulin A–mediated vasculitis characterized by some combination of nonthrombocytopenic palpable purpura, abdominal pain, arthritis/arthralgia, and renal manifestations. HSP is the most common vasculitis of childhood, with 75% of cases occurring between 2 and 11 years of age and a peak incidence at 5 years of age. Male subjects are affected twice as often as female subjects, and there is a seasonal predilection in the spring and fall. Although the precise etiology is unknown, most cases are preceded by upper respiratory tract infections caused by organisms such as group A *Streptococcus,* Epstein-Barr virus, *Mycoplasma,* and parvovirus B19.

Generally, HSP is a benign illness, and in most cases the symptoms resolve completely, but 1% to 2% can progress to renal failure.

Acute hemorrhagic edema of infancy (AHEI) is another small-vessel vasculitis that has clinical features similar to HSP. At presentation, AHEI appears with a classic triad of sudden development of large, palpable purpuric lesions that are distributed on the face, ears, and limbs; edema; and fever in a non–toxic-appearing child less than 24 months of age. Male subjects are affected more often than female subjects, and there is often a history of recent upper respiratory infection, immunization, or medication use. AHEI has a benign long-term prognosis.

Clinical Presentation

History

As noted earlier, there is usually a history of a preceding upper respiratory tract infection, often associated with malaise and low-grade fever. The classic symptoms then begin to appear simultaneously or sequentially, over a period of days to weeks. About three-quarters of patients complain of colicky, episodic, abdominal pain that is rarely associated with vomiting, hematemesis, and/or gross blood in the stools. About two-thirds of the time, the patient complains of pain and swelling of the large joints, such as the knees and ankles. Rarely, gross hematuria is noted. In as many as 50% of cases, the classic purpuric rash is not evident at presentation, although eventually all patients or parents report an erythematous rash on the buttocks and lower extremities.

Physical Examination

The order of presentation of physical examination findings can vary, but typically there is an erythematous, blanching, lacy, macular rash that quickly evolves into palpable purpura on the buttocks and lower extremities. The patient may also have a toxic appearance. There may be abdominal tenderness and, if intussusception is present, rebound and abdominal guarding. The patient can also present with warmth, tenderness, and swelling without erythema of the knees and ankles. Hypertension may be noted, but it is more common in a patient with renal involvement.

Laboratory Workup

There are no definitive or diagnostic tests for HSP. The remainder of the laboratory evaluation depends on the differential diagnosis.

Afebrile Patient With Classic Rash and No Signs of Sepsis

Perform a complete blood cell count (platelet count is normal), stool guaiac test, and urinalysis, but coagulation studies are unnecessary. While approximately 50% of patients develop microscopic hematuria, a minority have gross blood, white blood cells, and protein in the urine. If hematuria and/or proteinuria is found, obtain electrolyte, blood urea nitrogen, creatinine, and albumin levels. To quantify the degree of proteinuria (if present), calculate the spot urine protein/creatinine ratio to determine whether the patient has nephrotic range proteinuria (ratio >2).

Well-Appearing Patient Younger Than 2 Years of Age With Rapid Onset of Large, Tender Purpuric Lesions and Edema of the Face, Ears, and Limbs

Perform the same tests as for an afebrile patient with the classic rash and no signs of sepsis.

Ill-Appearing Patient With Classic Rash

In addition to the tests mentioned for an afebrile infant with the classic rash, perform blood and urine culture. If the patient has meningeal signs or an altered mental status, perform a lumbar puncture.

Arthritis Without Classic Rash

Obtain an erythrocyte sedimentation rate and/or C-reactive protein level and perform a rheumatologic workup (see Chapter 113, Juvenile Idiopathic Arthritis), including rheumatoid factor, antinuclear antibody, and complement levels.

Possible Intussusception (Crampy Abdominal Pain, Drawing Up of the Legs)

See Chapter 118, Acute Abdomen.

Differential Diagnosis

See Table 74-1 for the differential diagnosis of purpura. If diagnostic uncertainty persists, consult with a dermatologist to arrange a skin biopsy. In both HSP and acute hemorrhagic edema of infancy, leukocytoclastic vasculitis will be found.

Treatment

If the patient has widespread palpable purpura, along with fever and a toxic appearance, immediately perform a blood culture and treat with intravenous (IV) antibiotics, either ceftriaxone (100 mg/kg/d, divided into doses administered every 12 hours) or cefotaxime (200 mg/kg/d, divided into doses administered every 12 hours; 6-g/d maximum). Add doxycycline (2.2 mg/kg per dose; maximum, 100 mg per dose, every 12 hours) if Rocky Mountain spotted fever is suspected.

There is no specific treatment for HSP. In most cases the illness is benign and self-limiting, and symptoms usually resolve in 4 weeks. If the patient has joint swelling and pain, administer a nonsteroidal anti-inflammatory drug (NSAID) such as naproxen (10–20 mg/kg/d, divided into doses administered every 12 hours; 1,000-mg/d maximum) or ibuprofen (10 mg/kg per dose every 6 hours; 40-mg/kg/d maximum), although NSAIDs may be contraindicated with renal impairment.

Table 74-1. Differential Diagnosis of Purpura	
Diagnosis	**Clinical Features**
Coagulopathy	Ecchymoses Abnormal PT and/or PTT
Drug reaction	History of taking an offending agent (penicillin, sulfonamide, oral contraceptives)
Idiopathic thrombocytopenic purpura	Petechiae without purpura Mucosal bleeding Thrombocytopenia
Septicemia (bacterial, Rocky Mountain spotted fever)	Fever, toxicity Purpura not limited to lower extremities
Subacute bacterial endocarditis	Heart murmur or history of heart disease Osler nodes, Janeway lesions, splinter hemorrhages

Abbreviations: PT, prothrombin time; PTT, partial thromboplastin time.

Treat a patient with severe abdominal pain and normal ultrasonographic and/or radiologic findings or joint swelling and pain unresponsive to NSAIDs with methylprednisolone (1 mg/kg/d for 2 weeks, 80-mg/d maximum) and slowly taper over 1 to 2 weeks or longer, depending on the response. Use the IV route to start because oral absorption is poor secondary to the gastrointestinal vasculitis.

Indications for Consultation

- **Nephrology:** Hypertension, decreased renal function, nephrotic syndrome, or proteinuria for more than 1 week
- **Surgery:** Intussusception, intestinal hemorrhage, obstruction, or perforation

Disposition

- **Intensive care unit transfer:** Severe hypertension that requires continuous antihypertensive therapy
- **Discharge criteria:** Symptoms (abdominal pain, arthritis) are no longer incapacitating, and renal function is normal or improving

Follow-up

- **Primary care:** Blood pressure check and urinalysis in 1 week for an uncomplicated case (no hematuria or proteinuria and normal renal function); continue weekly for 3 weeks, then monthly until 6 months after presentation
- **Nephrology:** 1 week if the patient has proteinuria for more than 1 week; immediate consultation if the patient has renal failure or nephrotic syndrome

Pearls and Pitfalls

- In as many as 30% to 50% of patients, the classic rash will develop up to 2 weeks after other clinical manifestations.
- Renal disease can develop over the subsequent 6 months, despite normal initial urinalysis results.
- Intussusception in HSP is usually ileoileal and may resolve spontaneously. Otherwise, an air enema is not effective, and surgery will be required.
- Most patients with AHEI require symptomatic treatment only.

Bibliography

Bluman J, Goldman RD. Henoch-Schönlein purpura in children: limited benefit of corticosteroids. *Can Fam Physician.* 2014;60(11):1007–1010

Fiore E, Rizzi M, Simonetti GD, Garzoni L, Bianchetti MG, Bettinelli A. Acute hemorrhagic edema of young children: a concise narrative review. *Eur J Pediatr.* 2011; 170(12):1507–1511

Reid-Adam J. Henoch-Schönlein Purpura. *Pediatr Rev.* 2014;35(10):447–449

Sohagia AB, Gunturu SG, Tong TR, Hertan HI. Henoch-Schonlein purpura—a case report and review of the literature. *Gastroenterol Res Pract.* 2010;2010:597648

Trnka P. Henoch-Schönlein purpura in children. *J Paediatr Child Health.* 2013;49(12): 995–1003

Nephrolithiasis

Introduction

Nephrolithiasis accounts for about 1 in 1,000 pediatric hospitalizations in the United States, although the incidence has increased over the past 10 years. Consequences of untreated nephrolithiasis include severe pain, increased risk for infection, and, rarely, kidney injury.

Physiological risk factors for nephrolithiasis include low urine volume, low urine pH level, bacterial urinary tract infection, increased urinary concentrations of stone-forming metabolites, and reduced concentrations of inhibitors (eg, citrate, magnesium) of stone formation. Clinically, these risks typically manifest in the setting of metabolic derangements, anatomic abnormality of the urinary tract (eg, ureteropelvic obstruction), and infection. Metabolic factors are found to cause more than 50% of pediatric renal calculi, with hypercalciuria and hypocitrauria being the most common, especially in younger children.

Repeated infection, with or without anatomic abnormality, can also lead to nephrolithiasis in children. Urease-producing bacteria, such as *Proteus, Providencia, Klebsiella, Pseudomonas,* and enterococci, promote renal stone formation by lowering urinary pH level, leading to struvite precipitation and the "staghorn" type of renal stone. A history of surgical correction of genitourinary abnormalities or prolonged immobilization further increases the risk of nephrolithiasis.

Clinical Presentation

History

At presentation, nephrolithiasis usually appears with a combination of abdominal pain that may be generalized and not colicky, flank pain, back pain, vomiting, and gross hematuria. In the first few months of life, the presentation may seem consistent with infantile colic. Ask about a history of renal disease, urinary tract infections, and other chronic medical conditions. Determine if the patient is taking any medications, such as calcium supplements, loop diuretics, acetazolamide, prednisone, and adrenocorticotropic hormone, which can predispose the patient to renal stones. A first-degree relative affected by nephrolithiasis suggests a genetic etiology. Prolonged immobilization because of a lower-extremity fracture can result in hypercalciuria, leading to renal stones.

Physical Examination

Examination findings are inconsistent and nonspecific. Abdominal pain with palpation and costovertebral angle tenderness may be present. Usually there is no abdominal guarding or rebound tenderness. The acute pain of renal colic is classically writhing in nature, with the patient having difficulty finding a position of comfort.

Laboratory Workup

Perform urinalysis and urine culture to evaluate the patient for hematuria and markers of infection, such as pyuria, leukocyte esterase, nitrites, and bacteria. However, as many as one-third of pediatric patients with nephrolithiasis do not present with hematuria.

Once the presence of a stone is confirmed, it is important to identify the exact type before initiating specific treatment. Arrange for the nursing staff or the patient/parent to strain the urine and send any recovered stones for analysis. A 24-hour urine collection is the best way to identify any abnormal metabolites (calcium, oxalate, phosphate, citrate, magnesium, cysteine, xanthine, uric acid). Since this collection may be difficult to perform in a younger patient, send a random urine sample for calcium, citrate, cystine, oxalate, and uric acid evaluation, calculate the metabolite to creatinine ratio for each, and compare the ratios to standard values (most useful for calcium to creatinine ratio). For example, divide the spot calcium level in milligrams by the spot creatinine level in milligrams to determine the urinary calcium to creatinine ratio. (See Table 75-1 for reference values.)

Order further laboratory tests, such as serum electrolyte, calcium, phosphorous, and magnesium levels, on the basis of the clinical picture, stone composition, and urine metabolite evaluation. For example, in a patient with a calcium stone or high calcium to creatinine ratio, consider a broad differential

Table 75-1. Normal Values for Urine Metabolite to Creatinine Ratios			
Metabolite Ratio	**Age**	**Normal Range[a]**	**Diagnoses Associated With Increased Ratios**
Calcium to creatinine ratio	0–6 mo of age	<0.80	Bartter syndrome
	6–12 mo of age	<0.60	Distal renal tubular acidosis
	2–18 y of age	<0.20	Loop diuretics
Oxalate to creatinine ratio	0–6 mo of age	<0.30	Cystic fibrosis
	6 mo to 4 y of age	<0.15	Primary oxaluria
	>4 y of age to adult	<0.10	
Cystine to creatinine ratio	All ages	<0.02	Cystinuria
Citrate to creatinine ratio	All ages	<0.51	

[a] Urine metabolite to creatinine ratios are calculated with values in milligrams.

for hypercalciuria, including abnormal gastrointestinal absorption of calcium, renal tubular dysfunction, endocrine derangements, and metabolic disorders. This workup may be deferred to the outpatient setting.

Radiology Examinations

Order anteroposterior abdominal radiography (also known as "KUB") as the initial radiologic study, although many stones may be missed if they are small in size or composed of material that is less radio-opaque, such as uric acid or cystine. Ultrasonography (US) will most likely demonstrate a clinically significant stone or unilateral hydronephrosis, which provides indirect evidence of an obstructing calculus. The most accurate test is non–contrast-enhanced computed tomography, which is 96% sensitive and 98% specific, although it entails radiation exposure.

Differential Diagnosis

The differential diagnosis for renal colic is broad and includes most of the common causes of significant abdominal pain (Table 75-2).

Table 75-2. Differential Diagnosis of Nephrolithiasis	
Diagnosis	**Clinical Features**
Appendicitis	Fever, vomiting Periumbilical pain that migrates to the right lower quadrant Abdominal guarding and rebound tenderness
Cholelithiasis	Risk factors: hemolysis, postpartum status, rapid weight loss Right upper quadrant pain, hyperbilirubinemia (+) Abdominal ultrasonography
Glomerulonephritis	No colic Hypertension Tea-colored urine with red blood cell casts
Intussusception	Intermittent abdominal pain, drawing the legs up No hematuria (+) Guaiac test, currant jelly stools
Malrotation	Vomiting, abdominal distention, no colic No hematuria
Ovarian/testicular torsion	Intermittent lower abdominal pain No hematuria (+) Ultrasonography
Pancreatitis	Epigastric or left upper quadrant pain relieved by leaning forward ↑ Amylase and lipase levels
Pyelonephritis	Fever, toxicity Costovertebral angle tenderness but no colic ↑ White blood cell count Pyuria, bacteriuria, (+) nitrites and leukocyte esterase

"–" indicates a negative finding, "+" indicates a positive finding.

Treatment

The treatment of nephrolithiasis varies on the basis of the underlying cause of stone formation. However, the mainstays of therapy are aggressive intravenous hydration and adequate analgesia. Administer 5% dextrose one-half normal saline with 20 mEq/L (20 mmol/L) KCl at 1.5 to 2 times maintenance levels, provided there is no evidence of urinary obstruction and urine output is adequate. This will dilute the stone components and encourage excretion of excess metabolites. In addition, prescribe morphine (0.1–0.2 mg/kg every 2–4 hours; maximum dose, 2 mg for an infant, 4–8 mg for a child, and 15 mg for an adolescent). However, nonsteroidal anti-inflammatory drugs, such as ibuprofen (10 mg/kg every 6 hours; maximum, 800 mg per dose) and ketorolac (0.5 mg/kg per dose every 6 hours, 120-mg/d maximum) may suffice if there is no evidence of acute kidney injury or history of chronic kidney disease. If infection is suspected, start empirical antibiotic treatment with ceftriaxone (50 mg/kg/d, divided into doses administered every 12 hours; 4-g/d maximum), then tailor the antibiotics to the culture results.

A urology consult is indicated for significant hydronephrosis that causes obstruction, a stone larger than 5 mm, or recurrent pain. Among the treatment options are extracorporeal shock wave lithotripsy or surgical stone excision.

Once the underlying cause of nephrolithiasis is found, specific long-term pharmacologic treatments may be implemented in conjunction with a consulting nephrologist. For example, thiazide diuretics reduce calcium excretion and slow the formation of calcium stones.

Indications for Consultation

- **Metabolism/genetics:** Recurrent stones, abnormal urine metabolic profile (if performed)
- **Nephrology:** Recurrent stones, abnormal urine metabolic profile (if performed)
- **Urology:** Hydronephrosis or other stone-related obstruction, recurrent stones

Disposition

Discharge criteria: Adequate oral intake of both fluids and pain medication with normal urine output

Follow-up

- **Primary care:** 1 to 2 weeks
- **Urology and/or nephrology:** 1 week

Pearls and Pitfalls

- The absence of hematuria does not rule out nephrolithiasis.
- Consider anteroposterior abdominal radiography or US as the initial imaging study when nephrolithiasis is suspected.
- There may be an iatrogenic cause for nephrolithiasis, such as medications and prolonged immobilization.

Bibliography

Cambareri GM, Kovacevic L, Bayne AP, et al. National multi-institutional cooperative on urolithiasis in children: age is a significant predictor of urine abnormalities. *J Pediatr Urol.* 2015;11(4):218–223

Copelovitch L. Urolithiasis in children: medical approach. *Pediatr Clin North Am.* 2012; 59(4):881–896

Habbig S, Beck BB, Hoppe B. Nephrocalcinosis and urolithiasis in children. *Kidney Int.* 2011;80(12):1278–1291

Hoppe B, Kemper MJ. Diagnostic examination of the child with urolithiasis or nephrocalcinosis. *Pediatr Nephrol.* 2010;25(3):403–413

Tasian GE, Copelovitch L. Evaluation and medical management of kidney stones in children. *J Urol.* 2014;192(5):1329–1336

Nephrotic Syndrome

Introduction

Nephrotic syndrome (NS) is a consequence of increased glomerular permeability with resultant heavy proteinuria. This leads to hypoalbuminemia, hyperlipidemia, and hypercoagulability. The decreased plasma oncotic pressure and sodium retention predispose the patient to edema when the extravascular fluid increases to greater than 3% to 5% of the patient's body weight.

NS can be classified according to etiology as either primary (or idiopathic) or secondary. In 85% to 90% of patients, primary NS is caused by minimal-change NS (MCNS), occurring in school-aged children. Other primary diseases are focal segmental glomerulosclerosis (FSGS) and membranous nephropathy.

Secondary causes include infections (HIV, hepatitis C, hepatitis B, syphilis, malaria) and drugs (nonsteroidal anti-inflammatories, penicillamine, lithium, interferon-γ), as well as lymphoma, systemic lupus erythematosus (SLE), immunoglobulin A nephropathy, Henoch-Schönlein purpura, and membranoproliferative glomerulonephritis (MPGN), also known as *mesangiocapillary glomerulonephritis*.

Congenital NS appears within the first 3 months of life and can be suspected in the presence of a large placenta at prenatal ultrasonography (US). Other causes of congenital NS include syphilis, toxoplasmosis, cytomegalovirus, measles, and HIV.

Clinical Presentation

History

The most common presentation is gravity-dependent edema (periorbital, pedal, pretibial, labial/scrotal). Reduced oncotic pressure leads to a decrease in the effective circulatory volume, which can result in oliguria. Urinary loss of anticoagulant proteins can predispose the patient to venous thrombosis, while immunoglobulin losses can increase susceptibility to severe infections (peritonitis, pneumonia, sepsis) caused by encapsulated organisms (eg, *Streptococcus pneumoniae,* group B streptococci).

In chronic resistant NS, renal losses of thyroxin-binding proteins and vitamin D–binding protein predispose the patient to the development of hypothyroidism and vitamin D deficiency, respectively.

Physical Examination

The hallmark of NS is edema, which appears in areas of low tissue resistance, such as the periorbital, pedal, pretibial, scrotal, and labial regions, as well as the abdominal cavity (ascites). The edema is characteristically dependent, so that in the morning it is periorbital and later in the day localizes primarily to the lower extremities. It can generalize and evolve into anasarca.

Intravascular hypovolemia causes tachycardia and signs of peripheral vasoconstriction. More severe hypoalbuminemia may lead to pleural effusions and dyspnea, as well as ascites, with resultant abdominal pain, umbilical or inguinal hernias, peritonitis, and shock.

Laboratory Workup

If NS is suspected, perform urinalysis and a spot urine test for protein to creatinine ratio (normal ratio, <0.2; non–nephrotic-range proteinuria, 0.2–2.0; nephrotic-range proteinuria, >2). If the ratio is greater than 2 in an older child, order a 24-hour urine collection to confirm the diagnosis. Nephrotic-range proteinuria in a child is defined as greater than 50 mg/kg per 24 hours, or greater than 40 mg/m^2/h, or greater than 1 g/m^2 per 24 hours. For an adult, it is greater than 3 g per 24 hours.

Although gross hematuria is rare in NS, microscopic hematuria occurs in up to 20% of patients. MPGN can produce a nephritic-nephrotic picture, with hematuria and increased blood pressure, while gross hematuria is most often seen in MPGN or acute glomerulonephritis.

Other laboratory tests to perform include:

- Serum electrolyte levels, including calcium, phosphorous, and magnesium: Hyponatremia can occur secondary to antidiuretic hormone secretion. Hypoalbuminemia predisposes the patient to apparent hypocalcemia, although the ionized calcium level is normal.
- Blood urea nitrogen (BUN)/creatinine ratio: Intravascular volume depletion predisposes the patient to prerenal azotemia.
- Total protein and albumin levels: Hypoalbuminemia lower than 2.5 g/dL (25 g/L) is characteristic, with a low total protein level (<5 g/dL [<50 g/L]).
- Lipid profile: Hyperlipidemia is typical, with increased total serum cholesterol and triglyceride levels.

Additional laboratory testing, to be performed on an individualized basis, includes:

- Complement levels: These are normal in MCNS, while a low complement component 3 (C3) level is associated with glomerulonephritis.

- Viral serologic studies to determine an etiology: HIV antibody, hepatitis B surface antigen, hepatitis C antibody.
- Antinuclear antibodies (SLE), especially in a patient older than 10 years.

Radiology Examinations

During the initial workup, perform renal US to ensure the presence of bilateral normal kidneys while ruling out congenital malformations, renal masses, and renal vein thrombosis.

Differential Diagnosis

NS is the most common cause of edema in childhood and the only diagnosis associated with significant proteinuria (Table 76-1). A patient with MCNS usually has normal blood pressure, renal function, and complement levels (Table 76-2). Box 76-1 summarizes the differential diagnosis of periorbital edema.

Treatment

Initial Presentation

Because the most likely cause of NS is MCNS, initially treat all patients with steroids (after performing a purified protein derivative skin test to rule out tuberculosis). Use prednisone 60 mg/m2/d (administered once per day or divided into doses delivered twice a day; 80-mg/d maximum). For most

Table 76-1. Differential Diagnosis of Nephrotic Syndrome	
Diagnosis	**Clinical Features**
Edema	
Cirrhosis/liver disease	Abnormal liver function test results
	Signs of portal hypertension
Congestive heart failure	S3 gallop
	Pulmonary edema and/or hepatomegaly
	Abnormal echocardiogram findings
	↑ N-terminal pro-BNP
Protein-losing enteropathy	Diarrhea
	Failure to thrive
	↑ Stool α1-antitrypsin level
Dark-colored urine	
Acute glomerulonephritis	Gross hematuria
	Hypertension more likely
	Evidence of recent strep infection
	↓ C3 level, normal C4 level

Abbreviations: C3, complement component 3; C4, complement 4; pro-BNP, prohormone of brain natriuretic peptide.

Table 76-2. Differential Diagnosis of Primary Etiologies of Nephrotic Syndrome

Diagnosis	Clinical Features
Minimal change nephrotic syndrome	Patient age, 2–6 y Microscopic hematuria (20% of cases) Responsive to steroids (>80% of cases)
Focal segmental glomerulosclerosis	Hematuria (60%–80% of cases) Hypertension (20% of cases) Responsive to steroids (15%–20% of cases)
Membranous nephropathy	Patient age >18 y Hematuria (60% of cases) Venous thromboembolism
Membranoproliferative glomerulonephritis	Hematuria (80% of cases) Hypertension (35% of cases) ↓ C3 level

Abbreviation: C3, complement component 3.

Box 76-1. Differential Diagnosis of Periorbital Edema

Infectious	Noninfectious
Dacryocystitis (unilateral) Eyelid insect bite (unilateral or bilateral) Orbital or periorbital cellulitis/abscess (unilateral) Preseptal cellulitis (unilateral)	Angioedema (unilateral or bilateral) Neoplasm (unilateral or bilateral) Dacryocystitis (unilateral) Seasonal allergy (bilateral) Trauma (unilateral or bilateral)

patients with MCNS, the proteinuria will clear by the third week of oral prednisone treatment. However, proteinuria may persist for 7 to 10 days after initiation of steroids, so being proteinuria free is not a discharge criterion. Continue the daily steroids for 6 weeks, followed by alternate-day therapy (1.5 mg/kg/d; 40-mg/d maximum) for 6 weeks and then a gradual taper over 6 weeks.

Manage edema with dietary sodium restriction (<2 g/d or 1–2 mEq/kg/d [1 mEq = 23 mg sodium]). If the patient has pulmonary edema or severe edema that affects ambulation, administer a single dose of intravenous (IV) furosemide (1 mg/kg) and monitor the response. If there is no improvement, administer low-sodium 25% IV albumin (0.5–1.0 g/kg over 4 hours) concomitantly with the furosemide. This regimen can be repeated as frequently as every 8 hours for a responsive patient. However, be aware that albumin can cause pulmonary edema. Avoid diuretic use in a patient with evidence of significant intravascular volume depletion.

Closely monitor the patient's intravascular volume status and obtain daily electrolyte and BUN/creatinine ratios until there is satisfactory diuresis, with clinical improvement of edema. Monitor the patient's weight daily and the urine output per shift to confirm the response to treatment.

If the patient does not have a good clinical response or has persistent edema and proteinuria after 4 weeks of treatment with prednisone, consult a nephrologist to consider initiating other treatments, such as an angiotensin-converting enzyme inhibitor, angiotensin II receptor blocker, or immuno-suppressant agent (cyclosporine, tacrolimus, mycophenolate, etc).

A renal biopsy is indicated if there is no response to treatment within 4 to 6 weeks. Other indications include steroid-responsive NS with more than 2 relapses in a 6-month period or more than 4 relapses in any 12-month period, low serum C3 level at the time of initial presentation of the NS (not related to acute poststreptococcal glomerulonephritis), hypertension at presentation (higher likelihood of FSGS), renal failure with increased BUN/creatinine ratio, and age younger than 1 year.

Relapses

The baseline risk of relapse within 6 months of initial treatment with steroids is 60%. Consult a nephrologist and resume the same steroid regimen as detailed earlier. Continue until the urine is protein free for 3 consecutive days, and then taper the dose in the same fashion as described in the initial treatment.

Complications

A patient with NS is at increased risk of infections. Up to 15% of patients with ascites may develop bacterial peritonitis, usually caused by *S pneumoniae* or *Escherichia coli*. Suspect peritonitis if the patient has ascites and fever, abdominal pain, and/or vomiting, although the presentation may be subtle. Note that a patient taking steroids may be afebrile or have just a low-grade fever. Promptly arrange for abdominal paracentesis to obtain fluid for cell count, Gram stain, and culture. Infected fluid usually has more than 250 white blood cells/mm^3. Administer IV ceftriaxone (50 mg/kg every day, 4-g/d maximum) or cefotaxime (150 mg/kg/d, divided into doses administered every 8 hours; 8-g/d maximum) for 10 days. Ascites fluid culture findings may be negative in up to 50% of cases of primary peritonitis. Therefore, complete the course of antibiotics if the clinical presentation and ascites fluid cell count are consistent with peritonitis, regardless of a negative culture result.

Indications for Consultation

- **Genetics:** Congenital or infantile NS (<1 year old), if there is no clear etiology
- **Hematology:** Hypercoagulable event
- **Infectious diseases:** Peritonitis
- **Nephrology:** All patients

Disposition

- **Intensive care unit transfer:** Severe anasarca, acute pulmonary edema, deep venous thrombosis or pulmonary embolus
- **Discharge criteria:** No anasarca or respiratory distress and family education complete

Follow-up

- **Primary provider:** Outpatient dipstick monitoring of proteinuria once weekly, either in the office or at home
- **Nephrology:** 2 to 4 weeks

Pearls and Pitfalls

- The patient may not initially present with edema.
- NS is a risk factor for a hypercoagulable state, and venous thromboembolism prophylaxis is indicated for a patient with other concomitant risk factors.
- Most cases are caused by steroid-responsive MCNS, while most patients refractory to steroids will have FSGS.

Bibliography

Andolino TP, Reid-Adam J. Nephrotic syndrome. *Pediatr Rev*. 2015;36(3):117–126

Kerlin BA, Haworth K, Smoyer WE. Venous thromboembolism in pediatric nephrotic syndrome. *Pediatr Nephrol*. 2014;29(6):989–997

Lombel RM, Gipson DS, Hodson EM; Kidney Disease: Improving Global Outcomes. Treatment of steroid-sensitive nephrotic syndrome: new guidelines from KDIGO. *Pediatr Nephrol*. 2013;28(3):415–426

Rheault MN. Nephrotic and nephritic syndrome in the newborn. *Clin Perinatol*. 2014; 41(3):605–618

Samuel S, Bitzan M, Zappitelli M, et al. Canadian Society of Nephrology Commentary on the 2012 KDIGO clinical practice guideline for glomerulonephritis: management of nephrotic syndrome in children. *Am J Kidney Dis*. 2014;63(3):354–362

CHAPTER 77

Postinfectious Glomerulonephritis

Introduction

The term *acute glomerulonephritis (AGN)* encompasses the spectrum of diseases that leads to variable degrees of inflammation in the glomeruli. AGN can be an isolated, self-limited illness or the first presentation of chronic glomerulonephritis (GN). Clinical manifestations vary from asymptomatic microscopic hematuria to acute nephritic syndrome, characterized by abrupt onset of gross hematuria, proteinuria, and edema, often with hypertension and some degree of renal insufficiency.

Postinfectious AGN (PIAGN) is the classic example of AGN and the most frequent cause in children. It most commonly occurs after pharyngitis or skin infection with group A *Streptococcus,* although it can be seen after many other bacterial, mycobacterial, viral, fungal, or parasitic infections. PIAGN classically presents 7 to 14 days after pharyngitis or up to 3 to 12 weeks after pyoderma. It typically occurs in school-aged children and is rare before 2 years of age.

Berger disease, or immunoglobulin A (IgA) nephropathy, is the most common GN worldwide. It occurs most often in patients older than 10 years and can frequently appear as recurrent episodes of gross hematuria in childhood.

Other causes of pediatric AGN include membranoproliferative (mesangiocapillary) GN and vasculitic diseases, including Henoch-Schönlein purpura (HSP).

Clinical Presentation

History

Painless gross hematuria and edema are the most common presenting symptoms of PIAGN. The patient may report the abrupt development of puffy eyes or facial edema, accompanied by foamy, cola-colored urine and decreased urine volume. A patient with PIAGN will often develop hypertension, but hypertensive emergency with encephalopathy is uncommon. This appears with headaches, seizures, altered mental status, and visual disturbances at presentation. Other rare complaints include dyspnea or cough as a result of pulmonary edema. The gross hematuria and edema of PIAGN usually resolve within 3 to 7 days, with gradual normalization of urine output and blood pressure over the following 2 to 4 weeks.

Ask about recent or concurrent infections to determine the etiology of the AGN. Exacerbations of IgA nephropathy often occur concurrently with mild infections. Note any other preceding infections, particularly endocarditis, visceral abscess, osteomyelitis, and shunt infection.

Fever and systemic symptoms are typically absent in PIAGN. However, a history of fever, abdominal pain, arthralgia, arthritis, or rash may be present in a patient with systemic vasculitis, such as systemic lupus erythematosus (SLE) or HSP.

Physical Examination

With the possible exception of increased systolic and/or diastolic blood pressure, the physical examination findings may be normal, although pallor, edema (localized or generalized), and/or pulmonary rales may be noted. There may also be physical findings (eg, hair loss, epistaxis, joint swelling, and rash) specific to the systemic etiology. Also, carefully assess growth parameters, since chronic kidney disease may initially manifest as AGN.

Laboratory Workup

Hematuria is the hallmark of PIAGN and is defined by the presence of 5 or more red blood cells (RBCs) per high-power field. For any patient presenting with dark urine, perform a complete urinalysis with urine microscopy to distinguish among the various causes of red urine, including RBCs, hemoglobinuria, myoglobinuria, and discoloration from drugs or foods. Gross hematuria is turbid, while urine containing myoglobin or hemoglobin is dark, but clear. For further differentiation, examine the centrifuged serum, which will be clear in myoglobinuria but have a pink tinge with hemoglobinuria.

Once the presence of RBCs is confirmed, perform a urine culture, complete blood cell count, basic chemistry panel, and complement component 3 (C3) and 4 (C4) assessment. To screen for PIAGN, check the anti-streptolysin O (ASO) and anti-deoxyribonuclease (anti-DNase) titers. A positive ASO result does not confirm the diagnosis of PIAGN but only establishes that either colonization or infection (old or new) with *Streptococcus* has occurred. Moreover, PIAGN that is unrelated to streptococcal infection will feature negative results for both ASO and anti-DNase antibody responses. Perform renal/bladder ultrasonography if the patient presents with bright red blood (to rule out a mass) or has recurrent hematuria or a systemic disease.

In PIAGN, the urine will be reddish-brown or cola colored, with dysmorphic RBCs, RBC casts, and often white blood cells. Nonnephrotic-range proteinuria is commonly present. Anemia is usually hemodilutional, but PIAGN has been associated with autoimmune hemolytic anemia. Depending on the degree of renal dysfunction, the blood urea nitrogen (BUN)/creatinine ratio may be increased. The C3 level is decreased in 90% of patients, while the C4 level is typically normal. In general, the ASO level is increased in a patient with streptococcal pharyngitis, while the anti-DNAse titer is high in cases of pyoderma.

If the AGN does not seem to be postinfectious and/or the patient has acute and severe deterioration in renal function (ie, rapidly progressive GN), obtain antibodies to the glomerular basement membrane (anti-glomerular basement membrane; Goodpasture syndrome) or those associated with other forms of vasculitis (anti-neutrophil cytoplasmic antibodies).

Differential Diagnosis

The differential diagnosis of hematuria is extensive, but painless gross hematuria suggests a glomerular etiology. Potential causes can be further classified according to C3 and C4 levels. GN associated with normal C3 and C4 levels includes IgA nephropathy, Alport syndrome, and HSP, while low C3 level occurs in PIAGN, and low C3 and C4 levels occur in membranoproliferative GN, shunt nephritis, and SLE. Additional details for each of these conditions are summarized in Table 77-1.

Table 77-1. Differential Diagnosis of Painless Gross Hematuria	
Diagnosis	**Clinical Features**
Alport syndrome	X-linked dominant inheritance Sensorineural hearing loss Ocular disease: retinopathy, cataracts, lenticonus
Berger disease/IgA nephropathy	Patient >10 y of age Macroscopic hematuria concurrent with infections ↑ IgA level in 50% of cases; normal complement levels
Henoch-Schönlein purpura	Purpuric rash, arthritis, abdominal pain Normal complement levels
Lupus nephritis	Photosensitive malar rash, arthralgia, serositis ↓ C3 and C4 levels (+) ANA, anti-dsDNA
Membranoproliferative glomerulonephritis	Similar to PSAGN Persistent ↓ C3 level with or without ↓ C4 level
PSAGN	Patient 2–12 y of age Pharyngitis or skin infection 1–12 wk prior ↓ C3 level, normal C4 level (+) ASO/anti-DNase
Shunt nephritis	History of shunt Arthralgia, lymphadenopathy, hepatosplenomegaly ↓ C3 level

Abbreviations: ANA, antinuclear antibody; anti-DNase, anti-deoxyribonuclease; anti-dsDNA, anti–double-stranded DNA; ASO, anti-streptolysin O; C3, complement component 3; C4, complement component 4; IgA, immunoglobulin A; PSAGN, poststreptococcal glomerulonephritis; +, positive finding.

Chapter 77: Postinfectious Glomerulonephritis

Treatment

Treatment of PIAGN is largely supportive and focuses on control of hypertension and fluid overload. Since these are primarily caused by enhanced salt and water retention, fluid and salt restriction is the first-line treatment. Limit sodium to 1 to 2 mEq/kg/d (1–2 mmol/kg/d). Fluid restriction varies on the basis of the degree of edema and circulating volume but may be as strict as 1 to 2 times the amount needed to replace insensible losses (400–800 mL/m^2/d).

If further treatment is needed to control volume overload and/or mild to moderate hypertension, administer a loop diuretic (intravenous [IV] furosemide 0.5–1.0 mg/kg every 8 hours). If the hypertension persists, provide a calcium-channel blocker such as oral nifedipine (0.25–0.50 mg/kg, every 4–6 hours; maximum, 10 mg per dose) or oral amlodipine (0.05–0.40 mg/kg once daily, 10-mg maximum). Consult with a nephrologist before ordering an angiotensin-converting enzyme inhibitor because there is a risk of decreasing the glomerular filtration rate and causing hyperkalemia.

Initial IV treatment options for a hypertensive emergency include hydralazine (start at 0.1 mg/kg per dose, titrate to the desired blood pressure with 0.2–0.4 mg/kg per dose, 20-mg maximum) or labetalol (0.2–1.0 mg/kg per dose, 40-mg maximum; avoid use with significant acute respiratory disease or asthma). If these measures do not provide adequate control of blood pressure, options include nicardipine (0.5–5.0 μg/kg/min; start at 0.1–0.2 μg/kg/min), nitroprusside (0.3–0.5 μg/kg/min, 10-μg/kg/min maximum), or labetalol (0.25–3.00 mg/kg/h). If the patient has hypertension and volume overload, administer furosemide (1 mg/kg per dose, 6-mg/kg/d maximum). For any patient treated with IV antihypertensive medications, check the blood pressure at least every 5 to 15 minutes and titrate the infusion to reach the target blood pressure. There are a number of specific guidelines for safe blood pressure reduction. One approach is to target a normal blood pressure in a stepwise fashion by reducing the blood pressure by 25% over the first 8 hours, followed by another 25% over the next 8 to 12 hours, and the remaining 50% over the next 24 hours.

Indications for Consultation

Nephrology: Blood pressure difficult to control, renal insufficiency, need for biopsy, concern for a systemic disease

Disposition

- **Intensive care unit transfer:** Hypertensive emergency, need for dialysis or hemofiltration, need for ventilator support
- **Discharge criteria:** Blood pressure controlled, renal impairment improving

Follow-up

- **Primary care:** 1 week for blood pressure check, BUN/creatinine ratio assessment, and urinalysis
- **Nephrology:** 4 weeks to check C3 level (if it was low)

Pearls and Pitfalls

- Poststreptococcal AGN runs a typical course. Evaluate the patient for other etiologies of AGN if the presentation is unusual in terms of clinical and/or laboratory features.
- Up to 50% of patients with AGN and an abnormal urinalysis result are asymptomatic.
- A patient with hypertensive encephalopathy or acute renal failure may have a marginally abnormal urinalysis result.

Bibliography

Eison TM, Ault BH, Jones DP, Chesney RW, Wyatt RJ. Post-streptococcal acute glomerulonephritis in children: clinical features and pathogenesis. *Pediatr Nephrol.* 2011;26(2):165–180

Kambham N. Postinfectious glomerulonephritis. *Adv Anat Pathol.* 2012;19(5):338–347

VanDeVoorde RG 3rd. Acute poststreptococcal glomerulonephritis: the most common acute glomerulonephritis. *Pediatr Rev.* 2015;36(1):3–12

Zaffanello M, Cataldi L, Franchini M, Fanos V. Evidence-based treatment limitations prevent any therapeutic recommendation for acute poststreptococcal glomerulonephritis in children. *Med Sci Monit.* 2010;16(4):RA79–RA84

Urinary Tract Infection

Introduction

Urinary tract infection (UTI) is a common, serious bacterial infection of childhood that frequently leads to hospital admission. About 5% of febrile infants younger than 12 months have a UTI, although most can be treated on an outpatient basis. Indications for inpatient treatment include age younger than 1 to 2 months, dehydration, inability to tolerate oral antibiotics, and concern for a serious complication or anatomic abnormality (renal abscess, obstructive uropathy, or sepsis). The most common pathogen isolated is *Escherichia coli*, which is responsible for 80% of infections. Girls younger than 3 years are twice as likely as boys to have UTIs, although uncircumcised boys under 6 months of age are at least 4 times more likely than circumcised boys to have a UTI.

Clinical Presentation

History

Typically, the patient presents with fever and some combination of dysuria, urgency, frequency, incontinence, and malodorous urine. However, in an infant, the fever may be accompanied only by nonspecific complaints, such as irritability (infants), nausea, vomiting, diarrhea, abdominal pain, flank pain, and jaundice. Ask about risk factors, including prenatal urinary tract dilatation, history of previous UTIs, chronic constipation and stool-withholding behaviors, daytime wetting, underlying urinary tract anomaly, diseases predisposing the patient to neurogenic bladder, sexual activity (for an adolescent), and family history of renal anomalies.

Physical Examination

The patient is typically febrile and may have a toxic appearance, but hypertension is unusual in the absence of chronic renal disease. Check for abdominal tenderness, distention, or mass, as well as suprapubic and costovertebral angle tenderness. Examine the external genitalia for abnormalities and signs of irritation or local infection and note the presence of labial adhesions or the circumcision status, as appropriate. Check for other causes of the fever. Consider pyelonephritis in any patient, especially girls up to 2 years of age, who have high fever (>39.4°C [>103°F]) without a source.

Laboratory Workup

The diagnosis of a UTI requires both evidence of inflammation at urinalysis (UA) and growth of a single pathogen from a urine culture. Confirmation of a UTI in a patient 2 to 24 months of age now entails a positive culture of a single uropathogen (colony count >50,000 colony-forming units [CFU]/mL), along with pyuria (>5 white blood cells per high-power field) and/or bacteriuria at UA. Use a minimum of more than 100,000 CFU/mL for a clean-catch specimen in an older child. A positive UA finding for pyuria or nitrites is 99% sensitive, but only nitrites are highly specific for the diagnosis of UTI. Perform a urine culture prior to administration of antibiotics. If the patient is too young to effectively perform a clean catch, perform the urine culture via straight catheterization (see Chapter 33, Urinary Bladder Catheterization) or suprapubic aspiration (see Chapter 31, Suprapubic Bladder Aspiration). Suprapubic aspiration may result in less contamination but has a lower success rate than urethral catheterization, unless aided by direct visualization of a full bladder at ultrasonography (US). Do not rely on a bag specimen, which is frequently contaminated, for culture, although a negative finding is likely a true-negative finding. However, bag specimens are useful for UA.

Perform a complete sepsis evaluation (blood, urine, and possibly cerebrospinal fluid cultures) for a febrile infant younger than 2 months (see Chapter 64, Fever in Infants Younger Than 60 Days). Perform a blood culture for a toxic-appearing patient of any age.

Differential Diagnosis

Asymptomatic bacteriuria is likely if the urine culture result is positive, while the UA result is negative for leukocyte esterase. Other common causes of dysuria, urgency, frequency, and/or pyuria include dysfunctional voiding, viral cystitis, vaginitis, vaginal foreign body, and urethritis (such as from bath products), while glycosuria can cause polyuria. Sterile pyuria can occur with Kawasaki disease, Behçet syndrome, lupus, Sjögren syndrome, and chemical urethritis.

Treatment

Antibiotics

Choose the initial treatment based on local antibiogram results. Ultimately, use the urine culture identification and sensitivity to guide therapy. The dosing for some antibiotics may require adjusting if the patient has renal insufficiency.

Patient Younger Than 2 Months

Initially treat intravenously with the combination of intravenous (IV) ampicillin (50 mg/kg per dose every 6 hours) *and either* IV gentamicin (full-term neonates 0–7 days old with normal renal function, 2.5 mg/kg every 12 hours; >7 days old, 2.5 mg/kg every 8 hours) *or* a third-generation cephalosporin (IV cefotaxime 50 mg/kg every 12 hours if <7 days old or every 6–8 hours if >7 days old; *or* IV/intramuscular ceftriaxone 50 mg/kg every 12 hours).

Use this combination at least until bacteremia and/or meningitis is excluded, then continue monotherapy tailored to the sensitivity of the organism until the patient is afebrile for 24 hours and the blood culture result (if obtained) is negative. Complete a 10-day course with oral antibiotics.

Patient 2 Months and Older

If the patient fits the criteria for inpatient treatment of a UTI, start with IV antibiotics. Since most *E coli* bacteria are resistant to ampicillin, use ceftriaxone 50 mg/kg every day (2-g/d maximum) or cefotaxime 150 mg/kg/d, divided into doses administered every 8 hours (6-g/d maximum). If the patient is at increased risk for *Pseudomonas* infection (prior history of *Pseudomonas* UTI, chronic indwelling catheter, neurogenic bladder), administer IV ciprofloxacin 18 to 30 mg/kg/d, divided into doses administered every 8 hours (1.2-g/d maximum), or oral ciprofloxacin 20 to 30 mg/kg/d, divided into doses administered every 12 hours (1.5-g/d maximum). If there is a risk factor for *Enterococcus*, such as genitourinary instrumentation or renal anomaly, or if gram-positive rods are noted on the Gram stain, add ampicillin 100 mg/kg/d, divided into doses administered every 6 hours (4-g/d maximum) empirically. If *Staphylococcus aureus* grows from the urine culture, consider hematogenous spread. Confirm a negative blood culture result and perform a thorough physical examination to look for signs of soft-tissue, joint, pulmonary, or cardiac involvement.

Treat sepsis and complicated pyelonephritis, such as with a renal abscess or in a pregnant adolescent, with a 10- to 14-day course of therapy, based on bacterial identification and sensitivities.

Transition to oral antibiotics after the patient no longer meets criteria for inpatient treatment. Depending on the sensitivities of the identified organism (if available), use cephalexin 50 mg/kg/d, divided into doses administered every 8 hours (maximum, 500 mg per dose), cefixime 8 mg/kg/d (400-mg/d maximum), or sulfamethoxazole/trimethoprim (trimethoprim 10 mg/kg/d, divided into doses administered every 12 hours; maximum, 100 mg per dose). When sensitivities are available, choose the effective choice that has the narrowest antibiotic spectrum.

Treat for a total of 7 to 14 days, although a 2- to 4-day treatment course may suffice for a patient older than 3 months with a presumed infection of just the lower urinary tract.

Treat Constipation, If Present

Bowel/bladder dysfunction is associated with repeat UTIs. Treat with laxatives, such as polyethylene glycol 3350, 0.2 to 0.8 g/kg/d (maximum dose, 17 g/d) orally once daily, and behavioral interventions, such as timed voiding and double voiding.

Antibiotic Prophylaxis

Do not administer antibiotic prophylaxis after a first UTI. While prophylaxis may result in a small reduction in recurrent UTIs, there is no proven difference in future renal scarring. In addition, there is a risk of increased antibiotic resistance with subsequent UTIs. However, refer a child with grade IV or V vesicoureteral reflux (VUR) to a urologist to consider surgical and medical therapeutic options, including prophylaxis. If prophylaxis is recommended, use either sulfamethoxazole/trimethoprim (trimethoprim 2 mg/kg every day if patient is >2 months of age; 160-mg/d maximum) or nitrofurantoin 2 mg/kg every day if the patient is older than 1 month (100-mg/d maximum). Prescribe an initial 3- to 6-month course of treatment, since most recurrences are within 6 months of the initial infection.

Radiology Examinations

Screen patients with a first febrile UTI with renal/bladder US (RUS). Obtain a follow-up voiding cystourethrogram (VCUG) if the RUS finding is abnormal. For a patient who has not undergone any imaging but presents with a second or third febrile UTI, perform RUS and VCUG. While RUS is not sensitive for low-grade VUR, waiting for a second febrile UTI before performing VCUG balances prompt diagnosis of high-grade VUR with avoidance of invasive testing of these infants, most of whom do not have significant VUR. Also order VCUG if posterior urethral valves are suspected in a male infant (palpable bladder distention, dribbling urine). A technetium-99m dimercaptosuccinic acid scan is indicated only if recommended by a consulting nephrologist or urologist.

Indications for Consultation

- **Nephrology:** Renal insufficiency, recurrent UTIs, voiding dysfunction
- **Urology:** Renal abscess, urinary tract dilation, ureteropelvic obstruction, ureterovesical junction obstruction, neurogenic bladder, grade III–V VUR, posterior urethral valves

Disposition

- **Intensive care unit transfer:** Septic shock, multisystem organ failure, renal failure
- **Discharge criteria:** Adequate oral intake, effective outpatient treatment regimen available (eg, patient is tolerating oral antibiotics or has a peripherally inserted central catheter placed for multi–drug-resistant organisms that require extended IV antibiotics), complications resolved (shock, abscess, acute renal failure, etc), and radiologic workup arranged (if indicated)

Follow-up

- **Primary care:** Within 1 to 2 weeks to assess completion of the antibiotic course and assess the need for prophylaxis or radiologic studies
- **Urology:** 1 to 2 weeks if there is a known genitourinary abnormality
- **Nephrology (if the patient has renal insufficiency):** 1 to 2 weeks

Pearls and Pitfalls

- Instruct the family to seek medical care promptly for a UTI evaluation if there is a new febrile illness or a change in urine odor. This is more important than any follow-up imaging study.
- Test of cure with a repeat urine culture is not necessary if the patient has a prompt clinical response to the antibiotics.
- Lack of clinical response suggests bacterial resistance or an underlying obstruction, such as a renal abscess or obstructive stone.
- Reproductive health counseling is indicated for adolescents with new-onset, recurrent UTIs.

Bibliography

American Academy of Pediatrics Subcommittee on Urinary Tract Infection; Steering Committee on Quality Improvement and Management. Urinary tract infection: clinical practice guideline for the diagnosis and management of the initial UTI in febrile infants and children 2 to 24 months. *Pediatrics*. 2011;128:595–610

Brady PW, Conway PH, Goudie A. Length of intravenous antibiotic therapy and treatment failure in infants with urinary tract infections. *Pediatrics*. 2010;126(2):196–203

Hoberman A, Greenfield SP, Mattoo TK, et al. Antimicrobial prophylaxis for children with vesicoureteral reflux. *N Engl J Med*. 2014;370:2367–2376

Keren R, Shaikh N, Pohl H, et al. Risk factors for recurrent urinary tract infection and renal scarring. *Pediatrics*. 2015;136(1):e13–e21

Schroeder AR, Chang PW, Shen MW, Biondi EA, Greenhow TL. Diagnostic accuracy of the urinalysis for urinary tract infection in infants <3 months of age. *Pediatrics*. 2015;135(6):965–971

Shaikh N, Shope TR, Hoberman A, Vigliotti A, Kurs-Lasky M, Martin JM. Association between uropathogen and pyuria. *Pediatrics*. 2016;138(1):e20160087

Zee RS, Herbst KW, Kim C, et al. Urinary tract infections in children with prenatal hydronephrosis: a risk assessment from the Society for Fetal Urology Hydronephrosis Registry. *J Pediatr Urol*. 2016;12(4):261

Neurology

Acute Ataxia

Introduction

Ataxia is the inability to coordinate or modulate movements. It is commonly attributed to dysfunction of the cerebellum but may also be secondary to vestibular, sensory, epileptic, or psychogenic disorders. Acute ataxia implies that the symptoms evolved in less than 72 hours, often in a previously well child, which differentiates it from episodic, subacute, and progressive ataxias. These are rare in childhood and are often caused by genetic or metabolic disorders.

The common causes of acute ataxia in childhood can be divided by category: infectious or immune-mediated or caused by drug or toxin exposure, mass lesions, trauma, or paraneoplastic syndromes. The most common causes are acute postinfectious cerebellar ataxia (APCA, 30%–50% of cases), toxic exposure (30% of cases), and Guillain-Barré syndrome (GBS, 7%–15% of cases). APCA is an autoimmune phenomenon that leads to cerebellar demyelination. It is usually preceded by infection, such as varicella, Epstein-Barr virus, enterovirus, parvovirus B19, and *Mycoplasma pneumoniae*. Toxic exposure may be accidental (common in early childhood) or intentional (more often in adolescence). Agents that can cause ataxia include organic chemicals, heavy metals, and alcohols, as well as many medications (antiepileptic drugs, benzodiazepines, antihistamines, and antineoplastic drugs).

Ataxia associated with GBS is caused by a sensory derangement (Miller Fisher syndrome and other variants), or it may be simulated by ascending muscle weakness.

Clinical Presentation

History

Symptoms of ataxia may be subtle or profound and limited to focal disability or compromising coordination of all movements, including limb, trunk, ocular, and oropharyngeal. The patient usually presents to the hospital shortly after the onset of symptoms, which may include altered speech, clumsiness of extremity movements, abnormal eye movements, refusal to walk, and a wide-based, "drunken" gait. A detailed history of onset, timing, and progression of the ataxia and associated symptoms is essential. Ask about recent infection, immunizations, trauma, and possible toxin exposure. Other priorities are fever, rash, headache, diplopia, paresthesia, sensation of vertigo, and change in mental status. Focus on symptoms of life-threatening conditions, such as a mass lesion, central nervous system (CNS) infection, or hydrocephalus, to facilitate rapid identification.

APCA occurs primarily in children younger than 6 years. It presents days to weeks after an illness (most commonly varicella) and is characterized by the sudden onset of ataxia. Vomiting, visual disturbances, and slurred speech may also be seen, but fever, extreme irritability, and altered mental status are absent.

Physical Examination

Perform a thorough physical examination, including a funduscopic and detailed neurologic evaluation. Ataxia may appear with abnormalities of gait, trunk, extremity, tongue, and/or eye movements at presentation.

Dyssynergia (loss of smoothness of a motor activity), dysmetria (errors in range or force of limb movements), dysdiadochokinesia (errors in rate and regularity of rapid alternating movements), and dysarthria may accompany ataxia and are specific to a cerebellar etiology. Evaluate dyssynergia and dysmetria with finger-to-nose and heel-to-shin testing. Test for dysdiadochokinesia by having the patient repeatedly tap a foot or pat the examiner's hand. In the toddler or young child, assess these functions by having the patient reach for and use toys. Nystagmus can be attributed to a cerebellar disorder but may also be caused by abnormality in other locations, including the vestibular system. The differentiation of ataxia from vertigo can be difficult, especially in a nonverbal patient. Nausea and nystagmus often accompany vertigo and may be elicited or worsened by sudden changes in the patient's head position.

Ataxia caused by weakness can be determined by thorough manual muscle testing of suspected muscle groups. Muscle tone and reflexes are usually preserved in cerebellar disorders, whereas GBS often presents with ascending weakness and diminished reflexes. Decreased reflexes can also be seen in sensory disorders. Sensory ataxia can be determined by a positive Romberg sign (loss of standing balance once eyes are closed). Gait evaluation is essential in the ataxic patient who classically compensates for imbalance by widening the base of support. Evaluate variations of gait and single leg balance to uncover subtle degrees of ataxia.

Signs characteristic of APCA are exclusively cerebellar and include stance and gait ataxia, dysarthria, dysmetria, intention tremor, and nystagmus. If fever accompanies these signs, consider an infectious etiology, such as acute cerebellitis. Mental status integrity helps differentiate APCA from other conditions, such as toxic exposure, acute disseminated encephalomyelitis, mass lesions, and CNS infection (encephalitis, cerebellitis).

Ophthalmologic examination may help identify papilledema, which is indicative of an intracranial lesion, bleed, or hydrocephalus. Declining consciousness, Cushing triad, bulging of the fontanelle, and cranial nerve palsies are other signs of an emergent intracranial process. A fixed and dilated pupil may occur when a rapidly expanding intracranial hemorrhage causes compression of cranial nerve III and may also herald impending herniation. Constriction or dilatation of the pupils may be indicative of toxic ingestion. Rapid, multivectorial conjugate eye movements are the hallmark of opsoclonus-myoclonus syndrome.

Laboratory Workup

The diagnosis of APCA can often be assigned clinically. Imaging and cerebrospinal fluid (CSF) analysis are not indicated if the history and examination findings are clearly consistent with the diagnosis. If performed, magnetic resonance (MR) imaging findings are usually normal but may demonstrate bilateral diffuse abnormalities of the cerebellar hemispheres. Screening laboratory values, including a complete blood cell count, C-reactive protein level and/or erythrocyte sedimentation rate, glucose level, electrolyte level, and liver function test results, may assist in determining an infectious or inflammatory etiology. If the etiology is unclear or the history is suggestive of a toxic ingestion or exposure, perform urine and serum drug screens to determine a toxic exposure. Testing for specific agents may be necessary and directed by the most likely exposures, including the patient's medications, other drugs in the home, environmental toxins from food or water sources, or toxins associated with homeopathic treatments.

Ataxia associated with trauma requires emergent computed tomography (CT) of the head, neck, and/or spine. Emergent neuroimaging is also indicated when there is evidence of increased intracranial pressure, focal neurologic findings, or altered mental status. CT is generally readily available and can usually be used to detect conditions that require urgent intervention, such as hydrocephalus, traumatic injury, evolving hematoma, and many mass lesions. MR imaging is superior to CT for identifying posterior fossa disease, demyelinating disease, and intracranial tumors.

In the evaluation of ataxia, a lumbar puncture with opening pressure is not strictly indicated; however, it should be performed if CNS infection is suspected. Marked pleocytosis and a highly increased protein level are indicative of an active infectious process. In GBS, the CSF will often have an increased protein level without significant pleocytosis, while in APCA, the leukocyte count and protein level will be normal to mildly increased.

Electromyography and nerve conduction studies can help to confirm the diagnosis of GBS but may have normal findings early in the course of the disease. If ataxia is accompanied by opsoclonus or myoclonus, obtain urine and serum catecholamine levels because this constellation of symptoms may represent a paraneoplastic syndrome secondary to neuroblastoma.

Order a simple electroencephalogram (EEG) if the patient displays altered consciousness, a history consistent with seizure, or fluctuating clinical signs. Long-term EEG monitoring is indicated if symptoms persist and if simple EEG findings are nondiagnostic.

Differential Diagnosis

APCA, toxin exposure, and GBS are the most common causes of acute ataxia of childhood and account for most cases. An expanded differential diagnosis is summarized in Table 79-1.

Treatment

The priority is treatment of associated life-threatening symptoms, such as respiratory failure (GBS, toxic ingestion) and increased intracranial pressure (intracranial hemorrhage, mass, stroke). Consult with the appropriate sub-specialist (critical care, infectious disease, neurology, neurosurgery, oncology) to manage respiratory insufficiency, intracranial infection, tumor, or hemorrhage. In general, treatment of ataxia is supportive and includes physical and occupational therapy and emotional support.

The treatment for APCA is supportive. Monitor and support nutrition and hydration as needed. Up to 90% of patients will recover full function within 4 months, and recurrences are extremely rare.

The treatment of toxic exposure may require consultation with the local poison control center and depends on the specific agent and quantity of the exposure. Life-threatening complications to consider include respiratory compromise and/or cardiac arrhythmias.

The treatment of GBS is summarized in Chapter 81, Acute Weakness.

Indications for Consultation

- **Neurology:** Unclear etiology, consideration of treatment for neurologic disorder (GBS)
- **Physical medicine and rehabilitation:** Persistent, significant functional deficit
- **Neurosurgery, toxicology, infectious disease, oncology:** Depending on the etiology

Table 79-1. Differential Diagnosis of Ataxia	
Diagnosis	**Clinical Features**
Acute cerebellitis	Postinfectious or associated with current infection Cerebellar signs *and* fever, headache, vomiting, altered consciousness MR imaging findings limited to the cerebellum: global edema, signal intensity changes on T2-weighted images
Acute postinfectious cerebellar ataxia	Follows an acute febrile illness by days to weeks Sudden onset, afebrile, normal mental status Dysfunction limited to cerebellar signs
Acute disseminated encephalomyelitis	Altered mental status, possible lethargy or seizures Multifocal neurologic dysfunction MR images: multifocal, diffuse white matter demyelination
Bacterial meningitis	Fever, meningismus, ill appearance CSF: pleocytosis, ↑ protein level, ↓ glucose level
Encephalitis	Fever, headache, irritability, altered mental status Variable examinations, depending on affected CNS areas CSF: pleocytosis usual, moderately ↑ protein level
Guillain-Barré syndrome	Afebrile, normal mental status, paresthesia common Ascending weakness with diminished reflexes CSF: mild initial pleocytosis, moderately ↑ protein level
Intracranial hemorrhage	Patient often has a history of preceding head or neck trauma Afebrile, mental status usually altered; focal, evolving neurologic deficits CT: evidence of hemorrhage
Labyrinthitis	Fever variable, normal mental status, intense vertigo, vomiting Often occurs with associated otitis media, hearing loss, nystagmus Lack of other cerebellar signs
Miller Fisher variant of Guillain-Barré syndrome	Ophthalmoplegia with ataxia and areflexia Incomplete variants exist Contrast-enhanced MR images: cranial nerve enhancement
Postconcussive syndrome	Onset often acute after mild traumatic brain injury Afebrile, mental status normal, headache, unsteady gait Lack of other cerebellar signs
Posterior fossa tumor	Altered personality, headache, vomiting Head tilt, nuchal rigidity, cranial neuropathies Papilledema, diplopia MR imaging or CT evidence of tumor
Toxic ingestion	Acute onset, vomiting, seizures, altered mental status Patient usually afebrile, declining level of consciousness Pupillary changes Duration: hours to days

Abbreviations: CNS, central nervous system; CSF, cerebrospinal fluid; CT, computed tomography; MR, magnetic resonance.

Disposition

- **Intensive care unit transfer:** Compromised neurologic state affecting brain stem function, declining mental status, hemodynamic instability, respiratory insufficiency
- **Discharge criteria:** Stabilization and/or improvement of the ataxia, adequate oral intake

Follow-up

- **Primary care:** within 1 week and then close follow-up until ataxia resolves
- **Physical therapy, occupational therapy, physical medicine and rehabilitation:** 1 to 2 weeks (if functional deficit persists)
- **Pediatric neurology:** 1 to 2 weeks

Pearls and Pitfalls

- Delayed recovery of function can occur in up to 10% of children with APCA.
- Relapse is extremely rare in patients with APCA.
- Benzodiazepines and antiepileptic medications, such as phenytoin, are common causes of acute ataxia.

Bibliography

Poretti A, Benson JE, Huisman TA, Boltshauser E. Acute ataxia in children: approach to clinical presentation and role of additional investigations. *Neuropediatrics*. 2013;44(3): 127–141

Salas AA, Nava A. Acute cerebellar ataxia in childhood: initial approach in the emergency department. *Emerg Med J*. 2010;27(12):956–957

Whelan HT, Verma S, Guo Y, et al. Evaluation of the child with acute ataxia: a systematic review. *Pediatr Neurol*. 2013;49(1):15–24

Winchester S, Singh PK, Mikati MA. Ataxia. In: Dulac O, Lassonde M, Sarnat HB, eds. *Handbook of Clinical Neurology*. Vol 112 (3rd series). *Pediatric Neurology Part II*. Amsterdam, the Netherlands: Elsevier BV; 2013:1213–1217

Acute Hemiparesis

Introduction

Acute hemiparesis, or unilateral weakness, typically implicates the contralateral corticospinal tract, which travels from the cortex, through the internal capsule, to the medulla. In the medulla, it decussates to the contralateral side and descends in the lateral spinal cord. It then synapses on the anterior horn cells, which give rise to the peripheral nerves. Because unilateral spinal cord injury is rare, especially acutely, cerebral pathology is the most common cause for acute hemiparesis.

Clinical Presentation

History

The most likely causes of any acute neurologic symptoms fall into the categories of seizure, stroke, and migraine, with the most concerning being stroke. However, stroke mimics are frequent in children. Therefore, priorities in the patient's history include evidence for prior seizures (with subsequent Todd paralysis) or infection (meningitis, cerebral abscess), risk factors for stroke (especially trauma for arterial dissection and family history of hypercoagulability), and *gradual* progression of weakness over 1 hour in the setting of headache (suggestive of hemiplegic migraine). Ask about recent illness or immunization, followed by abrupt neurologic symptoms (including hemiparesis), which raises the concern for a demyelinating process (acute disseminated encephalomyelitis [ADEM]). Do not assume that decreased use of a limb is simply due to pain from trauma.

Physical Examination

The presence of fever suggests an infectious or inflammatory process. Hypertension is typical for stroke (ischemic or hemorrhagic), although normal blood pressure does not definitively exclude stroke. Attempt to determine if the weakness is central or peripheral. With rare exception, involvement of the corticospinal tract results in weakness in contiguous limbs or the face. That is, there will be weakness in the face/arm or arm/leg or face/arm/leg. Although a monoplegia implies a peripheral nervous system insult, an exception is an anterior cerebral artery infarct that causes unilateral leg weakness.

A patient younger than 12 months has immature myelination of the corticospinal tract and may present with subtle signs of weakness. Careful observation at the bedside is typically more revealing than overzealous examination.

Laboratory Workup

Laboratory testing includes screening tests, as well as more directed evaluations once a diagnosis is established. Perform a complete blood cell count and complete metabolic panel, including liver function tests, which may yield increased values with certain viral infections (herpes). See Chapter 70, Toxic Exposures, if the clinical presentation suggests a stroke or new-onset seizures. If an infectious etiology is a possibility, perform a lumbar puncture (LP) either before or after head computed tomography (CT), unless the patient has a platelet count lower than 20,000/mm³ (20×10^9/L). Do not defer administration of antibiotics if the LP will be delayed or is difficult to perform. If an intracranial hemorrhage (ICH) is suspected or confirmed, obtain a prothrombin time/partial thromboplastin time and urgently administer fresh frozen plasma or platelets as needed to correct a coagulopathy or thrombocytopenia. For ischemic and hemorrhagic strokes, evaluate the patient for systemic lupus erythematosus, vasculitis, or sickle cell disease, if the clinical picture is consistent with one of those conditions. Check for a family history of connective tissue disease or aneurysm, with or without kidney disease.

While the hematologic studies for ischemic stroke are not standardized, in the absence of a clear vascular or cardiac etiology, obtain homocysteine level, antiphospholipid antibodies, protein C and S levels, activated protein C resistance, lipoprotein(a) level, and ferritin level. If these are unremarkable, genetic studies, including factor V Leiden, PT G20201A, can be helpful. A tiered approach to diagnosis potentially limits unnecessary and expensive studies, and it is reasonable to defer genetic testing to the outpatient setting, except in the unlikely case that the results will change the acute management.

In addition, for an ischemic stroke, obtain an electrocardiogram and a transthoracic echocardiogram.

Radiology Examinations

Imaging is the most informative study when evaluating a patient with acute hemiparesis. Perform head CT if there is a concern for an ICH, which will be immediately evident. Arteriovenous malformation is by far the most common cause of ICH in children; discuss further imaging with a neurosurgeon and radiologist. After 3 to 6 hours, ischemic stroke may be visible at CT, although magnetic resonance (MR) imaging can be used to identify an ischemic stroke within minutes of symptom onset and is therefore the preferred modality. MR imaging is also more sensitive for encephalitis, brain dysplasia, and tumor. However, if MR imaging is not available, CT angiography (CTA) is a rapid way to evaluate the patient for thrombosis.

Contrast-enhanced MR angiography (MRA) of the head can be used to identify a vasculopathy, the most common cause of pediatric acute ischemic stroke. MRA of the neck with fat-suppressed imaging can be used to identify arterial dissections, particularly in the setting of trauma. CTA of the head and neck is also sensitive for dissection.

Differential Diagnosis

The initial priority is the diagnosis of an acute ischemic stroke or intracerebral hemorrhage (Table 80-1). Evaluation for an acute ischemic stroke includes looking for cardiac, vascular, infectious, immune-mediated, or hematologic causes.

The key to diagnosing a cerebral abscess is the identification of risk factors in a patient with new focal weakness, seizures, or change in level of alertness with or without fever. In a child, the infection is typically caused by contiguous spread of sinusitis, mastoiditis, or dental abscess. Other potential sources of bacteremia include cellulitis, pulmonary infection, and endocarditis.

Hemiplegic migraine is a diagnosis of exclusion, after alternative diagnoses such as stroke and seizure have been ruled out. The typical history involves the gradual spread of neurologic symptoms over 20 to 30 minutes, followed by headache. The development of symptoms, visual loss, numbness, and weakness correlates with the progression of cortical depression.

ADEM is a multifocal, monophasic, demyelinating illness that develops over hours to days. It is typically postinfectious or parainfectious, with multiple potential infectious causes (most often viral). The patient presents with the new onset of multifocal neurologic disease that consists variously of change in mental status, visual loss, ataxia, limb weakness, and sometimes seizures. Perform an LP and send cerebrospinal fluid (CSF) for blood cell count, glucose level, protein level, oligoclonal band screen, myelin basic protein level, and immunoglobulin G (IgG) index (requires simultaneous serum IgG testing). Typical findings are an increased blood cell count (>6 white blood cells/mm^3) and increased protein level (>25 mg/dL [>0.25 g/L] in a patient <18 years of age).

Treatment

Stroke and Increased Intracranial Pressure

Perform nonenhanced head CT. Transfer the patient to the intensive care unit (ICU) and then (if necessary) to a center with immediately available pediatric neurosurgery, as well as diagnostic imaging (MR imaging) and capability for monitoring intracranial pressure (ICP). Consult with a neurologist to

Table 80-1. Differential Diagnosis of Acute Hemiparesis		
Diagnosis	**Clinical Features**	**Radiologic Studies**
Acute disseminated encephalomyelitis	Abrupt onset of weakness Encephalopathy associated with a febrile illness	MR imaging with and without contrast material Demyelination on T2-weighted MR images
Acute ischemic stroke	Abrupt lateralizing limb weakness Sensory and/or language impairment Cranial neuropathies	Head CT (nonenhanced acutely) Brain MR imaging Head/neck MRA vs CTA
Brain tumor (complicated by intracranial hemorrhage or seizure)	Prior subtle signs of weakness and headache	MR imaging with and without contrast material
Cerebral abscess	Headache Penetrating trauma Contiguous infection Cyanotic congenital heart disease	MR imaging with and without contrast material
Complex migraine	May have a personal/family history of migraines Gradually migrating cortical depression over 30–60 min, followed by headache	Nonenhanced MR imaging MRA
Encephalitis (especially herpes)	Lateralizing weakness Fever, confusion May have seizures EEG: PLEDs (herpes)	CT acutely MR imaging with and without contrast material
Hypoglycemia	Focal weakness History of diabetes	MR imaging for persistent encephalopathy or limb weakness
Intracerebral hemorrhage	Headache, hypertension Altered mental status, seizures Limb weakness	Head CT (nonenhanced acutely) Brain MR imaging Head/neck MRA vs CTA
Meningitis (especially West Nile virus)	Fever, headache, vomiting Neck/back pain, meningismus	None (consider spine MR imaging)
Mitochondrial myopathy, encephalopathy, lactic acidosis, and stroke	Unexplained lateralizing weakness Headache and/or confusion Can appear with seizures	Brain MR imaging (signal intensity changes do not follow a vascular distribution)
Seizure/Todd paralysis	Acute history of paroxysmal movements Weakness or somnolence	MR imaging

Abbreviations: CT, computed tomography; CTA, CT angiography; EEG, electroencephalogram; MR, magnetic resonance; MRA, MR angiography; PLED, periodic lateralized epileptiform discharges.

determine whether to administer intravenous (IV) tissue plasminogen activator (tPA), which has limited use in children because of the frequency of stroke mimics. The adult neurology stroke service may be helpful in evaluation and treatment decision making.

Obtain urgent neurosurgical consultation if the patient has a posterior fossa ICH or an ICH with mass effect (displacement or compression of adjacent structures). Elevate the head of the bed to 30° but defer intubation if the patient is alert to avoid sedation and its subsequent effects on the neurologic examination. While there is no standardized goal blood pressure, to maintain an adequate cerebral perfusion pressure with acute ischemic stroke, permissive hypertension to 1½ times the normal value for the patient's age is the rule. More aggressive blood pressure control is indicated in the case of intracerebral hemorrhage. Discuss these parameters, as well as the need for invasive ICP monitoring for a patient with an ICH with both neurology and neurosurgery consults. Monitor closely for signs of deterioration, such as a change in mental status (becoming more difficult to arouse), anisocoria, or worsening limb weakness. An acute alteration in the neurologic examination warrants repeat head CT. If the patient had been receiving chronic anticoagulation therapy, consult with a hematologist to initiate reversal.

If ischemic stroke is either suspected or confirmed on images and hemorrhage is excluded, administer aspirin, 5 mg/kg (maximum dose, 325 mg) by mouth. Give the patient nothing by mouth and administer normal saline fluids at a maintenance rate until the child is evaluated by a speech-language pathologist. Control any fever with acetaminophen (15 mg/kg; maximum, 1,000 mg per dose) and/or cooling blankets. Monitor the blood sugar level and maintain it at less than 200 mg/dL (<11.1 mmol/L). Neurosurgical involvement is not usually necessary in the early management of ischemic stroke, with the exception of a large middle cerebral artery or posterior fossa infarction that is causing mass effect.

The evaluation for an acute ischemic stroke includes looking for cardiac, vascular, infectious, immune-mediated, or hematologic causes. Perform a thrombophilia evaluation, electrocardiogram, and transthoracic echocardiogram and consult a rheumatologist. Perform an LP to evaluate the patient for immune-mediated vasculitis or viral infections such as varicella, which are treatable causes of viral vasculopathy and strokes in children.

Seizures

The evaluation and treatment of seizures is detailed in Chapter 85.

Encephalitis

If there is any concern about herpes simplex virus (HSV) encephalitis, initiate acyclovir immediately (28 days to 12 years of age, 20 mg/kg every 8 hours for 21 days; >12 years of age, 10 mg/kg every 8 hours for 21 days). Note that while the sensitivity of HSV CSF polymerase chain reaction (PCR) is high, it is not 100%, so a patient with herpes encephalitis can have a negative PCR finding. Therefore, rely on both clinical suspicion and the HSV PCR results to determine whether to initiate and continue acyclovir. Also, the PCR result can remain positive for days after treatment has begun, so an LP performed after the initiation of acyclovir is still useful. The response to acyclovir is not immediate, so a patient who is back to baseline mental status within less than 24 hours of the initiation of treatment is unlikely to have HSV encephalitis. In contrast, the combination of normal CSF, the absence of periodic lateralized epileptiform discharges on the electroencephalogram, and a normal brain MR imaging finding essentially excludes HSV encephalitis. Another treatable form of viral encephalitis to consider is varicella zoster virus (VZV) encephalitis, particularly if there is prior history of a painful or dermatomal rash. Perform VZV PCR and VZV IgG assessment of the CSF.

Hemiplegic Migraine

See Chapter 84, Headache, but do not use sumatriptan, which causes vasoconstriction and might worsen the hemiplegic migraine.

Cerebral Abscess

Obtain an infectious disease consult and treat empirically with IV antibiotics for 6 to 8 weeks. The choice of antibiotic therapy is based on the presumed source of infection (oral flora, hematogenous spread, postneurosurgical procedure), but in some cases a brain biopsy is necessary for identification of pathogens. In the setting of significant mass effect, manage increased ICP and consult a neurosurgeon. A focal neurologic examination is a contraindication to LP.

Acute Disseminated Encephalomyelitis

IV steroid treatment is controversial, because it does not clearly affect outcome in mild to moderate cases but may speed the recovery. Consult with a neurologist to determine whether to treat with IV methylprednisolone (15–30 mg/kg every day for 15 days, 1-g/d maximum), IV immunoglobulin (2 g/kg, administered either as a single dose or over the course of 3-5 days), or plasmapheresis.

Indications for Consultation

- **Hematology:** Patient with stroke who requires thrombophilia evaluation and/or is receiving anticoagulation therapy
- **Neurology:** Acute hemiparesis
- **Neurosurgery:** Hemorrhagic stroke, brain tumor, cerebral abscess
- **Oncology:** Brain tumor
- **Rheumatology:** Acute ischemic stroke not caused by cardiac embolus or dissection

Disposition
- **ICU transfer:** Acute hemiparesis associated with acute encephalopathy (delirium), airway concerns, stroke, status epilepticus, or rapidly evolving neurologic changes
- **Discharge criteria:** Stable, nonevolving condition; action plan in place for recurrent events (eg, seizures, migraines); adequate plan for administration and monitoring of therapy and rehabilitation (if needed)

Follow-up
- **Primary care:** 1 to 2 weeks
- **Neurology:** 1 to 2 weeks

Pearls and Pitfalls
- If the patient has a history of recent trauma, consider embolic stroke caused by arterial dissection.
- New hypertension in the setting of hemiparesis is suggestive of stroke.
- Todd paralysis after a seizure implies a focal seizure and is often associated with a structural lesion, such as remote stroke, cortical dysplasia, or a brain tumor.
- Perform CT early if a stroke is suspected to identify a patient for whom tPA is a potential option (within 4.5 hours of symptom onset).
- For questions about thrombolysis therapy, consult 800/NO-CLOTS, a pediatric thromboembolic hotline staffed by Toronto Sick Kids.

Bibliography

Bhate S, Ganesan V. A practical approach to acute hemiparesis in children. *Dev Med Child Neurol*. 2015;57(8):689–697

Blumenfeld AE, Victorio MC, Berenson FR. Complicated migraines. *Semin Pediatr Neurol*. 2016;23(1):18–22

Jordan LC, Hillis AE. Challenges in the diagnosis and treatment of pediatric stroke. *Nat Rev Neurol*. 2011;7(4):199–208

Koelman DL, Chahin S, Mar SS, et al. Acute disseminated encephalomyelitis in 228 patients: a retrospective, multicenter US study. *Neurology*. 2016;86(22):2085–2093

Rivkin MJ, Bernard TJ, Dowling MM, Amlie-Lefond C. Guidelines for urgent management of stroke in children. *Pediatr Neurol*. 2016;56:8–17

Acute Weakness

Introduction

Acute muscle weakness is the decreased ability to move muscles against resistance. It can be the result of pathology anywhere in the neuromuscular system and may occur abruptly or evolve over the course of hours to days. Acute weakness can be life-threatening if it advances to include the respiratory muscles or is secondary to an intracranial process.

One of the most common causes of acute weakness in children is Guillain-Barré syndrome (GBS), also known as *acute inflammatory demyelinating polyneuropathy.* Other common etiologies of acute weakness include viral myositis, intracranial tumor, seizure, medication side effect, toxin exposure, and conversion disorder. Diseases that cause chronic weakness may appear acutely at presentation and must be considered in the differential diagnosis.

Clinical Presentation

History

Ask about the timing and severity of the weakness and whether there is any associated fever, rash, headache, double vision, altered mental status, changes in sensation, or bowel or bladder dysfunction. Other pertinent points include a history of trauma or travel, seizure, preceding viral or bacterial illness, possible medication or toxin exposure, and family history of childhood weakness.

Physical Examination

The first priorities are circulation, airway, and breathing. After the patient has been stabilized, perform a thorough neuromuscular examination, attempting to localize the affected portion of the neuromuscular system. Grade the muscle strength (grade 5, normal; grade 4, active movement against gravity and resistance; grade 3, active movement against gravity; grade 2, active movement with gravity eliminated; grade 1, flicker or trace of contraction; or grade 0, no contraction) and note the distribution of weakness. Perform a thorough neurologic examination, including assessment of mental status, cranial nerves, muscle tone, sensation, and reflexes.

Upper motor neuron lesions are caused by pathologic lesions of the cerebral cortex and spinal cord. These lesions typically appear with acute onset of weakness at presentation, either unilateral or bilateral. Other symptoms include spasticity, hypertonicity, hyperreflexia, and encephalopathy. However, in the early phase, the patient may have decreased muscle tone prior to the development of spasticity. Mental status changes are indicative of an intracranial process, while nuchal rigidity is caused by meningitis or an epidural abscess. Focal tenderness along the back is suggestive of spinal cord lesion, focal inflammation, or infection.

Lower motor neuron lesions include disorders of the anterior horn cell, neuromuscular junction, and peripheral nerve. Symptoms include absent or diminished reflexes, decreased muscle tone, muscle atrophy, and fasciculations. Primary disorders of the muscle typically appear with a subacute or indolent course of muscle weakness, associated with muscle pain, swelling, or tenderness at presentation. Muscle atrophy may be a late finding. Evaluate the skin to look for the heliotrope rash of dermatomyositis, attached ticks, or signs of trauma.

Laboratory Workup

Obtain a complete blood cell count, C-reactive protein level, and/or erythrocyte sedimentation rate if there is concern for an infectious or inflammatory disease. Check a basic metabolic panel, including electrolyte, calcium, creatinine, glucose, magnesium, and phosphate levels, because abnormalities can cause acute weakness. If there is proximal muscle weakness, muscle tenderness, or a history of dark, tea-colored urine, obtain a creatinine kinase (CK) level and perform urinalysis (dipstick and microscopic analysis). If urine is positive for blood on a dipstick and negative for red blood cells at microscopy, this is consistent with myoglobinuria, which is consistent with rhabdomyolysis. Perform a lumbar puncture if meningitis, encephalitis, GBS, or multiple sclerosis (MS) is suspected. Send the cerebrospinal fluid (CSF) for cell count and differential, total protein and glucose (with paired serum sample) level assessment, culture, and, if MS is a concern, oligoclonal band evaluation. Send CSF for viral testing and/or autoimmune panels if encephalitis is suspected. Order an electroencephalogram if a seizure is suggested by the history or physical examination findings.

Radiology Examinations

Emergent computed tomography (CT) of the head is indicated for abrupt onset of weakness with deterioration of mental status, focal neurologic deficits, or preceding trauma to look for acute intracranial hemorrhage or tumor. Perform magnetic resonance (MR) imaging of the brain in a clinically stable patient with symptoms of intracranial pathologic processes because this will provide more detail on an intracranial process. If a spinal cord pathology is suspected, perform emergent MR imaging of the spine to evaluate the patient for trauma, infection, transverse myelitis, or tumor.

Differential Diagnosis

Upper Motor Neuron Disorders

Pathologic findings located in the cerebral cortex appear with acute onset of unilateral weakness, headache, vomiting, seizure, and/or mental status changes at presentation. The persistence of neurologic deficits is an indication for an urgent evaluation to rule out an evolving process, such as stroke, intracranial abscess, and epidural hematoma. Spinal cord injury, spinal epidural hematoma, and other causes of spinal cord compression may predominantly affect the upper motor neurons. The symptoms associated with this mixed injury include unilateral or bilateral weakness, altered sensation below the level of the lesion, and bowel and/or bladder dysfunction. Focal back pain at the level of the lesion may be present, while reflexes below the level of the lesion are absent.

Lower Motor Neuron Disorders

With disorders of the anterior horn cell, the patient will have normal or decreased reflexes, muscle atrophy, and fasciculations. Diseases of the peripheral nerves cause diminished reflexes (bilateral or unilateral), paresthesia, and dysesthesia. The most common etiology is GBS, which is a group of diseases that result in an acute inflammatory demyelinating polyneuropathy. The classic presentation occurs 2 to 4 weeks after a benign febrile respiratory or gastrointestinal illness. Symptoms start with paresthesia of the distal extremities, followed by ascending symmetrical paralysis. The patient may also present with cranial neuropathies, such as bulbar weakness, ophthalmoplegia, and facial paralysis (Miller Fisher variant). Neuropathic pain and paresthesia may be absent or pronounced. There can also be associated autonomic dysfunction, with changes in blood pressure, cardiac arrhythmias, or bowel and bladder dysfunction. In up to 25% of patients, paralysis will ascend to include the respiratory muscles, necessitating patient observation in a unit capable of providing assistance with ventilation.

Disorders of the neuromuscular junction cause generalized weakness and hypotonia. These include botulism, tick paralysis, myasthenia gravis, and organophosphate toxicity.

Primary Muscle Disorders

Disorders of the muscle are often associated with a slower onset of weakness and an increased CK level.

Other Conditions

Suspect a conversion disorder when the physical examination findings are not consistent with an organic lesion. Often the patient has an inconsistent neuroanatomic constellation of symptoms, as well as a negative medical workup finding.

The differential diagnosis of acute weakness is summarized in Table 81-1.

Table 81-1. Differential Diagnosis of Acute Weakness	
Diagnosis	**Clinical Features**
Disorders of the cerebral cortex	
Acute disseminated encephalomyelitis (ADEM)	Acute encephalopathy Seizures, headache, vomiting Patient may have ataxia
Acute intracranial hemorrhage Cerebrovascular accident	Abrupt onset Altered mental status Headache, vomiting, seizure
Encephalitis Meningitis	Fever Altered mental status Weakness may be global
Alternating hemiplegia of childhood Hemiplegic migraine	Acute onset of hemiplegia and headache Family history of migraines
Multiple sclerosis	Presentation similar to that of ADEM Oligoclonal bands present in CSF Frequent relapses after remission
Todd paralysis	Unilateral weakness after seizure Typically rapid recovery of symptoms (<24 h)
Transient ischemic attack	Unilateral weakness Duration <24 h
Tumor	Headache, clumsiness, behavior changes Vomiting (especially in the morning)
Disorders of the spinal cord	
Anatomic abnormalities: atlantoaxial instability, Chiari malformation, tethered cord	History of chronic weakness Progressive worsening of symptoms
Diskitis Epidural abscess	Fever Back pain
Spinal cord concussion	History of trauma Symptoms resolve within a few hours
Transverse myelitis	Progressive symptoms Paresthesia Neck or back pain Typically preceded by an illness in the prior 3 wk
Traumatic injury: epidural hematoma, vertebral body compression fracture, dislocation, transection	History of trauma Abrupt onset of symptoms Paresthesia, bowel and bladder dysfunction

Table 81-1. Differential Diagnosis of Acute Weakness, continued

Diagnosis	Clinical Features
Disorders of the spinal cord, continued	
Tumor	Focal back pain
	Weight loss
Disorders of the anterior horn cell	
Paralytic poliovirus	Preceded by fever, malaise, sore throat
	Typically unilateral weakness
	Extremely rare in the United States
	Other non-polio enteroviruses can also cause weakness
Spinal muscle atrophy	Tongue fasciculations in an infant
	Motor delay
Disorders of the peripheral nerves	
Acute intermittent porphyria	Abdominal pain, sensory changes
	Family history of porphyria
Guillain-Barré syndrome (GBS)	Ascending weakness (usually symmetrical)
	↑ CSF protein level (>2× normal levels)
	Patient may have mild CSF pleocytosis
Toxins: heavy metals	History of exposure
	Weakness typically distal
Disorders of the neuromuscular junction	
Botulism	*Patient <6–12 mo of age*
	Exposure to honey
	Poor feeding, constipation, lethargy
	Patient >6–12 mo of age
	Direct ingestion of toxin
	Dry mouth, blurred vision, nausea, vomiting
	Symptoms can rapidly progress to weakness of the bulbar and skeletal muscles
Myasthenia gravis	Ptosis, diplopia
	Extraocular muscle weakness
	Weakness worsens with activity
Organophosphate toxicity	Diarrhea, emesis
	Miosis, bradycardia
Tick paralysis	GBS-like ascending weakness and paresthesia
	Tick usually found on scalp
Primary muscle disorders	
Inflammatory myopathies: dermato-myositis, polymyositis	Fever, heliotrope rash in dermatomyositis
	Proximal muscle weakness
	↑ CK level
Congenital myopathies Metabolic myopathies Mitochondrial disease Muscular dystrophies	Slowly progressive weakness
	Muscle tenderness and wasting
	Patient may have hypertrophy in advanced stages
	↑ CK level

Continued

Table 81-1. Differential Diagnosis of Acute Weakness, continued	
Diagnosis	**Clinical Features**
Primary muscle disorders, continued	
Periodic paralysis	Episodic weakness Associated with potassium abnormalities May also occur with sodium abnormalities
Pyomyositis	Multifocal muscle abscesses Patient typically immunocompromised
Rhabdomyolysis	Myalgia Dark, tea-colored urine (+ for hemoglobin/myoglobin without RBCs) Markedly ↑ CK level (typically >5× the upper limit of normal) Altered mental status, chills, malaise may be present
Viral myositis	Preceding viral illness, commonly caused by influenza B Myalgia
Other conditions	
Conversion disorder	Inconsistent neurologic examination findings (-) Medical workup findings
Toxic exposure: antineoplastics, ciguatoxin, isoniazid, nitrofurantoin, paralytic shellfish toxin, zidovudine	Paresthesia History of possible exposure

Abbreviations: ADEM, acute disseminated encephalomyelitis; CK, creatinine kinase; CSF, cerebrospinal fluid; GBS, Guillain-Barré syndrome; RBC, red blood cell; -, negative finding; +, positive finding.

Treatment

General management of all patients with acute weakness includes close observation of respiratory status, nutritional status, and functional abilities. Closely follow bulbar function by assessing the strength of the gag reflex and monitoring the patient for the onset of drooling, dysarthria, and decrease in oral motor integrity. Follow the respiratory status closely with oxygen saturations, forced vital capacity, and negative inspiratory forces (NIFs). These measures provide an early warning of impending respiratory compromise. If respiratory compromise is suspected, perform a blood gas analysis. (See Chapter 105, Acute Respiratory Failure.) Immobilize the neck if there is concern for head or neck trauma.

Early in the hospitalization, institute a bowel regimen of stool softeners daily and suppositories as needed. Monitor pre- and postvoid bladder volumes to evaluate urinary retention. If volumes are consistently greater than those predicted for age (normal bladder volume in ounces = [patient's age in years] + 2), initiate a catheterization program every 4 to 6 hours as needed and consult with a urologist. Prophylaxis for deep venous thrombosis may be necessary if a patient is unable to ambulate (see Chapter 5, Deep Venous Thrombosis).

Immediate neurosurgery consultation is imperative in the case of acute intracranial or spinal cord mass, abscess, or hemorrhage. An epidural abscess will require decompression and culture from the wound, followed by broad-spectrum intravenous (IV) antibiotics, including coverage for methicillin-resistant *Staphylococcus aureus*. Acute intracranial hemorrhage may require immediate evacuation. If an intracranial tumor is suspected, consult with a pediatric oncologist. If meningitis or encephalitis is suspected, start empirical antibiotics and/or antivirals while awaiting culture and viral testing results.

If MS, myasthenia gravis, botulism, muscular dystrophy, peripheral neuropathy, or a disorder of the neuromuscular junction is suspected, consult a neurologist, who may recommend nerve conduction velocities, electromyography, or, rarely, muscle biopsy. If myasthenia gravis is suspected, arrange for a Tensilon test, which involves administering a short-acting acetylcholinesterase inhibitor. The diagnosis is confirmed if the symptoms resolve.

If GBS is suspected on the basis of clinical examination findings, consult a neurologist. Additional confirmatory testing, including nerve conduction velocities and electromyography, may be required. First-line treatment is IV immune globulin (0.4 mg/kg daily for 2, 3, or 5 days) or plasma exchange. A patient with GBS requires close inpatient observation until the nadir of the illness has been reached, typically within 4 weeks of the onset of symptoms. Follow the respiratory status closely with oxygen saturations, forced vital capacity, and NIFs. Transfer to a pediatric intensive care unit (ICU) is indicated if the weakness is rapidly progressing, NIFs are less than 30 cm H_2O, oxygen saturations are consistently less than 90%, vital capacity is declining, or advancing bulbar muscle weakness is advancing. Monitor the patient for signs of autonomic dysfunction and treat pain promptly. Start rehabilitation as soon as the patient is medically stable, in conjunction with physical medicine. Assessments by a physical therapist, occupational therapist, and speech therapist are essential to determine the functional impairment of the patient, assist with strength and range of motion exercises, and prescribe adaptive equipment as needed.

Treat tick paralysis with immediate removal of the tick. Symptoms will typically resolve within several days. Consult a neurologist and treat transverse myelitis, acute disseminated encephalomyelitis, or other demyelinating diseases with high-dose IV pulse methylprednisolone (0.5–1.0 mg/kg/d, 1,000-mg/d maximum, for 3–5 days) and intensive rehabilitation. If a patient continues to have symptoms, plasma exchange and/or IV immune globulin may be necessary. Treat viral myositis with rest, analgesia, and hydration. However, if there is dark, tea-colored urine and markedly increased CK level consistent with rhabdomyolysis, administer IV hydration and perform serial assessments of renal function and output. Treat electrolyte abnormalities with replacements, but the patient may require monitoring in a unit with central telemetry, particularly if IV replacements are delivered.

If conversion disorder is suspected, limit the medical workup. Assess the psychological status of the patient and consult with a psychiatrist and/or psychologist.

Indications for Consultation
- **Neurology:** All patients with acute weakness
- **Neurosurgery:** Tumor, abscess, or hemorrhage of the brain or spinal cord
- **Physical, occupational, and/or speech and swallow therapy:** Significant functional impairment

Disposition
- **Discharge criteria:** Depending on the primary process, the weakness has improved or stabilized, and an adequate plan is in place to meet functional needs
- **ICU transfer:** Rapid escalation of weakness, respiratory compromise or worsening bulbar muscle weakness, signs of increased intracranial pressure

Follow-up
- **Primary care:** 1 to 2 weeks
- **Neurology:** 1 to 2 weeks

Pearls and Pitfalls
- A thorough history and physical examination are key to determining the location of the pathologic origin along the neuromuscular pathway.
- Prompt diagnosis of the etiology of weakness is critical, because treatments are specific and tailored to pathologic findings.
- Perform emergent MR imaging if a spinal process is suspected.
- Ongoing observation and evaluation are essential to monitor respiratory status in patients with acute weakness, because patients can progress to respiratory failure.

Bibliography

Huber AM. Idiopathic inflammatory myopathies in childhood: current concepts. *Pediatr Clin North Am.* 2012;59(2):365–380

Hughes RA, Swan AV, van Doorn PA. Intravenous immunoglobulin for Guillain-Barré syndrome. *Cochrane Database Syst Rev.* 2012;CD002063

Morgan L. The child with acute weakness. *Clin Pediatr Emerg Med.* 2015;16(1):19–28

Ness JM. Demyelinating disorders of the central nervous system. In: Kliegman RM, Stanton BF, St Geme JW III, Schor NF. *Nelson Textbook of Pediatrics.* 20th ed. Philadelphia, PA: Elsevier; 2016: 2919–2925

Willison HJ, Jacobs BC, van Doorn PA. Guillain-Barré syndrome. *Lancet.* 2016; 388(10045):717–727

Wolf VL, Lupo PJ. Lotze TE. Pediatric acute transverse myelitis overview and differential diagnosis. *J Child Neurol.* 2012;27(11):1426–1436

Altered Mental Status

Introduction

Altered mental status (AMS) is a derangement in consciousness, which is defined as arousal and awareness of one's self and environment. Awareness is determined by the cerebral hemispheres, whereas arousal is controlled by the ascending reticular activating system. Although derangements in either or both systems may alter mental status, there is a spectrum of decreasing states of consciousness, ranging from confusion (loss of clear thinking) to coma (no response to pain and the eyes remain closed).

The etiology of AMS can be either structural (eg, mass, hemorrhage) or medical (eg, infection, ingestion, intoxication, inborn error of metabolism, diabetic ketoacidosis [DKA]). Structural causes of AMS may be associated with focal neurologic deficits, while medical etiologies generally are not.

While there are numerous possible etiologies for AMS, a rapid, thorough assessment of the patient's history and a physical examination are crucial for determining the appropriate initial interventions to target the underlying cause. Persistent AMS is more worrisome than transient AMS (ie, syncope), because the former is associated with increased morbidity and mortality. An age-based approach is helpful for identifying the most common diagnoses.

Clinical Presentation

History

Ask about the onset of the change in consciousness (acute vs subacute), along with a history of recent illnesses, behavioral changes, and specific associated symptoms, such as focality. For an infant, determine whether there are symptoms suggestive of an inborn error of metabolism, such as poor feeding, lethargy, failure to thrive, and seizures. In an older child, a careful review of the patient's medical history may yield clues, such as diabetes (DKA) and kidney (uremia) or liver disease (encephalopathy). Inquire about contact with sick persons, recent travel, immunization status, and any potential immunodeficiency. Key information to collect for both suspected accidental ingestion in toddlers and intentional overdose in adolescents includes a current medication list and the availability of medications, illegal drugs, and toxins in the home or environment. Also inquire about any recent history of accidental or inflicted trauma, particularly head trauma.

A patient with sickle cell anemia or congenital heart disease may develop AMS because of a thrombotic or ischemic stroke. A patient with a seizure disorder can be postictal or have nonconvulsive status epilepticus (subclinical seizures) and present with AMS. A patient with ventriculoperitoneal shunt (VPS) malfunction will complain of acute headache and/or vomiting, while a patient with a brain tumor may present with headaches and vomiting over weeks to months. Such tumors can cause mass effect that leads to focal neurologic deficits (such as eye deviation, pupillary changes, and motor weakness) or hydrocephalus with increased intracranial pressure (ICP).

Physical Examination

Immediately assess the vital signs, address the CABs (chest compressions, airway, and breathing), and evaluate the patient for signs of trauma (ecchymoses, hematomas). Priorities in a focused physical examination include features that can help differentiate between structural and medical etiologies. Perform a thorough neurologic examination to evaluate the pupillary response, fundi, cranial nerves, reflexes, upper and lower motor neuron functions, and sensory responses. Specific findings associated with structural lesions include abnormal pupillary light reflexes (either asymmetrical or dilated pupils), abnormalities in extraocular movements, asymmetry of motor response, and decorticate or decerebrate posturing.

As a result of the relatively fixed volume within the skull, insults that cause a mass effect can increase ICP, which is characterized by irritability, headache, and vomiting. In addition, downward eye deviation ("setting sun"), papilledema, and cranial nerve palsies (particularly cranial nerves III, IV, and VI) may be seen. Cushing triad (hypertension, bradycardia, and irregular respirations) are late signs of increased ICP and signify impending herniation. Uncal herniation affects cranial nerve III, causing a dilated pupil on the ipsilateral side. Central herniation leads to a progression of symptoms from small but reactive pupils with intact extraocular movements to pinpoint fixed pupils, absent extraocular movement, and flaccid paralysis.

If the neurologic examination is nonfocal and structural lesions are not suspected, a more thorough physical examination may elucidate the underlying medical etiology. Classic signs of infection include fever, nuchal rigidity, lymphadenopathy, and rash. For metabolic derangements, the focused physical examination varies with the specific organ system that is responsible. Liver disease may appear with hepatomegaly, ascites, and jaundice at presentation. DKA may appear with signs of dehydration, Kussmaul breathing, and fruity breath odor.

A patient with an ingestion or intoxication can present with varied symptoms and altered vital signs; thus, knowledge of common toxidromes (see Chapter 70, Toxic Exposures) is essential for identification, intervention, and treatment.

Laboratory Workup

Initial laboratory tests include an immediate bedside serum glucose level determination, complete blood cell count, serum electrolyte and calcium levels, liver function studies, ammonia level, and coagulation profile, as well as a venous blood gas analysis if the patient is breathing abnormally or a toxic ingestion is suggested. If an intracranial infection is suspected in a patient with signs of increased ICP, treat with appropriate antibiotics (see Chapter 68, Sepsis) and defer the lumbar puncture until the patient is clinically stable and can tolerate the procedure. Culture additional sites as indicated. Perform serum and urine toxicology to guide management of a suspected ingestion or intoxication. A stool guaiac test may have a positive finding in cases of intussusception.

Radiology Examinations

If the patient is comatose, order head computed tomography (CT) (without contrast material) to immediately rule out a central nervous system bleed, mass lesion, or hydrocephalus. Also perform CT if there are signs or symptoms of increased ICP or focal neurologic findings.

Differential Diagnosis

While there are many causes of AMS (Table 82-1), a focused history, physical examination, laboratory tests, and imaging will help narrow the differential diagnosis. Structural causes of AMS are often associated with focal neurologic findings, such as abnormal pupils, extraocular movements, focal weakness, asymmetrical reflexes, and posturing. Medical etiologies cause global cerebral dysfunction and generally do not produce focal neurologic deficits. In addition, a gradual change in mental status is more suggestive of a medical etiology, while an abrupt onset may indicate a structural lesion.

AMS accompanied by fever, photophobia, headache, and vomiting suggests an infectious etiology. Acute onset of behavioral changes, seizures, and sleep disturbances is suspicious for autoimmune encephalitis, which has recently been recognized as a more prevalent cause of encephalitis.

Intoxications and ingestions may appear with similar symptoms at presentation, such as temperature derangements and vomiting. Maintain a high level of clinical suspicion, because often there is no reported history of ingestion. In addition to exogenous toxins, there are numerous metabolic derangements that can result in AMS, including electrolyte imbalance, hypoxia, thyroid and adrenal disease, acid-base disturbance, and extremes of temperature.

Consider nonconvulsive status epilepticus, in which there are electrographic seizures without motor movements, in a patient who experiences AMS for more than 60 to 90 minutes after a seizure.

Any mechanism of injury that is inconsistent with the clinical findings or is unlikely, given the patient's developmental capability, raises the concern for non-accidental trauma (see Chapter 102, Child Abuse and Neglect).

Intussusception (see Chapter 118, Acute Abdomen) is an unusual cause of AMS in a young infant who may also present with vomiting and guaiac-positive stools.

Table 82-1. Differential Diagnosis of AMS	
Diagnosis	**Clinical Features**
Acute demyelinating encephalomyelitis	Recent infection or vaccination Fever, headache, vomiting Weakness, vision loss, discoordination
Autoimmune encephalitis	Viral prodrome Behavioral changes, sleep disturbances Seizures, abnormal movements
Brain tumor/↑ ICP	Headache, vomiting Cushing triad: bradycardia, hypertension, Cheyne-Stokes respiration Asymmetrical pupils, cranial nerve VI palsy
CNS infection	Fever, photophobia, headache, vomiting Nuchal rigidity
Concussion/head trauma	(+) History Confusion, headache, memory loss Scalp/skull hematoma or ecchymoses
Confusional migraine	History of migraines Headache, confusion, aphasia
Diabetic ketoacidosis	Abdominal pain, vomiting, polyuria Fruity breath odor Kussmaul breathing Hyperglycemia, ketonuria, anion gap acidosis
Hemorrhagic stroke	Headache, vomiting Signs of ↑ ICP Focal neurologic deficits
Hypertension	Headache
Hypoglycemia	Dizziness, tremor, diaphoresis ↓ Glucose level
Hypotension	Dizziness Poor perfusion

Table 82-1. Differential Diagnosis of AMS, continued	
Diagnosis	**Clinical Features**
Inborn errors of metabolism	Lethargy, poor feeding Seizures Hypoglycemia, acidosis
Ingestion/intoxication	Confusion, slurred speech, hallucinations Hyper- or hypothermia, respiratory depression Seizures
Intussusception	Episodic abdominal pain, currant jelly stools
Ischemic stroke	Headache, vomiting, focal neurologic deficits Signs of ↑ ICP
Liver failure	Jaundice Easy bleeding Ascites
Nonaccidental trauma	Story inconsistent with injuries Fracture in a nonmobile infant Retinal hemorrhages
Psychiatric conditions	Catatonia (can maintain posture) Echolalia Resists eye opening
Seizure	Shaking, twitching, eye rolling Incontinence
Sepsis	Fever, tachycardia, poor perfusion, widened pulse pressure Source of infection
Subarachnoid hemorrhage	Headache, photophobia, irritability Meningismus
Uremia	Anorexia, lethargy, fatigue
Venous thrombosis	Headache, seizures Signs of ↑ ICP
VPS malfunction	History of hydrocephalus and shunt Headache, vomiting Signs of ↑ ICP

Abbreviations: AMS, altered mental status; CNS, central nervous system; ICP, intracranial pressure; VPS, ventriculoperitoneal shunt; +, positive finding.

Treatment

Initial management of AMS involves addressing the CABs and restoring and ensuring stable respiratory and hemodynamic status. Continuously monitor the patient's vital signs and provide oxygen via facemask or non-rebreather mask until normal oxygenation is documented. Arrange for intubation if there is a loss of airway reflexes and/or a concern for airway protection. Secure large-bore intravenous (IV) access for the administration of medications and isotonic fluids. Correct hypoglycemia (<40 mg/dL [<2.22 mmol/L]) with 5 mL/kg of 10% dextrose (0.5 mg/kg). Administer a 20-mL/kg bolus of isotonic fluid (0.9% sodium chloride or lactated Ringer solution) for hypotension, poor perfusion, or signs of dehydration. Monitor the clinical response and repeat as necessary. Identify and treat abnormalities in temperature, blood pressure, and electrolyte levels.

In a case of known or suspected trauma, stabilization of the cervical spine is essential until a fracture can be ruled out. Assess the patient for other signs of injury and perform imaging as indicated. Perform emergent head CT and consult a neurosurgeon for any intracranial hemorrhage, because surgical intervention may be necessary.

Once the patient is intubated and the airway protected, allow hyperventilation to a $PaCO_2$ of 35 to 40 mm Hg. Also elevate the head of the bed to 45°, with the head maintained midline. Administer mannitol (0.5–1.0 g/kg) or hypertonic (3%) saline (3–5 mL/kg) for treatment of suspected cerebral edema and consult with an intensivist and a neurosurgeon.

After consultation with a neurologist, treat acute demyelinating encephalomyelitis with a 5-day course of IV methylprednisolone (30 mg/kg/d; maximum, 1,000 mg) followed by a 4- to 6-week oral prednisone taper.

There are specific antidotes (see Chapter 70, Toxic Exposures) for some ingestions or intoxications. Treat a suspected opiate intoxication with IV naloxone (0.1 mg/kg, 2-g maximum) and repeat every 2 to 3 minutes as needed. Note that the opiate antagonist has a shorter half-life than the opiate, so multiple doses or a continuous infusion of naloxone may be required.

The management of seizures (see Chapter 85) and intussusception (see Chapter 118, Acute Abdomen) is discussed elsewhere.

Indications for Consultation

- **Intensivist:** AMS that requires intubation, mechanical ventilation, severe electrolyte disturbances, or end-organ dysfunction
- **Neurology:** New-onset seizures, focal seizures
- **Neurosurgery:** Head trauma, increased ICP, VPS malfunction, brain tumor, intracranial hemorrhage
- **Poison control:** Ingestion or overdose
- **Surgery:** Intussusception

Disposition

- **Intensive care unit transfer:** AMS, unstable airway, intracranial bleed, severe electrolyte disturbances, or end-organ dysfunction
- **Discharge criteria:** Patient's mental status is at or near baseline and underlying cause has been addressed

- **Subacute rehabilitation:** Once the mental status change plateaus or begins to improve

Follow-up
- **Primary care:** 1 to 2 weeks
- **Neurology:** 1 week

Pearls and Pitfalls
- Lethargy may be the only presenting symptom in a child with intussusception.
- Consider child abuse in an infant with AMS, regardless of whether bruising is present or absent.
- Kernig and Brudzinski signs may be absent in a comatose patient with meningitis.
- Structural lesions, such as hydrocephalus or bilateral subdural hematomas, may cause a nonfocal examination.
- Acute onset of psychosis usually has an organic etiology, even with a history of psychiatric illness.

Bibliography

Conway EE. Altered states of consciousness. In: Fisher MM, Alderman EM, Kreipe RE, Rosenfeld WD, eds. *Textbook of Adolescent Health Care.* Elk Grove Village, IL: American Academy of Pediatrics; 2011:1321–1332

Kochanek PM, Carney N, Adelson PD, et al. Guidelines for the acute medical management of severe traumatic brain injury in infants, children, and adolescents—second edition. *Pediatr Crit Care Med.* 2012;13(Suppl 1):S1–S82

Piña-Garza JE. Altered states of consciousness. In: Piña-Garza JE, ed. *Fenichel's Clinical Pediatric Neurology.* 7th ed. Philadelphia, PA: Saunders/Elsevier; 2013:47–75

Pomeranz AJ, Sabnis S, Busey SL, Kliegman RM. Altered mental status. In: *Pediatric Decision-Making Strategies.* 2nd ed. Philadelphia, PA: Saunders/Elsevier; 2016:208–211

Cerebrospinal Fluid Shunt Complications

Introduction

Cerebrospinal fluid (CSF) shunts are named for the positions of the proximal and distal catheters. Proximal catheters are in the lateral, third, or fourth ventricles or in an intracranial cyst and exit the skull via a burr hole. Distal catheters are tunneled under the skin to their final location, which can be in the peritoneal space, right atrium, and pleural space, among others. Most commonly, ventriculoperitoneal shunts are placed.

Between the proximal and distal catheters is a one-way valve system that allows drainage of CSF at a predetermined pressure differential. Some valves have adjustable pressure settings, and these must be reset after any magnetic resonance (MR) imaging. All CSF shunts include an inline reservoir, which is located proximal to the valve and exterior to the skull to allow CSF withdrawal or medication infusion if necessary. Rarely, anti-siphon devices are spliced inline to prevent overdrainage.

The most common acute complications of CSF shunts are shunt malfunctions and shunt infections. CSF shunt malfunction is most frequent and occurs in 40% of new or revised shunts within 2 years of placement, secondary to debris, fibrosis, choroid plexus, or parenchymal occlusion of the proximal catheter. Delayed malfunctions (>2 years after insertion) are frequently caused by obstruction, breaking of the catheter, migration of the distal catheter, and, rarely, kinking or knotting. A CSF shunt infection is the second most common complication, most of which occur within 6 months of shunt surgery. The most common pathogens include *Staphylococcus epidermidis*, *Staphylococcus aureus*, and gram-negative bacilli.

A rare complication is slit-ventricle syndrome (slit-like ventricles on brain images, with poor ventricular compliance). If CSF shunt malfunction then develops, the patient's intracranial pressure (ICP) can increase quickly and without radiologic evidence of ventricular expansion, making the diagnosis difficult.

Less acute complications of CSF shunts include an abdominal pseudocyst, which is a loculated fluid mass within the peritoneum around the catheter tip. It can appear with signs of shunt malfunction at presentation, along with decreased appetite, abdominal pain, tenderness, distention, mass, guarding, inguinal hernia, and intractable hiccups.

CSF overdrainage can also occur, generally within 1 month after either shunt insertion or revision. Symptoms include positional headaches and vomiting, which is worse when upright and improved when recumbent.

Clinical Presentation

History

With a CSF shunt malfunction, the symptoms are highly variable and age dependent. Infants usually present with irritability, poor feeding, and lethargy, while older children usually present with persistent headache, nausea, vomiting, blurred vision, and parental suspicion from previous malfunctions. The presentation of a CSF shunt infection is similar to a shunt malfunction, with or without infectious symptoms, such as fever, wound erythema or exudate, abdominal pain, and peritonitis and recent revision (within 6 months).

Physical Examination

A patient with a CSF shunt malfunction may have altered mental status, irritability, nonerythematous swelling around the shunt tract, a bulging or full fontanel, increased head circumference, cranial nerve VI palsy, papilledema, and ataxia. Rarely, a patient will present with signs of severe increased ICP, including the sunset eye sign, hypertension, bradycardia, and irregular respirations. If the shunt is infected, there may be nonspecific signs of a shunt malfunction, fever, or cellulitis or signs of a wound infection around the shunt tract and signs of peritonitis.

Laboratory Workup and Radiology Examinations

Shunt Malfunction

If a patient presents with signs and symptoms consistent with shunt malfunction, immediately obtain a shunt series and preferably perform fast MR imaging or computed tomography (CT) of the brain. A shunt series includes plain radiographs of the skull, neck, chest, and abdomen and will demonstrate disconnections, kinks, and migration of catheters. While proximal and distal catheters are radio-opaque, reservoirs and connectors can be radiolucent; therefore, the images must be reviewed carefully. CT or MR images of the brain will show the location of the proximal catheter tip and size of the ventricles. Comparison to a prior study is critical, but if these images are unavailable, evidence of transependymal flow and sulcal effacement are suggestive of malfunction. Order abdominal ultrasonography (US) if an abdominal pseudocyst is suspected.

Less commonly, immediate cranial US can be used, but only for a patient with an open anterior fontanelle.

Shunt Infection

If a patient presents with signs or symptoms of a shunt infection, immediately order a shunt series and fast MR imaging of the brain (or head CT or cranial US) to rule out coincident malfunction. Also obtain a complete blood cell count, C-reactive protein level and/or erythrocyte sedimentation rate, and blood and urine cultures to rule out other infectious etiologies. If these workup findings are negative and the patient is within 6 months of a previous shunt surgery or if a shunt infection is highly suspected, consult with a neurosurgeon to arrange a shunt tap or, in rare circumstances, a lumbar puncture. Send the CSF for Gram stain, culture, cell count, and assessment of glucose and protein levels and measure the opening pressure, if possible.

Differential Diagnosis

The differential diagnosis of shunt complications is summarized in Table 83-1.

Table 83-1. Differential Diagnosis of CSF Shunt Complications	
Diagnosis	**Clinical Features**
CSF shunt infection	Shunt operation within the past 6 mo Purulent wound Erythema along the shunt tract
CSF shunt malfunction	Symptoms similar to those of previous malfunction Headache and vomiting without diarrhea Disconnection on the shunt series Increase in ventricle size on CT/MR images
Gastroenteritis	Contact with sick persons May have diarrhea
Meningitis	Meningismus, fever, decreased level of consciousness No change in ventricle size on CT/MR images
Urinary tract infection	No shunt operation within the past 6 mo Dysuria (+) Urinalysis
Viral syndrome	Contact with sick persons May have rhinorrhea, cough, conjunctivitis, pharyngitis

Abbreviations: CSF, cerebrospinal fluid; CT, computed tomography; MR, magnetic resonance; +, positive finding.

Treatment

Shunt Malfunction

For the rare patient who presents with signs of severe increased ICP, start emergent treatment, including elevating the bed to 30°, intubating and hyperventilating to a Pco_2 level of 28 to 33 mm Hg, and administering a bolus of either intravenous (IV) mannitol (0.5–1.0 g/kg) or 3% saline (5 mg/kg). If the patient is moribund, consult with a neurosurgeon to arrange an emergency shunt tap or ventricular tap through the burr hole or open fontanelle, prior to urgent definitive shunt revision. For most other patients who are ambulatory and have headaches and vomiting over several days, urgent neurosurgery consultation is indicated to plan a shunt revision within 24 hours.

Shunt Infection

Urgent neurosurgery consultation is necessary. Surgical approaches to hardware removal vary among neurosurgeons, but most will completely remove the shunt and place an external ventricular drain (EVD). However, with small ventricles or in medically complex patients, the distal end of the existing shunt may instead be externalized at the level of the clavicle or abdomen. Treat with IV vancomycin (20 mg/kg every 8 hours, 1-g maximum) and IV ceftriaxone (50 mg/kg every 12 hours, 2-g maximum). Tailor the antibiotic coverage once the culture and sensitivity results are available. Generally, the course of antibiotics is 7 to 21 days, with 14 days being typical, followed by shunt reinsertion.

Indications for Consultation

- **Infectious disease:** CSF shunt infection
- **Neurosurgery:** Any suspicion for a CSF shunt malfunction or infection

Disposition

- **Intensive care unit transfer:** Severely increased ICP, meningitis, and/or sepsis; depending on the institution, externalized shunts and EVDs
- **Pediatric center with neurosurgical services:** Shunt complication is highly suspected and services are not available locally; preferably, transfer to the pediatric neurosurgical center actively following up the patient
- **Discharge criteria:** No further symptoms/signs of the acute complication and recovery from surgical treatment of the hydrocephalus (eg, repaired CSF shunt after malfunction, reinternalized CSF shunt after infection)

Follow-up

- **Primary care:** 1 to 2 weeks
- **Neurosurgery:** 2 to 4 weeks

Pearls and Pitfalls

- In general, CSF shunt malfunctions appear in a consistent fashion at presentation for a given patient. Ask the family how the patient's shunt failure usually appears.
- In a symptomatic patient, an increase in ventricle size on brain images is the most specific finding for shunt malfunction.
- Fast MR imaging is rapidly replacing CT for shunt malfunction to prevent excessive long-term radiation exposure.
- Shunt infection is unlikely if the patient has not undergone shunt surgery within the past 6 months and/or is presenting with diarrhea. Neurosurgery services are therefore reluctant to tap the shunt in these circumstances.

Bibliography

Kulkarni AV, Riva-Cambrin J, Butler J, et al. Outcomes of CSF shunting in children: comparison of Hydrocephalus Clinical Research Network cohort with historical controls: clinical article. *J Neurosurg Pediatr*. 2013;12(4):334–338

Riva-Cambrin J, Kestle JR, Holubkov R, et al. Risk factors for shunt malfunction in pediatric hydrocephalus: a multicenter prospective cohort study. *J Neurosurg Pediatr*. 2016;17(4):382–390

Simon TD, Butler J, Whitlock KB, et al. Risk factors for first cerebrospinal fluid shunt infection: findings from a multi-center prospective cohort study. *J Pediatr*. 2014: 164(6):1462–1468

Stone JJ, Walker CT, Jacobson M, Phillips V, Silberstein HJ. Revision rate of pediatric ventriculoperitoneal shunts after 15 years. *J Neurosurg Pediatr*. 2013;11(1):15–19

Tamber MS, Klimo P Jr, Mazzola CA, Flannery AM; Pediatric Hydrocephalus Systematic Review and Evidence-Based Guidelines Task Force. Pediatric hydrocephalus: systematic literature review and evidence-based guidelines. Part 8: Management of cerebrospinal fluid shunt infection. *J Neurosurg Pediatr*. 2014;14(Suppl 1):60–71

Chapter 83: Cerebrospinal Fluid Shunt Complications

Headache

Introduction

Although headache is a common presenting complaint in pediatrics, it rarely requires inpatient workup and management. However, admission is indicated when headache is associated with altered mental status/level of consciousness, seizures, or an abnormal neurologic examination finding. Examples include severe migraine or migraine variants and headaches secondary to intracranial infection (encephalitis, meningitis) and increased intracranial pressure (ICP) secondary to mass effect, trauma, hemorrhage, or thrombosis.

Clinical Presentation

History

Ask about the onset of the headache (including any aura) and its intensity, frequency, location/focality, and associated symptoms, such as fever, nausea, vomiting, visual changes, photophobia, seizures, and neck stiffness. Inquire about medication use, possible toxin exposure, and significant medical problems (ventriculoperitoneal shunt, immunodeficiency or immunosuppression, coagulopathy). Finally, perform a thorough psychosocial assessment, including a substance abuse history.

Physical Examination

Priorities in the physical examination include vital signs (to look for hypertension alone or as part of a Cushing triad), growth parameters, pupillary responses and extraocular movements, and neurocutaneous findings, such as hamartomas, neurofibromas, café au lait macules, or hemangiomas. Perform ophthalmoscopy to look for the absence of venous pulsations and blurring of the disk margins and a comprehensive neurologic examination to look for signs of increased ICP, focal neurologic findings, and meningismus. If none of these signs are present, the likelihood of a secondary headache related to significant central nervous system (CNS) pathology is quite low.

Laboratory Workup

If the clinical presentation is suspicious for a primary CNS condition, obtain a complete blood cell count, erythrocyte sedimentation rate, and/or C-reactive protein level to screen for an infection or inflammatory process. If meningitis is a concern, also perform a blood culture and obtain cerebrospinal fluid for

Gram stain and culture, cell count, and protein and glucose level assessment. Always measure the opening pressure when a lumbar puncture (LP) is performed during the evaluation of a headache. In general, if signs of increased ICP are absent, head computed tomography (CT) is not necessary prior to LP. If increased ICP is suspected, delay the LP, regardless of the CT results.

If a focal neurologic deficit exists, neuroimaging is usually indicated to rule out secondary intracranial causes of headache. Since there is no consensus of opinion over the routine use of CT and/or magnetic resonance (MR) imaging for headache, undertake a careful analysis of the benefits and probable yield prior to exposing patients to the risks associated with each (radiation, contrast material, sedation, anesthesia). CT is indicated if acute bleeding or thrombosis is suspected, but perform MR imaging if there is concern about an intracranial mass or inflammatory condition.

Differential Diagnosis

The priority is to rule out an intracranial mass lesion, hemorrhage, thrombosis, and meningitis/encephalitis (Table 84-1).

A positive family history of headache in a first- or second-degree relative is suggestive of a primary headache, while recurrent, chronic, severe, progressive, or unconventional headaches are more likely with a secondary headache. Headaches that raise a concern for primary CNS pathology include those that wake a child from sleep, are worse in the morning or improve over the course of the day, or are worse when recumbent or with a Valsalva maneuver. Sudden onset of severe headache, the so-called thunderclap headache, demands urgent evaluation to rule out subarachnoid hemorrhage or venous sinus thrombosis.

Treatment

Treat a migraine with sumatriptan (5 mg intranasally, 25 mg orally, or 0.1 mg/kg per dose intradermally) and repeat in 2 hours, if necessary. A migraine cocktail, consisting of a combination of ketorolac (0.5 mg/kg; 15-mg maximum if the patient weighs <50 kg; 30-mg maximum if the patient weighs >50 kg), an antiemetic (prochlorperazine 0.10–0.15 mg/kg, 10-mg maximum), an antihistamine (diphenhydramine 0.5 mg/kg, 25–50-mg maximum), and intravenous fluids, may be effective if sumatriptan therapy fails. Consult a pediatric neurologist for status migrainosus or migraine variants.

Treat the underlying cause of a secondary headache. For a headache associated with a systemic infection or inflammatory condition, administer acetaminophen (10–15 mg/kg per dose every 4–6 hours) or ibuprofen (5–10 mg/kg every 6 hours). See Chapter 68, Sepsis, for the treatment of suspected meningitis.

Table 84-1. Differential Diagnosis of Headaches	
Diagnosis	**Clinical Features**
Central nervous system infection (meningitis)	Fever, altered mental status Nuchal rigidity, photophobia (+) Kernig and/or Brudzinski signs Patient may have petechiae and/or purpura
Idiopathic intracranial hypertension (pseudotumor)	Patient overweight/obese Visual disturbances Papilledema
Inflammatory conditions	Fever, malaise, myalgia, fatigue, weight loss Rash/skin changes Arthralgia/arthritis
Intracranial mass	Headache awakens the patient at night, is worse in the morning Abnormal neurologic examination finding Signs of ↑ intracranial pressure
Migraine	(+) Family history Multiple previous episodes Nausea and/or vomiting Phonophobia, photophobia Possible pattern, such as menses related
Non–central nervous system infection	Patient may have an upper respiratory infection, pharyngitis, or facial pain Fatigue, myalgia, abdominal pain
Posttraumatic origin	Antecedent history of trauma (acute or chronic)
Vascular origin	Abnormal headache character Focal neurologic findings, especially cranial nerve deficits
Viral meningitis	Fever Headache with or without photophobia Patient may not have meningeal signs

"+" indicates a positive finding.

Venous sinus thrombosis often requires anticoagulation therapy (see Chapter 5, Deep Venous Thrombosis) with low–molecular weight heparin, such as enoxaparin (1 mg/kg every 12 hours) unless significant bleeding has occurred, as well as treatment of the cause of the thrombosis. Obtain emergent consultation with a pediatric neurosurgeon for intracranial bleeding and treat with platelets, fresh frozen plasma, cryoprecipitate, and/or other clotting factors, as indicated for any underlying coagulopathy.

Diagnostic and therapeutic LP is often adequate in the acute setting of idiopathic intracranial hypertension, but long-term treatment requires identification of the underlying cause. In addition, a headache secondary to enteroviral meningitis is often relieved by the LP.

Indications for Consultation

- **Infectious diseases:** Unusual organism causing a systemic or CNS infection
- **Neurology:** Status migrainosus, migraine variants, seizure
- **Neurosurgery:** Intracranial hemorrhage, intracranial mass, increased ICP
- **Ophthalmology:** Possible papilledema or assessment of eye involvement in systemic illness, especially inflammatory conditions
- **Rheumatology:** Systemic inflammatory conditions affecting the CNS

Disposition

- **Intensive care unit transfer:** Signs of impending herniation/increased ICP, hemodynamic instability associated with systemic illness/infection
- **Discharge criteria:** Baseline mental status and neurologic examination findings

Follow-up

- **Primary care:** 4 to 7 days
- **Subspecialists involved in care during hospitalization:** 1 week

Pearls and Pitfalls

Risk factors for a serious cause of a headache include a new headache in a preschool-aged patient, occipital headache, inability to characterize the quality of headache, atypical headache pattern, and abnormal neurologic findings.

Bibliography

Choe MC, Blume HK. Pediatric posttraumatic headache: a review. *J Child Neurol.* 2016;31(1):76–85

Gofshteyn JS, Stephenson DJ. Diagnosis and management of childhood headache. *Curr Probl Pediatr Adolesc Health Care.* 2016;46(2):36–51

Jacobs H, Singhi S, Gladstein J. Medical comorbidities in pediatric headache. *Semin Pediatr Neurol.* 2016;23(1):60–67

Kabbouche M. Pediatric inpatient headache therapy: what is available. *Headache.* 2015;55(10):1426–1429

Rothner AD, Parikh S. Migraine variants or episodic syndromes that may be associated with migraine and other unusual pediatric headache syndromes. *Headache.* 2016; 56(1):206–214

CHAPTER 85

Seizures

Introduction

Approximately 5% of children will have a seizure by 16 years of age. The goals of the initial evaluation are to identify whether the seizure has stopped or if there is concern for status epilepticus, identify potential treatable causes, decide whether to start seizure medications, and determine when the patient can be discharged or if further diagnostic evaluation and management are indicated.

Generally, the patient and family want to know why the seizure occurred, what tests are necessary, if medication is required, and if a seizure will happen again.

Clinical Presentation

History

The context in which the seizure occurs is crucial and guides management. Is there evidence of recent illness, trauma, systemic infection, or disease? Is the child appropriately vaccinated according to age, or is the patient immunocompromised? Is the child taking medications, or are there potential toxic/metabolic causes? Does the child have an abnormal neurologic examination finding or a history of neurologic impairment or developmental delay? Is there a family history of febrile seizures or epilepsy?

Physical Examination

First, obtain the patient's vital signs and address chest compressions, airway, and breathing (CABs). Pay close attention to any airway obstruction caused by the postictal state, benzodiazepines, or other medications used to stop seizure activity.

After a brief initial assessment, evaluate the patient for ongoing seizure activity. Clonic jerks or tonic stiffening of the trunk or limbs may be present. Subtler signs of seizure include tachycardia; dilated, poorly reactive pupils; sustained eye deviation; oral or hand automatisms; and increased salivation. Look for any evidence of pupillary asymmetry, lateralized facial or limb weakness, and alterations in tone or reflexes. Note worrisome signs, such as sustained hypertension or the presence of bradycardia, which could indicate increased intracranial pressure (ICP).

Perform a thorough neurologic examination. In addition to recognizing persistent seizures, the goal is to look for evidence of underlying structural, vascular, infectious, or neoplastic processes. Check for upper motor neuron signs, such as arm drift, asymmetrical differences in limb tone, movement and reflexes, up-going toes (Babinski sign), or finger flexor reflex (Hoffman reflex; flexion of distal thumb when the third or fourth fingernail is tapped). Also assess the patient for the Chvostek sign (for hypocalcemia). Perform a funduscopic examination to look for signs of increased ICP, such as absent venous pulsations and papilledema.

Differential Diagnosis

There are 4 categories to consider when evaluating the patient with seizures: a provoked seizure (eg, electrolyte abnormalities, ingestion), acute symptomatic process (eg, stroke or encephalitis), remote symptomatic cause (pre-existing structural brain abnormality), or idiopathic cause.

A combination of protocol and clinical judgment determines the diagnostic workup. Guidelines from the American Academy of Neurology (AAN) recommend emergent imaging (computed tomography [CT]) if there is concern for a clinically significant abnormality. This applies to a patient with an abnormal neurologic examination finding, significant trauma, history of anticoagulation therapy, altered mental status, persistent vomiting or headache, or history of cancer. When compared to adults in whom seizures are frequently caused by cortical tumors or stroke, the yield of routine CT for a first seizure in a child is much lower. This is also true of routine laboratory tests. Clinically significant abnormalities in each typically range from 5% to 10%.

A patient who is not awakening or who has subtle, rhythmic oral or eye movements may have persistent electrographic seizures, which require an electroencephalogram (EEG) for confirmation.

Laboratory Workup

Febrile Seizure

An EEG, lumbar puncture (LP), and neuroimaging are not indicated for a patient with a simple febrile seizure and a normal, nonfocal neurologic examination finding. However, perform an LP when the clinical presentation is suspicious for bacterial meningitis. Other indications for an LP are a patient 6 to 12 months of age who is immunocompromised or fully unimmunized or whose status is deficient in immunizations for *Haemophilus influenzae* type b (Hib) or *Streptococcus pneumoniae*. In addition, have a low threshold for performing an LP in a patient who has had recent antibiotic exposure that may affect the physical examination so that meningeal signs are not evident. Other tests will be dictated by the need to find the source of fever.

Afebrile Seizure

Neonatal seizures, defined as seizures in the first month of life, are a distinct entity that require a high index of suspicion for infectious and metabolic disorders. Measure serum glucose level, chemistry values, ammonia level, and complete blood cell count (CBC) and perform urgent imaging, either nonenhanced CT or magnetic resonance (MR) imaging. Perform an LP if there are signs suggestive of associated sepsis or meningitis. Observe an afebrile, well-appearing infant 1 to 6 months of age for 24 hours. Also, consider an inborn error of metabolism in a young infant with altered mental status or acidosis.

In an older infant or child, the history and physical examination guide the choices for laboratory testing, especially if there is a prior illness, concern about an ingestion, or dehydration. Otherwise, routine laboratory testing is of limited value in the alert, well-appearing patient or a child with known epilepsy who has a breakthrough seizure. However, if the patient has had a first afebrile seizure, obtain at a minimum a set of electrolyte levels to help identify potential causes of a provoked seizure. Chemistry values are also helpful for children with chronic encephalopathy, those receiving gastrostomy tube feedings, and/or those whose neurologic examination findings have changed from baseline.

Serum levels of antiepileptic drugs are not needed to guide therapy unless an overdose is suspected, but they can be helpful when evaluating the patient for adherence.

If the patient has persistent alteration in mental status after the seizure activity has ceased, order an EEG to rule out subclinical status epilepticus. Also obtain an EEG if infantile spasms are a concern. While brief afebrile seizures are an indication for a follow-up outpatient EEG, do not order one for a patient with a simple febrile seizure.

Status Epilepticus

The most common cause of status epilepticus is low seizure medication level(s) in a patient with known epilepsy, although acute symptomatic processes account for approximately 20% of cases. Emergent nonenhanced head CT is indicated, as are bedside glucose level, CBC, and complete metabolic profile. Perform an LP and treat appropriately if meningitis is a concern. See Chapter 70, Toxic Exposures, if an ingestion is a possibility. If the CT findings are normal, MR imaging is more sensitive for parenchymal processes, especially for a patient who presents with status epilepticus without pre-existing epilepsy or someone with known epilepsy with a change in seizure morphologic appearance.

Radiology Examinations

Guidelines from the AAN recommend emergent imaging (CT) when there is concern for a clinically significant abnormality, specifically blood or mass effect. This applies to a patient with an abnormal neurologic examination finding, significant head trauma, history of anticoagulation therapy, altered mental status, persistent vomiting or headache, or history of a malignancy. In contrast, the yield of routine head CT for a patient with a first afebrile seizure is low (5%–10%), especially in a child over 6 months of age. MR imaging is the preferred imaging modality if there is concern about parenchymal disease or pathology at the base of the skull or in the posterior fossa. Consult with a neurologist to determine if MR imaging is not necessary during the acute inpatient stay.

Differential Diagnosis

Differentiation of a seizure from nonepileptiform events can be difficult in a young child. The history often provides adequate details to detect characteristics of the nonepileptiform events described in Table 85-1. Otherwise, direct observation or video recording of the events allows the most accurate assessment. Episodes that can be extinguished with a change in position or immobilization of extremities are unlikely to be epileptiform. Atypical movements during sleep in infants are most often benign sleep myoclonus.

Treatment

First-Time Seizure—Febrile

A simple febrile seizure does not require daily seizure medication or abortive medication with rectal diazepam. This is also generally true for a patient with complex febrile seizures. However, a child with a history of febrile status epilepticus has a higher chance that future seizures will progress to status epilepticus. Therefore, offer the parents rectal diazepam (0.5 mg/kg), with instructions to administer the medication to the patient for any seizure that lasts 3 minutes or longer.

First-Time Seizure—Afebrile

In general, the definition of epilepsy is 2 unprovoked seizures separated by 24 hours. This is based on the risk of a second unprovoked seizure, which is approximately 1 in 3. Therefore, most children do not require seizure

Table 85-1. Differential Diagnosis of Seizures	
Diagnosis	**Clinical Features**
Benign sleep myoclonus	Migrating, multifocal repetitive limb jerks during sleep Jerks extinguished when aroused
Breath-holding spell	Occurs when child is upset or after occipital head trauma Two types: pallid or cyanotic
Migraine	Patient may have an aura Associated with headache, nausea, photophobia
Reflux (Sandifer syndrome)	History of spitting up Generalized stiffening and opisthotonic posturing Occurs within 30 min of a feeding
Shuddering spell	Often occurs with excitement, urination, or feeding; no associated regression or encephalopathy (helps to distinguish it from infantile spasms)
Syncope	Episodes occur when standing or overheated Preceded by nausea and/or darkening of vision with light-headedness No postictal period

medication after a single unprovoked seizure. Potential exceptions include the presence of pre-existing structural brain abnormalities, such as stroke or cortical dysplasia. In such a patient, the risk of recurrent seizure may be as high as 70%. Consult with a pediatric neurologist to assist in deciding whether to initiate antiepileptogenic medication. Seizure counseling also requires discussions regarding safety, a seizure action plan, potential medication side effects, and approximate duration of medication therapy.

A patient who presented with afebrile status epilepticus is at increased risk for subsequent status epilepticus. Offer rectal diazepam, as described earlier.

Status Epilepticus—Febrile and Afebrile

Status epilepticus is a neurologic emergency that requires immediate treatment, with the hospitalist simultaneously evaluating the patient for potential causes. Address the CABs and obtain intravenous (IV) access, bedside glucose level, comprehensive metabolic panel, and CBC. Perform an LP and neuroimaging (if indicated), but the patient must be stable enough for the procedures.

Emergent first-line therapy is IV lorazepam 0.1 mg/kg (maximum, 4 mg per dose) or diazepam 0.2 mg/kg (maximum, 12 mg per dose). Repeat if the seizure activity persists after 5 minutes. If IV access is not available, administer rectal diazepam, 0.5 mg/kg if 6 months to 11 years of age or 0.2 mg/kg if over 12 years of age (20-mg maximum); or midazolam (intranasal 0.2 mg/kg; intramuscular 5 mg if the patient weighs 13–40 kg or 10 mg if the patient weighs >40 kg).

If the seizures persist, deliver a loading dose of IV fosphenytoin, 20 to 30 mg phenytoin equivalents per kilogram, administered slowly over 10 to 15 minutes (1.5 mg fosphenytoin sodium is equivalent to 1 mg phenytoin sodium and is referred to as *1 mg phenytoin sodium equivalents*; maximum, 1.4 g per dose). IV phenytoin is an alternative (20–30 mg/kg administered slowly over 20–30 minutes).

If the patient has refractory seizures, consult with a neurologist. Options include a loading dose of a second control medication or transfer to an intensive care unit (ICU) for initiation of a pharmacologic coma. Second medication options include IV levetiracetam (30–60 mg/kg), IV valproic acid (20–40 mg/kg; contraindicated if the patient has thrombocytopenia or a possible metabolic disease), or IV phenobarbital (20 mg/kg; maximum, 1 g per dose; monitor the patient for respiratory depression and hypotension).

Indications for Consultation
- **Neurology:** Focal neurologic findings, persistent altered mental status, status epilepticus, febrile seizure in an infant younger than 6 months, afebrile seizure in a patient younger than 24 months, concern for infantile spasms, recurrent seizures
- **Neurosurgery:** Signs of increased ICP or abnormal head imaging findings

Disposition
- **ICU transfer:** Status epilepticus, respiratory depression secondary to antiepileptics, persistent altered mental status
- **Video EEG monitoring unit:** Concern for nonepileptic disorder mimicking seizures, ruling out subclinical seizures, capturing events that have not been witnessed by medical providers
- **Discharge criteria:** Baseline neurologic examination findings

Follow-up
- **Primary care:** 2 to 3 days
- **Neurology:** 1 to 2 weeks

Pearls and Pitfalls
- Rapidly consider all of the possible treatable causes of seizure.
- Perform a limited workup for a child with simple febrile seizure.
- Excessive benzodiazepine use can cause respiratory failure.

Bibliography

Abend N, Loddenkemper T. Management of pediatric status epilepticus. *Curr Treat Options Neurol.* 2014;16(7):301–316

Freilich ER, Schreiber JM, Zelleke T, Gaillard WD. Pediatric status epilepticus: identification and evaluation. *Curr Opin Pediatr.* 2014;26(6):655–661

Gupta A. Febrile seizures. *Continuum (Minneap Minn).* 2016;22(1 Epilepsy):51–59

Kimia AA, Bachur RG, Torres A, Harper MB. Febrile seizures: emergency medicine perspective. *Curr Opin Pediatr.* 2015;27(3):292–297

Kimia AA, Ben-Joseph E, Prabhu S, et al. Yield of emergent neuroimaging among children presenting with a first complex febrile seizure. *Pediatr Emerg Care.* 2012; 28(4):316–321

Subcommittee on Febrile Seizures, American Academy of Pediatrics. Clinical practice guideline—febrile seizures: guideline for the neurodiagnostic evaluation of the child with a simple febrile seizure. *Pediatrics.* 2011;127:389–394

Nutrition

Failure to Thrive

Introduction

Failure to thrive (FTT) is generally defined as a weight lower than the third or fifth percentile on a growth chart or a change in weight that has crossed down 2 major percentile lines over 3 to 6 months.

FTT is caused by inadequate calorie intake, excessive calorie losses, or increased calorie requirements. The most common cause, found in 85% of cases in the United States, is inadequate calorie intake, which may be associated with significant psychosocial issues. However, this view is too rigid, because often, inadequate nutrition reflects a complex interaction among a child's medical, nutritional, emotional, and social issues. Therefore, a thorough psychosocial evaluation is an important part of patient and family assessment.

Indications for hospitalization include failure of outpatient therapies, severe FTT or malnutrition, serious infections, neglect or a concern for the patient's safety, or the need for a multidisciplinary team approach and/or services for parental education, support, and coordination of care that are best performed in the inpatient setting.

Clinical Presentation

History

Obtaining a detailed history is critical to assigning the diagnosis. Compile a thorough dietary history, including foods and formulas (preparation, frequency), feeding/breastfeeding patterns, juice/water intake, behaviors at mealtime, and the duration of feedings. Quantify the daily caloric intake. It is best to do a 24-hour diet recall or to have the family keep a 3-day diet log. Inquire about gastrointestinal (GI) symptoms (vomiting or spitting up, rumination, difficulty swallowing or eating), stool production (pattern, frequency, consistency, diarrhea, bloody, mucoid), respiratory issues (difficulty breathing, chronic cough, snoring), and recurrent infections. Pregnancy and birth history, including birth weight, as well as a complete medical history and review of symptoms, are essential. Document the developmental milestones for an infant and confirm the newborn screening results.

As noted earlier, there is often a psychosocial component to FTT. A complete assessment of the family and social situation is important, including who is caring for the child during the day. Assess the parents' economic status, mental health and intellectual capacity, and parent-child interaction. Try to determine whether there are other stressors in the home, family dysfunction, prior involvement with social services, and behavior consistent with child maltreatment, including Munchausen syndrome by proxy. Obtain a complete family history, focusing on systemic diseases (inflammatory bowel disease, asthma, cystic fibrosis, renal tubular acidosis), FTT, and short stature (note the height and weight of both parents).

Review the growth chart trends. Inadequate nutrition leads to poor weight gain, which will be followed, over time, by decreased height velocity. Head circumference is typically normal unless the problem is severe.

Physical Examination

The vital signs and general appearance (dysmorphic features, cachexia, general activity) are priorities. Examine the oropharynx for a cleft palate, poor suck or swallow, dental caries, and enlarged tonsils. Assess the work of breathing, auscultate for a murmur, and palpate the abdomen for hepatomegaly. Note any loose skin, edema, poor hygiene, rash, or bruises or evidence of trauma. Perform a neurologic examination for muscle tone, reflexes, social interaction, and developmental milestones. One final, important part of the physical examination is observation of the parent/child interaction and feeding routine.

Laboratory Workup

Limit the use of laboratory tests and evaluations to those suggested by the history and physical examination, because without specific evidence for organic disease, laboratory testing is rarely helpful in determining the etiology of FTT. When indicated, screening tests may include a complete blood cell count; comprehensive chemistry evaluation (including electrolyte levels, blood urea nitrogen/creatinine ratio, and calcium, phosphorus, magnesium, and albumin levels); liver function tests; erythrocyte sedimentation rate; urinalysis; and stool samples for occult blood, pH level, and reducing substances (Table 86-1). Other tests to consider, *only if indicated* by the findings in the history and physical examination, are thyroid function tests, ammonia level, lactate level, HIV, tuberculosis testing, and bone age.

Differential Diagnosis

The diagnosis of FTT is primarily a clinical endeavor. Perform a comprehensive review of the growth chart trends and identify chronic illnesses and syndromes that alter growth. In contrast to a patient with an endocrinologic or chromosomal disorder, a child with FTT will "fall off" the weight curve before "falling off" the height/length curve, with the weight being lower down on the curve than the height/length.

Table 86-1. Differential Diagnosis of Failure to Thrive		
Diagnosis	**Clinical Features**	**Initial Laboratory Tests and Evaluations**
Inadequate caloric intake		
Breastfeeding failure Feeding problem	Uncoordinated suck/swallow Mother feels milk supply is inadequate	Observe infant feeding Weigh infant pre- and postfeeding Consult lactation counselor (if breastfeeding)
Excess juice consumption	Dietary history	None
Incorrect formula preparation	Dietary history History of economic pressures	CBC, electrolyte levels
Oromotor dysfunction	Observation of feeding	Speech/swallow consult
Psychosocial—insufficient food	Stressors in the home	CBC, electrolyte levels Family psychosocial screening
Inadequate caloric absorption/usage		
Celiac disease	Family history Diarrhea	CBC, albumin levels Anti-tissue transglutaminase level Stool pH level, reducing substances, fecal fats
Cystic fibrosis	Family history Abnormal newborn screening results Respiratory symptoms Diarrhea	Review newborn screening results Sweat test Stool pH level, reducing substances, fecal fats
Gastroesophageal reflux	Vomiting history	Response to treatment with/without swallowing study or pH level probe
Increased intracranial pressure	Vomiting history Cushing triad Abnormal neurologic examination finding	Head CT Neurology consult
Inflammatory bowel disease	Family history Diarrhea, bloody stools	CBC, ESR/CRP level, albumin level Stool occult blood
Liver disease	Jaundice Diarrhea	Liver function tests Hepatitis serologic studies
Milk protein allergy	Family history Vomiting history Diarrhea, bloody stools Eczema	Stool occult blood GI consult Possible endoscopy
Increased caloric requirements		
Adrenal diseases	Vomiting, diarrhea Hyperpigmentation Hypotension	Chemistry assessment Glucose level
Blood disorders	Fatigue Pallor	CBC

Continued

Table 86-1. Differential Diagnosis of Failure to Thrive, continued		
Diagnosis	**Clinical Features**	**Initial Laboratory Tests and Evaluations**
Increased caloric requirements, continued		
Cardiopulmonary diseases	Fatigue, especially with feedings Respiratory illnesses	Chest radiography ECG and echocardiogram
Diabetes mellitus	Polydipsia, polyuria, polyphagia	Chemistry assessment, fasting glucose level Urinalysis
Genetic diseases	Family history Dysmorphic features	Specific for suspected diseases
Hyperthyroidism	Fatigue, increased sweating, polyphagia Nervousness, sleep disturbance Diarrhea Tachycardia, exophthalmos	Thyroid studies
Renal tubular acidosis	Normal anion gap metabolic acidosis	Venous blood gas analysis and urinalysis (compare serum and urine pH levels)

Abbreviations: CBC, complete blood cell count; CRP, C-reactive protein; CT, computed tomography; ECG, electrocardiogram; ESR, erythrocyte sedimentation rate; GI, gastrointestinal.

Base the differential diagnosis on caloric intake and expenditure (Table 86-1). The etiology may be secondary to inadequate caloric intake, inadequate caloric absorption/usage, or increased caloric requirements (excess metabolic demand as occurs in chronic diseases). Inadequate caloric intake is by far the most common cause of FTT. However, some diseases, such as congenital heart disease or bronchopulmonary dysplasia, appear with a mixed picture of inadequate intake and a hypermetabolic condition at presentation.

Physiological causes of short stature and symmetrically small growth that are not considered to be FTT include a history of prematurity or small size for gestational age, familial short stature, and constitutional growth delay.

Treatment

The treatment for FTT is to provide adequate nutrition for catch-up growth (Box 86-1). Therefore, the patient will require 150% or more of the usual maintenance calories to transition from a negative to a positive nitrogen balance.

Box 86-1. Nutrition for Catch-up Growth
$$\text{kcal/kg required} = \frac{[\text{IBW in kg (50th percentile wt/ht)}] \times [\text{kcal/kg/d (DRI for age)}]}{[\text{actual weight (kg)}]}$$

Abbreviations: DRI, Dietary Reference Intake (available at http://fnic.nal.usda.gov/interactiveDRI/); ht, height; IBW, ideal body weight; wt, weight.

Once adequate nutrition is delivered, typical rates of weight gain are as follows: 0 to 4 months of age, 23 to 34 g/d; 4 to 8 months of age, 10 to 16 g/d; 8 to 12 months of age, 6 to 11 g/d; and 12 to 24 months of age, 4 to 9 g/d. However, there may be a lag of several days before weight gain finally begins. Close, continued outpatient follow-up is essential.

Before stopping breastfeeding, encourage the mother to continue breast-feeding, with efforts made to increase the milk supply and/or improve the milk transfer. Consult with a breastfeeding-trained pediatrician and/or a lactation consultant. The severity of the poor weight gain will determine if and how much supplementation is needed for the breastfeeding infant.

When an infant does not gain weight with a regular formula (20 kcal/oz), first change to a hypercaloric one (24–30 kcal/oz). For an exclusively breastfed infant, use expressed breast milk if the breast milk volume is adequate. If the supply is poor or milk transfer is inadequate, supplement with formula. If weight gain remains low despite adequate intake, add fortification. As a general estimate, adding a teaspoon of a powdered formula (Similac NeoSure Advance, Enfamil EnfaCare Lipil Powder, Nestle Good Start Gentle Plus, etc) to 100 mL of breast milk will increase the caloric density to about 24 cal/oz. If a formula concentration greater than 24 kcal/oz is needed, request a nutrition consult. One option is to add 0.4 mL of medium-chain triglycerides (MCT oil) to 1 ounce of the 24-kcal/oz formula.

For a patient older than 1 year, consult with a nutritionist and use behavioral modification and high-calorie foods. The "rule of 3s" is helpful (3 meals, 3 snacks, and 3 choices), as is the use of high-calorie liquids (fortified whole milk or commercial formulas that contain >20 kcal/oz). Hypercaloric feedings are usually, but not always, hyperosmolar, which may cause side effects, such as osmotic diarrhea, if the feedings are advanced too quickly.

Reintroduce nutrition slowly to avoid refeeding syndrome, which occurs when a malnourished patient begins to receive adequate nutrition too quickly. This triggers insulin release, thereby causing intracellular shifts of phosphate, potassium, and magnesium. Although refeeding syndrome is rare except in severe malnutrition, marasmus, or kwashiorkor, manifestations may include hypophosphatemia (most common), hypokalemia, and hypomagnesemia. Insulin secretion can also cause renal sodium resorption, leading to edema and volume overload. To prevent refeeding syndrome in a patient at risk, consult a nutritionist and begin feeding slowly, starting with 50% of the caloric needs, then increase the intake by 25% of the daily calories every 3 to 4 days. Closely monitor the vital signs, daily weights, and physical examination (for edema). Check the electrolyte levels (comprehensive chemistry assessment with magnesium and phosphorus levels) daily at first, but if refeeding syndrome is suspected, evaluate electrolyte levels 2 to 3 times a day and correct any abnormalities. If there are serious derangements, transfer the patient to an intensive care unit (ICU) for closer monitoring.

Assess growth with calorie counts and daily weights. Nasogastric or transpyloric tube feedings are indicated when a patient cannot manage adequate oral intake because of increased energy needs and/or physiological impairment, while at the same time, the GI tract is fully or partially functioning. Transplyoric or pyloric (nasoduodenal or nasojejunal) tube feeding is useful when a nasogastric feeding is not indicated, such as when there are congenital upper GI anomalies, inadequate gastric motility, high aspiration risk, severe gastroesophageal reflux, or upper GI obstruction.

See Table 86-2 for the details on starting continuous tube feeding. The overall rate is determined by the kilocalories per day necessary, based on the catch-up growth formula described in Box 86-1. Transition to bolus nasogastric feedings (Table 86-3) once continuous maintenance intake is tolerated, but do not use bolus feeding with a nasoduodenal or nasojejunal tube. Make one change, either volume or concentration, when adjusting enteral feedings and monitor the patient for tolerance. If the patient does not tolerate a full-strength formula, decrease the volume and slowly increase as tolerated. If the patient will be on a combination bolus and continuous feeding schedule (day/nocturnal feedings), wait 2 hours from the end of the continuous schedule to initiate the bolus schedule.

Table 86-2. Continuous Feeding Guidelines[a]

Age	How to Start	How to Advance	Tolerance Volume
0–12 mo	1–2 mL/kg/h	1–2 mL/kg every 2–8 h	6 mL/kg/h
1–6 y	1 mL/kg/h	1 mL/kg every 2–8 h	1–5 mL/kg/h
>7 y	25 mL/h	25 mL every 2–8 h	100–150 mL/h

[a] Adapted from Courtney E, Grunko A, McCarthy T. Enteral nutrition. In: Hendricks KM, Duggan C, eds. *Manual of Pediatric Nutrition.* 4th ed. Hamilton, Ontario, Canada: BC Decker; 2005.

Table 86-3. Bolus Feeding Guidelines[a]

Age	How to Start	How to Advance	Tolerance Volume
0–2 mo	10–15 mL/kg every 2–3 h	10–30 mL per feeding	20–30 mL/kg every 4–5 h
1–6 y	5–10 mL/kg every 2–3 h	30–45 mL per feeding	15–20 mL/kg every 4–5 h
>7 y	90–120 mL every 3–4 h	60–90 mL per feeding	330–480 mL every 4–5 h

[a] Adapted from Courtney E, Grunko A, McCarthy T. Enteral nutrition. In: Hendricks KM, Duggan C, eds. *Manual of Pediatric Nutrition.* 4th ed. Hamilton, Ontario, Canada: BC Decker; 2005.

Indications for Consultation

- **Child Protection Team:** Concern for child abuse or neglect
- **Gastroenterology:** Severe gastroesophageal reflux or milk protein allergy, inflammatory bowel disease, cystic fibrosis, celiac disease
- **Lactation specialist:** Breastfeeding failure
- **Nutritionist:** All patients admitted for FTT
- **Social work:** Assessment of family dynamics, emotional health, and ability to adhere to outpatient plan
- **Speech therapy:** Cleft palate, oromotor dysfunction

Disposition

- **ICU transfer:** Critical malnutrition (bradycardia, hypothermia, severe dehydration, altered mental status), severe electrolyte disturbances (hypophosphatemia, hypokalemia, hypomagnesemia, hypocalcemia) secondary to refeeding syndrome
- **Discharge criteria:** Adequate, consistent weight gain demonstrated for 2 to 3 consecutive days; any underlying disease identified and treated; feeding regimen with adequate calories established; family demonstrates understanding of nutrition recommendations, proper feeding techniques, and growth expectations; relevant social and emotional issues have been adequately addressed

Follow-up

Primary care: Weekly to monitor long-term weight gain and development

Pearls and Pitfalls

- Hospitalizing a patient does not necessarily contribute to identifying the cause of FTT, and a planned weekend admission for FTT may significantly increase health care costs.
- FTT is often a multifactorial illness that requires a multidisciplinary approach.
- Most cases of FTT are failure to (adequately) feed, so compiling a detailed feeding history is critical.
- Use a disease-specific growth curve to plot data for a child with a congenital or genetic disease.
- Laboratory testing is usually not helpful in determining an etiology.
- Careful and thorough documentation is especially important in a suspected case of child neglect or abuse.

- Red flags for possible child abuse or neglect include multi-organ system involvement, previous evaluations at multiple institutions or providers, a convoluted history, or numerous reported allergies.
- Suggested management algorithms may lead to quicker diagnosis, improvement in nutrition, and shorter lengths of stay.

Bibliography

American Academy of Pediatrics Committee on Nutrition. Failure to thrive. In: Kleinman RE, Greer FR, eds. *Pediatric Nutrition.* 7th ed. Elk Grove Village, IL: American Academy of Pediatrics; 2014:663–700

Jaffe AC. Failure to thrive: current clinical concepts. *Pediatr Rev.* 2011;32(3):100–107

Mash C, Frazier T, Nowacki A, Worley S, Goldfarb J. Development of a risk-stratification tool for medical child abuse in failure to thrive. *Pediatrics.* 2011;128(6):e1467–e1473

Thompson RT, Bennett WE Jr, Finnel SM, Downs SM, Carroll AE. Increased length of stay and costs associated with weekend admissions for failure to thrive. *Pediatrics.* 2013;131(3):e805–e810

CHAPTER 87

Feeding Tubes and Enteral Nutrition

Introduction

Feeding tubes are commonly used in children as an alternative means of providing nutrition, hydration, and medication. Although feeding tubes can be used to manage acute self-limiting illnesses, this chapter's focus is on the patient with a chronic feeding problem. Feeding tube management in such a child is best served by a multidisciplinary team of specialists, including nurses, dietitians, therapists, and equipment suppliers.

Types of Feeding Tubes

There are 2 types of feeding tubes.

- Enterostomy tubes are inserted endoscopically, surgically, or percutaneously (institutionally dependent). Examples include gastrostomy tubes (G-tubes), gastrojejunal tubes (GJ-tubes), and jejunal tubes (J-tubes). All of these are indicated for longer-term use (>8–12 weeks).
- Oronasal tubes include nasogastric (NG), orogastric, and nasojejunal tubes. These are generally reserved for short-term use or as a bridge to a more permanent enterostomy tube. They are associated with an increased risk of dislodgment and migration.

Enterostomy Tubes

- Enterostomy tubes have 3 main components (Figure 87-1).
- An internal portion (balloon, mushroom, bulb, pigtail) within the stomach prevents inadvertent tube withdrawal.
- The external stabilizing portion is often a disk or bar near the skin.
- A feeding port is either close to the stabilizer in low-profile devices or attached to a longer tube in traditional tubes.

Typically, traditional tubes are initially placed and then replaced with a low-profile device after 6 to 12 weeks. However, the timing is dependent on local practice.

Indications for G-Tubes

- Chronic oral-motor feeding problem (ie, neuromuscular disease, brain injury) with resultant inability to maintain hydration orally, prolonged feeding times, and risk of pulmonary aspiration

Figure 87-1. Types of Enterostomy Tubes

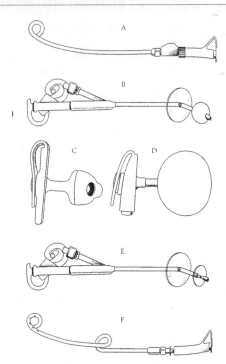

Low profile (button tubes): Device is flush to the skin.

C: Gastrostomy tube with a mushroom-shaped dome tip.

D: Gastrostomy tube with a silicone balloon tip that can be inflated with saline.

Non–low profile: Device has a long external portion.

A: Gastrostomy tube with an internal pigtail loop and an external locking device.

B: Gastrostomy tube with an internal balloon tip and an external port for inflating/deflating the balloon.

E: Gastrostomy tube with a mushroom or wing tip to secure the tube to the stomach.

F: Gastrojejunal tube with a gastric loop and a distal loop that sits in the jejunum.

- Failure to thrive as a result of inadequate caloric intake due to a specific disease process (cystic fibrosis, congenital heart disease, chronic renal failure, malignancy)
- Delivery of an elemental diet or essential medications for the treatment of disease processes (inflammatory bowel disease, eosinophil esophagitis, metabolic disease)

Indications for Jejunal Feedings (GJ- and J-Tubes)

GJ-tubes, which bypass the stomach and pyloric sphincter, are used selectively because they are associated with more mechanical problems, such as clogging and migrating. They also present a greater inconvenience for families.

- Used for treatment of severe gastroesophageal reflux (GER) that is inadequately controlled medically and/or surgically, these tubes are especially useful in a patient who is at risk for aspiration while receiving G-tube feedings and is already receiving maximal treatment for GER.
- G-tubes are used with gastrointestinal anatomic anomalies, such as superior mesenteric artery syndrome.

Complications Associated With G-, GJ-, and J-Tubes

Complications related to enteral tubes are best divided into early (<30 days of the procedure) and late. Complication rates depend on the technique of placement. Late, minor complications are common with all techniques.

Early (Procedure-Related)

Early complications include bleeding, infection (peristomal or systemic), puncture of other intra-abdominal organs (colon), misplacement of the tube (into the small or large bowel), peritonitis (about 2%), esophageal tear (percutaneous endoscopic gastrostomy [PEG]), aspiration, anesthetic-related complications, and death (rare).

Late

Late complications include tube problem (blockage, dislodgment, breakage), peristomal wound infections, stomal enlargement with leakage around the tube, buried bumper syndrome (PEG), peritonitis caused by replacement of the tube into the peritoneum (rare), and intussusception around the distal portion of tube (GJ-tube).

Management of Enterostomy Tube Placement Complications

Peritonitis (All Tubes)

Peritonitis usually occurs within 48 hours after insertion or during the first weeks after, when the tract between the stomach wall and skin is not yet formed. Causes include gastric leakage of contents into the peritoneal space, dislodgment of the tube into the peritoneum, and perforation of other organs or vessels during the procedure. The patient presentation is similar to other causes of peritonitis, with fever, irritability, vomiting, and peritoneal signs.

Management involves general measures, including discontinuing feedings, placing an NG-tube for gastric drainage, and administering broad-spectrum antibiotics (see Chapter 118, Acute Abdomen), as well as aggressive fluid management. In addition, obtain a radiograph or fluoroscopic study with contrast material (tube check) to confirm tube placement and the presence of pneumoperitoneum. If there is a concern about intra-abdominal collections or bleeding, perform ultrasonography (US) or computed tomography. In some cases, an emergent laparotomy will be necessary to investigate and manage a possible perforation.

Vomiting (All Tubes)

Always consider non–tube-related causes, including GER, which may worsen after the placement of an enterostomy tube. G-tubes, particularly those with a long internal portion or without a securing mechanism (Mac-Loc [Cook Medical], Foley catheter), can migrate into the duodenum or esophagus. Perform a contrast-enhanced study (G-tube check). GJ-tubes can also migrate, becoming malpositioned, or promote reflux (duodenal gastric). In addition, a common complication in these tubes is intussusception (see the following).

Clogging (All Tubes)

Obstruction or clogging of an enteral tube is usually caused by a medication (Box 86-1), thickened feeding materials, or failure to flush the tube after feedings. A tube with a thinner outside diameter is also more prone to blockage. To relieve the obstruction, gently flush with warm water by using a 1- to 3-mL syringe. If this is ineffective, repeat with a carbonated beverage or cranberry juice. However, in some cases, as a last resort, the tube may have to be removed.

Box 87-1. Medications and Substances That Commonly Block Enterostomy Tubes	
Cholestyramine resin	Kayexalate
Ciprofloxacin	Lactulose
Clarithromycin	Magnesium oxide
Cornstarch	Nelfinavir mesylate
Cotazym	Pyridoxine (vitamin B)
Iron (liquid)	

Intussusception (GJ-Tubes Primarily)

Intussusception has been reported with (pigtail) Mac-Loc (Cook Medical) catheters, as the distal portion of the tube acts as a lead point for a small-bowel intussusception. The highest risk is in an infant younger than 1 year, who can present with bilious vomiting and irritability. Diagnosis is assigned with abdominal US, and management includes tube removal and placing a temporary Foley catheter into the stomach. Recurrences may be prevented by shortening the tube. However, recurrences are an indication for discontinuing the GJ feedings and trying other options, such as fundoplication and continuous gastric feedings.

Dislodged Tube (All Tubes)

If tube dislodgement occurs more than 8 weeks after the initial insertion, when the tract has been formed, insert a temporary Foley catheter as soon as possible, because the stoma can close within 1 to 2 hours. Use a Foley catheter that is the same size or one size smaller than the G-/GJ-tube. Wet the Foley catheter with some lubricating jelly and insert it 1.5 to 2 inches (4–6 cm) into the stoma, fill the balloon of the Foley catheter with 3 mL of sterile or distilled water, then tape the catheter to the patient's abdomen. Confirm the position in the stomach by withdrawing the stomach contents through a syringe connected to the end of the Foley catheter. The Foley catheter can then be used for feeding or medications until a replacement tube is inserted for a child who is G-tube fed. For a patient with GJ-tube dislodgement, initiate temporary gastric feedings only if it is medically safe (the patient is not at a high risk of aspiration).

However, if the dislodgement occurs within 8 weeks of initial insertion, when the tract is not completely formed, do not insert a temporary Foley catheter. The patient is at risk of peritoneal placement of the tube and subsequent peritonitis. Obtain a contrast-enhanced study of the tract prior to inserting the Foley catheter or any other replacement tube.

Skin Infection (All Tubes)

Several steps in the care of G-tube sites can help prevent site infections, including cleaning the stoma daily with soap and water, keeping the stoma dry, and avoiding covering the stoma site with dressings. An infection appears with redness around the site and/or pus. Consider other causes of redness around the G-tube site, which may be confused for infection (Table 87-1).

Feeding Via an Enterostomy Tube

Decisions regarding the type and route of feedings are best made in consultation with a nutritionist. Basic considerations include the following.

Bolus Versus Continuous Feedings

Generally speaking, bolus feedings are safe because they represent physiological stomach function, although there is controversy as to whether continuous feedings are safer. A general recommendation is to calculate the daily caloric requirement and deliver one-eighth of the total every 3 hours, with each feeding delivered over 1 hour. Adjustments can be made accordingly. However, if the patient is receiving transpyloric feedings, do not use boluses because the small intestine (unlike the stomach) is not capable of receiving fluids in this manner.

Caloric and Fluid Needs

Calories and fluids will vary widely, depending on the patient and the indication(s) for the tube. For example, a patient with severe neurologic delay and a decreased metabolic rate will have a lower caloric need than an otherwise active patient with cystic fibrosis. As a general rule, calculate a

Table 87-1. Differential Diagnosis of Peristomal Erythema

Diagnosis	Presentation	Management
Bacterial infection	Rarely complicated by abscess formation	Topical bacitracin/polymyxin Oral antibiotics (cephalexin)
Fungal infection	Erythema with satellite lesions May have coexisting oral thrush or diaper candidiasis	Topical antifungal cream Oral nystatin for coexistent oral candidiasis
Granulation tissue	Pinkish-red, moist tissue May bleed May be painful	Warm saline compresses No dressings or creams Silver nitrate cautery
Irritation secondary to leakage of gastric contents	Erythema, breakdown, or ulceration	Keep area dry Barrier cream (zinc oxide) Consider application of a topical antacid
Skin sensitivity/contact dermatitis	Red, scaly, dry skin	Remove all dressings Change the adhesive tape

fluid/calorie estimate, then track the patient over a period of 3 to 5 days to ensure adequate tube function, adequate weight gain, and appropriate hydration.

Types of Formula

There is nothing particularly unique about a tube-fed patient in terms of the choice of nutrition, although this may depend somewhat on the reason(s) why the tube was placed. Allow the gut physiology to drive the choice of breast milk or formula. As an example, initially order that the patient be fed with one of the standard formulas or breast milk (for an infant) or one of the higher-calorie products (for a toddler), if there is no underlying condition suggesting otherwise.

Discharge Planning

Discharge planning is an area where pediatric hospitalists will need some expertise and experience to anticipate the patient's needs. In most situations, a case manager or social worker will assist in the transition of the patient and family from the inpatient to the outpatient setting in terms of medical equipment and formula delivery. One useful, common strategy for facilitating the transition to the home environment is to implement daytime bolus feedings (allowing the patient time off the feeding pump) and overnight continuous feedings, then monitor the patient for a day or two.

Pearls and Pitfalls

The delivered tube feeding volume is often less than what was ordered because the feedings are frequently stopped, delayed, or withheld for multiple reasons. Base calorie counts on volume delivered, not ordered.

Bibliography

Kazmierski M, Jordan A, Saaed A, Aslam A. The benefits and management of gastrostomy in children. *Paediatr Child Health*. 2013;23(8):351–355

McSweeney ME, Smithers CJ. Advances in pediatric gastrostomy placement. *Gastrointest Endosc Clin N Am*. 2016;26(1):169–185

Rahnemai-Azar AA, Rahnemaiazar AA, Naghshizadian R, Kurtz A, Farkas DT. Percutaneous endoscopic gastrostomy: indications, technique, complications and management. *World J Gastroenterol*. 2014;20(24):7739–7751

The Royal Children's Hospital Melbourne. Gastrostomy acute replacement of displaced tubes. http://www.rch.org.au/clinicalguide/guideline_index/Gastrostomy_Acute_replacement_of_displaced_tubes/. Accessed February 22, 2017

Soscia J, Friedman JN. A guide to the management of common gastrostomy and gastrojejunostomy tube problems. *Paediatr Child Health*. 2011;16(5):281–287

Fluids and Electrolytes

Introduction

Volume depletion (dehydration) and electrolyte disturbances are common in hospitalized children. While most instances are relatively mild, in severe cases they can result in shock, seizures, coma, and death. Hypovolemia can occur with an increased, normal, or decreased serum sodium (Na^+) level (hypertonic, isotonic, or hypotonic hypovolemia), and abnormalities in serum Na^+ level can be seen in patients without hypovolemia (eg, syndrome of inappropriate antidiuretic hormone secretion [SIADH]).

Clinical Presentation: Dehydration

History

Usually there is a history of emesis, diarrhea, decreased oral intake and urinary output, malaise, and central nervous system (CNS) depression. High fever, high-pitched cry, and irritability can occur with hypernatremic dehydration. Markedly decreased urinary output implies greater than 10% dehydration. Assess the patient's intake (volume and specific fluid) and losses (vomitus, stool, urine).

Physical Examination

Evaluate the child's general appearance and look for signs of dehydration, including sunken eyes, dry mucous membranes, and absence of tears. Tachycardia (pulse >95th percentile for age) and orthostatic pulse changes are early signs of hypovolemia. However, fever can be a confounder because it increases the heart rate by about 10 beats per minute for each degree above 37°C (98.6°F). Overt hypotension is a late finding in hypovolemic shock in children, and its absence does not preclude the diagnosis of significant hypovolemia. Check the capillary refill by raising the extremity to be tested slightly above the heart and briefly pressing the nail bed on a finger or toe to compress the underlying capillaries (blanching). Observe as the skin returns to a normal color when the pressure is released. Moderate to severe dehydration and most types of shock cause a sluggish or prolonged capillary refill time greater than 2 seconds, although this can also occur as a consequence of simple exposure to a cold external environment.

Laboratory Workup

Obtain a set of electrolyte levels, if not previously done, and conduct a urinalysis. The serum Na^+ level is not a reflection of volume status and must be interpreted in the context of whether the patient is hypovolemic, euvolemic, or hypervolemic. Investigate causes of abnormal glucose level, acidosis, and increased anion gap (normal <12 mEq/L [<12 mmol/L]). Assess the urine for ketone bodies, which are products of fatty acid oxidation during fasting or hypoglycemia.

$$\text{Anion gap} = [Na^+ - (\text{chloride} + \text{bicarbonate})]$$

Suspect acute kidney injury (AKI) if the patient is oliguric or polyuric despite clinical signs of dehydration or has a blood urea nitrogen/creatinine ratio that is disproportionately high or continues to increase despite proper management. Suspect SIADH (postoperative, pulmonary or CNS disease, malignancies, medications) if the patient presents with hyponatremia and increased urine osmolality, without clinical signs of dehydration. If AKI or SIADH is suspected, calculate the serum/urine ratios and the fractional excretion of Na^+ (FE_{Na}), which will generally be less than 1% in a patient with normal renal function, greater than 1% in a patient with renal disease, and less than 1% to 2% in a patient with SIADH, depending on Na^+ intake (Table 88-1):

$$FE_{Na} = (\text{urine } Na^+ \times \text{plasma creatinine})/(\text{plasma } Na^+ \times \text{urine creatinine}) \times 100$$

When the plasma osmolality is low, suggesting SIADH, use the urine/serum osmolality ratios as shown in Table 88-1. Repeat the electrolyte assessments 4 to 6 hours later if the patient is not improving or has significant abnormalities in serum Na^+ or potassium (K^+) level, severe acidosis, or signs of possible renal dysfunction. If the child has persistent ongoing losses and is primarily or exclusively receiving intravenous (IV) fluids, check the electrolyte levels daily for the first 2 to 3 days, then as warranted by the clinical condition. The causes of Na^+ and K^+ level abnormalities are summarized in Table 88-2.

Treatment: Fluid and Electrolyte Therapy

Calculate a patient's fluid and electrolyte requirements based on the clinical presentation and underlying diagnosis. Take into consideration the severity of illness, as well as the basal metabolic needs, initial hydration and electrolyte status (deficits), and ongoing losses. Acute changes in body weight reflect fluid losses. For example, a 20-kg patient who is 10% dehydrated has lost 2 kg, equal to 2 L of fluid.

Table 88-1. Laboratory Values in Oliguria			
	Prerenal	**Renal**	**SIADH**
Urine			
Sodium level (mEq/L)	<20	>40	>40
Specific gravity	>1.020	~1.010	>1.020
Osmolality (mOsm/kg)	>500	<350	>500
Urine/serum ratios			
Urine/serum osmolality	>1.3	<1.3	>2
Urine/serum urea level	>20	<10	>15
Urine/serum creatinine level	>40	<20	>30
FE_{Na} (%)	<1	>2	<1–2

Abbreviations: FE_{Na}, fractional excretion of sodium; SIADH, syndrome of inappropriate antidiuretic hormone secretion.

To convert milliequivalents per liter to millimoles per liter for sodium level, multiply by 1.0. To convert milliosmoles per kilogram to millimoles per kilogram for osmolality, multiply by 1.0.

Table 88-2. Causes of Sodium and Potassium Level Abnormalities	
Diagnosis	**Causes**
Hyponatremia	
Pseudo/fictitious	Hyperlipidemia, hyperproteinemia, hemolysis
Factitious	Hyperglycemia (diabetic ketoacidosis) Na^+ level ↓ 1.6 mEq/L (1.6 mmol/L) for each ↑ 100 mg/dL (5.55 mmol/L) of glucose
Euvolemic	Syndrome of inappropriate antidiuretic hormone secretion (central nervous system or pulmonary disease, medications, postoperative, malignancy)
Hypovolemic	Burns, dietary, cerebral salt wasting, gastrointestinal losses, iatrogenic
Hypervolemic	Cardiac impairment, edema, renal disease (nephrotic syndrome), iatrogenic origin, liver failure
Hypernatremia	
With ↓ total body Na^+ level	Diarrhea, renal disease, sweat
With normal total body Na^+ level	Diabetes insipidus (central, nephrogenic), heat
With ↑ total body Na^+ level	Hyperaldosteronism, iatrogenic, renal disease
Hypokalemia	
	Dietary issues (chronically ill), gastrointestinal losses, medications (β-agonists, diuretics), renal disease
Hyperkalemia	
	Acidosis, Addison disease, congenital adrenal hyperplasia, iatrogenic origin, medications, renal disease, rhabdomyolysis

Maintenance therapy is required to preserve intravascular volume in a euvolemic, otherwise healthy patient who does not have any abnormal deficits or ongoing losses, such as an infant with pre- or postoperative status. Add glucose, Na^+, and K^+ (only if the patient is voiding, without hyperkalemia) requirements to prevent iatrogenic hypoglycemia, hyponatremia, and/or hypokalemia. Overnight maintenance IV fluid is typically not needed in a euvolemic older child without ongoing losses who is receiving nothing by mouth (nil per os, or NPO) for next-day surgery. However, avoid prolonged fasting prior to surgery.

Maintenance Fluid

Use the Holliday-Segar method (Table 88-3) for a patient weighing more than 3.5 kg. If the child is obese, use the ideal body weight or the 50th percentile weight for the child's height. These calculations are for an otherwise healthy child. For a patient who is ill or dehydrated, adjust the fluids to take into account the volume deficit, maintenance requirements, and clinical course (changes in oral intake, urine output, ongoing losses, etc). Use 5% dextrose to minimize catabolism, because this will provide 2 to 4 mg/kg/min of glucose infusion, equivalent to the liver glucose production rate.

Maintenance Electrolytes

Replace the daily Na^+ and K^+ losses in the sweat, urine, and stool. Use a solution that is at a minimum 0.45 normal saline (NS) and has 1 to 2 mEq/kg/d (1–2 mmol/kg/d) of K^+ (generally, 20 mEq/L [20 mmol/L] of K^+ will suffice). Defer administering K^+ if the patient has hyperkalemia, marked oliguria/anuria, or suspected renal insufficiency. Avoid concentrations of K^+ greater than 20 mEq/L (>20 mmol/L) in a peripheral IV catheter to prevent phlebitis.

If a patient will be receiving NPO and IV maintenance fluids for more than 48 hours, use an isotonic solution (NS, lactated Ringer [LR] solution). This will prevent iatrogenic hyponatremia, possibly because of antidiuretic hormone production. NS can also be used as the initial IV maintenance fluid.

Table 88-3. Holliday-Segar Method	
Body Weight	Water (mL/kg per 24 h)
First 10 kg of body weight	100
Second 10 kg of body weight	50
Each additional kilogram (>20 kg)	20

Volume Depletion

Calculate the fluid deficit and add that volume (as NS) to the daily maintenance fluids to be infused over 24 hours. However, correct significant volume
depletion with urgent bolus infusions of NS.

Ongoing Losses

Always consider ongoing losses of both volume and Na^+ (emesis Na^+ level:
60–155 mEq/L [60–155 mmol/L]; diarrhea Na^+ level: 40–120 mEq/L
[40–120 mmol/L]; third-spacing Na^+ level: 140 mEq/L [140 mmol/L]).
Measure volume losses and assess replacement needs every 4 hours.

Severe Hyponatremia With Seizures (Na^+ Level <120 mEq/L [<120 mmol/L])

Use 3% NaCl (513 mEq/L [513 mmol/L]) through a central venous line until
the seizures stop (1.2 mL/kg will increase serum Na^+ levels about 1 mEq/L
[1 mmol/L]). Administer the NaCl slowly if only a peripheral IV catheter
is available.

For nonemergent correction, increase the serum Na^+ level by no more
than 0.5 mEq/L/h (0.5 mmol/L/h) to prevent central pontine myelinolysis.

Hypernatremia (Na^+ Level >145 mEq/L [>145 mmol/L])

$$\text{Free water deficit} = 4 \text{ mL/kg} \times \text{weight} \times (Na^+_{plasma} - Na^+_{desired})$$

Decrease the serum Na^+ level by no more than 0.5 mEq/L/h (0.5 mmol/L/h)
to prevent cerebral edema.

Hypokalemia (K^+ Level <3 mEq/L [<3 mmol/L])

To properly interpret the serum K^+ level, consider the effect of blood pH level
on the intracellular-extracellular movement of K^+. A decrease of 0.1 in blood
pH level increases the serum K^+ level by approximately 1 mEq/L (1 mmol/L),
while an increase of 0.1 in blood pH level decreases the serum K^+ level by
approximately 1 mEq/L (1 mmol/L). In addition, take into account that only
2% of the total body K^+ (TBK) level is found in plasma, with most being in the
intracellular space. Each 1-mEq/L (1-mmol/L) decrease in serum K^+ level represents a decrease in TBK level of approximately 12%. Therefore, in general,
hypokalemia implies marked TBK depletion.

Symptoms of moderate hypokalemia include muscular weakness, myalgia,
and muscle cramps. Severe hypokalemia leads to depressed muscle function,
flaccid paralysis, diminished reflexes, respiratory depression, and, potentially,
rhabdomyolysis. Severe hypokalemia is characterized by electrocardiogram

(ECG) abnormalities, such as a prominent U wave after the T wave, ST segment depression, and atrioventricular conduction abnormalities.

Whenever possible, correct a K^+ deficiency enterally, because this is much safer. Mild hypokalemia will usually resolve with just oral repletion. However, severe symptomatic hypokalemia requires IV K^+ correction with 0.5 mEq/kg (0.5 mmol/kg) per dose (20-mEq [20-mmol] maximum). A rapid infusion of K^+ is rarely needed and requires close monitoring, preferably in an intensive care unit (ICU). Correct a significant K^+ deficit slowly over 3 to 5 days with an IV solution containing 30 to 40 mEq/L (30–40 mmol/L) of KCl or K- acetate (if the patient is acidotic). Do not exceed an infusion rate of 0.5 mEq/kg/h (0.5 mmol/kg/h) or 4 to 5 mEq/kg/d (4–5 mmol/kg/d) and do not use a K^+ concentration greater than 40 mEq/L (>40 mmol/L) through a peripheral IV catheter because it can cause acute phlebitis.

Hyperkalemia (K^+ Level >6 mEq/L [>6 mmol/L])

Recheck the electrolyte levels to confirm the K^+ level, check the bicarbonate level to assess for acidosis (which causes a K^+ shift into the extracellular fluid), look for hemolysis of the sample (spurious hyperkalemia), and obtain an ECG. If there are findings consistent with hyperkalemia (peaked T waves, shortening of the QT interval, prolonged PR interval, widened QRS complex) or if the K^+ level is greater than 7 mEq/L (>7 mmol/L), initiate treatment, preferably in an ICU. Discontinue the administration of exogenous K^+ and use therapeutic agents that can transiently redistribute K^+: 25% dextrose (2 mL/kg over 30 minutes and repeat every 30 minutes), along with regular insulin (1 unit/kg/h), as well as nebulized albuterol. Also administer 10% calcium gluconate to protect the myocardium: 1 mL/kg = 100 mg/kg per dose over 5–10 minutes (500-mg/kg/d maximum) and repeat in 6 hours, if necessary. To enhance K^+ excretion, use a loop diuretic (IV furosemide 1–2 mg/kg every 6 hours) and polystyrene sulfonate (1 g/kg). Dialysis is indicated for life-threatening hyperkalemia.

Ongoing Losses

Gastrointestinal (emesis, diarrhea, ileus, third-spacing), renal, and insensible water losses affect fluid maintenance requirements. Assess ongoing losses frequently, because they may change rapidly (Table 88-4).

Table 88-4. Changes in Maintenance Fluid Requirements		
	Increase	**Decrease**
Activity (eg, seizures)	30%	NA
Anuria/oliguria	NA	50%
Diabetes insipidus	≥200%–400%	NA
Diarrhea	≥10%–50%	NA
Humidified oxygen	NA	25%–40%
Hyperventilation	50%–65%	NA
Polyuria (eg, diabetic ketoacidosis)	100%	NA
Sweat	5%–50%	NA
Temperature	12% per degree Celsius >37°	12% per degree Celsius <37°

Abbreviations: NA, not applicable.

Resuscitation Fluids Practical Guidelines

What follows is a safe, simplified method to minimize common iatrogenic fluid and electrolyte disturbances. Compare the calculated rehydration plan to MedCalc, which provides in-depth electronic fluid and electrolyte calculations (www.medcalc.com/pedifen.html). However, this plan is not a substitute for clinical judgment and assessing and reassessing the status of the patient.

Start Fluid Resuscitation With an Isotonic Solution (NS or LR)

1. Administer 20-mL/kg IV boluses over 15 to 20 minutes.
2. Reassess and repeat boluses as needed, up to 60 mL/kg in 60 minutes. Always consider possible life-threatening conditions that require a different approach, especially if more than 80 mL/kg is needed. These include sepsis (fever and hypotension), congestive heart failure (CHF) or myocarditis (respiratory distress, gallop rhythm, hepatomegaly), intracranial hypertension (history of hydrocephalus; bradycardia, altered mental status), and adrenal crisis (unresponsive shock). When CHF or myocarditis is a concern, administer multiple small boluses of 10 mL/kg rather than larger boluses and monitor the response closely to avoid fluid overload. Follow the changes in pulse, blood pressure, urine output, and pulmonary auscultation and change the fluid management as necessary.
3. If the patient is in shock, rapidly secure intraosseous access if IV access appears suboptimal.

Subsequent Fluid and Electrolyte Therapy

1. Calculate the maintenance (Holliday-Segar method) and deficit fluid volumes (as detailed earlier), while monitoring ongoing losses.
   a. Isonatremic/hyponatremic dehydration: Use 5% dextrose one-half NS or NS with 20-mEq/L (20-mmol/L) KCl. This will provide additional NaCl to slowly compensate for the deficit, as well as the K^+ and glucose requirements (2–4 mg/kg/min).
   b. Hypernatremic dehydration: Use 5% dextrose one-quarter to one-half NS with 20-mEq/L (20-mmol/L) KCl over *48 hours.*
   c. Confirm that the patient has voided before adding K^+ to the IV fluids.
   d. Resume oral feeding as early as possible.
   e. Monitor the patient's pulse, blood pressure, and urine output.
2. If the patient is stable and well hydrated (postrehydration, NPO)
   a. Weight less than 10 kg: 5% dextrose one-quarter NS with 20-mEq/L (20-mmol/L) KCl
   b. Weight greater than 10 kg: 5% dextrose one-half NS or 5% dextrose NS with 20-mEq/L (20-mmol/L) KCl

Indications for Consultation

- **Endocrinology:** Possible adrenal crisis or urine output greater than 5 mL/kg/h (diabetes insipidus)
- **Metabolism:** Laboratory findings suggestive of a metabolic disorder (severe acidosis, unexplained increased anion gap, and/or hypoketotic hypoglycemia)
- **Nephrology:** Anuria or signs of renal disease (increased creatinine level), severe hypo- or hypernatremia or hypo- or hyperkalemia

Disposition

- **ICU transfer:** Shock not responding to resuscitation fluids, acute kidney injury, hyperkalemia requiring IV medications, severe hypokalemia, severe hypo- or hypernatremia
- **Discharge criteria:** Patient back to premorbid weight, tolerating maintenance oral fluids, with adequate urine output ($\geq$1 mL/kg/h)

Follow-up

Primary care: 1 to 3 days

Pearls and Pitfalls

- To avoid fluid overload, use the patient's ideal body weight or the 50th percentile weight for height for an obese patient.
- Assume greater than 10% dehydration if the patient is anuric/oliguric or has hypernatremic dehydration.
- As a result of reperfusion, severe metabolic acidosis can worsen immediately after rehydration.
- In the context of oliguria, FE_{Na} less than 1% suggests prerenal azotemia, rather than intrarenal injury/acute tubular necrosis.
- Proteinuria and glucosuria can falsely increase the urine specific gravity and thereby mask renal insufficiency.
- Always consider the possibility of acute adrenal insufficiency in a hypotensive, unresponsive patient with hyponatremia and/or hyperkalemia.
- Monitor ongoing losses and add them to maintenance and replacement fluids. These can be significant, especially with secretory diarrhea.

Bibliography

Favia I, Garisto C, Rossi E, Picardo S, Ricci Z. Fluid management in pediatric intensive care. *Contrib Nephrol*. 2010;164:217–226

Foster BA, Tom D, Hill V. Hypotonic versus isotonic fluids in hospitalized children: a systematic review and meta-analysis. *J Pediatr*. 2014;165(1):163–169

Friedman A. Fluid and electrolyte therapy: a primer. *Pediatr Nephrol*. 2010;25(5): 843–846

Hanna M, Saberi MS. Incidence of hyponatremia in children with gastroenteritis treated with hypotonic intravenous fluids. *Pediatr Nephrol*. 2010;25(8):1471–1475

Peruzzo M, Milani GP, Garzoni L, et al. Body fluids and salt metabolism—part II. *Ital J Pediatr*. 2010;36:78

Simpson JN, Teach SJ. Pediatric rapid fluid resuscitation. *Curr Opin Pediatr*. 2011;23(3): 286–292

Wang J, Xu E, Xiao Y. Isotonic versus hypotonic maintenance IV fluids in hospitalized children: a meta-analysis. *Pediatrics*. 2014;133(1):105–113

Obesity

Introduction

Nearly 1 in 5 American children and teenagers are obese, and another 1 in 3 are overweight. In addition, the prevalence of extreme obesity, defined as a body mass index (BMI) at or above 120% of the 95th percentile for children of the same age and sex, is estimated at 3% to 5% of the population. Extreme obesity is associated with higher incidences of cardiovascular disease (CVD) and type 2 diabetes mellitus (T2DM), which are more likely to persist into adulthood.

Most obese children will not have a specific genetic or metabolic cause detected. Rare syndromic causes of obesity, such as Prader-Willi syndrome, Bardet-Biedl syndrome, and McCune-Albright syndrome, are associated with some combination of short stature, hypogonadism, developmental delay, and dysmorphic features. In general, most endocrinologic causes (hypothyroidism, Cushing syndrome) will have other symptoms at the time of presentation. Some psychotropic medications, such as risperidone and quetiapine, can cause weight gain as a side effect.

Definition

For children 2 years of age and older, the definition of obesity relies on calculating the BMI as follows: BMI = (mass in kilograms)/(height in meters)^2. A patient with a BMI greater than the 95th percentile is classified as obese, while a child with a BMI greater than the 85th percentile is classified as overweight.

Clinical Presentation

History

Ask about diet history, physical activity, sleep history, and early growth trajectory, if known, as well as development and menstrual history in female subjects. Check the family history for T2DM, thromboembolic events, hypertension, and dyslipidemias. Assess the patient for psychological comorbidities (depression, bullying, anxiety, disordered eating). Review past and current medication use.

Physical Examination

Priorities at the physical examination include BMI, blood pressure, and skin inspection for acanthosis nigricans (associated with hyperinsulinemia and diabetes), abdominal striae, and intertrigo. While hirsutism and acne are relatively common in overweight female adolescents, the presence of these signs suggests the possibility of polycystic ovary syndrome (PCOS). Perform a musculoskeletal examination to look for a limp, hip and/or knee pain, and pes planus.

Comorbidities

As with adults, there are significant comorbidities associated with childhood obesity that may affect inpatient management.

Endocrine

Type 2 Diabetes

Obesity leads to insulin resistance and abnormal glucose tolerance, which are common precursors to T2DM, which is now the most common form of diabetes in children. Institute screening at 10 years of age for any overweight child who has 2 or more of the following risk factors: family history positive for T2DM (first- or second-degree relative); African American, Hispanic American, American Indian, or Asian/South Pacific Islander ethnicity; or physical findings or signs of insulin resistance (acanthosis nigricans, hypertension, dyslipidemia, PCOS). For such patients, obtain a hemoglobin A1c level (a level increased >5.7% is prediabetic), although a fasting blood glucose level greater than 100 mg/dL (>5.55 mmol/L) may also be used. The hemoglobin A1c level is preferred for inpatients, since acute illness, intravenous fluids, and corticosteroid use can all temporarily cause hyperglycemia.

Metabolic Syndrome

Metabolic syndrome is a complex disorder defined by a cluster of interconnected risk factors that increase the likelihood of developing CVD and T2DM. While metabolic syndrome is well defined in adults, its identification in childhood and adolescents remains somewhat controversial. Adult criteria include increased fasting plasma glucose level greater than 100 mg/dL (>5.55 mmol/L), central (abdominal) obesity, increased triglyceride levels at or above 150 mg/dL (≥1.695 mmol/L), decreased high-density lipoprotein (HDL) cholesterol level (<40 mg/dL [<1.036 mmol/L] in male subjects; <50 mg/dL [<1.295 mmol/L] in female subjects), and blood pressure of 130/85 mm Hg or higher. Early identification of these risk factors is important because they tend to track relatively well throughout adulthood and suggest an increased risk of CVD and T2DM.

Polycystic Ovary Syndrome

Clinical history and findings include menstrual irregularity, hirsutism, acne, and increased insulin levels. However, oligomenorrhea independent of PCOS is common in the first 2 years after menarche, and there are other conditions that may mimic PCOS. If PCOS is suspected, obtain a free testosterone level and luteinizing and follicle-stimulating hormone levels, as well as an early morning 17-OH progesterone level. Depending on the clinical picture, a total testosterone, dehydroepiandrosterone sulfate, sex hormone–binding globulin, prolactin, and/or free thyroxine and thyroid-stimulating hormone levels may be indicated to exclude other conditions.

Cardiovascular

Hypertension

An obese child has a fourfold greater risk of increased systolic blood pressure and a twofold greater risk of increased diastolic blood pressure. Persistent increased blood pressure is an indication for renal and cardiac assessment. Be aware that falsely increased blood pressure readings may occur in an obese patient if an undersized cuff is used.

Dyslipidemia

In general, obese children and adolescents are more likely to have increased levels of total cholesterol, triglycerides, and low-density lipoprotein cholesterol and reduced levels of HDL cholesterol. If feasible, obtain a fasting lipid profile in a patient older than 2 years of age with a BMI in the 85th percentile or above, if not performed previously.

Respiratory

Almost half of obese children can develop obstructive sleep apnea (OSA) and chronic hypoxemia, which may contribute to insulin resistance and low-level inflammation, independent of BMI. Nocturnal polysomnography is the standard of reference for diagnosing OSA. In addition to OSA, hypoventilation syndrome may occur in extremely obese individuals, when both awake and asleep. The association with obesity and asthma has also been long recognized, although the relationship between these two disorders continues to be elucidated. Consult with a pediatric pulmonologist if the patient has dyspnea, because pulmonary function test results can help distinguish between obstructive lung disease and poor conditioning.

Neurologic

An obese child is at risk for developing idiopathic increased intracranial pressure and pseudotumor cerebri, which may appear with severe headache and papilledema at presentation. Cerebrospinal fluid cell count and chemistry values will be normal.

Gastrointestinal

Non-Alcoholic Fatty Liver Disease

Up to 10% of overweight children have histologic evidence of hepatic steatosis, which may progress to steatohepatitis and, eventually, cirrhosis. Risk factors for non-alcoholic fatty liver disease (NAFLD) include Mexican and Asian ethnicities, as well as male sex. Though alanine transaminase (ALT) and aspartate aminotransferase levels are often increased, they have low sensitivity and specificity for detection of NAFLD. An ALT level increased 2 times the upper limit of normal, as well as a value greater than 100 U/L (>1.67μkat/L), are indications for consultation with a pediatric gastroenterologist.

Gallstones

As many as 2% of obese adolescents may develop gallstones. The risk is greatest in older teens, female subjects, Latinos, extremely obese subjects, and girls using oral contraceptives.

Musculoskeletal

Blount Disease

Blount disease is characterized by abnormal growth of the proximal tibial physis and is most common in African American and male subjects, occurring in up to 3% of obese preadolescent boys. It appears with progressive bowing (genu varum), gait disturbance, and arthritis at presentation.

Slipped Capital Femoral Epiphysis

An obese child is at increased risk for this condition, which requires immediate surgical correction. Consider a slipped capital femoral epiphysis (SCFE) in any overweight patient who presents with limp, hip pain, or referred knee pain (commonly medial).

Fractures

Obese children may be at increased risk of fractures, and they are also more prone to physeal fractures. Obesity is a risk factor for fractures that require external fixation.

Pharmacologic

Most pediatric medications are dosed on the basis of body weight, so that some obese children may require more than an adult dose of a particular drug. In addition, there may be significant variations in drug distribution and metabolism. In such cases, consultation with a clinical pharmacologist may be helpful.

Considerations Specific to Obesity in the Inpatient Setting

Obesity is associated with inflammation, weakened immune response, and increased length of stay after surgery. Obesity is a risk factor for higher mortality in children with critical illness, oncologic diagnoses, and transplants. Obese patients are at specific risk for encountering difficulties with airways and anesthesia, as well as developing venous thromboembolisms.

Airway

An obese patient is at increased risk for airway obstruction after administration of general anesthesia. Previously undetected obstructive sleep apnea or hypopnea may manifest, and incomplete ventilation during or after anesthesia may lead to ventilation/perfusion mismatch, hypoxemia, and hypercapnia. Although oximetry may be useful, a formal nocturnal polysomnography evaluation and consultation with a pulmonologist or otolaryngologist may be necessary. Extremely obese patients are also at risk for obesity hypoventilation syndrome (Pickwickian syndrome), in which the normal central response to hypercapnia is blunted, significantly increasing postanesthetic complications.

Infection

An obese child may be at increased risk for postinfectious complications as a result of the underlying metabolic derangement and the relatively avascular condition of adipose tissue. Give careful attention to skin hygiene and the potential presence of candidal infection (intertrigo).

Venous Thromboembolism

Venous thromboembolism seems to be increasing among pediatric patients (although there is currently no universally accepted screening tool for children). Risk factors include BMI greater than 30, surgery or trauma, smoking, prolonged immobility or length of stay (≥3 days), malignancy, respiratory disease, inflammatory bowel disease, hypercoagulable states (use of oral contraceptives), current or previous indwelling central venous catheter, history of thrombotic events, family history of hypercoagulability or thrombosis (eg, factor V Leiden), and musculoskeletal sepsis, osteomyelitis, or staphylo-coccal infections. See Chapter 5, Deep Venous Thrombosis, for determining when to screen or administer prophylaxis.

Pharmacologic

As noted earlier, most pediatric medications are dosed on the basis of body weight, so that obese children may require more than an adult dose. There may also be significant variations in pharmacokinetics in children when com-pared to adults, particularly for drugs that have a narrow therapeutic window. In contrast, the Broselow tape, which is frequently used in emergency settings, may lead to underestimation of weight in obese children.

Ergonomics

Standard-sized hospital equipment (blood pressure cuffs, wheelchairs, scales, etc) may be inadequate to meet the needs of an extremely obese patient. Infrequently, such patients may be unable to undergo routine procedures such as magnetic resonance imaging (due to weight or size limits) or echocardiography (due to thoracic diameter). Imaging modalities such as ultrasonography for appendicitis may also be more difficult to perform, which may then increase the need for abdominal computed tomography and its radiation exposure.

Approach to the Hospitalized Overweight or Obese Child

Management of acute illness often takes precedence over treating obesity. However, always consider the comorbidities and potential complications associated with obesity.

An important first step is to calculate the BMI, enter it into the patient's chart, and document whether the child is overweight or obese. Hospitaliza-tion for an acute illness may provide a "teachable moment" or motivation for a family or patient to consider lifestyle modification, particularly if the child is hospitalized for an obesity-related complication.

Obesity is emotionally charged. Approaching the child and family in a non-judgmental and empathetic manner can often begin a constructive discussion. Simply asking for the family or patient's permission to discuss weight (a prime tenet of motivational interviewing) may offer a more patient-centered approach and facilitate providing assistance with nutrition and exercise counseling. Consultation with a registered dietitian or physical therapist may be more accessible in the inpatient setting for some families and patients, particularly at tertiary centers. At discharge, there may also be opportunities to refer patients to a pediatric weight management program, if available.

Adolescent bariatric surgery is becoming more available and has generally been shown to be well tolerated and effective. However, challenges related to access and insurance coverage remain. Although weight loss medications continue to be introduced and prescribed for adults, only orlistat has been approved by the U.S. Food and Drug Administration for use in adolescents, and despite its relative safety, its minimal effectiveness and substantial side effects (steatorrhea) have generally limited its use.

Ample evidence exists that many health care professionals may be biased against overweight patients. Obese individuals report feeling stigmatized in health care settings, which can amplify vulnerability to depression and low self-esteem and dampen motivation to change. Unkind or insensitive comments made by hospital staff in the hospital environment and during procedures can affect the experience of the obese individual in the hospital setting. Having correct instruments and equipment is vital, while focusing on the patient, rather than the obesity, will ensure a more positive interaction.

Options for the Morbidly Obese Patient

Modalities available for this population include low-calorie diets, typically administered in liquid form, and bariatric interventions (such as gastric bypass and laparoscopic gastric banding). Refer the patient to an obesity center.

Indications for Consultation

- **Cardiology or nephrology:** Severe hypertension
- **Endocrinology:** PCOS, diabetes
- **Gastroenterology/liver:** Dyslipidemia, NAFLD
- **Neurology:** Increased intracranial pressure
- **Orthopedics:** Blount disease, SCFE
- **Psychiatry:** Disordered eating, depression, suicide
- **Pulmonology:** Obstructive sleep apnea, obesity hypoventilation syndrome
- **Surgery:** Gallstones

Pearls and Pitfalls

- Do not visually categorize a patient as overweight or obese without calculating the BMI.
- Do not overlook the opportunity to address lifestyle changes while the patient is admitted.

- Obese children cannot tolerate receiving nothing by mouth for a longer duration than a normal-weight patient.

Bibliography

Bechard LJ, Rothpletz-Puglia P, Touger-Decker R, Duggan C, Mehta NM. Influence of obesity on clinical outcomes in hospitalized children: a systematic review. *JAMA Pediatr*. 2013;167(5):476–482

Doyle SL, Lysaght J, Reynolds JV. Obesity and post-operative complications in patients undergoing non-bariatric surgery. *Obes Rev*. 2010;11(12):875–886

Estrada E, Eneli I, Hampl S, et al. Children's Hospital Association consensus statements for comorbidities of childhood obesity. *Child Obes*. 2014;10(4):304–317

Halvorson EE, Irby MB, Skelton JA. Pediatric obesity and safety in inpatient settings: a systematic literature review. *Clin Pediatr (Phila)*. 2014;53:975–987

King MA, Nkoy FL, Maloney CG, Mihalopoulos NL. Physicians and physician trainees rarely identify or address overweight/obesity in hospitalized children. *J Pediatr*. 2015;167(4):816–820

Rosenfeld RL. The diagnosis of polycystic ovary syndrome in adolescents. *Pediatrics*. 2015;136(6):1154–1165

Parenteral Nutrition

Introduction

Parenteral nutrition (PN) is a form of complete intravenous (IV) nutrition that bypasses the gastrointestinal tract. It is indicated for a patient who is unable to receive or tolerate adequate nutrition through an oral or enteral route, such as a child who has undergone bowel surgery, was born prematurely, or has short gut syndrome, severe pancreatitis, Stevens-Johnson syndrome, burns, or trauma. Nutrition is then provided in an IV solution that contains dextrose, protein, lipids, electrolytes, vitamins, and trace elements.

In comparison to an adult, a child has fewer energy and protein stores and can develop nutritional deficiencies more rapidly. In addition, the calorie and protein requirements for growth can significantly increase the nutrient demands, so that the need for PN often arises sooner in a child. If a patient will be receiving nil per os (NPO, nothing by mouth) for more than 3 days, some sort of nutritional support is indicated (enteral or parenteral). However, enteral feedings should resume as soon as the patient is able to tolerate adequate oral caloric intake.

Access

Ideally, achieve IV access selection well in advance of PN order writing. The delivery route will depend on the duration of PN therapy, calorie needs, and nutritional goals. *Peripheral* generally means that the catheter tip is in a vein other than the superior or inferior vena cava. Peripheral and midline catheters are not appropriate for vesicant chemotherapy, central PN solutions, medications with pH levels less than 5 or greater than 9, and solutions/medications with an osmolarity greater than 900 mOsm/L. Most institutions have policies and procedures regarding the osmolarity of a solution that may be delivered via peripheral vein. In general, peripheral PN solutions range from 10% to 12.5% dextrose and 2% to 2.5% amino acids. Electrolytes and minerals contribute to the final osmolarity of the solution, as well. Consult with a clinical pharmacist if there are any questions regarding the suitability of a solution for a peripheral line.

A central venous catheter is for long-term use in a patient who requires a PN solution with an osmolarity greater than 900 mOsm/L. In general, there are 4 types of catheters: peripherally inserted central catheter, nontunneled catheter, tunneled catheter, and totally implanted venous access (ports). The tips of these catheters reside in the superior or inferior vena cava and are therefore considered central. Discuss with the surgeon or interventional radiologist the goals of PN and the other needs for the central line to determine if a single, double, or triple lumen line is required. Advance planning can then save a patient from needless discomfort.

History and Physical Examination

The goals of PN and the patient's nutritional and medical status guide the decisions made regarding nutrient needs, mixture, and rate of delivery. First, assess whether or not the patient can tolerate enteral (oral or tube) feedings. If not, determine the patient's medical history, current nutritional status, expected duration of receiving NPO, and percentage of the total daily caloric requirement to be administered parenterally. Look for oral lesions, a murmur, hepatomegaly, and old surgical scars, because these may be important clues for ongoing medical problems, liver dysfunction, or need for fluid restriction. Next, assess the overall nutritional status and determine if the patient is malnourished or overweight.

Calculating PN

Minimum amounts of glucose, fat, and protein are required to prevent hypoglycemia, essential fatty acid deficiency, and hypoproteinemia, respectively. However, feeding the child an excess of these nutrients can be a factor in the development of hepatic steatosis, excessive carbon dioxide production, increased infection risk, or prerenal azotemia. In general, consider protein requirements first and then energy needs when determining PN (Table 90-1). A patient with a significant fluid restriction, for example, may need protein intake provided at the expense of decreasing energy intake. There are larger gains in protein accretion with increases in protein intake than with increases in energy intake. Unless a patient has renal or liver impairment or disease, there is no reason to limit initial protein intakes to less than calculated needs.

There can be considerable variation in intra- and interindividual, as well as day-to-day, energy needs. Energy requirements for the hospitalized child can be difficult to define accurately. With critically ill patients, in most cases the provision of resting energy is sufficient. The Dietary Reference Intake (DRI) values (Table 90-1) may lead to overestimation of the caloric requirements for a given patient. Thus, an initially conservative approach to calorie delivery will minimize overfeeding or excessive weight gain. Use the tables as a starting point, to be adjusted on the basis of the pediatric dietitian's assessment and the patient's response to treatment.

PN calculations are often complex; therefore, it is important to have a consistent and reproducible system. Although each hospital uses a

Table 90-1. Estimated Energy and Protein Requirements for Infancy Through Adolescence[a]

	Age	Reference Weight (kg)[b]	Reference Height (cm)[b]	Basal Metabolic Rate (kcal/kg/d)[c]	DRI: Energy Based on EER With PAL = Sedentary		DRI: Protein	
					kcal/d	kcal/kg/d		DRI: Protein
Infants	0–2 mo	NA	NA	NA	NA	NA	NA	1.52[d]
	2–3 mo	6	62	54	610	102	9.1	1.52[d]
	4–6 mo	6	62	54	490	82	9.1	1.52[d]
	7–12 mo	9	71	51	720	80	11	1.2[e]
	13–35 mo	12	86	56	990	82	13	1.05[e]
Young boys	3 y	12	86	57	1019	85	13	1.05[e]
	4–5 y	20	115	48	1405	70	19	0.95[e]
	6–7 y	20	115	48	1279	64	19	0.95[e]
	8 y	20	115	48	1186	59	19	0.95[e]
Young girls	3 y	12	86	55	986	82	13	1.05[e]
	4–5 y	20	115	45	1291	65	19	0.95[e]
	6–7 y	20	115	45	1229	61	19	0.95[e]
	8 y	20	115	45	1183	59	19	0.95[e]

Continued

Chapter 90: Parenteral Nutrition

Table 90-1. Estimated Energy and Protein Requirements for Infancy Through Adolescence[a], continued

	Age	Reference Weight (kg)[b]	Reference Height (cm)[b]	Basal Metabolic Rate (kcal/kg/d)[c]	DRI: Energy Based on EER With PAL = Sedentary		DRI: Protein	
					kcal/d	kcal/kg/d		
Older male subjects	9–11 y	36	144	36	1756	49	34	0.95[e]
	12–13 y	36	144	36	1601	45	34	0.95[e]
	14–16 y	61	174	29	2385	39	52	0.85[e]
	17–18 y	61	174	29	2230	37	52	0.85[e]
	>18 y	70	177	28	2550	36	56	0.8[e]
Older female subjects	9–11 y	37	144	33	1550	42	35	0.95[e]
	12–13 y	37	144	32	1491	40	35	0.95[e]
	14–16 y	54	163	26	1890	33	46	0.85[e]
	17–18 y	54	163	26	1684	31	46	0.85[e]
	>18 y	57	163	22	1939	34	46	0.8[e]

Abbreviations: DRI, Dietary Reference Intake; EER, estimated energy requirement; NA, not applicable; PAL, physical activity level.

[a] This table is meant to be a quick-reference guide because calculations are based on reference heights and weights. Therefore, some calculations reflect the average between sex and age groups.

[b] Reference weights and heights were taken from Institute of Medicine. *Dietary Reference Intakes: The Essential Guide to Nutrient Requirements Divided Into Smaller Groupings*. Washington, DC: Institute of Medicine; 2006.

[c] Estimates are based on Schofield equations for calculating basal metabolic rate in children.

[d] Adequate intake.

[e] Recommended daily allowance.

somewhat different system to calculate PN, there are a number of key steps for ensuring that the appropriate PN is delivered to the patient. Contact the nutrition service to get assistance with the local ordering system.

PN Order Writing

1. Assess protein and energy requirements: Estimate the energy requirements by using the resting energy expenditure or DRI listed in Table 90-1. If the patient is adequately nourished, use the actual weight in kilograms. Use the ideal body weight (weight for patient length or BMI at the 50th percentile) if the patient is malnourished and needs additional energy for catch-up growth. For an obese patient (>150% ideal body weight), use an adjusted or ideal weight to determine energy needs. The protein requirement may range from the DRI (Table 90-1) to a greater value, depending on the individual requirements (Table 90-2).

2. Maintenance fluid requirements: Calculate the maintenance IV fluid requirement based on the patient's weight, body surface area, medical condition, and any ongoing losses.

3. Determine contribution of energy from fat, dextrose, and amino acids: Order a solution that delivers 20% to 30% of the calories from fat and 60% to 70% from the dextrose and amino acid solution. In general, an appropriate solution has 40% to 60% of the calories from dextrose and a glucose infusion rate (GIR) of 6 to 14 mg/kg/min.

4. Volume of lipid: Divide the energy required from fat (in kcal/d) by 2 kcal/mL to determine the milliliters per day of lipid. This will usually result in an initial fat delivery rate of 2 to 5 mL/kg/d. Increase in a stepwise fashion to a goal of 5 to 10 mL/kg/d, or approximately 30% of the daily caloric intake. Generally, a patient will tolerate 20% to 40% of total calories supplied by the fat emulsion, but avoid more than 50% to 60%, which may result in ketosis. One determinant of the rate of fat clearance is the amount infused per unit time. Thus, the longer the infusion time, the less likely the patient will experience intolerance (hypertriglyceridemia). IV fat may be administered on the same day as amino acid and dextrose initiation.

5. Determine the energy density for amino acid–dextrose solution: From Table 90-3, choose the desired concentrations of amino acids and dextrose.

6. Volume for amino acid–dextrose solution: Divide the energy from amino acids and dextrose (from Step 3) by the energy density of the solution (Table 90-3). Compare the protein provided with estimated protein needs (grams per day).

7. Total protein (grams) $\times$ 100 = % protein (milliliters of amino acid/% dextrose)

8. Determine electrolyte dosages (Table 90-4).

9. The addition of the vitamins, minerals, and trace elements is body weight based. Most hospitals will automatically add these to PN.

10. For advancing PN, see Table 90-5.

Table 90-2. Protein Needs Are Estimated on the Basis of ASPEN Clinical Guidelines[a]

Age	Protein Recommendations (g/kg/d)
0–2 y	2.5–3.0
2–13 y	1.5–2.0
13–18 y	1.5

Abbreviation: ASPEN, American Society for Parenteral and Enteral Nutrition.

[a] Adapted from Mehta NM, Compher C; A.S.P.E.N. Board of Directors. A.S.P.E.N. clinical guidelines: nutrition support of the critically ill child. *JPEN J Parenter Enteral Nutr.* 2009;33(3):260–276.

Table 90-3. Energy Density of Solution[a]

Percentage Dextrose	Percentage Amino Acids								
	1.0%	2.2%	2.4%	2.8%	3.0%	3.5%	4.0%	5.0%	6.0%
7.5%	0.30	0.34	0.36	0.37	0.38	0.40	0.42	0.46	0.50
10%	0.38	0.43	0.44	0.45	0.46	0.48	0.50	0.54	0.58
12.5%	0.47	0.51	0.51	0.54	0.55	0.57	0.59	0.63	0.67
15%	0.55	0.60	0.61	0.62	0.63	0.65	0.67	0.71	0.75
17.5%	0.64	0.68	0.69	0.71	0.72	0.74	0.89	0.80	0.84
20%	0.72	0.77	0.78	0.79	0.80	0.82	0.84	0.88	0.92
25%	0.89	0.94	0.95	0.96	0.97	0.99	1.01	1.05	1.09
30%	1.06	1.11	1.1	1.13	1.14	1.16	1.18	1.22	1.26
35%	1.23	1.28	1.29	1.30	1.31	1.33	1.35	1.39	1.43
40%	1.40	1.45	1.46	1.47	1.48	1.50	1.52	1.56	1.60

Values are kilocalories per milliliter of total PN.

[a] Adapted from Texas Children's Hospital. *Pediatric Nutrition Reference Guide.* 9th ed. Houston, TX: Texas Children's Hospital; 2010.

Table 90-4. Parenteral Nutrition Electrolyte Dosing Guidelines[a,b]

Electrolyte	Preterm Neonate	Full-Term Neonate, Infant, and Child	Child or Adolescent >50 kg
Sodium	2–5 mEq/kg	2–5 mEq/kg	1–2 mEq/kg
Potassium	2–4 mEq/kg	2–4 mEq/kg	1–2 mEq/kg
Calcium	2–4 mEq/kg	0.5–4.0 mEq/kg	10–20 mEq/d
Phosphorus	1–2 mmol/kg	0.5–2.0 mmol/kg	10–40 mmol/d
Magnesium	0.3–0.5 mEq/kg	0.3–0.5 mEq/kg	10–30 mEq/d
Acetate	As needed to maintain acid-base balance		
Chloride	As needed to maintain acid-base balance		

To convert milliequivalents to millimoles for sodium and potassium levels, multiply by 1.0. To convert milliequivalents to millimoles for calcium and magnesium levels, multiply by 0.5.

[a] Adapted from Mirtallo J, Canada T, Johnson D, et al. Safe practices for parenteral nutrition. *JPEN J Parenter Enteral Nutr.* 2004;28(6):S39–S70. © 2004 by SAGE Publications. Reprinted by permission of SAGE Publications, Inc.

[b] Assumes normal organ function and losses.

Table 90-5. Recommendations for Initiation and Advancement of Parenteral Nutrition[a]					
	Initiation		**Advancement**		**Goals**
Neonates and Infants (<1 y of age)					
	Preterm	Term	Preterm	Term	Preterm	Term
Protein	1.5–3.0 g/kg/d	1 g/kg/d	1 g/kg/d	1 g/kg/d	3–4 g/kg/d	2–3 g/kg/d
Carbohydrate	5–7 mg/kg/min	6–9 mg/kg/min	1.0%–2.5% dextrose/d	1–2 mg/kg/min or 2.5%–5.0% dextrose/d	8–12 mg/kg/min; maximum, 14–18 mg/kg/min	12 mg/kg/min; maximum, 14–18 mg/kg/min
Fat	1–2 g/kg/d	1–2 g/kg/d	0.5–1.0 g/kg/d	0.5–1.0 g/kg/d	3.0–3.5 g/kg/d; maximum, 0.17-g/kg/h	3 g/kg/d; maximum, 0.15-g/kg/h
Children (1–10 y of age)					
Protein	1–2 g/kg/d		1 g/kg/d		1.5–3.0 g/kg/d	
Carbohydrate	10% dextrose		5% dextrose/d		8–10 mg/kg/min	
Fat	1–2 g/kg/d		0.5–1.0 g/kg/d		2–3 g/kg/d	
Adolescents					
Protein	0.8–1.5 g/kg/d		1 g/kg/d		0.8–2.5 g/kg/d	
Carbohydrate	3.5 mg/kg/min or 10% dextrose		1–2 mg/kg/min or 5% dextrose per day		5–6 mg/kg/min	
Fat	1 g/kg/d		1 g/kg/d		1.0–2.5 g/kg/d	

[a] Adapted from Corkins MR, ed. *The A.S.P.E.N. Pediatric Nutrition Support Core Curriculum.* Silver Spring, MD: American Society for Parenteral and Enteral Nutrition; 2010. Republished with permission of American Society for Parenteral and Enteral Nutrition; permission conveyed through Copyright Clearance Center, Inc.

Complications

The exact rate of PN-related complications is unknown, but there are several factors that increase the risk: intestinal resection, recurrent episodes of infection, lack of enteral feedings, or overfeeding of carbohydrate or protein. These complications can be categorized as metabolic, mechanical, and infectious. Metabolic complications include electrolyte abnormalities related to refeeding syndrome (significant decreases in potassium, phosphorous, and magnesium), liver disease (varies from minimal, with transient increases in liver-related blood tests, to biliary cirrhosis to liver failure), drug nutrient interactions (furosemide, amphotericin B), or metabolic acidosis. The risk of developing refeeding syndrome is higher in younger patients and those who have gone more than 5 to 10 days with little or no nutritional intake. Mechanical problems include line occlusions related to precipitants (calcium and phosphorus, drug or lipid), blood clots, line fractures (caused by excessive pressure), and kinks in the line.

Monitoring PN

Monitoring PN includes the routine assessment of metabolic factors, as well as growth, developmental, and psychological parameters (Table 90-6). Initial laboratory assessment is based on the patient's nutritional status, medical condition, and medications. Subsequently, measure the serum electrolyte and blood sugar levels daily until full PN is achieved and the electrolyte levels are stable. Pay meticulous attention to blood-drawing procedures. Discontinue all fluid infusions prior to phlebotomy, minimize the blood volumes withdrawn, and time these measurements with the middle or latter end of the PN infusion to minimize spurious results. In addition, limiting entry into the line will decrease the risk of developing iatrogenic bloodstream infections.

An initial or baseline measurement of serum protein, calcium, magnesium, phosphorous, and triglyceride levels may be helpful in some patients (eg, malnutrition, liver or renal disease, sepsis). A patient with significant malnutrition or liver or metabolic diseases or a patient at risk for refeeding syndrome may require more frequent monitoring of some electrolyte and mineral levels.

Glucose

Monitoring the urine glucose and blood glucose levels, as well as calculating the GIR (milligrams of glucose per kilogram of body weight per minute) is important for minimizing the potential complications of overfeeding with this nutrient. Insulin increases potassium, magnesium, and phosphorous uptake by the cells. Therefore, these minerals will also need to be monitored frequently with insulin use. Measure blood glucose level in a patient receiving cyclic (<24 hours) PN at the beginning, middle, and end of the cycle to assess tolerance.

Fat

A malnourished patient will have a decreased capillary mass and, as a result, less lipoprotein lipase, which resides there. Therefore, a malnourished patient will have a slower rate of lipid clearance. IV fat tolerance may need to be monitored more frequently than suggested in Table 90-6 in such a patient.

Protein

Traditional protein monitors (albumin, prealbumin, transthyretin, transferrin) can be influenced by inflammation, end-stage liver disease, or renal disease. Therefore, every patient receiving PN requires an individualized monitoring regime based on the disease state and nutritional goals. For example, in liver disease, the serum ammonia level may need to be followed if the patient has increased direct bilirubin and transaminase levels. In a patient with short gut,

Table 90-6. Monitoring Parenteral Nutrition in Pediatrics[a]

Parameter	Initial	Follow-up
Growth		
Weight	Daily	Daily to monthly
Length/stature	Weekly to monthly	Monthly
Head circumference	Weekly	Weekly to monthly
Body composition	Monthly	Monthly to annually
Metabolic: serum		
Electrolytes	Daily to weekly	Weekly to monthly
BUN/creatinine ratio	Weekly	Weekly to monthly
Ca, PO$_4$, Mg	Twice weekly	Weekly to monthly
Acid/base	As indicated until stable	Weekly to monthly
Albumin/prealbumin	Weekly or every other week	Every 2 wk to monthly
Glucose	Daily to weekly	Weekly to monthly
Triglyceride	Daily with changes	Weekly to monthly
Liver function	At 2 wk	Weekly to monthly
CBC	Weekly	Weekly to monthly
PT/PTT and platelets	Weekly	Weekly to monthly
Iron indices	As indicated	Every 3–4 mo
Trace elements	Monthly	Every 6–12 mo
Fat-soluble vitamins	As indicated	Every 6–12 mo
Carnitine	As indicated	Every 6–12 mo
Folate/vitamin B$_{12}$	As indicated	Every 6–12 mo
Ammonia	As indicated	As indicated
Metabolic: urine		
Glucose/ketones	2–6 times per day	Daily to weekly
Specific gravity Urea nitrogen	As indicated	As indicated
Other		
Bone density	As Indicated	As indicated
Verify line placement	As indicated with growth	Every 6–12 mo
Developmental	Monthly	Every 6–12 mo
Occupational therapy Physical therapy	At 1 mo, as indicated	Annually

Abbreviations: BUN, blood urea nitrogen; Ca, calcium; CBC, complete blood cell count; Mg, magnesium; PO$_4$, phosphate; PT, prothrombin time; PTT, partial thromboplastin time.

[a] Adapted with permission from Davis AM. Initiation, monitoring, and complications of pediatric parenteral nutrition. In: Baker RD Jr, ed. *Pediatric Parenteral Nutrition.* New York, NY: Springer; 1997:212–237.

malabsorption, or protein-losing enteropathy, there may be an increased loss of enteric protein, so that monitoring fecal α1-antitrypsin excretion may be useful in assessing protein losses and determining whether the patient would benefit from additional protein intake. The blood urea nitrogen level can also be used if renal function and hydration are normal.

Liver Function Tests

Liver injury is associated with PN therapy. Monitor liver function (aspartate transaminase, alanine transaminase, γ-glutamyltransferase, and bilirubin levels; prothrombin time; and partial thromboplastin time) if the patient receives PN for 2 weeks or longer. A patient with liver disease or no enteral intake will need more frequent assessments (weekly or more frequently).

Pearls and Pitfalls

- Vitamin, mineral, and amino acid shortages make PN order writing a challenge. Maintain an ongoing dialogue with the nutrition support team and clinical pharmacist to be informed about product unavailability. The American Society for Parenteral and Enteral Nutrition (http://www. nutritioncare.org/) has up-to-date guidelines for all PN product shortages.
- Iron is not routinely added to PN solutions. A patient receiving long-term (>1 month) PN may need IV iron infusions if unable to tolerate oral intake.
- Sodium bicarbonate is contraindicated in PN solutions because it will change the pH level of the solution and may result in calcium/phosphorous precipitation. Sodium or potassium acetate may be added, but some patients may require additional bicarbonate administration through a separate line.

Bibliography

American Academy of Pediatrics Committee on Nutrition. Enteral nutrition. In: Kleinman RE, Greer FR, eds. *Pediatric Nutrition*. 7th ed. Elk Grove Village, IL: American Academy of Pediatrics; 2014:591–608

Boullata JI, Gilbert K, Sacks G, et al; and American Society for Parenteral and Enteral Nutrition. A.S.P.E.N. clinical guidelines: parenteral nutrition ordering, order review, compounding, labeling, and dispensing. *JPEN J Parenter Enteral Nutr*. 2014;38(3):334–377

Corkins MR, ed. Parenteral nutrition support. In: Corkins MR, ed. *The A.S.P.E.N. Pediatric Nutrition Support Core Curriculum*. 2nd ed. Silver Spring, MD: American Society for Parenteral and Enteral Nutrition; 2015:593–614

Gargasz A. Neonatal and pediatric parenteral nutrition. *AACN Adv Crit Care*. 2012;23(4):451–464

Singla S, Olsson JM. Enteral nutrition. In: Perkin RM, Swift JD, Newton DA, Anas NG, eds. *Pediatric Hospital Medicine.* 2nd ed. Philadelphia, PA: Lippincott Williams & Wilkins; 2008:797–808

Texas Children's Hospital. Pediatric nutrition support (infants-adolescents). In: Bunting DK, Mills J, Ramsey E, Rich S, Trout S. *Pediatric Nutrition Reference Guide.* 10th ed. Houston, TX: Texas Children's Hospital; 2013

Verger J. Nutrition in the pediatric population in the intensive care unit. *Crit Care Nurs Clin North Am.* 2014;26(2):199–215

Ophthalmology

Acute Vision Loss

Introduction

Acute vision loss may be secondary to intrinsic (cornea, lens, anterior chamber, vitreous, retina) or extrinsic (optic nerve, optic chiasm, visual cortex) eye pathologic conditions. The most likely causes include trauma, infection, inflammation, and mass effect. Specific etiologies range from the relatively benign (eg, migraine) to the life-threatening (eg, hemorrhage into intracranial tumor). Visual deficits may be readily reversible if managed properly or potentially permanent if the patient does not receive expeditious treatment. True ophthalmologic emergencies that appear with acute vision loss at presentation and require immediate ophthalmologist consultation include alkali or acid burns, ruptured globe, and central retinal artery occlusion.

Clinical Presentation

History

Ask about any recent trauma, conjunctival injection, ocular discharge, photophobia, monocular versus binocular symptoms, and presence and quality of pain. Assess the patient for systemic symptoms, including fever, headache, and nausea/vomiting, as well as any neurologic changes (concurrent or past). Relevant past medical history includes sickle cell disease, hypercoagulable states, and migraines. Very young children may have difficulty verbalizing vision loss, but parents may be able to detect subtle acute visual changes based on the patient's behavior.

Physical Examination

If there is a concern for a ruptured or lacerated globe, place a hard shield over the affected eye and obtain an emergent ophthalmologic evaluation. Otherwise, first check the visual acuity in each eye by using a near-vision card. If testing is unsuccessful, check the ability to discern light or fingers at a close distance. In the hospital setting, check the visual acuity daily to monitor the patient for changes.

Evaluate the external structures for trauma, periorbital swelling, proptosis, and conjunctival injection. Assess the patient for full and painless extraocular movements, as well as pupillary appearance and reaction to light. A Marcus Gunn pupil, or relative afferent pupillary defect, is seen with optic nerve damage or severe retinal disease. Evaluation of the visual fields is important to diagnose a homonymous defect seen in retrochiasmal pathologic processes. Perform a funduscopic examination to evaluate the patient for papilledema, vitreous or retinal hemorrhage, retinal detachment, or general pallor (as seen in central retinal artery occlusion). Perform a slit lamp examination to assess the clarity of the cornea, anterior chamber, lens, and vitreous.

Perform a thorough neurologic examination to assess the patient for concurrent deficits.

Laboratory Workup

In many cases, routine laboratory testing and imaging are not indicated. If uveitis or retinitis is diagnosed at physical examination, order laboratory testing to evaluate the patient for an underlying etiology, including syphilis serologic testing, Lyme titers, purified protein derivative, and antinuclear antibodies. A lumbar puncture with opening pressure is indicated if there is a concern for a central nervous system (CNS) disease, such as meningitis or idiopathic intracranial hypertension.

Radiology Examinations

Perform contrast-enhanced computed tomography of the brain and orbits in cases of orbital trauma and orbital cellulitis; image only the orbits if there is global trauma or a suspected intraocular foreign body. Perform contrast-enhanced magnetic resonance (MR) imaging of the brain and orbits if an extrinsic cause of vision loss (optic neuritis, optic or CNS tumor) is a concern.

Differential Diagnosis

There are 3 primary clinical distinctions to differentiate among the causes of acute vision loss: traumatic versus atraumatic, monocular versus binocular, and painful versus painless. Traumatic vision loss may be related to traumatic iritis, hyphema, optic nerve avulsion, vitreous hemorrhage, retinal detachment, or a perforated globe.

Vision loss does not always appear with ocular abnormalities at presentation, because it may represent a neurovisual pathway disorder, ranging from optic chiasmal pathologic conditions to other CNS diseases. In the absence of trauma, binocular vision loss suggests a retrochiasmal lesion.

Acute vision loss can often be associated with a red eye, which can be painful or painless. Uveitis can be secondary to an underlying systemic illness, such as juvenile idiopathic arthritis. In addition, conjunctivitis (from various etiologies), chemical burns, keratitis, acute glaucoma, and endophthalmitis can present similarly.

Common and emergent causes of acute vision loss are summarized in Table 91-1.

Table 91-1. Common and Emergent Causes of Acute Vision Loss	
Diagnosis	**Clinical Features**
Central retinal artery occlusion	Painless monocular vision loss Retinal pallor Relative afferent pupillary defect
Chemical injury	Photophobia, blepharospasm Ischemia of the conjunctiva Altered pH level of the ocular surface
Endophthalmitis	Painful, red eye Hypopyon (exudate in the anterior chamber) seen at slit lamp examination
Glaucoma	Painful, red eye; photophobia Corneal clouding Buphthalmos (enlarged eye)
Idiopathic intracranial hypertension	Headache worse in the morning and with the Valsalva maneuver Papilledema Intermittent visual loss
Intracranial tumor	Acute vision loss typically caused by hemorrhage into tumor Lack of ocular abnormalities May have other neurologic deficits at examination
Keratitis	Painful, red eye Ocular discharge Corneal opacity Foreign-body sensation
Migraine	Headache, aura Nausea and vomiting
Optic neuritis	Monocular painful eye Papillitis Associated with multiple sclerosis and neuromyelitis optica Relative afferent pupillary defect
Orbital cellulitis	Fever, toxic appearance Proptosis, chemosis Decreased and painful extraocular motility
Retinal detachment	Typically occurs after trauma Floaters and flashes of light (photopsia) Painless Elevated retinal folds at funduscopic examination
Ruptured globe	Occurs after direct trauma Teardrop-shaped pupil distortion
Uveitis	Painful or painless, depending on the location Constricted and irregular pupil Leukocytes seen in the anterior chamber at slit lamp examination
Vitreous hemorrhage	Typically occurs after trauma Obscuration of red reflex or retina at funduscopic examination

Treatment

Treatment will generally be determined by the consulting ophthalmologist, along with neurology and/or neurosurgery consults, depending on the underlying etiology. Acute vision loss caused by an intracranial mass may be life threatening and requires urgent neurosurgical consultation and management.

The treatment of a perforated globe (see Chapter 92, Ocular Trauma), orbital cellulitis (see Chapter 18, Orbital and Periorbital Cellulitis), and chemical burns (see Chapter 92, Ocular Trauma) is detailed elsewhere in this text.

Indications for Consultation

- **Neurology:** Migraines, optic neuritis (multiple sclerosis, neuromyelitis optica)
- **Neurosurgery:** Suspected intracranial mass, subdural hematoma or abscess
- **Ophthalmology:** Acute vision loss
- **Otolaryngology:** Orbital cellulitis with sinusitis

Disposition

- **Intensive care unit transfer:** Increased intracranial pressure, need for acute neurosurgical intervention
- **Transfer to tertiary care hospital**: Immediate ophthalmology consult not available
- **Discharge criteria:** Visual acuity stable or improving with oral (or no) medication

Follow-up

- **Ophthalmology:** Daily or weekly, depending on the etiology
- **Other subspecialists (otorhinolaryngology, neurosurgery, neurology):** Depending on the etiology

Pearls and Pitfalls

- The 3 primary distinctions to make in determining the cause of acute vision loss are traumatic versus atraumatic, monocular versus binocular, and painful versus painless.
- True ophthalmologic emergencies that cause acute vision loss and require immediate consultation include alkali or acid burns, ruptured globe, and central retinal artery occlusion.
- Vision loss does not always appear with ocular abnormalities at presentation, particularly with lesions of the CNS.
- Atraumatic binocular vision loss typically represents a lesion in the retrochiasmal visual pathway.

Bibliography

Bagheri N, Mehta S. Acute vision loss. *Prim Care*. 2015;42(3):347–361

Beran DI, Murphy-Lavoie H. Acute, painless vision loss. *J La State Med Soc*. 2009;161(4): 214–216, 218–223

Cheng KP, Biglan AW. Opthalmology. In: Zitelli BJ, McIntire SC, Nowalk AJ, eds. *Zitelli and Davis' Atlas of Pediatric Physical Diagnosis*. 6th ed. Philadelphia, PA: Saunders/Elsevier; 2012:731–773

Dull KE. Eye: visual disturbances. In: Shaw KN, Bachur RG, eds. *Fleisher & Ludwig's Textbook of Pediatric Emergency Medicine*. 7th ed. Philadelphia, PA: Wolters Kluwer; 2016:170–175

Patel KN. Acute vision loss. *Clin Pediatr Emerg Med*. 2010;11(2):137–142

CHAPTER 92

Ocular Trauma

Introduction

Ocular trauma is the leading cause of noncongenital unilateral vision loss in children. Traumatic injury to the eye is classified as either open or closed globe. Open-globe injury refers to full-thickness injury to the cornea, sclera, or both. Open-globe injury can be further classified as laceration (penetrating, perforating, or intraocular foreign body) or rupture. The closed-globe category consists of contusion or lamellar (partial thickness) laceration.

Ocular injuries that require urgent care include ocular burns, an open globe, traumatic optic neuropathy, extraocular muscle entrapment (secondary to orbital fracture), rhegmatogenous (traumatic tear) retinal detachment, and retrobulbar hemorrhage.

In terms of chemical injuries, acids cause coagulation necrosis, resulting in corneal scarring and ulceration. Alkalis, which tend to be more severe injuries, lead to saponification of phospholipid layers, epithelial cell death, and caustic penetration of the cornea.

Clinical Presentation

History

With the exception of chemical injuries, where immediate treatment is the priority, obtain a detailed account of the injury, including time, location (periorbital, head), mechanism of injury, extent (how hard any impact was and how many times it occurred), and whether eye protection was in place, and screen for other associated injuries. Determine the patient's visual function prior to injury and inquire about prior head, periorbital, or ocular trauma and surgery.

Assess the pain level and qualifiers, changes in vision (decreased acuity, flashes, floaters, curtain), diplopia (monocular or binocular, variation with gaze), foreign-body sensation, tearing, and photophobia.

Obtain the patient's current medication list and past medical history, with special attention paid to history of hemoglobinopathies, bleeding disorders, and anticoagulation medications.

Physical Examination

Ocular trauma has a highly variable presentation and requires a comprehensive examination. Start with visual acuity, followed by general inspection, noting any injury to the eyelids or orbit, as well as the presence of asymmetry, proptosis, or a foreign body. Note ecchymoses and edema of periorbital soft tissues, subcutaneous emphysema, palpable step-off along the orbital rim, enophthalmos/hypoglobus, or lacerations of the globe or periorbital tissues. For lacerations external to the globe, assess whether there is lid margin or canalicular (medial to the puncta) involvement or violation of the septum (prolapsed orbital fat).

Examine the pupil, looking for an irregular shape consistent with globe rupture, or an afferent pupillary defect via the swinging light test, indicating significant retinal or optic nerve pathology. Check the extraocular movements, examine the anterior chamber (to look for blood), and if a ruptured globe is not suspected, perform a fluorescein test to look for corneal abrasions. If multiple linear abrasions are noted, evert the eyelids to check for a foreign body; a topical anesthetic may be necessary. If the patient cannot cooperate for a comprehensive examination, arrange for one to be performed with anesthesia.

One of the few true ocular emergencies is an open globe. This is a potentially sight-threatening and organ-threatening injury. However, at examination, a full-thickness violation of either the sclera or cornea is not always evident. Signs of a potential open globe include prolapse of uveal tissue, severe subconjunctival hemorrhage, deep or shallow anterior chamber, hyphema (blood in the anterior chamber), peaked or irregular pupil, laceration of the cornea or sclera, and an intraocular foreign body. If the clinical picture is suspicious for an open globe, cover it with an eye shield but *do not* place pressure on the globe during examination, check ocular pressure or motility, or dilate the pupil.

Children may present with a white-eyed orbital blowout fracture, in which the eye is relatively well appearing and without obvious hemorrhage. Watch for symptoms of nausea, vomiting, and bradycardia, which may indicate the oculocardiac reflex, a sign of orbital injury. Greenstick fractures, or incomplete fractures of the orbit, are common in children because of increased elasticity of the bones. These orbital floor fractures create a trapdoor phenomenon, in which the bone bends and then retracts, entrapping and incarcerating soft tissue, causing decreased range of motion. Restriction in extraocular movements secondary to tissue entrapment is an urgent condition. Arrange for surgical correction within 48 hours to prevent ischemia and fibrosis.

Arrange for a slit lamp and dilated funduscopic examination to assess the anterior and posterior segments. This can be essential for diagnosing a variety of closed-globe injuries, including corneal abrasion, traumatic iritis, hyphema, commotio retinae, choroidal rupture, nonaccidental trauma, vitreous hemorrhage, and retinal detachment. Note that with nonaccidental trauma, external eye findings are frequently absent and should be considered in any infant who presents with persistent crying of unknown etiology.

Laboratory Workup

Obtain prothrombin time and partial thromboplastin time in any patient for whom a history cannot be obtained. If hyphema is observed, order a screen for sickle cell disease or trait. Sickle cell disease places the patient at greater risk of the complications of hyphema, such as increased intraocular pressure, nonclearing hyphema, and corneal blood staining.

Radiology Examinations

Imaging of choice for acute ocular trauma is unenhanced axial and coronal computed tomography (CT) of the face and orbits, with 1- to 2-mm sections. CT is helpful for assessing an open globe, traumatic optic neuropathy, entrapment secondary to orbital fracture, and retrobulbar hemorrhage. CT can also demonstrate the integrity and shape of the globe and the presence and location of intraocular foreign bodies. Magnetic resonance (MR) imaging is contraindicated if a metallic retained foreign body is suspected, but MR imaging may be helpful in the case of nonmetallic foreign body, once metallic exposure has been ruled out. Bedside ultrasonography may also be helpful if the patient is too unstable to undergo other radiologic examinations.

Diagnosis

The diagnosis of ocular trauma is summarized in Table 92-1.

Table 92-1. Diagnosis of Ocular Trauma	
Diagnosis	**Clinical Features**
Corneal abrasion	Pain, tearing, photophobia (+) Fluorescein test
Ocular burn	Corneal perforation ↓ Visual acuity
Open globe	Irregularly shaped or peaked pupil Uveal tissue prolapse Patient may have associated hyphema
Orbital fracture	Patient may have limitation of upward gaze and/or diplopia Numbness of cheek, upper lip, teeth (floor fracture) Numbness of scalp and forehead (roof fracture) Oculocardiac reflex
Retinal detachment, lens dislocation	Floaters, flashes of light, photophobia Blurred vision
Retrobulbar hemorrhage	Proptosis Afferent pupillary reflex defect

"+" indicates a positive finding.

Treatment

In general, consult an ophthalmologist for any ocular trauma, except for a superficial corneal abrasion and if there is no concern for herpes simplex infection.

If there is an ocular burn, immediately perform a prolonged irrigation of the eye. Use normal saline or lactated Ringer solution for irrigation. Obtain a pH level of the eye 5 to 10 minutes after the initial 30 minutes of irrigation. Stop the irrigation if the pH level is neutral (7.0) and recheck in 10 minutes. If the pH level is not neutral, perform another 30 minutes of irrigation. Use a Morgan Lens if no foreign body is suspected; otherwise, use intravenous (IV) tubing to flush fluids into the affected eye. If topical anesthesia is needed, administer 1 to 2 drops of proparacaine 0.5% to the affected eye.

If the clinical picture is suspicious for an open globe, place a Fox Eye Shield *(do not patch or apply pressure)* over the traumatized eye. Determine the time of the patient's last meal, give the child nothing by mouth, raise the head of the bed to 30°, administer anti-emetics (ondansetron 0.1 mg/kg per dose as needed every 6 hours; maximum, 8 mg per dose) and IV analgesia (morphine, see Chapter 115, Pain Management), and update the patient's tetanus status. Perform orbital CT to rule out intraocular foreign body. Administer IV antibiotics, vancomycin (15 mg/kg every 6 hours; maximum, 1.5 g per dose) *and* ceftazidime (50 mg/kg every 8 hours; maximum, 2 g per dose), for antimicrobial coverage of *Bacillus,* coagulase-negative *Staphylococcus, Staphylococcus aureus, Streptococcus,* and gram-negative bacteria. Consult with an ophthalmologist, because urgent surgery is necessary.

Entrapment secondary to orbital fracture requires urgent surgery within 48 hours to avoid ischemia and fibrosis. Other indications for orbital fracture repair include enophthalmos greater than 2 mm, greater than 50% floor fracture, and functional diplopia secondary to restriction with positive forced duction test findings.

Retrobulbar hemorrhage requires emergent intervention within 60 to 120 minutes if it causes changes in vision or pupils or increased intraocular pressure. Consult an ophthalmologist about performing lateral canthotomy and inferior cantholysis.

Consult an ophthalmologist for recommendations of medical management of both traumatic iritis and hyphema. Patients with hyphema will be followed up closely because of the risk of secondary complications, such as rebleeding, increased intraocular pressure, and corneal blood staining.

Remove a superficial corneal foreign body with irrigation, a moistened cotton-tip swab, or a needle tip under slit lamp guidance. However, always assess the patient for a full-thickness penetration prior to foreign body removal. Also evert the eyelids and sweep the fornices for particulate matter. Treat a simple corneal abrasion with topical antibiotics and a topical nonsteroidal anti-inflammatory, such as 1 drop of ketorolac 4 times a day. Treat corneal abrasion in patients who do not wear contact lenses with erythromycin ointment 0.5%, 4 times a day for 3 to 5 days. Treat corneal abrasion in patients who wear contact lenses with antipseudomonal coverage, such as ofloxacin 0.3%, 1 to 2 drops every 2 hours while awake, and refer the patient to an ophthalmologist for daily follow-up.

A lid laceration, especially involving the lower lid canaliculus, requires surgical intervention. Depending on the time of the injury and macular involvement, a retinal detachment may also require urgent surgical intervention.

If there is suspicion for nonaccidental trauma, as evidenced by retinal hemorrhages, for example, assess the patient for other potential injuries, contact the local child protective services agency (see Chapter 102, Child Abuse and Neglect), and admit the patient to the hospital pending investigation.

Indications for Consultation

- **Child protection services:** Inflicted or suspected nonaccidental trauma
- **Facial trauma surgical team (may be oral and maxillofacial surgery, otolaryngology, or plastic surgery):** Orbital or facial fractures
- **Neurosurgery:** Orbital roof fracture
- **Ophthalmology:** Acute vision loss with any cause, open globe, orbital fracture with entrapment, lid laceration, retrobulbar hemorrhage

Disposition

- **Interinstitutional transfer:** Subspecialty services not immediately available
- **Discharge criteria:** Vision stable, surgical issues resolved, appropriate follow-up arranged

Follow-up

- **Primary care:** 1 to 2 days
- **Ophthalmology:** Varies, depending on the nature of the injuries

Pearls and Pitfalls

- An open globe, entrapment secondary to orbital fracture, retinal detachment, and retrobulbar hemorrhage all require urgent surgical intervention.
- Maintain a high index of suspicion for open-globe injury and order CT to confirm.

- Watch for white-eyed blow-out fracture and carefully assess the patient for motility restriction, decreased pulse, and other signs of parasympathetic surge in the context of orbital fracture.
- Investigate any abnormality or any change in the ocular vitals: vision, pupils, and intraocular pressure.
- Corneal abrasion in a contact lens wearer requires antipseudomonal coverage and daily ophthalmology follow-up.

Bibliography

Al Shetawi AH, Lim CA, Singh YK, Portnof JE, Blumberg SM. Pediatric maxillofacial trauma: a review of 156 patients. *J Oral Maxillofac Surg*. 2016;74(7):1420

Broyles JM, Jones D, Bellamy J, et al. Pediatric orbital floor fractures: outcome analysis of 72 children with orbital floor fractures. *Plast Reconstr Surg*. 2015;136(4):822–828

Hammond D, Grew N, Khan Z. The white-eyed blowout fracture in the child: beware of distractions. *J Surg Case Rep*. 2013;2013(7):rjt054

Kanski JJ, Bowling B. *Clinical Ophthalmology: A Systematic Approach*. 7th ed. New York, NY: Elsevier Saunders; 2011:871–896

Lipke KJ, Gümbel HO. Emergency treatment of ocular trauma. *Facial Plast Surg*. 2015;31(4):345–350

Messman AM. Ocular injuries: new strategies in emergency department management. *Emerg Med Pract*. 2015;17(11):1–21

Ophthalmoplegia

Introduction

Opthalmoplegia, or paralytic strabismus, is a disorder of ocular motility. It is caused by abnormalities of the ocular motor nerves, ocular muscles, or neuromuscular transmission. Opthalmoplegia may be congenital or acquired.

Clinical Presentation

Acute ophthalmoplegia reaches maximum intensity within 1 week of onset. The key symptom is diplopia.

History

Obtain a thorough history, including onset of symptoms, associated symptoms, precipitating events, and underlying medical conditions, if any. Specifically ask about fever, emesis, headache, pain with eye movements, eyelid redness and swelling, recent infections, possible drug/toxin ingestion, confusion, and history of eye trauma or sinus disease.

Physical Examination

Signs can vary, depending on etiology, and may include limitation of and painful extraocular eye movements, mydriasis, proptosis, facial nerve palsy, signs of meningeal irritation, and altered mental status. Look for cranial nerve palsy, including oculomotor nerve palsy (cranial nerve III; mydriasis, eye deviated down and out, ptosis), trochlear nerve palsy (cranial nerve IV; vertical diplopia that may be corrected by a head tilt), and abducens nerve palsy (cranial nerve VI; esotropia or limited lateral gaze). Perform a funduscopic examination for papilledema.

Laboratory Workup/Imaging

Choose laboratory testing based on the history and physical examination findings.

- Infectious process: Complete blood cell count and differential, C-reactive protein level and/or erythrocyte sedimentation rate, and, in the proper clinical context when central nervous system (CNS) disease is suspected, collection of cerebrospinal fluid for cell count, chemistry assessment, and culture
- Vascular diseases, including hemorrhage and thrombosis: Coagulation

studies and, in the proper clinical context, hypercoagulability panel
- Myopathies: Creatine kinase and other muscle enzymes (lactate dehydrogenase, alanine aminotransferase, aspartate aminotransferase, aldolase)
- Drug/toxic ingestion: Electrocardiogram and urine and plasma toxicologic evaluation
- Increased intracranial pressure (ICP): Lumbar puncture for opening pressure; when the physical examination is concerning for increased ICP, perform neuroimaging first

Radiology Examinations

Neuroimaging is indicated. Most aneurysms will be seen on contrast-enhanced magnetic resonance (MR) images or MR angiography images. MR imaging will demonstrate brainstem glioma and orbital tumors. MR venography is useful for demonstrating absence of flow into cerebral venous sinuses. Contrast-enhanced computed tomography of orbit and paranasal sinuses will demonstrate orbital cellulitis and a subperiosteal abscess.

Differential Diagnosis

Causes of acute ophthalmoplegia include pathologic processes of the brainstem (encephalitis, intoxication, multiple sclerosis, subacute necrotizing encephalopathy, tumor, vascular abnormality) or ocular motor nerves (increased intracranial pressure, infectious process, inflammatory process, postinfectious origin, trauma, tumor, vascular abnormality). Other causes include abnormalities of neuromuscular transmission (botulism, myasthenia gravis, tick paralysis) and myopathies (Kearns-Sayre syndrome, mitochondrial myopathies, orbital inflammatory disease, thyroid disease).

Treatment

Obtain urgent ophthalmology consultation, especially if the patient has painful ophthalmoplegia. Neurologist (for CNS or neuromuscular disease) and otolaryngologist (for orbital cellulitis, subperiosteal abscess) involvement may also be necessary. Treatment depends on the etiology and findings at neuroimaging.

For infectious processes, begin empirical antibiotic therapy with vancomycin (40–60 mg/kg/d, divided into doses administered every 6–8 hours; 4-g/d maximum) *plus* ceftriaxone (100 mg/kg/d, divided into doses administered every 12 hours; 4-g/d maximum). Add metronidazole (30–40 mg/kg/d, divided into doses administered every 8 hours; 2-g/d maximum) if anaerobic coverage is indicated. An alternative regimen is the combination of vancomycin (as detailed herein) *plus* ampicillin/sulbactam (300 mg/kg/d, divided into doses administered every 6 hours; 8-g/d maximum). If an abscess or fluid collection is identified, arrange for urgent surgical drainage.

If an orbital tumor or other oncologic disease is possible, also consult with a hematologist-oncologist. Emergent neurologist and/or neurosurgeon involvement is necessary for a patient with a vascular disease, including vascular malformations, hemorrhage, infarction, and thrombosis.

Disposition

- **Intensive care unit transfer:** Hemodynamic instability, worsening altered mental status
- **Discharge criteria:**
  - **Infectious process:** Diplopia has resolved, fluid collection (if any) has been surgically drained, length and route of outpatient antibiotic administration has been determined
  - **Increased ICP, tumors, vascular diseases, and disorders of neuro-muscular transmission:** There is no new neurologic deficit (establishing new baseline mental status is important), appropriate inpatient surgical and medical treatment is completed, and, if neurologic deficits resulted in loss of function or diminished physical capability, appropriate consultation with physical medicine and rehabilitation service are arranged

Follow-up

- **Primary care:** 1 week
- **Surgical specialist, neurology, hematology-oncology:** Within 1 to 2 weeks

Pearls and Pitfalls

- The history and physical examination will dictate laboratory and imaging studies in patients who present with acute ophthalmoplegia.
- For most patients, involvement of a multidisciplinary team will be necessary.

Bibliography

Gerstenblith AT, Rabinowitz MP. *The Wills Eye Manual: Office and Emergency Room Diagnosis and Treatment of Eye Disease*. 6th ed. Philadelphia, PA: Lippincott Williams & Wilkins; 2012:153–176

Kaiser PK, Friedman NJ. *The Massachusetts Eye and Ear Infirmary: Illustrated Manual of Ophthalmology*. 4th ed. Philadelphia, PA: Saunders/Elsevier; 2014:1–32

Piña-Garza JE. Disorders of ocular motility. In: Piña-Garza JE, ed. *Fenichel's Clinical Pediatric Neurology*. 7th ed. Philadelphia, PA: Saunders/Elsevier; 2013:295–312

Red Eye

Introduction

Pediatric "red eye" is one of the most common inpatient ophthalmologic diagnoses. It describes a large range of infectious or inflammatory conditions that may originate from the lids, conjunctiva, cornea, iris, sclera, or other internal ocular tissues. Serious etiologies of red eye include infectious conjunctivitis in a newborn, keratoconjunctivitis, foreign body, orbital trauma, and systemic or autoimmune diseases. Recognition of the need for emergent referral to an ophthalmologist is critically important.

Clinical Presentation

History

Obtain a thorough history of ocular and systemic symptoms, including onset and duration of symptoms, associated trauma, visual changes, photophobia, discharge, burning, pain, itching, and constitutional symptoms. Also ask about contact lens use, ocular medications, prior ophthalmologic surgery, and past episodes of red eye.

Physical Examination

First, observe the patient's spontaneous eye movements. Note areas of color change, edema, or discharge in the periorbital region, conjunctiva, and sclera. Use a light source to directly evaluate the pupil size and reactivity. Assess the presence, symmetry, and color of the red reflex with a direct ophthalmoscope in a dimly lit room. Assess visual acuity, if the patient is able. Perform a fluorescein stain examination to rule out a corneal abrasion/ulcer or herpes keratitis. Evert the lid to look for the presence of a foreign body.

Differential Diagnosis

The priority is to expeditiously diagnose eye- or vision-threatening conditions. Warning signs include altered visual acuity, ocular pain, severe photophobia, excessive tearing, and a ciliary flush (Table 94-1).

Table 94-1. Differential Diagnosis of Red Eye	
Diagnosis	**Clinical Features**
Allergic conjunctivitis	Itching and tearing Conjunctival bogginess and injection
Blepharitis	Most common among school-aged children Chronic burning and itching but no discharge Can be associated with a chalazion
Chemical conjunctivitis	Starts in the first 24 h of life Bilateral watery discharge and bulbar injection
Congenital glaucoma	Photophobia, blepharospasm Buphthalmos (enlargement of the eyeball) ↑ Intraocular pressure
Corneal abrasion/ulcer	Pain, tearing, blepharospasm (+) Fluorescein test ↓ Visual acuity
Dacryocystitis	Fever Erythema, swelling, and tenderness lateral to the medial canthus
Herpes keratoconjunctivitis	Pain, photophobia Vesicles on the eyelids (+) Fluorescein test
Hyphema	Pain and photophobia History of blunt ocular trauma
Infectious conjunctivitis	Bacterial: copious purulence at the lid margin Viral: watery discharge, upper respiratory infection prodrome
Keratitis	Pain, photophobia Conjunctival hyperemia (+) Fluorescein test
Ophthalmia neonatorum (chlamydial)	Starts in the first 5–14 d of life Watery to mucopurulent discharge (+) Direct fluorescent antibody or enzyme-linked immunosorbent assay
Ophthalmia neonatorum (gonococcal)	Starts in the first 2–5 d of life Hyperacute purulent discharge Chemosis, eyelid edema Gram stain: gram-negative diplococci
Orbital cellulitis	Fever Pain, proptosis, chemosis, impaired ocular movements, ↓ vision or optic nerve dysfunction
Preseptal cellulitis	Fever Pain, swelling
Scleritis	Pain, ↓ vision Violet discoloration of the globe Anterior chamber inflammation
Subconjunctival hemorrhage	Confluent, bright red patch Does not extend past the limbus
Systemic disease related	Features are related to the specific disease, such as erythema multiforme, Kawasaki disease, Stevens-Johnson syndrome, Reiter syndrome, sarcoidosis, tuberculosis, etc
Uveitis	Pain, photophobia, redness with ciliary flush Constricted and irregular pupil ↓ Visual acuity

"+" indicates a positive finding.

Laboratory Workup

Routine laboratory testing is unhelpful in most cases of red eye. If there is a purulent discharge, particularly in the first 2 weeks of life, swab for culture and Gram stain. If gonococcal ophthalmia neonatorum is suspected, perform a full sepsis workup, including a lumbar puncture. In cases of uveitis or scleritis, obtain a complete blood cell count with differential, C-reactive protein level or erythrocyte sedimentation rate, antinuclear antibody level, rheumatoid factor, and uric acid level. When a systemic disease is being considered, perform the appropriate tests for assigning that diagnosis.

If herpes infection is suspected in an infant younger than 6 weeks, obtain herpes simplex virus DNA via polymerase chain reaction from the serum and cerebrospinal fluid. In addition, obtain swabs of the mouth, oropharynx, conjunctiva, rectum, and any surface lesions. Also perform liver function tests and obtain urine for herpes culture.

Treatment

Because of the highly specialized nature of treatment, consult an ophthalmologist prior to initiating therapy for glaucoma, uveitis, scleritis, or infectious/noninfectious corneal disease. If ocular herpes infection is suspected, immediately initiate intravenous (IV) acyclovir (60 mg/kg/d, divided into doses administered 3 times a day) for 14 days. Add a topical ophthalmic antiviral agent (1% trifluridine, 0.1% iododeoxyuridine, 3% vidarabine).

Neonatorum ophthalmia is an ocular emergency and warrants urgent ophthalmology consult. Treat with either IV or intramuscular (IM) ceftriaxone (25–50 mg/kg every day, 125-mg maximum) or IV or IM cefotaxime (50 mg/kg every 12 hours if patient is <7 days old, every 8 hours if patient is >7 days old). Order sterile saline eye irrigations every 2 hours to keep the eye surface clear of debris, discharge, and obstruction. Treat chlamydia with oral erythromycin (50 mg/kg/d, divided into doses administered every 6 hours) for 14 days.

Treat acute dacryocystitis with either ampicillin/sulbactam (150 mg/kg/d, divided into doses administered every 6 hours; 8-g/d maximum) or cefuroxime (100 mg/kg/d, divided into doses administered every 8 hours; 4.5-g/d maximum). If methicillin-resistant *Staphylococcus aureus* is a concern, add clindamycin (40 mg/kg/d, divided into doses administered every 6 hours; 4.8-g/d maximum) or vancomycin (40 mg/kg/d, divided into doses administered every 6 hours; 4-g/d maximum) after performing cultures of the discharge. Warm compresses may help with disease resolution. Immediate ophthalmology consultation is indicated.

Treat conjunctivitis with a topical antibiotic ointment (bacitracin, polymyxin B, tobramycin) or solution (ciprofloxacin, ofloxacin, polymixin B, tobramycin) applied 3 times a day. Use a fluoroquinolone (ciprofloxacin, ofloxacin) when treating a *Pseudomonas* corneal ulcer or conjunctivitis in a contact lens wearer.

See Chapter 18 for the treatment of preseptal and orbital cellulitis.

Indications for Consultation

Ophthalmology: Moderate or severe ocular pain, abnormal pupil size, altered visual acuity, severe photophobia, excessive tearing, ciliary flush, corneal opacity, ophthalmia neonatorum, ocular herpes, dacryocystitis

Disposition

Discharge criteria: Good response to treatment, identification and sensitivity of infection (if any) known, close ophthalmology follow-up arranged

Pearls and Pitfalls

- Proceed with caution when adding steroids to the treatment regimen for infectious conjunctivitis because herpes keratitis will worsen.
- Antibiotic ointment is preferred in children because of difficulty with achieving appropriate antibiotic levels with drops.
- If drops are prescribed, apply them to the inner canthus (eye closed for best dosing).
- Suspect a bleeding disorder or nonaccidental trauma if a patient has recurrent or large subconjunctival hemorrhages.

Bibliography

Beal C, Giordano B. Clinical evaluation of red eyes in pediatric patients. *J Pediatr Health Care*. 2016;30(5):506–514.

Palejwala NV, Yeh S, Angeles-Han ST. Current perspectives on ophthalmic manifestations of childhood rheumatic diseases. *Curr Rheumatol Rep*. 2013;15(7):341

Seth D, Khan FI. Causes and management of red eye in pediatric ophthalmology. *Curr Allergy Asthma Rep*. 2011;11(3):212–219

Wong MM, Anninger W. The pediatric red eye. *Pediatric Clin N Am*. 2014;61(3):591–606

White Eye (Leukocoria)

Introduction

The red reflex is a simple, yet imperative, screening test for pediatric ocular disease. Leukocoria is a white pupillary light reflex caused by pathologic processes in the lens, vitreous, or retina. It may represent significant ocular pathology and warrants urgent ophthalmologic referral.

Clinical Presentation

History

Leukocoria is predominantly diagnosed at physical examination. The abnormal red reflex, however, may first be noticed on a photograph of the child, when one pupil appears red while the other is darker or white. Ask about prenatal and postnatal exposures (infections, medications), eye trauma, exposure to animals, and family history of ocular tumors or cataracts.

Physical Examination

Check the red reflex in a dimly lit room by using the largest white light of an ophthalmoscope from a distance of 2 to 3 feet. Visualize both eyes and compare the red reflex size and color. With leukocoria, the center of one or both eyes will have a bright white appearance, although in some patients this may appear dull, gray, or black. In addition, there may be racial differences in the appearance of the red reflex, so that in a deeply pigmented patient a normal finding may be a lighter or silver reflex.

Differential Diagnosis

The most common causes of leukocoria are cataracts, persistent fetal vasculature, Coat disease, and retinoblastoma. Cataracts lead to partial or total blindness if not treated and may be caused by infection (rubella, toxoplasmosis, cytomegalovirus, syphilis), medications (corticosteroids), genetic syndromes, and galactosemia. Retinoblastoma, the most common intraocular tumor of childhood, appears at 1 to 2 years of age and has an excellent survival rate if diagnosed early. Less common causes of leukocoria include retinopathy of prematurity, toxocariasis, traumatic or atraumatic vitreous hemorrhage, and coloboma.

Treatment

Immediately consult an ophthalmologist if there is any suspicion of leukocoria.

Indications for Consultation

- **Pediatric ophthalmologist:** All patients
- **Pediatric hematologist/oncologist:** Any suspicion of retinoblastoma

Disposition

Discharge criteria: Evaluation complete and appropriate treatment plan arranged

Pearls and Pitfalls

- Failure to dim the lights in the examination room may yield false-negative red reflex results.
- Racial differences in the pupillary light reflex may lead to a false-positive leukocoria test result.
- Immediately consult an ophthalmologist for leukocoria.

Bibliography

Cheng KP, Biglan AW. Opthalmology. In: Zitelli BJ, McIntire SC, Nowalk AJ, eds. *Zitelli and Davis' Atlas of Pediatric Physical Diagnosis*. 6th ed. Philadelphia, PA: Saunders/Elsevier; 2012:731–773

Damasco VC, Dire DJ. A child with leukocoria. *Pediatr Emerg Care*. 2011;27(12):1170–1174

Olitsky SE, Hug D, Plummer LS, Stahl ED, Ariss MM, Lindquist TP. Disorders of the retina and vitreous. In: Kliegman RM, Stanton BF, St Geme JW III, Schor NF, eds. *Nelson Textbook of Pediatrics*. 20th ed. Philadelphia, PA: Elsevier; 2016:3049–3057

Patel N, Salchow DJ, Materin M. Differentials and approach to leukocoria. *Conn Med*. 2013;77(3):133–140

Varughese R, Frith P. Fifteen minutes consultation: a structured approach to the child with a white red reflex. *Arch Dis Child Educ Pract Ed*. 2014;99(5):162–165

Orthopedics

Fractures

Introduction

The 3 main causes of fractures are accidental trauma (most common), non-accidental trauma (child abuse), and abnormal bone (pathologic fractures). The most common fractures that necessitate inpatient treatment involve the femur, tibia-fibula, elbow (supracondylar fracture), and pelvis.

Fractures are categorized as displaced or nondisplaced and open or closed. In a displaced fracture, the bone snaps into 2 or more parts, which may be angulated and not aligned. If the bone is in many pieces, it is called a *comminuted fracture,* and future misalignment is a concern. In a nondisplaced fracture, the bone either partially or completely breaks but maintains its proper alignment. An open fracture is one in which the bone breaks through the skin, creating a portal of entry for infection. A closed fracture is when the bone breaks but there is no open wound in the skin.

The most serious direct complications of a fracture are infection, neurovascular compromise (most common with a supracondylar fracture), fat embolism, and compartment syndrome, which is secondary to ischemia caused by tissue pressure that exceeds the arteriolar and capillary pressures. The causes of compartment syndrome include hematoma, soft-tissue swelling, and crushing or high-energy injuries.

Clinical Presentation

History

Attempt to determine the mechanism of injury. Ask about the type and direction of the injuring force, the position of the involved body part(s) at that time, and the events immediately following the incident. Other important information includes whether there was any treatment in the field, ongoing medical conditions, previous orthopedic injuries (particularly at the same site), and chronic medication use. Also ask about any underlying disorders that could predispose the patient to pathologic fractures, such as known bone cysts, osteogenesis imperfecta, chronic steroid use, and other causes of osteopenia. Finally, an inflicted injury or child abuse is a concern when the mechanism of injury does not adequately explain the type or severity of the fracture found, the fracture is inconsistent with the patient's developmental capabilities, there was an unusual delay in seeking medical care, or the patient has a history of previous unexplained fractures.

Physical Examination

Most often, the patient is status post an attempt at reducing the fracture or awaiting either a surgical reduction or resolution of the swelling to allow for optimal reduction. Whether the attempt was successful or not, there will be swelling at the fracture site, which raises the risk for compartment syndrome. Perform a thorough neurovascular examination, including strength and capillary refill distal to the fracture site, which in some cases may be very distal because of the presence of a cast or splint. Check the skin under the edges of a cast for any possible areas of friction. Also check active and passive ranges of movement because pain may be elicited with passive stretching of the muscles within the swollen compartment. Note, however, that pulselessness and pallor can also be secondary to a vascular injury without compartment syndrome, although pain out of proportion to the injury or increasing pain despite adequate analgesia is particularly concerning for the development of compartment syndrome.

A femur fracture has the additional risk of significant loss of blood into the thigh. Measure the circumference at a fixed point on the thigh at admission, then repeat every 8 hours.

If the patient is status post fracture reduction, address the resultant rotation, length, and angulation. Although these are usually assessed by the orthopedic team, the postreduction examination must include evaluation for correction of any rotational displacement. Length can be assessed with radiography, while angulation of the long bones is rarely an issue because angles less than 20° to 30° will self-resolve.

Laboratory Workup

If the patient has a femur fracture, obtain a complete blood cell count as a baseline value to monitor for continuing blood loss. The need for other laboratory testing for underlying bone abnormalities is dictated by the clinical circumstances, with the possible exception of an evaluation for inflicted trauma (see Chapter 102, Child Abuse and Neglect). Do not perform a wound culture of an open fracture before surgical intervention.

Radiology Examinations

Although imaging is usually performed prior to hospital admission, it is important to review the pre- and postreduction images. Further imaging may be necessary if there is ongoing severe pain at the fracture site, since most pain is relieved by reduction and stabilization.

Computed tomography (CT) may be useful in cases of displaced or angulated fractures, complex intra-articular fractures (especially of the ankle), and vertebral and pelvic fractures.

Diagnosis

As noted earlier, consider possible inflicted injury or child abuse if the mechanism of injury does not adequately explain the type or severity of the fracture found, if there was an unusual delay in seeking medical care, if there are unexplained fractures in different stages of healing, or if a patient younger than 1 year presents with rib fractures, spinous process fractures, or a fracture of the sternum. Other concerns include epiphyseal and metaphyseal fractures of the long bones and corner or "chip" fractures of the metaphysis in a patient under 1 year of age.

A nondisplaced fracture may not be evident on initial plain radiographs. If there is significant suspicion for a fracture because of extreme pain, limited use of the affected extremity, or mechanism of injury, perform CT or magnetic resonance imaging acutely or follow-up radiography in 10 to 14 days to look for callous formation.

Complications

Some complications are particularly associated with certain types of fractures—for example, nonunion of tibial fractures, thromboembolism and hemorrhagic shock with pelvic fractures, and neurovascular compromise secondary to brachial artery or median nerve injury with supracondylar fractures. Persistence of intense pain after fracture reduction may be an indication of ischemia, compartment syndrome, or neurovascular compromise.

Compartment Syndrome

The signs of compartment syndrome are reduced pulse or capillary refill time, paresthesia, pain out of proportion to the severity of injury, pallor of the distal part of the affected extremity, reduced sensation, and increasing need for analgesia. The most reliable signs are hyperesthesia and increasing pain with passive stretching of the muscles within the compartment. Decreased pulse may not manifest until late in the process, although the absence of a pulse is not necessarily a danger sign, and the presence of a pulse does not guarantee that ischemia will be avoided. Maintain a high index of suspicion because not all of these signs need to be present to diagnose compartment syndrome.

Fat Embolism

Fat embolism and respiratory distress syndrome can occur in a patient with a femur or significant pelvic fracture. The risk increases if surgical repair is delayed more than 24 hours.

Treatment

Analgesia

For moderate to severe pain in a patient with no cardiovascular or central nervous system contraindications, administer intravenous (IV) or subcutaneous morphine (0.1 mg/kg per dose every 4 hours to start, then increase the dose or frequency as needed; maximum, 2 mg per dose for an infant, 4–8 mg per dose for a child, and 15 mg per dose for an adolescent). If a patient 5 to 7 years of age requires morphine more frequently than every 2 hours, either change to patient-controlled analgesia (see Chapter 115, Pain Management) or add IV ketorolac (1 mg/kg per dose every 6 hours; maximum, 15 mg per dose for 8 doses). Effective analgesia will not obscure physical findings and may increase cooperation during the examination.

Fever and Infection

The risk of a surgical site infection (SSI) increases when surgical hardware (nails and fixator pins) is placed into the area or when the patient has an open fracture. For this reason, irrigation and debridement are vitally important. Often the orthopedist will request skin prophylaxis (per local preference) for open reductions or hardware placement. See Chapter 97, Osteomyelitis, for the antibiotic treatment of an SSI.

"Bone fever" can occur in the hours immediately after reduction, then spontaneously resolve. High fever or subsequent spikes, increased pain and swelling, and discharge from the wound or hardware sites are signs of potential infection. Although pin sites can have some serosanguinous discharge initially, it is never purulent. Discourage the patient from using any devices to scratch under the cast, which can create abrasions. Order use of an incentive spirometer to promote respiratory expansion in a postoperative or sedated patient.

Neurovascular Monitoring

The key to preventing neurovascular injury is frequent neurovascular checks. Correct mild edema by maintaining elevation of the affected extremity above the level of the heart, although this will not prevent true compartment syndrome. Urgent management consists of removal of any splint or cast.

Continued or worsening symptoms are an emergency that requires surgical consultation and intervention.

Fat Embolism

The treatment for fat embolism is supportive care, possibly in an intensive care unit (ICU).

Deep Venous Thrombosis

Deep venous thrombosis prophylaxis remains controversial but is indicated for at-risk patients. (See Chapter 5, Deep Venous Thrombosis.)

Pressure Ulcers and Immobilization

In general, children tolerate immobilization well because they do not have underlying peripheral vascular disease and they continue to move as much as possible. Nevertheless, skin ulcers can occur. Pay particular attention to the areas underneath the ends of a hard cast and attempt to relieve other pressure spots by using special mattresses and frequently turning the nonmobile patient.

Other risks of prolonged immobilization are constipation and hypercalciuria. If a prolonged period of immobilization is expected, immediately begin a bowel regimen. In addition, ensure that the patient is undergoing appropriate physical therapy.

Hypercalciuria is a common cause of microscopic hematuria in an immobilized child. Obtain a weekly spot calcium/creatinine ratio (see Chapter 75, Nephrolithiasis) to screen for hypercalciuria, defined as a calcium/creatinine ratio greater than 0.21.

A problem unique to a patient in a hip spica cast is hypertension, thought to be caused by pressure on autonomic ganglia. Ensure that the cast is scooped off of the abdomen.

Indications for Consultation

- **Child abuse team:** Suspected nonaccidental trauma
- **Orthopedics:** Urgently for any fracture at risk for or with the symptoms of neurovascular compromise
- **Pain team/anesthesiology:** Difficulty providing adequate analgesia
- **Physical therapy:** As needed, for crutch training and help with other activities of daily living that may be limited by casts or hardware
- **Vascular surgery:** Any concern about vascular compromise

Disposition

- **ICU transfer:** Compartment syndrome, respiratory distress due to fat emboli
- **Interinstitutional transfer:** Pediatric orthopedic specialist not available locally for a patient with a complex fracture
- **Discharge criteria:** Fracture reduced, no risk for neurovascular compromise, pain controlled with oral medication

Follow-up

- **Primary care:** 1 to 2 weeks
- **Orthopedics:** 1 to 2 weeks

Pearls and Pitfalls

- Persistence of intense pain after fracture reduction may be an indication of ischemia from compartment syndrome.
- Always obtain a repeat radiograph after reduction.
- Properly treated physeal injuries are still at risk for longitudinal or angular abnormalities. This is particularly true for the distal femur, proximal tibia, and radial head or neck.
- In a case where nonaccidental trauma is strongly suspected, reporting it to the state child protective services agency is mandatory.
- After crutch training has been performed, document that the patient has demonstrated safe crutch use.
- Document neurovascular check results before and after surgery.

Bibliography

Arora R, Fichadia U, Hartwig E, Kannikeswaran N. Pediatric upper-extremity fractures. *Pediatr Ann.* 2014;43(5):196–204

Brousil J, Hunter JB. Femoral fractures in children. *Curr Opin Pediatr.* 2013;25(1):52–57

Chasm RM, Swencki SA. Pediatric orthopedic emergencies. *Emerg Med Clin North Am.* 2010;28(4):907–926

Flaherty EG, Perez-Rossello JM, Levine MA, Hennrikus WL; American Academy of Pediatrics Committee on Child Abuse and Neglect; Section on Radiology, American Academy of Pediatrics; Section on Endocrinology, American Academy of Pediatrics; Section on Orthopaedics, American Academy of Pediatrics; Society for Pediatric Radiology. Evaluating children with fractures for child physical abuse. *Pediatrics.* 2014;133(2):e477–e489

Flynn JM, Skaggs, DL, Waters PM. *Rockwood and Wilkins' Fractures in Children.* 8th ed. Wolters Kluwer; 2015

Wall CJ, Lynch J, Harris IA, et al; Liverpool (Sydney) and Royal Melbourne Hospitals. Clinical practice guidelines for the management of acute limb compartment syndrome following trauma. *ANZ J Surg.* 2010;80(3):151–156

Weinstein SL, Flynn JM. *Lovell and Winter's Pediatric Orthopaedics.* 7th ed. Lippincott Williams & Wilkins; 2014

Osteomyelitis

Introduction

Osteomyelitis is most often caused by hematogenous seeding of bacteria into the bone matrix. Other mechanisms include trauma or presence of foreign material (eg, spinal rods). In an older child, the thick periosteum may contain the infection and result in a subperiosteal abscess. In contrast, the thin periosteum of an infant allows inflammation to spread to surrounding tissues (myositis). In a patient under 18 months of age, end-loop capillaries feeding the immature epiphyses increases the risk of epiphyseal osteomyelitis and contiguous septic arthritis.

Approximately 90% of cases occur in the metaphyses of long bones (femur, tibia, humerus), 6% to 8% in the pelvis (ischium, ilium), and 1% to 3% in the vertebrae. Chronic osteomyelitis (>3 weeks in duration) results from insufficiently treated acute osteomyelitis, infection with an unusual pathogen, or a predisposing mechanism of injury (pressure ulcers, trauma). Complications of osteomyelitis include subperiosteal abscess, myositis, secondary bacteremia, pathologic fracture, growth disturbance, and fistula.

Methicillin-sensitive *Staphylococcus aureus* (MSSA) and methicillin-resistant *S aureus* (MRSA) are together the most common pathogen in all age groups, followed by group A β-hemolytic *Streptococcus* (*Streptococcus pyogenes*) in children and group B *Streptococcus* (*Streptococcus agalactiae*) in infants. Coagulase-negative staphylococci are associated with foreign bodies and implants.

Gram-negative and atypical pathogens are less common and are usually implicated in specific clinical situations: unvaccinated subjects (*Haemophilus influenzae* type b); toddlers (*Kingella kingae*); cat scratches or bites (*Bartonella henselae*); rat bites (*Streptobacillus moniliformis* or *Spirillum minus*); reptile or fowl exposures (*Salmonella* species); sickle cell disease (*Salmonella* species); neonates, diabetics, or intravenous (IV) drug users (*Enterobacteriaceae*, yeast, *Listeria monocytogenes*); mammalian bites (*Pasteurella, Capnocytophaga, Eikenella* species); and foot puncture wounds (*Pseudomonas aeruginosa*).

Clinical Presentation

History

In acute long-bone osteomyelitis, the patient presents with a few days of fever and either a limp or decreased use of the limb, although an infant or disabled child may only have subtle pseudoparalysis of the affected limb.

Pelvic osteomyelitis causes buttock or deep perineal pain and refusal to bear weight or sit. Vertebral osteomyelitis leads to back or abdominal pain, decreased back flexion and extension, and decreased weight bearing. Mandibular osteomyelitis presents with localized swelling and trismus. In contrast, chronic osteomyelitis at any site progresses over weeks and may not significantly affect function.

Ask about exposure to *S aureus* and possible MRSA risk factors, unpasteurized milk, tuberculosis, and animals (kittens, puppies, rodents, reptiles, amphibians, fowl). Ask about a history of furuncles, trauma, bite wounds, contaminated wounds, pressure ulcers, foreign material, travel, recent dental work, asplenia, and whether any family members are health care workers or have had a MRSA infection. Check the patient's vaccination status.

Physical Examination

Acute osteomyelitis presents with point tenderness, erythema, warmth, and/ or swelling over the bone. These classic symptoms can be subtle or absent, particularly when the affected limb is large because of muscle mass or obesity. Pelvic osteomyelitis causes hip tenderness, in addition to localized bone pain. At presentation, vertebral osteomyelitis appears with leg pain, focal bone back tenderness, and neurologic signs of the lower extremities that may suggest spinal cord irritation. Referred pain is common in a child, so examine the joint above and below the affected area. Indolent progression in a minimally weight-bearing, nontoxic preschooler suggests *K kingae* infection. Chronic osteomyelitis appears with point tenderness at presentation but may lack swelling or warmth, although a draining fistula is sometimes present. Finally, carefully examine all other bone sites to exclude a multifocal infection.

Laboratory Workup

If osteomyelitis is suspected, obtain a complete blood cell count, erythrocyte sedimentation rate (ESR), C-reactive protein (CRP) level, and blood culture prior to starting antibiotics (yield 30%–55% in acute osteomyelitis). Leukocytosis is present in about one-third of cases, while CRP level and ESR are increased in more than 90% of cases of acute osteomyelitis but may be normal in chronic osteomyelitis. In acute, febrile osteomyelitis, blood cultures obtained prior to treatment are positive for infection in up to 50% of patients. If possible, arrange for a bone aspirate for culture (65%–70% positive) prior to starting antibiotics. A bone biopsy sample sent for culture and pathologic evaluation is indicated if there is an unusual history (penetrating trauma, foreign body, treatment failure, mandibular involvement) or unusual risk factors (gram-negative organism, tuberculosis, immunocompromised host).

Radiology Examinations

Obtain plain radiographs to look for a fracture, neoplasm, and signs of inflammation. Deep soft-tissue inflammation is evident on plain radiographs at more than 3 to 10 days; periosteal increase at more than 10 days; and cortical changes at 14 to 21 days. Adjacent joint space widening suggests effusion from contiguous septic arthritis. Magnetic resonance (MR) imaging is the most sensitive (82%–100%) and specific (75%–96%) modality for imaging bone marrow changes in acute and chronic osteomyelitis. Computed tomography (CT) is less sensitive and specific and involves ionizing radiation, although CT can be helpful when MR imaging is not an option or in cases of chronic osteomyelitis to identify cortical bone thickening, sclerotic changes, encroachment of the medullary cavity, and chronic draining sinuses.

A bone scan can be helpful when occult osteomyelitis is suspected but difficult to localize (eg, fever of unknown origin) or when MR imaging is not an option. Focal hyperperfusion, hyperemia, and bone uptake are present in osteomyelitis, although inadequate ossification limits its usefulness in young infants.

Ultrasonography (US) may be useful for guided aspiration of a subperiosteal abscess. In addition, US is not impeded by orthopedic implants.

Differential Diagnosis

Once osteomyelitis has been ruled out, consider other infectious and noninfectious causes (Table 97-1). Vaso-occlusive crises in sickle cell disease (see Chapter 50) may be difficult to distinguish from infection, so that dual therapy may be necessary. Often sickle cell pain occurs at multiple or "typical" sites. Otherwise, multiple, simultaneous sites of involvement suggest a common source (endocarditis) or a systemic inflammatory process (juvenile idiopathic arthritis; chronic recurrent multifocal osteomyelitis [CRMO]; synovitis, acne, pustulosis, hyperostosis, and osteitis [SAPHO]; psoriatic arthritis).

At presentation, CRMO appears with recurrent episodes of focal bone pain and swelling at different sites, bone inflammation at biopsy, and negative bone culture findings. SAPHO is an inflammatory syndrome that has recurrent bone involvement, in addition to skin findings. The typical patient is a young female subject who presents with associated palmoplantar pustulosis, psoriasis vulgaris, or acute neutrophilic dermatosis.

Table 97-1. Differential Diagnosis of Osteomyelitis	
Diagnosis	**Clinical Features**
Infectious osteomyelitis	
Brodie abscess or sequestrum	Chronic history Abnormal imaging finding
Septic arthritis	Erythema, warmth, and decreased range of motion of the affected joint Decreased range of motion Joint effusion
Noninfectious osteomyelitis	
Sickle cell vaso-occlusive crisis	At-risk patient Presence or absence of fever Pain in "typical" location(s) Pain may be diffuse rather than point tenderness
Trauma	(+) History No fever History of trauma can precede bacterial osteomyelitis
Bone neoplasm	Gradual onset Constitutional symptoms: weight loss, fatigue, fever Pain may be worse at night (+) Imaging (onion skin sign, starburst pattern)
Chronic recurrent multifocal osteomyelitis	Recurrent episodes of focal bone pain and swelling Multiple sites (-) Culture results, (+) inflammatory markers
Juvenile idiopathic arthritis	Prolonged, cyclic fevers Recurrent arthralgia/arthritis Morning stiffness (-) Culture results with (+) inflammatory markers
Langerhans cell histiocytosis	Failure to thrive Patient may have chronic seborrheic-like rash and/or otorrhea Lytic skull lesions
Leukemia	Abnormal complete blood cell count Patient may have pallor or bleeding Constitutional symptoms: weight loss, fatigue
Synovitis, acne, pustulosis, hyperostosis, and osteitis	Acne and pustulosis Synovitis, hyperostosis, osteitis (-) Cultures

"-" indicates a negative finding, "+" indicates a positive finding.

Treatment

If osteomyelitis is suspected, consult an orthopedic surgeon for diagnostic biopsy and therapeutic aspiration because identifying the causative pathogen will facilitate definitive treatment decisions. In a stable patient, performing a bone culture prior to administering antibiotics is preferred, although it is often not practical or feasible. Sterilization of bone in significant *S aureus* osteomyelitis is unlikely with 24 to 48 hours of antibiotic therapy. Therefore, antibiotic therapy may be initiated if treatment cannot be delayed, either because of the severity of the illness or the unavailability of a timely bone biopsy. Perform a blood culture prior to starting antibiotics.

For uncomplicated acute hematogenous osteomyelitis, choose empirical IV treatment based on local bacterial resistance. When MRSA prevalence is greater than 10%, start with IV clindamycin (40 mg/kg/d, divided into doses administered every 8 hours; 2.7-g/d maximum). Monotherapy with a first-generation cephalosporin or an anti-staphylococcal penicillin is *not an option* in areas where MRSA is prevalent.

The increased prevalence of clindamycin-resistant MSSA makes first-generation cephalosporin or anti-staphylococcal penicillin the preferred initial option in some areas, but use dual IV treatment with one of these agents *plus* clindamycin in severe cases. Options include oxacillin (150–200 mg/kg/d, divided into doses administered every 6 hours; 12-g/d maximum [but recent manufacturer labeling suggests a maximum daily dose of 6 g/d]) *or* cefazolin (100–150 mg/kg/d, divided into doses administered every 8 hours; 6-g/d maximum) *or* vancomycin (40–60 mg/kg/d, divided into doses administered every 6 hours; 4-g/d maximum; goal trough, 15–20 µg/mL). Do not use ceftriaxone as monotherapy for culture-positive *S aureus*.

Since an infant aged 2 months or younger is at risk for infection with gram-negative organisms, initiate empirical therapy with IV cefotaxime *and* (depending on the concern for MRSA) either vancomycin *or* an anti-staphylococcal penicillin (oxacillin or nafcillin).

Reassess the patient daily, provide adequate analgesia, and monitor improvement in clinical symptoms and resolution of inflammatory markers. Improvement typically begins within 48 hours and is significant in 3 to 5 days. A delay in resolution of inflammatory factors is associated with a poorer prognosis and suggests an ongoing focus of infection or antibiotic failure.

Transition the patient to oral therapy, guided by final susceptibilities, once the patient is afebrile, bearing weight, or using the affected extremity and has significantly decreased inflammatory markers (eg, 50% decrease from peak value or CRP level <2 mg/L [19.05 nmol/L]). Use a dose that is 2 to 3 times higher than that used for minor infections to achieve adequate blood levels and bone penetration.

Common choices for definitive oral therapy include clindamycin (40 mg/kg/d, divided into doses administered every 8 hours; 2.7-g/d maximum), cephalexin (150 mg/kg/d, divided into doses administered every 6 hours; 4-g/d maximum), penicillin VK (120 mg/kg/d, divided into doses administered every 4–6 hours; 3-g/d maximum), and amoxicillin (100–200 mg/kg/d, divided into doses administered every 6 hours; 3-g/d maximum).

Oral options without culture guidance include a first-generation cephalosporin, clindamycin, dicloxacillin (100 mg/kg/d, divided into doses administered every 6 hours; 2-g/d maximum), or linezolid (<12 years of age, 10 mg/kg every 8 hours; ≥12 years of age, 600 mg every 12 hours; maximum, 600 mg per dose). Doxycycline and trimethoprim-sulfamethoxazole may be less effective for *S aureus* osteomyelitis. *K kingae* is susceptible to cefazolin or ampicillin.

Treat chronic osteomyelitis with oral antibiotics (clindamycin or first-generation cephalosporin) or tailor the therapy to the results of any deep bone cultures. Obtain an infectious diseases consult to determine the treatment of complicated osteomyelitis (penetrating injury, pressure ulcer, or prosthetic material). Return of osteomyelitis symptoms warrants re-evaluation for repeat cultures, imaging, and possible debridement of bone sequestrate by an orthopedic surgeon.

Treat acute osteomyelitis for 4 weeks, but 6 weeks of therapy may be needed if the patient has extensive disease or a slow clinical response. Treat chronic osteomyelitis for 6 to 8 weeks or more, based on clinical improvement and resolution of laboratory test abnormalities. At follow-up, confirm that the CRP level and ESR have normalized (ESR will lag behind the CRP level) prior to discontinuing treatment.

Indications for Consultation

- **Orthopedics:** Suspected or confirmed osteomyelitis
- **Infectious diseases:** Unusual risk factors or failure to respond to empirical therapy

Disposition

- **Interinstitutional transfer:** Urgent orthopedic consultation not available, especially if there is a subperiosteal abscess
- **Intensive care unit transfer:** Possible bacterial sepsis, toxic appearance
- **Discharge criteria:** Patient afebrile for 24 hours or more, surgical issues resolved, return of baseline functioning of the extremity, antibiotics narrowed (if sensitivities known), home treatment arranged (if needed), and CRP level and ESR improving; oral antibiotics are preferred

Follow-up

- **Primary provider:** 1 week
- **Orthopedics:** 1 to 2 weeks
- **Infectious diseases:** 2 to 4 weeks, if involved
- **Physical therapy/rehabilitation:** As indicated

Pearls and Pitfalls

- Whenever possible, perform a biopsy and culture prior to initiating treatment.
- If there are multiple sites of suspected osteomyelitis, consider a common source (endocarditis) or a noninfectious etiology (rheumatologic, CRMO, SAPHO).
- Consider *K kingae* in toddlers and preschoolers who are in child care.
- Given the risks associated with peripherally inserted central catheters, oral therapy at discharge is preferred when an oral agent equivalent is available and tolerated.

Bibliography

Dodwell ER. Osteomyelitis and septic arthritis in children: current concepts. *Curr Opin Pediatr.* 2013;25(1):58–63

Keren R, Shah SS, Srivastava R, et al. Comparative effectiveness of intravenous vs oral antibiotics for postdischarge treatment of acute osteomyelitis in children. *JAMA.* 2015;169(2):120–128

Martin AC, Anderson D, Lucey J, et al. Predictors of outcome in pediatric osteomyelitis: 5 years experience in a single tertiary center. *Pediatr Infect Dis J.* 2016;35(4):387–391

Montgomery NI, Rosenfeld S. Pediatric osteoarticular infection update. *J Pediatr Orthop.* 2015;35(1):74–81

Peltola H, Pääkkönen M. Acute osteomyelitis in children. *N Engl J Med.* 2014;370(4): 352–360

Schallert EK, Kan JH, Monsalve J, Zhang W, Bisset GS 3rd, Rosenfeld S. Metaphyseal osteomyelitis in children: how often does MRI-documented joint effusion or epiphyseal extension of edema indicate coexisting septic arthritis? *Pediatr Radiol.* 2015;45(8): 1174–1181

Septic Arthritis

Introduction

Septic arthritis is a bacterial infection of the joint space and synovium, usually secondary to hematogenous seeding of bacteria into the joint capsule. Other mechanisms are contiguous extension from an adjacent osteomyelitis (10%–15%) and direct inoculation by penetrating trauma. In the infant, transepiphyseal vessels, present until 18 months of age, allow hematogenous extension of the infection from the epiphysis into the joint capsule. In older children and adolescents, septic arthritis may complicate osteomyelitis after rupture of a subperiosteal abscess, where the articular capsule extends over the periosteum (shoulder, elbow, hip, knee). About 50% of patients are 2 years or younger, and more than 90% of cases are monoarticular; the knee and hip are the most common sites, followed by the elbow, ankle, shoulder, wrist, and sacroiliac joints.

Staphylococcus aureus is the most common pathogen in all age groups, accounting for more than 50% of positive culture findings. Other common organisms are age related: in neonates, group B *Streptococcus, Escherichia coli,* and, rarely, *Listeria monocytogenes;* in infants, *Streptococcus pneumoniae;* in children, group A *Streptococcus, Haemophilus influenzae,* and *Kingella kingae;* and in adolescents, *Neisseria gonorrhoeae* and group A *Streptococcus.*

Consider other etiologies based on known or suspected risk factors: tick exposure (*Borrelia burgdorferi*); unvaccinated subject (*H influenzae* type b); exposure to reptiles, amphibians, or fowl (*Salmonella* species); sickle cell disease (*Salmonella* species); complement deficiency (*Neisseria meningitidis, Salmonella* species); mammalian bites (*Pasteurella multocida, Pasteurella canis, Capnocytophaga* species, *Fusobacterium* species, *Eikenella corrodens*); rodent bites (*Streptobacillus moniliformis, Spirillum minus);* puncture wounds *(Pseudomonas aeruginosa)*; joint prosthesis *(Staphylococcus epidermidis,* non-tuberculous mycobacteria*)*; travel *(Mycobacterium tuberculosis,* chikungunya virus, brucellosis, coccidioidomycosis, blastomycosis*)*; central line or immunosuppression (yeast, multidrug-resistant gram-negative bacilli, *S epidermidis, L monocytogenes).*

Septic arthritis requires urgent diagnosis, arthrocentesis, and treatment to prevent permanent limitation of joint mobility. If septic arthritis is complicated by osteomyelitis of the epiphysis and growth plate, long-bone growth can be impaired. A patient with hip or shoulder septic arthritis is at risk for femoral or humeral head ischemic necrosis, respectively, because joint capsule inflammation occludes blood flow.

Clinical Presentation

History

At presentation, septic arthritis typically appears with acute onset of a painful joint, decreased range of motion, and inability to bear weight, often associated with fever (>38.4°C [101.1°F]). Septic arthritis in an infant or disabled child can appear as a subtle pseudoparalysis of the affected joint at presentation. *N gonorrhoeae* appears in sexually active adolescents as either an arthritis-dermatitis syndrome or a disseminated infection (polyarthritis, polyarthralgia, tenosynovitis) at presentation. Arthritis is a late manifestation of disseminated Lyme disease; the patient may not recall an earlier manifestation of Lyme disease, such as erythema migrans. Atypical organisms (eg, *K kingae)* can have an indolent presentation.

Ask about exposures and risk factors for unusual pathogens, including vaccination status, trauma, travel, immune status, asplenia, sickle cell disease, sexual activity, ingestion of unpasteurized dairy products, tick exposure, tuberculosis, exposure to animals, and recent pharyngitis or enteritis.

Physical Examination

In most cases, joint swelling, erythema, warmth, and tenderness are readily apparent. Range of motion is significantly decreased, and minimal manipulation of the joint or the extremity causes severe pain. However, the sole abnormality with a deep joint infection (hip, sacroiliac) can be decreased range of motion. The patient will guard the affected joint in the position of least pain (hip flexed and externally rotated; knee and elbow held carefully in neutral position). Referred pain is common (especially knee pain with a septic hip), so examine the joint above and below the presumed focus. Examine the remaining joints and palpate the long bones for point tenderness.

Polyarticular involvement can occur with *N gonorrhoeae, N meningitidis,* or *Salmonella* species. Other causes of polyarticular disease include acute rheumatic fever, Lyme arthritis, chikungunya virus, and juvenile idiopathic arthritis (JIA). A patient with Lyme arthritis often complains of a subacute, monoarticular, swollen ("boggy"), nonerythematous joint (most often the knee) but maintains weight bearing and range of motion with minimal discomfort.

Laboratory Workup

Obtain a complete blood cell count, erythrocyte sedimentation rate (ESR) and/or C-reactive protein (CRP) level, and blood culture (yield 20%–40%). Order additional tests if a specific organism is suspected: Lyme enzyme-linked immunosorbent assay with reflex to Western blot, nucleic acid amplification tests from urine and cervicovaginal samples for gonococcus and *Chlamydia*, chikungunya virus immunoglobulin (Ig) G and IgM, or tuberculin skin testing or interferon-γ release assay for *M tuberculosis*. The white blood cell count is typically increased with a left shift in bacterial arthritis. ESR and CRP level are increased (ESR >30 mm/h and CRP level >3 mg/L [>28.57 nmol/L]), although an ESR greater than 100 mm/h suggests autoimmune arthritis.

If septic arthritis is suspected, arrange for an *immediate* percutaneous diagnostic joint aspiration; ultrasonographic (US) guidance may be warranted, particularly if the hip is involved. Send joint fluid specimens for cell count, Gram stain, and culture (Table 98-1). To improve culture yields and detect fastidious organisms such as *K kingae,* some laboratories will inoculate synovial fluid into an aerobic blood culture bottle and incubate for 7 days. Request special cultures for mycobacteria, *S moniliformis, S minus,* and fungal pathogens, if suspected. Polymerase chain reaction testing is available for synovial fluid for *B burgdorferi, N gonorrhoeae,* and *K kingae.* Reserve remaining synovial fluid for additional testing. Immediate surgical irrigation by an orthopedist is indicated if the preliminary results are suggestive of bacterial infection. Some local experience in well-resourced, non–methicillin-resistant *S aureus* (MRSA)–endemic regions have favored less invasive surgical irrigation after diagnostic arthrocentesis; however, this experience may not be generalizable.

Chapter 98: Septic Arthritis

Table 98-1. Interpretation of Synovial Fluid Cell Count		
WBC Count	**% PMNs**	**Interpretation**
<200 WBCs/mm³	<25%	Normal
200–2,000 WBCs/mm³	<25%	Noninflammatory (osteoarthritis)
2,000–50,000 WBCs/mm³	>50%	Inflammatory, possibly noninfectious (reactive arthritis, JIA, Lyme disease, gonorrhea, tuberculosis, brucellosis)
>50,000 WBCs/mm³	>75%	Probably infectious (*Staphylococcus aureus*, group A *Streptococcus*, Lyme disease, gram-negative rods)

Abbreviations: JIA, juvenile idiopathic arthritis; PMN, polymorphonuclear neutrophil; WBC, white blood cell.

Radiology Examinations

Obtain plain radiographs to evaluate the presence of effusion, fracture, and other noninfectious causes, such as bone cyst or neoplasm. In suspected septic hip, US is rapid and diagnostic for joint fluid and facilitates therapeutic drainage. If primary contiguous osteomyelitis or a complication is suspected, perform magnetic resonance imaging. Computed tomography, while less sensitive, can be used if other imaging modalities are not readily available. Bone scintigraphy can be useful if multiple sites are suspected or if other imaging modalities are unavailable. Alternatively, repeat plain radiography 2 to 3 weeks after diagnosis to detect underlying osteomyelitis (see Chapter 97, Osteomyelitis). However, do not delay diagnostic arthrocentesis and empirical antimicrobial therapy while awaiting imaging.

Differential Diagnosis

First, confirm that the patient has arthritis and not merely arthralgia. At presentation, an arthritic joint appears with some combination of erythema, warmth, effusion, and limited range of motion. Once septic arthritis has been ruled out, consider other infectious and noninfectious causes of arthritis (Table 98-2).

Table 98-2. Differential Diagnosis of Septic Arthritis	
Diagnosis	**Clinical Features**
Infectious causes of arthritis	
Acute rheumatic fever	Preceding group A streptococcal pharyngitis Migratory polyarthritis Severe pain out of proportion to examination findings Patient may have carditis (+) GAS antibodies (anti-streptolysin O, anti-DNase B)
Gonorrhea	Patient sexually active Multiple smaller joints and knees affected (+) Urine/cervical nucleic acid amplification test
Lyme disease	History of tick bite or erythema migrans Swollen, boggy, nonerythematous knee (+) Lyme serologic testing 50% of knee arthritis in endemic areas; 3% in nonendemic areas
Osteomyelitis	Point tenderness of long bone No joint swelling or erythema
Parvovirus	Viral prodrome: fever, fatigue, headache, pharyngitis Typical rash: slapped cheeks followed by lacy appearance on trunk and extremities
Tuberculosis	(+) Risk factors (+) Purified protein derivative and/or interferon-γ release assay Joint fluid: lymphocytic predominance, acid-fast bacilli

Table 98-2. Differential Diagnosis of Septic Arthritis, continued	
Diagnosis	**Clinical Features**
Noninfectious causes of arthritis	
Henoch-Schönlein purpura	Palpable purpura of the lower extremities Abdominal pain Patient may have (+) stool guaiac and/or hematuria
Inflammatory bowel disease	Poor growth or weight loss Diarrhea, possibly guaiac (+) Iritis, rash
Juvenile idiopathic arthritis	Pain and stiffness worse in the morning (+) Serologic testing
Postinfectious/ postvaccination or reactive arthritis (formally Reiter syndrome)	Subacute onset over 2–3 weeks Patient may not have fever Less dramatic examination findings: ↓ erythema, swelling, pain Urethritis, uveitis, iritis, conjunctivitis, rash Preceding *Chlamydia trachomatis, Campylobacter jejuni,* streptococcal infection
Sickle cell disease vaso-occlusive crisis	(+) History Previous episodes with pain in typical location(s) Patient may be afebrile
Systemic lupus erythematosus	Symmetrical arthritis of the hands and feet Other features: malar rash, proteinuria, laboratory findings, etc (+) Serologic testing
Transient synovitis	Recent viral illness (eg, parvovirus) Less dramatic joint examination findings, bland arthrocentesis Responds to analgesics
Trauma	(+) History (+) Radiographic findings

Abbreviations: GAS, group A *Streptococcus*; -, negative finding; +, positive finding.

Treatment

Arrange for an immediate percutaneous diagnostic joint aspiration and culture by an orthopedic surgeon or other skilled personnel. Effective treatment involves initial intravenous (IV) antimicrobial therapy (Table 98-3) and urgent orthopedic surgical consultation for possible arthrotomy or arthroscopy. Surgical intervention is based on synovial fluid appearance, cell count and gram stain findings, clinical course, laboratory results, and suspected pathogen. In non-hip, non-shoulder arthritis in a well-appearing child, delay of antibiotic therapy for a few hours can be considered to perform preantibiotic cultures.

Consider a bacterial infection of a hip or shoulder to be a medical/surgical emergency and include vancomycin in the initial antibiotic regimen; perform baseline and weekly renal function testing. For non-hip, non-shoulder joints, include empirical MRSA coverage when community prevalence is greater than 10%; clindamycin is the preferred agent. However, an increased local prevalence of clindamycin-resistant strains of methicillin-sensitive *S aureus* (MSSA) makes a first-generation cephalosporin or an antistaphylococcal penicillin the preferred empirical option in non-hip, non-shoulder joints. Add ampicillin or cefazolin for *K kingae* while awaiting culture results. Obtain an infectious diseases consult for a contaminated wound, joint prosthesis, or unusual or resistant organisms.

Administer the initial IV antibiotics, provide adequate analgesia (acetaminophen, or ibuprofen if JIA is not a diagnostic consideration), and reassess the patient daily to look for resolution of clinical symptoms and inflammatory markers. Improvement begins within 72 hours and is significant by 5 to 7 days. Use the clinical course and organism identification and sensitivity to tailor antibiotic choice and transition to oral therapy. There is no absolute minimum duration of IV antibiotic treatment.

The total (IV plus oral) duration of antibiotics for uncomplicated *S aureus* septic arthritis is typically 3 weeks. In a Finnish study, rapidly resolving, uncomplicated MSSA septic arthritis was successfully treated with as little as 2 weeks of IV antibiotics plus oral treatment; however, it is unclear if this experience is generalizable to areas where MRSA is prevalent. Treatment can be as short as 10 to 14 days for *K kingae, S pneumoniae, H influenzae,* or culture-negative non–*S aureus* arthritis with rapid resolution. *Salmonella* (42 days) and other gram-negative organisms can require longer durations of therapy; consult an infectious diseases expert for atypical pathogens. Treat Lyme arthritis for a total of 28 days. Gonococcal arthritis warrants susceptibility testing and evaluation and treatment for other sexually transmitted infections.

If there is coexistent osteomyelitis, treat for at least 4 weeks (see Chapter 97, Osteomyelitis). Recommended treatment for culture-negative septic arthritis is 3 weeks; oral antibiotics are preferred when an oral agent with comparable spectrum to empirical therapy is available and tolerated. Concurrent therapy with IV dexamethasone has undergone trials. However, further research is needed to determine whether corticosteroid exposure and related adverse effects are worth any potential benefit to long-term outcomes. In reactive arthritis, treat the primary process.

Table 98-3. Empirical IV Antibiotic Treatment of Septic Arthritis

Infection	Empirical IV Treatment
Hip or shoulder	Vancomycin[a]: 40–60 mg/kg/d, divided into doses administered every 6–8 h: Maximum, 1 g per dose and 2 g/d; trough goal, 10–15 µg/mL Evaluate baseline and weekly renal function *PLUS* Oxacillin: 150–200 mg/kg/d, divided into doses administered every 6 h; 12-g/d maximum *or* Cefazolin: 100–150 mg/kg/d, divided into doses administered every 8 h; 3-g/d maximum
Other joints	Clindamycin[a]: 40 mg/kg/d, divided into doses administered every 6–8 h; 2.7-g/d maximum *If Kingella kingae or clindamycin-resistant Staphylococcus aureus is suspected, add cefazolin:* Cefazolin: 100–150 mg/kg/d, divided into doses administered every 8 h; 3-g/d maximum *If severe clindamycin-resistant S aureus is suspected, add vancomycin to cefazolin:* Vancomycin[a]: 40–60 mg/kg/d, divided into doses administered every 6–8 h: Maximum, 1 g per dose and 2 g/d; trough goal, 10–15 µg/mL Evaluate baseline and weekly renal function
Suspected gram-negative or unvaccinated child	*In addition to antistaphylococcal therapy,* Add ceftriaxone: 100 mg/kg/d, divided into doses administered every 12 h; 2-g/d maximum
Neonate	Nafcillin *or* oxacillin[b] (as detailed herein) *plus* gentamycin *or* cefotaxime (doses for both depend on age and weight)
Immunocompromised host	Cefepime: 150 mg/kg/d, divided into doses administered every 8 h; 6-g/d maximum
Penicillin allergy	Clindamycin or vancomycin or ceftriaxone or cefazolin
Lyme arthritis	Ceftriaxone: 50–75 mg/kg every 24 h; 2-g/d maximum
Gonococcal arthritis[c]	Patient weight ≤45 kg: IM or IV ceftriaxone 50 mg/kg/d every 24 h; maximum, 1 g per dose for 7 d Patient weight >45 kg: IM or IV ceftriaxone 1 g every 24 h for 7 d *For adolescents and adults, dual therapy is recommended for gonococcal arthritis:* Add oral azithromycin 1 g, once

Abbreviations: IM, intramuscular; IV, intravenous.

[a] For methicillin-resistant *S aureus* coverage if local community prevalence is >10% of *S aureus* isolates.

[b] If *Listeria monocytogenes* is suspected because of maternal risk factors, consider adding IV ampicillin.

[c] Per 2015 U.S. Centers for Disease Control and Prevention guidelines at http://www.cdc.gov/std/tg2015/gonorrhea.htm. Dual therapy not indicated in children.

Indications for Consultation

- **Orthopedics:** All cases of suspected septic arthritis
- **Infectious diseases:** Patient with unusual risk factors, organism, or failure to respond to empirical therapy
- **Physiatry/physical therapy:** As tolerated, once surgical issues are resolved

Disposition

- **Intensive care unit transfer:** Possible bacterial sepsis or toxic appearance
- **Interinstitutional transfer:** If orthopedic management is not available, especially if there is a concern about a septic hip
- **Discharge criteria:** Patient afebrile more than 24 hours, surgical issues resolved, significant improvement of joint function, antibiotic regimen narrowed (if sensitivities are known), and improving CRP level and/or ESR

Follow-up

- **Primary provider:** 3 days and at periodic intervals for 1 year to monitor the patient for growth arrest; obtain plain radiographs 2 to 3 weeks after diagnosis to identify concomitant osteomyelitis if osteomyelitis was suspected but diagnostic evaluation was not performed
- **Orthopedics:** 1 to 2 weeks; obtain plain radiographs 2 to 3 weeks after diagnosis to identify concomitant osteomyelitis if osteomyelitis was suspected but diagnostic evaluation was not performed
- **Infectious diseases:** 1 to 2 weeks (if involved)
- **Physiatry/physical therapy:** 1 to 2 weeks; coordinate with orthopedics because timing depends on severity of infection and joint involved (eg, more likely necessary with hip or shoulder)

Pearls and Pitfalls

- If septic arthritis is suspected, arrange for urgent arthrocentesis.
- Consider adjacent osteomyelitis of the epiphysis in a young infant.
- Ensure that at least one blood culture (and ideally a synovial culture) is performed prior to the first dose of antibiotics.
- Hip and shoulder septic arthritis are emergencies; begin empirical IV vancomycin.
- Review epidemiologic exposures to identify atypical pathogens and local antibiograms to determine prevalence of MRSA and clindamycin-resistant MSSA.
- In preschool children, consider *K kingae* in the case of a poor response to empirical vancomycin or clindamycin.
- Transition to oral antibiotics as soon as clinical examination findings are improving (increased range of motion, bearing weight, decreased pain, patient afebrile) and laboratory values support resolution.
- Given the risks associated with peripherally inserted central catheters, oral therapy at discharge is preferred when an equivalent oral agent is available and tolerated.

Bibliography

Deanehan JK, Nigrovic PA, Milewski MD, et al. Synovial fluid findings in children with knee monoarthritis in Lyme disease endemic areas. *Pediatr Emerg Care.* 2014;30(1): 16–19

Heyworth BE, Shore BJ, Donohue KS, Miller PE, Kocher MS, Glotzbecker MP. Management of pediatric patients with synovial fluid white blood-cell counts of 25,000 to 75,000 cells/mm³ after aspiration of the hip. *J Bone Joint Surg Am.* 2015;97(5):389–395

Monsalve J, Kan JH, Schallert EK, Bisset GS, Zhang W, Rosenfeld SB. Septic arthritis in children: frequency of coexisting unsuspected osteomyelitis and implications on imaging work-up and management. *AJR Am J Roentgenol.* 2015;204(6):1289–1295

Pääkkönen M, Peltola H. Management of a child with suspected acute septic arthritis. *Arch Dis Child.* 2012;97(3):287–292

Russell CD, Ramaesh R, Kalima P, Murray A, Gaston MS. Microbiological characteristics of acute osteoarticular infections in children. *J Med Microbiol.* 2015;64(Pt 4):446–453

Workowski KA, Bolan GA; Centers for Disease Control and Prevention. Sexually transmitted diseases, treatment guidelines, 2015. *MMWR Recomm Rep.* 2015;64(RR-03): 1–137

Bibliography

Psychiatry

Acute Agitation

Introduction

Agitation is a state of behavioral dyscontrol that manifests as excessive motor and verbal activity. It is the final common pathway for a broad range of medical and psychiatric conditions. Early recognition and effective management of agitation can prevent escalation and potential harm to patients, family members, and health care workers. The identification of the underlying etiology guides intervention that will diminish agitation and prevent restrictive treatment measures.

Clinical Presentation

History

The severity of agitation ranges from restlessness, irritability, crying, or confusion to loud speech, psychomotor agitation, and combative behavior. Ask how the patient's current state of behavioral control differs from baseline. What was the timing of the onset of agitation, and what are the associated factors? If agitation is reactive, ask what happens before, during, and after the episodes to delineate any triggers or secondary gain.

Obtain a biopsychosocial history, including past treatments for medical, neurologic, psychiatric, and behavioral disorders. Explore the possibility of toxin exposure, ingestion, or overdose. For a patient with a developmental disorder, ask about sensory preferences, modes of communication, and what irritates and soothes him or her. Ask about sleep-wake cycles and identify potential iatrogenic disruptions of sleep. Before selecting a pharmacologic agent for treatment of agitation, inquire about past paradoxical reactions to benzodiazepines or antihistamines. Additionally, inquire about relatives with sudden cardiac death or possible long QT syndrome (congenital hearing loss, seizures, syncope), which may affect the choice of antipsychotic medication. Identify the patient's allergies, prescribed and over-the-counter medications, and any other medications in the household.

During the interview, use nonpharmacologic de-escalation strategies: introduce yourself clearly, speak in a soft tone, offer frequent reassurance, respect the patient's autonomy, honor reasonable requests, use nonthreatening body language, avoid prolonged eye contact, leave the examination door open, and conduct the interview while seated. If feasible, offer the patient any available comforts, such as warm blankets, food, or drink, and directly integrate trusted family, friends, and staff members into the discussion.

Physical Examination

Priorities in the physical examination include autonomic instability, fever, signs of inadequate perfusion consistent with shock or sepsis, and Cushing triad, suggestive of increased intracranial pressure. Perform a detailed neurologic examination and evaluate pupillary size and reflex, focal neurologic deficit, muscle tone, reflexes, and abnormal movements. At mental status examination, assess the patient for orientation and attention to screen for delirium. Attention can be assessed in a verbal adolescent by asking them to say the months of the year backwards. Assess thought process and content for stigmata of mania and psychosis. The patient seeming to respond to stimuli that others do not perceive suggests visual or auditory hallucinations.

Laboratory Workup

If the patient is delirious and an underlying cause has not been determined, obtain a complete blood cell count, electrolyte and glucose levels, liver function test results, thyroid panel, ammonia level, folate level, vitamin B_{12} level, thiamine level, antinuclear antibody panel, acetaminophen level, salicylate level, and routine electroencephalogram and perform urinalysis. Perform urgent nonenhanced head computed tomography (CT) if the patient has demonstrated recent head trauma, partial seizure, known intracranial lesion, immunosuppression, suspected subarachnoid hemorrhage, progressive headache, papilledema, visual field deficit, or other focal neurologic findings. Perform a lumbar puncture with opening pressure with prior CT images if indicated (mental status changes accompanied by fever, headache, or focal neurologic deficit; physical examination signs of meningeal irritation; no reasonable alternative explanation for the agitation). Send the cerebrospinal fluid for cell count, glucose and protein level evaluation, Gram stain, and culture, and save an additional tube of fluid for possible serologic testing or polymerase chain reaction testing (herpes simplex virus, encephalitis panel, enterovirus, etc).

Differential Diagnosis

In a hospitalized child, there are 6 etiologic categories for agitation: toxic, metabolic, central nervous system (CNS) functional or traumatic/structural, infectious, psychiatric or developmental, and behavioral (Table 99-1). Of note, the first 4 categories (toxic, metabolic, CNS, and infectious) may appear as delirium at presentation. Deficits in orientation and a waxing and waning

Table 99-1. Etiologic Considerations for Agitation in the Hospitalized Child

Examples	Common Causes
Toxic etiology	
Adverse medication effects	Anticholinergics
Medication interaction	Baclofen withdrawal
Withdrawal	Benzodiazepines
	Corticosteroids
	Intoxication with illicit drugs
	Neuroleptic malignant syndrome
	Polypharmacy
	Serotonin syndrome
	Withdrawal from opiates or benzodiazepines
Metabolic etiology	
Electrolyte disturbance	Hepatic encephalopathy
Endocrinopathy	Hyper-, hypoglycemia
End-organ failure	Hyper-, hyponatremia
Hypoxia	Hypercarbia
Inborn error of metabolism	Hypertensive encephalopathy
	Renal failure
	Thyroid or parathyroid dysfunction
	Vitamin deficiencies (B_{12}, thiamine)
CNS functional, traumatic, structural etiologies	
CNS injury	Autoimmune encephalitis
↑ Intracranial pressure	Confusional migraine
Primary neurologic disorder	Hematoma
	Hemorrhage
	Hydrocephalus
	Parenchymal injury
	Seizure/postictal state
	Stroke
	Tumor or space-occupying lesion
Infectious etiology	
CNS infection	Brain abscess
Systemic infection	Meningitis
	Sepsis
	Viral or bacterial encephalitis
Exacerbation of primary psychiatric or developmental disorder	
Frustration	Anxiety disorder
Inclination towards aggression	Attention-deficit/hyperactivity disorder
Poor communication interfering with reporting of symptoms or needs	Autism
Natural exacerbation in course of illness	Bipolar disorder
Noncompliance with treatment regimen	Communication disorder
	Intellectual disability
	Posttraumatic stress disorder
	Schizophrenia and other psychoses
	Untreated pain or unmet hunger in a patient with a developmental or communication disorder

Continued

Table 99-1. Etiologic Considerations for Agitation in the Hospitalized Child, continued	
Examples	**Common Causes**
Behavioral etiology	
Secondary gain Situational response	Avoidance (procedures, therapies) Disruptive behavior disorder Interpersonal or family conflict Maladaptive response to limit setting Poor coping ability Psychosocial stress

Abbreviation: CNS, central nervous system.

pattern differentiate delirium from primary psychiatric or behavioral disturbances. The acute onset of hallucinations in a medically hospitalized patient with no past psychiatric history is delirium until proven otherwise.

Treatment

Maximize nonpharmacologic interventions for agitation before prescribing psychotropic medications. Yet, with severe agitation, physical and chemical restraints may be necessary to maintain safety.

If the patient is delirious, first aggressively pursue and treat the medical condition, ensure appropriate cardiorespiratory monitoring and airway support, reduce stimulation, reorient the patient frequently, and mimic night-day light cycles. Arrange for staff members to work consistently with the patient so they can develop familiarity and rapport. Avoid anticholinergic medications and benzodiazepines in a delirious patient because they can worsen and prolong the patient's agitation. For moderate agitation in delirium, use low doses of an oral atypical antipsychotic medication, such as risperidone, quetiapine, or olanzapine, on an as-needed basis or as scheduled in the evening to prevent sundowning. If there has been a toxin or substance ingestion, agitation will diminish with time in a controlled environment, but benzodiazepines are preferred as a first-line treatment, followed by antipsychotics. For a patient in withdrawal from opiates or benzodiazepines, carefully taper these medications while monitoring vital signs and symptoms of withdrawal.

For any agitated patient, arrange an adequate staff-to-patient ratio and remove all potentially harmful items from the room. Attempt to verbally de-escalate the episode, remove any agitating family members, decrease stimulation, and provide distraction and comfort. Offer the patient an orally dispensed medication to help them calm. If these efforts fail and agitation has escalated to threats or overt violence, a physical or chemical restraint is the least restrictive means to maintain safety for everyone involved.

Medication

When the underlying cause of agitation is a known psychiatric disorder, treat the patient with a medication that is U.S. Food and Drug Administration indicated for that disorder, whenever possible. When the underlying cause of agitation is behavioral, consult a psychologist or social worker for further evaluation and to implement psychotherapeutic, social, and behavioral interventions.

If the patient will not accept oral medications and if intravenous (IV) access is not secured, certain medications can be administered intramuscularly (Table 99-2). In such a case, prescribe monotherapy, followed by evaluation of the response, rather than administering multiple medications simultaneously.

<table>
<tr><th colspan="5">Table 99-2. Medications for the Treatment of Acute Agitation</th></tr>
<tr><th>Medication</th><th>Delivery Route</th><th>Initial Dose</th><th>Maximum Dose (mg)</th><th>Side Effects</th></tr>
<tr><td colspan="5">Antihistamines</td></tr>
<tr><td>Diphenhydramine</td><td>PO</td><td>1.25 mg/kg</td><td>50</td><td rowspan="4">Anticholinergic
CNS and/or respiratory depression
May worsen airway reactivity
Worsens delirium
Paradoxical disinhibition</td></tr>
<tr><td>IM/IV</td><td>1.25 mg/kg</td><td>50</td></tr>
<tr><td>Hydroxyzine</td><td>PO</td><td>0.6 mg/kg</td><td>100</td></tr>
<tr><td>IM</td><td>0.5–1.0 mg/kg</td><td>100</td></tr>
<tr><td colspan="5">Benzodiazepines</td></tr>
<tr><td rowspan="4">Lorazepam</td><td>PO</td><td>0.02–0.10 mg/kg</td><td>4</td><td rowspan="4">Habituation/tolerance
Paradoxical disinhibition
Respiratory depression
Worsens delirium</td></tr>
<tr><td>IV</td><td>0.02–0.10 mg/kg</td><td>4</td></tr>
<tr><td>IM</td><td>0.02–0.10 mg/kg</td><td>4</td></tr>
<tr><td>PR</td><td>0.5 mg/kg (using the IV formulation)</td><td>20</td></tr>
<tr><td colspan="5">Atypical antipsychotics (no weight-based dosing)</td></tr>
<tr><td rowspan="2">Ziprasidone (atypical antipsychotic)</td><td>PO</td><td>Not recommended</td><td>NA</td><td rowspan="2">Akathisia
Dystonic reactions[a]
Risk of NMS
Sedation
↑ QTc interval</td></tr>
<tr><td>IM</td><td>5 mg per dose</td><td>20 mg (40-mg/d maximum)</td></tr>
<tr><td>Risperidone (atypical antipsychotic)</td><td>PO or ODT</td><td>0.125–0.250 mg per dose</td><td>1 mg</td><td>Dystonic reactions[a]
Least seizure threshold reduction among atypical antipsychotics
Risk of NMS
↑ QTc interval</td></tr>
</table>

Continued

| | **Delivery** | | **Maximum** | |
Medication	Route	Initial Dose	Dose (mg)	Side Effects
Table 99-2. Medications for the Treatment of Acute Agitation, continued				
Atypical antipsychotics (no weight-based dosing), continued				
Olanzapine (atypical anti-psychotic)	PO or ODT	2.5–5.0 mg per dose	10 mg (30-mg/d maximum)	Can exacerbate hypotension or bradycardia induced by concomitant agents
	IM	2.5–5.0 mg per dose	10 mg (30-mg/d maximum)	Hypotension (at high doses) ↑ QTc interval ↓ Risk of EPS and NMS

Abbreviations: CNS, central nervous system; EPS, extrapyramidal symptoms; IM, intramuscular; IV, intravenous; NA, not applicable; NMS, neuromalignant syndrome; ODT, orally dissolvable tablet; PO, per os (oral); PR, per rectum; QTc, corrected QT interval.

ᵃ Treat dystonia (oculogyric crisis, torticollis, opisthotonus) with IV, IM, or oral diphenhydramine (1.25 mg/kg) every 30 minutes or with IV, IM, or oral benzotropine (0.02–0.05 mg/kg).

Restraint

Restraints are interventions that restrict patient movement and are categorized into physical and chemical (or pharmacologic) methods. There is variation among the states in terms of allowed and preferred physical restraints. In addition, safety is dependent on appropriate staff training and adherence to an individual hospital's monitoring protocols. A chemical restraint is any medication administered on an involuntary basis to sedate the patient and thus restrict movement. Do not use restraints as punishment, as a means of compensating for inadequate staff-to-patient ratio, or for convenience. The goals of restraint are to reduce further escalation, maintain safety, protect the patient and staff members from injury, and facilitate performing physical examinations, diagnostic tests, and essential medical interventions. Before initiating either method, carefully document all antecedent measures taken to calm the patient, as well as indications for escalating to restraint, and adhere to all of the institution's restraint policies and procedures.

If chemical restraint is used, start with the lowest dose necessary to calm the patient, and then titrate to the behavioral severity and urgency of the sedation. Always offer the patient an oral sedative. This can give the patient a sense of control and maintains rapport, while having a lower risk of side effects than parenteral medications. Be aware of any potential drug interactions that can cause QT interval prolongation or exacerbate respiratory or CNS depression. Provide continuous cardiorespiratory monitoring.

Therapeutic options for chemical restraint (Table 99-2) generally fall into 3 pharmacologic categories: antihistamines, benzodiazepines, and antipsychotics. Selection of the agent is determined by the underlying etiology.

Benzodiazepines are best for a medical illness or substance intoxication or for when the cause is unknown. For exacerbation of a mood or a psychotic disorder, use atypical (second-generation) antipsychotics. They have favorable short-term side effect profiles when compared with typical (first-generation) antipsychotics. Specifically, atypical antipsychotics are less likely to cause dystonia and neuroleptic malignant syndrome (NMS) than are high-potency typical antipsychotics.

Prevention

There are a number of basic measures that can lower the risk of agitation in an inpatient. Minimize the use and duration of indwelling catheters, implement venous thromboembolism prophylaxis in high-risk patients, reduce polypharmacy, and be vigilant for drug interactions. Training staff members in patient-centered preventive and de-escalation strategies effectively diminishes the use of restrictive interventions. Calling for security or additional staff members at the earliest sign of agitation may prevent escalation. In addition, the presence of security staff could also allow the patient to take a walk or change their surrounding environment.

Indications for Consultation

- **Child life specialist:** Most cases of agitation (once stabilized)
- **Neurology:** Stroke, NMS, serotonin syndrome, pre- or postictal state, confusional migraine, encephalitis
- **Psychiatry:** Moderate or severe agitation, exacerbation of a primary psychiatric disorder, NMS, serotonin syndrome, psychotropic polypharmacy
- **Psychology or social work:** Interpersonal or family conflict, psychosocial stress, poor coping ability, maladaptive response to limit setting, and when agitation yields secondary gain or functions to avoid treatment engagement
- **Occupational therapy and speech therapy:** As needed, for a patient with developmental, intellectual, or communication disorders

Disposition

- **Intensive care unit transfer:** NMS, severe serotonin syndrome, moderate/severe traumatic brain injury
- **Discharge criteria:** Agitation resolved and behavior returned to baseline or the family feels competent to manage at home and there are no safety concerns

Follow-up

- **Primary care provider:** 1 week
- **Mental health professional:** If indicated by any underlying mental health diagnosis

Pearls and Pitfalls

- Identification of the underlying cause of agitation is the first step in successful management.
- Delirium is common in medically ill children and can be differentiated from a primary psychiatric disorder by evaluating orientation, attention, and a waxing/waning pattern of symptoms.
- Document all de-escalation efforts and use restraint only when these less intrusive means of intervention have failed.

Bibliography

Bultas MW, Johnson NL., Burkett K, Reinhold J. Translating research to practice for children with autism spectrum disorder: part 2: Behavior management in home and health care settings. *J Pediatr Health Care.* 2016; 30(1):27–37

Carubia B, Becker A, Levine BH. Child psychiatric emergencies: updates on trends, clinical care, and practice challenges. *Curr Psychiatry Rep.* 2016;18(4):41

Marzullo LR. Pharmacologic management of the agitated child. *Pediatr Emerg Care.* 2014;30(4):269–275

Sonnier L, Barzman D. Pharmacologic management of acutely agitated pediatric patients. *Pediatr Drugs.* 2011;13(1):1–10

Turkel SB, Hanft A. The pharmacologic management of delirium in children and adolescents. *Pediatr Drugs.* 2014;16(4):267–274

Depression

Introduction

Depression is a psychiatric disorder with a wide spectrum of severity that affects up to 2% of children and about 10% of adolescents. In the most severe form, depression can lead to suicide, which is the third-leading cause of death among adolescents in the United States. Risk factors for depression are both genetic and environmental and include a family history of depression in a first-degree relative, personal history of anxiety disorders or attention-deficit/hyperactivity disorder, family dysfunction, low socioeconomic status, chronic illness, substance abuse, a history of physical or sexual abuse, and lesbian, gay, bisexual, and transgender identification. In addition, a hospital stay itself can promote depressive symptoms, while some medications are also risk factors (steroids).

Clinical Presentation

History

A patient with depression may present with recurrent somatic complaints (abdominal pain, headaches, myalgia) for which no organic cause can be found. The patient may have recently developed a loss of interest in friends or activities once found to be enjoyable. There may be a history of irritability, oppositional behavior, aggression, running away, stealing, fire setting, or being accident prone. Ask about suicidal ideation and whether the patient has formulated a plan. The parents may be concerned about a loss of appetite, poor school performance, increased isolation, or change in sleep pattern. Inquire about a family history of depression or suicide. *SIGE-CAPS* is a useful mnemonic for the signs of depression: Changes in **S**leep, loss of **I**nterest in activities, **G**uilt, decreased **E**nergy, reduced **C**oncentration, loss of **A**ppetite, **P**sychomotor (agitation or lethargy), and **S**uicidal ideation.

As a part of the review of systems, perform a mental health screening for any adolescent admitted to the hospital, regardless of the admitting diagnosis. In addition, a chronically ill patient will often have a psychological overlay to their illness, even if it does not meet the *Diagnostic and Statistical Manual of Mental Disorders, Fifth Edition,* threshold for inpatient hospitalization or medical therapy.

Physical Examination

Use the physical examination to screen for abnormalities associated with organic causes of depression. In a patient with depressive symptoms, poor hygiene and eye contact, flattened affect, and psychomotor depression or agitation may be present. Often, there are significant abnormalities in mood, thought content, and quality of speech.

Laboratory Workup

The goal of laboratory testing is to attempt to rule out organic causes of depression in a patient who is presenting with the disorder for the first time. Obtain blood for a complete blood cell count, chemistry assessment, thyroid function testing, and syphilis serologic testing and obtain urine for toxicologic evaluation.

Differential Diagnosis

Except for an acutely suicidal patient, the priority is to exclude medical conditions that can mimic the clinical presentation of depression. In addition, consider recent stressors (procedures, prolonged clinical course, "bad news") that may be contributing to the patient's depressive symptoms.

The definitive diagnosis of depression requires the input of a psychologist or psychiatrist, on the basis of a carefully assembled clinical history and mental status examination finding (Table 100-1). Screening tools, such as the Children's Depression Inventory, the RADS (Reynolds Adolescent Depression Scale), the Beck Depression Inventory, and the CES-DC (Center for Epidemiological Studies Depression Scale for Children), are helpful supplements for the evaluation of depressive symptoms.

Table 100-1. Psychiatric Conditions That Mimic Depression	
Diagnosis	**Clinical Features**
Adjustment disorder with depressed mood	Depressive symptoms start within 3 mo of a significant stressor and resolve within 6 mo Stressor can be chronic (ongoing abuse), leading to symptoms lasting >6 mo
Bipolar disorder	Episodes of mania alternating with depression At presentation, manic episodes may appear with decreased need for sleep, flight of ideas/distractibility, increased interest in pleasurable activities, or pressured speech
Medication- or substance-related mood disorder	Clinical findings of a pre-existing medical condition May not fulfill all *Diagnostic and Statistical Manual of Mental Disorders, Fifth Edition,* depressive disorder criteria Higher risk of suicide with chronic or terminal illness
Posttraumatic stress disorder	Depressive symptoms follow a traumatic event Flashbacks, recurrent dreams, reliving the event

Treatment

Consult a child psychiatrist to develop a comprehensive treatment plan. On the basis of the degree of depression and underlying medical conditions, the psychiatrist may recommend a regimen of pharmacologic intervention, psychotherapy, or a combination of both. Selective serotonin reuptake inhibitors are first-line pharmacologic treatments, but fluoxetine (in patients >8 years of age) and escitalopram (in patients >12 years of age) are the only U.S. Food and Drug Administration–approved antidepressants for use in children. Defer initiating pharmacologic treatment, including "off-label" uses of other common antidepressants (citalopram, sertraline, venlafaxine, bupropion), to the psychiatrist.

Since inpatient mental health resources for children are limited, a patient who requires inpatient psychiatric care may be admitted to a general pediatric ward until an appropriate inpatient psychiatric bed becomes available. The most frequent such indication is a suicide attempt, in which case the patient must be placed under continuous (one-on-one) observation.

Indications for Consultation

Psychiatrist, clinical psychologist, or therapeutic social worker: All patients

Disposition

- **Inpatient psychiatric service transfer:** Active suicidal ideation, attempt, or symptoms are having a severe effect on daily life
- **Discharge criteria:** A care plan is in place, with medication being tolerated, outpatient management arranged, and no active suicidal or homicidal ideation; potentially lethal items (firearms, medications) have been removed from the home

Follow-up

- **Mental health professional:** 1 week
- **Primary care provider:** 1 week

Pearls and Pitfalls

- Depression may appear with psychotic features at presentation, such as auditory and/or visual hallucinations and delusions.
- Little evidence exists that "contracting for safety" reduces suicide.
- Discharge planning can be challenging in view of the relative paucity of inpatient and outpatient pediatric psychiatry services.

Bibliography

Cox GR, Callahan P, Churchill R, et al. Psychological therapies versus antidepressant medication, alone and in combination for depression in children and adolescents. *Cochrane Database Syst Rev*. 2014;11:CD008324

Forman-Hoffman V, McClure E, McKeeman J, et al. Screening for major depressive disorder in children and adolescents: a systematic review for the U.S. Preventive Services Task Force. *Ann Intern Med*. 2016;164(5):342–349

Forti-Buratti MA, Saikia R, Wilkinson EL, Ramchandani PG. Psychological treatments for depression in pre-adolescent children (12 years and younger): systematic review and meta-analysis of randomised controlled trials. *Eur Child Adolesc Psychiatry*. 2016; 25(10):1045–1054

Lewandowski RE, Acri MC, Hoagwood KE, et al. Evidence for the management of adolescent depression. *Pediatrics*. 2013;132(4):e996–e1009

Southammakosane C, Schmitz K. Pediatric psychopharmacology for treatment of ADHD, depression, and anxiety. *Pediatrics*. 2015;136(2):351–359

Stockings E, Degenhardt L, Lee YY, et al. Symptom screening scales for detecting major depressive disorder in children and adolescents: a systematic review and meta-analysis of reliability, validity and diagnostic utility. *J Affect Disord*. 2015;174:447–463

CHAPTER 101

Suicide

Introduction

Suicide is the second leading cause of death among youth between 15 and 24 years of age, with approximately 4,600 deaths per year. However, for every suicide death in youth, there are at least 25 unsuccessful attempts. While girls are 3 times more likely to attempt suicide than boys, boys are 4 times more likely to succeed because they often choose more violent means of suicide (eg, guns or hanging).

Clinical Presentation

Risk factors for suicide include lesbian, gay, bisexual, or transgender identification; previous suicide attempts; history of psychological or mental disorder (particularly depression, schizophrenia, or social anxiety); history of abuse; history of substance abuse; impulsive or aggressive tendencies; or family history of suicide. Suicidal patients often have feelings of hopelessness, are isolated or lack social support, and are more likely to have a comorbid psychiatric condition and/or a chronic medical condition. As a part of the review of systems, perform a depression screening for any child or adolescent admitted to the hospital, regardless of the admitting diagnosis. Screen for personal or family history of suicide, as well as access to firearms, medications, and illegal drugs.

If the patient expresses suicidal ideation or suicidal threats, this needs to be taken seriously. "Red flags" or warning signs include

Expressing suicidal ideation
- Talking about suicide
- Making statements such as, "I'm going to kill myself," "I wish I were dead," or "I wish I hadn't been born"
- Mood changes, such as dysphoria, irritability, or self-reports of feeling "numb," although the patient might be irritable or cranky, rather than sad or dejected
- Preoccupation with death, dying, or violence
- Feeling trapped or expressing hopelessness

Demonstrating at-risk behaviors
- Social withdrawal
- Change in normal routine, including self-care and eating or sleeping habits
- Risky or self-destructive behaviors, such as substance use or reckless driving

- Giving away belongings, cleaning up a messy room, or discarding cherished items when there is no other logical explanation for doing this
- Change in school performance or refusal to go to school
- At-risk behaviors may include excessive crying spells, somatic complaints, decreased energy, or extreme sensitivity within the peer group, family, and/ or academic setting

Mental Status Assessment

The following screening tools and questions can be used (by the hospitalist team or the psychiatry/psychology/social work team) when assessing the patient:

- Clinical interview
- Patient Health Questionnaire 9 (PHQ-9, ages 11–17)
- Children's Depression Inventory II (ages 7–17)
- Columbia Suicide Severity Rating Scale

Assessing the Patient for Suicidal Ideation

- "Do you have any thoughts of hurting yourself? Have you had a plan of what you would do to hurt yourself?"
- "Have you considered ending your life?"
- "Do you want to die?"

Assessing Risk Factors

- "Have you ever attempted suicide or self-harm?"
- "Do you have a family history of mental illness?"
- "Do you have a family history of suicide attempts?"
- "Have you ever received a diagnosis of mental illness?"
- "Do you use alcohol or other substances?"
- "Have you recently started a new medication?" (eg, antidepressants may increase the patient's risk of suicidal ideation)
- "Do you have any other stressors in your life?" (eg, bullying, home environment, peer pressure, medical conditions, recent loss)

Assessing the Patient for a Suicide Plan

- "Do you have a plan or have you considered how you would hurt/harm/ kill yourself?"
- If yes, assess lethality:
  — "How, when, and where would you carry out this plan? What did you think would happen to you? Would there be anybody else physically with you when you started this plan?"

— "Do you have the means to take your own life?" (eg, hoarding of medications or gaining access to firearms or other lethal means, such as cleaning products)

Assessing Protective Factors

- Individual strengths, such as coping skills
- Psychosocial situation, for support (eg, friends, family, religion)
- Reasons for living
- Motivation and hopefulness
- Future-oriented thinking and planning

Physical Examination

There may not be any physical signs of suicidal ideation. In a patient with depression or other mood disorder, there may be signs of poor hygiene, poor eye contact, flattened affect, weight change, lack of energy, or disturbances in mood, thought, or speech. Use the physical examination to screen the patient for abnormalities associated with organic causes of depression, such as hypothyroidism, diabetes, active substance use, neurologic disorders, and infections. During the physical examination, there may be signs of self-injury or cutting behavior. These may be hidden under clothes in the groin, upper thigh, and forearm areas. Although self-injury is not a specific risk factor for suicidal ideation, it may reflect significant emotional distress.

Laboratory Workup

The goal of laboratory testing is to determine if there were any toxic ingestions (see Chapter 70, Toxic Exposures), organic causes of depression (see Chapter 100, Depression), or altered mental status (see Chapter 82, Altered Mental Status). Otherwise, routine tests are not indicated, with the exception of a pregnancy test in a postpubertal female patient.

Treatment

The safety of the patient is the priority, while the level of suicidal ideation/intent determines the best course of action. If the patient is suicidal with a detailed plan and intent to kill her- or himself, urgently consult a psychiatrist or psychologist for further evaluation and to develop a course of treatment. Arrange for one-on-one supervision and monitoring. If the patient remains suicidal but is medically stable for discharge, the psychiatrist will conduct a thorough suicide/risk assessment to determine if admission (involuntarily or voluntarily) to an inpatient psychiatric unit/hospital is warranted.

If the patient is expressing suicidal ideation but does not have a clear plan or intent, consider developing a safety plan, ideally with the psychiatrist or psychologist. While this is not a safety contract or legal document, it can help patients and parents develop a clear plan of action for hospital discharge. This safety plan often includes a list of coping strategies, reasons to live, and people or resources the patient would contact during times of crisis or if he/she felt suicidal. The plan is often a structured document written in outline form in the patient's own words (but with family input). Coping skills can include activities the patient can do alone or with others, including going for a walk, listening to music, taking a hot shower, journaling, or engaging in relaxation exercises, like diaphragmatic breathing. Additional coping skills may include the support of friends or family, including calling a friend, going to the mall, seeing a movie, or going out for a snack with others. A safety plan does not replace treatment or continued assessment, which is a necessity if the patient is expressing any plans or intent to self-harm.

If the patient is expressing suicidal gestures, self-injurious behavior that does not result in death, or self-harm behaviors (such as cutting various body parts [eg, wrists, thighs] but not deep enough to result in significant blood loss), the patient may be trying to achieve emotional relief via physical pain. There may be no intent or desire to die and no plan to commit suicide, but arrange an evaluation for depression or other psychiatric illness that could possibly lead to future suicide attempts. Conduct this assessment during hospitalization to help determine disposition and the appropriate outpatient plan. Bring behavior such as cutting to the parents' attention, as it indicates a high degree of emotional distress and could accidentally result in death. Remove any items in the patient's room that could be used for self-injury (eg, sharps, medicines, razors). In the hospital, this will require a room search of the patient's belongings.

Consultation

Arrange a consultation with a psychiatrist, psychologist, or therapeutic social worker. It is important to communicate with parents if you believe that the patient is at moderate to high risk of suicide or self-harm. Discuss these concerns with the parents and obtain collateral information that can be used to develop a safe and appropriate discharge plan. Before discharge, review the safety plan with the parents so they understand what coping skills the patient may find useful, whom the patient feels comfortable talking to in times of crisis, and whom to contact for additional resources. This will also help the family understand the severity of the symptoms, identify warning signs that the patient is in distress, and ensure outpatient follow-up. Breaching confidentiality is permitted if the patient is considered to be suicidal, although expressing suicidal ideation is not necessarily sufficient to warrant a breach. Use the consultative service to help make this determination.

Disposition

- **Transfer to an inpatient psychiatric facility:** The patient has active suicidal ideation or a plan or is experiencing severe symptoms that are affecting daily life
- **Discharge criteria:** The patient is deemed safe (no active suicidal or homicidal ideation, no active plans for suicide) by the psychiatry or psychology team, with appropriate outpatient psychiatry/psychology follow-up arranged; safety planning has been conducted with the psychiatry/psychology team, and the parents/caretakers are aware of this plan

Follow-up

- **Mental health professional:** As soon as possible, ideally within 1 to 3 days (up to 1 week maximum)
- **Provide additional referrals for the patient/family to use if needed:**
  — 911 or a local emergency service that can be called in an emergency
  — The national U.S. Suicide Hotline number: 800/273-TALK (800/273-8255)
  — A specific crisis line for the local county
- **Primary care provider:** 1 week

Pearls and Pitfalls

- Developing a safety plan does not guarantee that the patient will not initiate another suicide attempt in the future.
- Assessing the patient for a suicidal plan or ideation will not cause a patient to want to commit suicide. These questions are key to determining the seriousness of the situation.
- Discharge planning can be challenging because of the lack of outpatient pediatric psychiatric and psychological resources in the community. Start this process at admission with the help of the psychiatry/psychology/social work team.
- Appropriate family involvement, patient protective factors, and good communication between the treatment team and family/patient are keys for safe discharge planning and transition to an outpatient team of providers.

Bibliography

Bongar B. *The Suicidal Patient: Clinical and Legal Standards of Care*. Washington, DC: American Psychiatric Association; 1991

Centers for Disease Control and Prevention. Suicide prevention. http://www.cdc.gov/violenceprevention/suicide. Accessed May 2016

Dilillo D, Mauri S, Mantegazza C, Fabiano V, Mameli C, Zuccotti GV. Suicide in pediatrics: epidemiology, risk factors, warning signs and the role of the pediatrician in detecting them. *Ital J Pediatr*. 2015;41:49

Hawton K, Saunders KE, O'Connor RC. Self-harm and suicide in adolescents. *Lancet*. 2012;379(9834):2373–2382

Soole R, Kõlves K, De Leo D. Suicide in children: a systematic review. *Arch Suicide Res*. 2015;19(3):285–304

Psychosocial Issues

Child Abuse and Neglect

Introduction

Child maltreatment encompasses neglect, physical abuse, sexual abuse, and psychological maltreatment. Neglect is the most prevalent form of child maltreatment, though because of its very nature, it is the aspect seen least frequently by health care professionals. Failure to thrive (FTT) is the most common medical presentation of neglect. Neglect may also manifest as a lack of supervision, such as when a patient ingests a toxic substance or sustains a preventable injury. *Medical care neglect* refers to failing to continue critical treatment or management of a child's medical condition, such as not refilling prescriptions or missing medical appointments.

Physical abuse is any punishment that is excessive or causes a risk of or actual bodily injury to a child, although definitions may vary between individual states. Risk factors related to the parent include an adolescent mother, substance abuse, single parenthood, employment instability or overcommitment, and family violence, which is also associated with maternal depression and a history of abuse of the parent. Patient risk factors include prematurity, low birth weight, and disabilities. Child abuse is not limited to one societal group but cuts across all cultural and socioeconomic strata.

Identification of abused children is critical because they may be repeatedly victimized. As many as 35% of the patients who receive diagnoses of physical abuse have evidence of old injury at the time of diagnosis, with the most likely perpetrator being a parent.

Clinical Presentation

History

Accurate and detailed documentation is critical; use direct quotations when possible.

Ask about social support at home and any family stressors. In addition, assess the parent's affective behavior toward the patient by gently asking questions about how the parent responds to the patient when a need is expressed. How does the caregiver typically discipline the child or deal with difficult behaviors? To build trust and rapport, acknowledge stressors, frustration, poverty, and the medical problems that the parents may face.

It is critically important to carefully review the child's medical, developmental, birth, family, and social histories, including the nature and number of previous reports to the local child protective services (CPS) agency. Determine who, other than the parents, are regular caregivers, as well their relationship to the family, how long family has known them, and if other children are cared for along with the patient (other children may also be at risk). In addition, inquire about the child's global development, speech, temperament, sleep schedule, and behavioral issues.

Trauma may not be part of the chief complaint or history. The patient may instead present with apnea, an altered level of consciousness, new-onset afebrile seizures, vomiting, change in feeding pattern, or simply an unexplained or unwitnessed injury. If emesis or increased sleep is reported, can it be differentiated from the patient's usual condition (eg, reflux) or an acute viral illness? Has any swelling or bruising occurred or coloration changed?

In a case of trauma, obtain and document a step-by-step mechanism of injury from the caregiver and the child, if verbal, although the patient may be reticent to talk about the events. With physical abuse, the mechanism of injury is often inconsistent with the physical examination findings, so determining the exact mechanism is a priority. Important questions include: "What was the patient doing just before and just after the event? Who saw the patient last before the event, and what was the patient's status? Who saw the patient most immediately after the event, and what was the status then? Can anyone speak to if or how the patient's status changed over time after the event?" If the patient has fallen, inquire about the pre- and post-fall position, the reported fall distance, and the type of surface that the child's body hit.

Obtaining an accurate history can be particularly challenging when the parent/caregiver has a developmental disability, communication difficulties, behavioral issues, or mental illness. In such a case, consult with a trained interviewer, such as a child abuse pediatrician, social worker, psychologist, or psychiatrist.

Physical Examination

Measure and plot the patient's height, weight, and, if age appropriate, head circumference. Chronic abuse or neglect can be reflected in abnormal growth parameters, especially reduced weight (neglect) and increased head circumference (chronic subdural hematomas). The approach to a patient with FTT is summarized in Chapter 86, Failure to Thrive. A patient with a known genetic syndrome may have abnormal growth parameters that have persistently been below the standard curve values, but in the event of child abuse, the patient may have recently shown a further decrease in growth velocity.

Document bruising, petechiae, and other skin findings with a body diagram and/or digital camera if abuse is suspected; include any patterns.

Suspicious sites for inflicted skin injury include the head, ears, neck, jaw, and soft-tissue prominences, such as the cheeks, abdomen, and buttocks. Any bruise in a nonambulatory child is concerning for abuse. Also perform a thorough oral examination of the palate, the gum plates/teeth, and the frenula of the lips and tongue.

After 1 to 2 days, re-examine areas that are tender but do not have visible signs of injury, because these may be sites of deep bruising. A patient with abdominal injury may have equivocal abdominal examination findings, most often without visible bruising. In contrast to long bones, rib and metaphyseal fractures may not have tenderness with palpation at presentation.

Laboratory Workup

For physical abuse, use Table 102-1 to guide the choice of laboratory tests and radiology examinations. See Chapter 86, Failure to Thrive, for the workup of FTT.

Obtain a complete blood cell count to look for acute anemia (acute trauma) or an abnormal smear result to identify mimics of abuse, such as leukemia. Also obtain liver enzyme levels and perform urinalysis to evaluate the patient for possible occult abdominal injury, but amylase and lipase determinations are less helpful. Liver injury is the most common abdominal injury and manifests as transient increase of enzyme levels, decreasing hemoglobin levels, and vital sign changes. A prothrombin time and partial thromboplastin time are useful to screen for a bleeding diathesis if the patient presents with bruising or central nervous system hemorrhage, although these tests will not necessarily allow detection of von Willebrand disease or disorders of platelet aggregation.

Table 102-1. Laboratory Evaluation of Suspected Abuse			
	<12 Months of Age	12–35 Months of Age	>3 Years of Age
CBC with peripheral smear, AST/ALT levels, urinalysis	Always	Always	Per history or physical examination findings
Abdominal CT	Per history, physical examination findings, and laboratory test results		
Dilated indirect funduscopic examination	For all patients with intracranial bleeding or external ocular injury		
Head CT (to rule out intracranial bleed)	With signs or symptoms of head trauma	With signs of inflicted trauma	
Brain MR imaging (a first choice for infants in some centers)	Follow-up for an abnormal head CT as needed		
Skeletal survey (when stable)	Always	Always	Per history or physical examination findings

Abbreviations: ALT, alanine transaminase; AST, aspartate transaminase; CBC, complete blood cell count; CT, computed tomography; MR, magnetic resonance.

A bone metabolism workup may be indicated for a formerly premature patient to determine if the patient's osteopenia could predispose him or her to fracture(s).

Head computed tomography (CT) can provide evidence of an intracranial bleed, and magnetic resonance (MR) imaging can further demonstrate the extent of the bleed, as well as offer good detail on associated parenchymal injury. Most pediatric centers now use low-dose radiation for head CT in accordance with the Image Gently protocol (www.imagegently.org). Order a skeletal survey in a patient younger than 2 years of age when the patient cannot communicate pain because of developmental status or when the patient has a history of trauma with a disabling injury. Since this is not an urgent study, defer it until the patient is clinically stable and skilled pediatric radiology personnel are available. In many cases, a repeat skeletal survey conducted 2 weeks later will show missed occult fractures that subsequently demonstrate callus formation.

Although up to 80% of infants with abusive head trauma have retinal hemorrhages, funduscopy is not a useful screening study for occult head injury. Rather, arrange a dilated funduscopic examination to evaluate the patient for comorbid retinal hemorrhage, retinal detachment, or vitreous hemorrhage if there is either intracranial or external ocular injury.

Differential Diagnosis

There is more concern for abuse if the caretaker's explanations are absent, vague, variable (from the same historian or between caretakers), or inconsistent with the pattern of injuries or the developmental capabilities of the patient. Consider the use of complementary or alternative medicines, cultural practices, and healing traditions that may harm the child by leaving marks, burns, or bruises, such as coining, spooning, holding the child upside down to hit the feet, and treatment for sunken fontanelle (or "caida de mollera"). The intention of these cultural practices is to heal or treat a perceived illness rather than to inflict injury and should therefore be addressed in a manner sensitive to the caretakers' beliefs.

Finding a child unconscious without an explanation is suspicious for abuse. Consider inflicted trauma if a nonambulatory infant has any bruising. In contrast, a cruising toddler will typically have bruising on extensor surfaces (shins) or over prominences of bone, such as the forehead. Recurrent injuries are suspicious for maltreatment if there is no clear and consistent explanation from the caregiver. Injuries that are also concerning for abuse include multiple, complex, diastatic, or occipital skull fractures, as well as hematomas on brain images. Some fracture types in infants, such as posterior rib fractures or metaphyseal fractures, are highly specific for inflicted injury.

New-onset seizures require neuroimaging, usually MR imaging. If there is persistent altered mental status (AMS), CT images can be used to confirm the diagnosis of trauma. Infections, such as meningitis or encephalitis, can cause AMS or seizures, as well as vomiting. There may be a history of fever, headache, cold symptoms, or a rash. Ingestion and purposeful administration of a toxic substance are other etiologies of AMS and seizures.

Above-average weight gain while the patient is receiving observed care and large amounts of ad lib intake is suspicious for nutritional neglect. Consider food insecurity, poverty, and domestic violence, which may contribute to nutritional problems and access to appropriate foods.

See Table 102-2 for differential diagnosis of child abuse and neglect.

Table 102-2. Differential Diagnosis of Child Abuse and Neglect	
Diagnosis	**Clinical Features**
Failure to thrive: See Chapter 86 for the differential diagnosis.	
Bleeding	
Glutaric aciduria type 1	Macrocranium Subdural hematoma, frontotemporal atrophy Sparse retinal hemorrhages
Hemophilia	(+) Family history Hemarthrosis ↑ Partial thromboplastin time
Hemorrhagic disease of the newborn	History of no vitamin K prophylaxis or home birth Patient exclusively breastfed Parenchymal cerebral hemorrhage and mucosal bleeding
Idiopathic thrombocytopenic purpura	Petechiae Thrombocytopenia
Cutaneous findings	
Coining	Erythematous, linear abrasions over the patient's back/extremities
Cupping	Bruises are circular and appear in a pattern
Mongolian spots	Nontender macules No change in appearance when re-examined
Fractures	
Osteogenesis imperfecta	Patient may have (+) family history Transverse long-bone and rib fractures Blue sclerae (not seen in all types) Macrocephaly, numerous Wormian bones
Rickets	History of prematurity History of poor vitamin D and/or calcium intake ↓ Calcium, ↑ alkaline phosphatase levels Patient exclusively breastfed; minimal sun exposure Uniform changes at costochondral junctions and of all long bones on radiographs Frontal bossing (severe)

Continued

Table 102-2. Differential Diagnosis of Child Abuse and Neglect, continued	
Diagnosis	**Clinical Features**
Abdominal injury	
Volvulus with malrotation	Bilious vomiting Surgical abdomen

"+" indicates a positive finding.

Treatment

Stabilization of circulation, airway, and breathing is always the priority. Ensure that the patient is hemodynamically stable before being sent for neuroimaging. If there is concern for head injury or other trauma, consult the appropriate surgical services, and for all other injuries, treat according to the standards of care. Carefully document all findings and management decisions by using objective language. Provide appropriate emotional and psychological support.

Caring for a maltreated child is emotionally unsettling and can lead to strong protective feelings in medical staff that may compromise objectivity. The role of the medical team is to focus on the health and support of the child, not to investigate a potential crime or judge a perceived perpetrator. Consult with the local CPS agency, social workers, and the appropriate hospital administration to limit family visitation if the hospital staff are threatened by a caretaker or if the safety of other patients is jeopardized. However, parental visitation cannot be broadly denied unless CPS agents decide it is necessary for the protection of the child.

Child Safety and Protection

If there is any *reasonable basis to suspect* abuse or neglect, report the case to the local CPS agency. It is not necessary to have a specific perpetrator or hypothesis in mind. In addition, the Health Insurance Portability and Accountability Act has specific exclusions in child maltreatment cases so that it defers to state laws regarding reporting and patient confidentiality. Know your state laws, which can be found on the U.S. Department of Health and Human Services Web site at www.childwelfare.gov/topics/systemwide/laws-policies/state/.

Indications for Consultation

- **Child protection team:** All patients
- **Dietitian:** FTT
- **Genetics:** Suspected glutaric academia type 1 or osteopenic bone disease, such as osteogenesis imperfecta

- **Hematology:** Suspected coagulopathy
- **Neurosurgery:** Intracranial injury or displaced skull fracture
- **Ophthalmology:** If a dilated funduscopic examination is indicated, evaluation and management of eye injuries
- **Orthopedics:** Evaluation and management of fractures
- **Surgery:** Suspected intra-abdominal injury

Disposition

- **Intensive care unit transfer:** Unstable vital signs or altered mental status
- **Discharge criteria:** Injuries stable or improved; CPS has identified a safe environment into which the child may be discharged; follow-up plan established

Follow-up

- **Primary care:** 2 weeks for repeat skeletal survey for a patient younger than 2 years, biopsychosocial follow-up, vaccine catch-up, etc
- **Developmental-behavioral pediatrician:** As needed for problems with regression, fears, tantrums, aggression, and sleep problems
- **Early intervention or Head Start program:** As needed for developmental delay
- **Mental health services:** As needed for signs of depression, posttraumatic stress

Pearls and Pitfalls

- A short fall (<3 ft [<.9 m]) can result in a simple, linear skull fracture with scalp bruising and swelling but rarely causes multiple, complex, diastatic, or occipital skull fractures or a significant intracranial injury.
- A reasonable basis to suspect abuse is sufficient to report the case to the local child protection authorities. A useful strategy is to file a report if just one member of the team believes it is necessary.
- Maintain a high index of suspicion, particularly with infants, because many abused children are treated for their injuries by medical professionals prior to abuse being diagnosed. One bruise in a nonambulatory infant strongly correlates with other concomitant injuries.
- The age of a bruise cannot be determined by physical examination or color of the bruise.

Bibliography

Christian CW; Committee on Child Abuse and Neglect, American Academy of Pediatrics. The evaluation of suspected child physical abuse. *Pediatrics*. 2015;135(5):e1337–e1354

Flaherty EG, Perez-Rossello JM, Levine MA, Hennrikus WL; American Academy of Pediatrics Committee on Child Abuse and Neglect; Section on Radiology, Section on Endocrinology, and Section on Orthopaedics, American Academy of Pediatrics; and Society for Pediatric Radiology. Evaluating children with fractures for child physical abuse. *Pediatrics*. 2014;133(2):e477–e489

Hibbard R, Barlow J, Macmillan H; The Committee on Child Abuse and Neglect and American Academy of Child and Adolescent Psychiatry, Child Maltreatment and Violence Committee; American Academy of Child and Adolescent Psychiatry; and Child Maltreatment and Violence. Psychological maltreatment. *Pediatrics*. 2012;130(2):372–378

Piteau SJ, Ward MG, Barrowman NJ, Plint AC. Clinical and radiographic characteristics associated with abusive and nonabusive head trauma: a systematic review. *Pediatrics*. 2012;130(2):315–323

Sheets LK, Leach ME, Koszewski IJ, Lessmeier AM, Nugent M, Simpson P. Sentinel injuries in infants evaluated for physical abuse. *Pediatrics*. 2013;131(4):701–707

U.S. Department of Health and Human Services, Administration for Children and Families, Children's Bureau. *Child maltreatment*. http://www.acf.hhs.gov/programs/cb/research-data-technology/statistics-research/child-maltreatment/. Accessed March 24, 2016

CHAPTER 103

Sexual Abuse

Introduction

Sexual abuse is defined as sexual activities that the child cannot comprehend, activities for which the child is developmentally unprepared and cannot give consent, and/or activities that violate the law or social taboos of society. Most perpetrators are male, with adolescents implicated in at least 20% of cases.

Clinical Presentation

History

At presentation, sexual abuse appears in variable ways, ranging from parental concern alone to nonspecific physical symptoms to the demonstration of sexualized behaviors and even frank disclosure of the abuse by the child. If there are signs or symptoms concerning for abuse, interview the caregiver and the patient separately. Ask open-ended questions, which will facilitate obtaining a full history and explanation. For example, ask the patient, "Has anyone ever touched you in a way you didn't like or didn't want?" Respond calmly and without strong emotions.

If the patient has recently arrived in the United States, ask how he or she traveled here and what happened after arrival. Questions that can help screen for human trafficking include, "Can you tell me about what happened to you when you traveled to the United States? Did you have to do anything so that they would help you? Have you been threatened or harmed if you try to quit or leave your situation? Did anyone where you stay ever make you feel scared or unsafe?"

A thorough review of systems is necessary, including asking questions about abdominal pain, dysuria, enuresis, encopresis, bleeding, discharge, phobias, difficulty sleeping, possible physical trauma, and exposure to adult or pornographic material. Also ask about homicidal or suicidal ideation. Specific symptoms of sexual abuse include rectal or genital bleeding and developmentally unusual sexualized behavior.

If there is enough information to raise a concern that inappropriate contact has occurred, arrange for a separate, detailed interview to be conducted by a trained professional. This can occur in the hospital by contacting the child protection team or a social worker. Occasionally, it may be appropriate to delay the interview until the child can be seen at an advocacy center if follow-up can be arranged within a short period of time, if the patient is safe from the perpetrator after discharge, if the disclosure is of remote contact, and if the child has no physical complaints. Regardless, the hospital team must obtain a history pertinent to the diagnosis and treatment of any medical diagnoses secondary to the abuse. This includes the type of abuse, when the last incident occurred, the type of contact that happened, any signs or symptoms of sexually transmitted infections (STIs), and date of menarche in female subjects. Do not interview a patient younger than 3 years, but document any spontaneous utterances in quotation marks, such as, "You won't hurt my pee-pee like John did, will you?"

Physical Examination

If the incident(s) occurred more than 4 days prior to presentation and there are no genitourinary symptoms, the examination may be deferred until the patient can be seen at a children's advocacy center equipped with trained examiners and a colposcope. Collection of forensic evidence is warranted when the last episode of abuse occurred within 72 to 96 hours, if the child is acutely injured, and if the history includes the potential for exposure to bodily fluids. Perform the examination in accordance with the protocols for sexual assault victims to properly collect the evidence. Many institutions have a pediatric sexual assault nurse examiner (SANE-P) or child abuse pediatrician available to perform the genital and rectal examination with colposcopic viewing and photography. Ideally, arrange for the presence of a supportive adult who is not involved in the allegations of abuse.

If no designated examiner is available, start with explaining the examination to the patient and parent/guardian, if present. Inspect the oropharynx and skin for signs of trauma or infection. Note the child's affect and development; however, there is no standard victim reaction to sexual assault. The patient may be poorly interactive, sad, withdrawn, or, in contrast, smiling and engaged with the examiner.

During the genitourinary examination, note the patient's sexual maturity rating and describe each part of the genitalia, breasts, perineal region, anus, and buttocks as necessary, with accompanying drawn diagrams or photographs. The best way to visualize the hymen and female genitalia is by means of labial traction. Place the patient in the frog-leg or lithotomy position, grasp each of the labia majora with the thumb and forefinger, and gently pull toward the examiner (as if pulling up a sock). If performed correctly, the examination is painless, and the hymen will become more three-dimensional in relation to the introitus and vaginal canal. However, the hymen can have a variety of normal configurations that may require specialized training to recognize.

It is uncommon to discover physical examination findings that are diagnostic of sexual abuse, even among victims of chronic sexual abuse. Concerning findings include abrasions or bruising of the inner thighs and labia; tears or scars of the labia minora, fossa navicularis, posterior fourchette or posterior hymen; interruption of the posterior hymen; or absent hymeneal tissue. In the assessment for genital injury, anal injury is the most rarely identified. Anal bruising, lacerations, or scars can also be consistent with an acute sexual assault.

Laboratory Workup

Complete a forensic evidence collection kit, if not already performed in the emergency department, if the abuse has occurred in the past 72 to 96 hours or if there is a possibility of direct contact with blood or body fluids. To decide on testing for STIs, consider the following:

- Was there oral, genital, or rectal contact with bodily secretions? Digital fondling alone is unlikely to transmit an STI.
- How common are STIs in the community?
- Is the child symptomatic? Do not perform testing in an asymptomatic prepubertal child, given the low prevalence of STIs in this population. Exceptions include a patient who shares the environment with a child or alleged perpetrator who is symptomatic or known to be infected.

Typical STI testing includes obtaining samples to test for gonorrhea, chlamydia (throat swab for culture and urine nucleic acid amplification testing), Venereal Disease Research Laboratory or rapid plasma reagin screening for syphilis, and HIV. Also perform a pregnancy test for a postmenarchal girl. Pregnancy or the presence of sperm or semen is diagnostic of sexual contact. A positive test result for gonorrhea, chlamydia, syphilis, or HIV is diagnostic of child abuse when vertical transmission has been excluded. Since it is unusual for a prepubertal victim to present immediately after the abuse occurred, select tests on a case-by-case basis in consultation with a child abuse expert.

Differential Diagnosis

Normal behavior surrounding genitalia is playful, driven by curiosity, and sometimes involves other children of the same age range. Sexually reactive behaviors may include a child who attempts to force another child, whether younger or an age peer, to engage in sexual behaviors or a child who performs insertive acts on him- or herself, on toys, or on playmates. As with many medical conditions, a diagnosis of sexual abuse does not rely solely on the physical examination findings. Often, a clear and consistent history is sufficient to assign the diagnosis.

In the case of genital abnormalities, consult a child abuse specialist or pediatric gynecologist who has the expertise to categorize abnormalities.

Reporting

A reasonable suspicion of sexual abuse is sufficient to report the case to the local child protection authorities. Health care providers are mandatory reporters for any reasonable suspicion. See Table 103-1 for guidance.

Treatment

Antibiotics

Treatment for STIs depends on the type of contact with the alleged perpetrator. Order prophylactic antibiotics if there was a possible exposure to bodily fluids in a pubertal (or older) patient, but prophylaxis is rarely indicated for a prepubertal victim.

Table 103-1. Guidelines for Making the Decision to Report Sexual Abuse of Children[a]					
Data Available				**Response**	
History	Behavioral Symptoms	Physical Examination Finding	Diagnostic Test Finding	Level of Concern about Sexual Abuse	Report Decision
Clear statement	Present or absent	Normal or abnormal	(+) or (−)	High	Report
None or vague	Present or absent	Normal or nonspecific	(+)[b]	High	Report
None or vague	Present or absent	Concerning or diagnostic finding	(+) or (−)	High[c]	Report
Vague or history given by parent only	Present or absent	Normal or nonspecific	(−)	Indeterminate	Refer when possible
None	Present	Normal or nonspecific	(−)	Indeterminate	Possible report[d], refer or follow up

"−" indicates a negative finding, "+" indicates a positive finding.

[a] Adapted from Kellogg N; American Academy of Pediatrics Committee on Child Abuse and Neglect. The evaluation of sexual abuse in children. *Pediatrics.* 2005;116(2):506–512.

[b] Positive test result for *Chlamydia trachomatis*, gonorrhea, *Trichomonas vaginalis*, HIV, syphilis, or herpes if nonsexual transmission is unlikely or excluded.

[c] Confirmed with various examination techniques and/or peer review with expert consultation.

[d] If behaviors are rare or unusual in normal children.

Administer

> Intramuscular ceftriaxone 250 mg once *or oral* cefixime 400 mg once
>
> *plus* oral metronidazole 2 g once
>
> *plus* oral azithromycin 1 g once *or* oral doxycycline 100 mg twice a day for
> 7 days
>
> If the patient is not fully vaccinated for hepatitis B, complete the series.

HIV Prophylaxis

If there is concern for HIV, contact a retrovirologist or infectious diseases expert for guidance with postexposure prophylaxis (PEP) because the regimen may vary, depending on regional viral profiles. An additional useful resource is the PEPline (888/448-4911; nccc.ucsf.edu/clinician-consultation/pep-post-exposure-prophylaxis/).

Emergency Contraception

Postpubertal female adolescents should be offered emergency contraception. If the patient presents within 72 hours of the assault, she can be offered oral levonogestre, 1.5 mg in 1 dose or 0.75 mg in 1 dose, followed by a second dose of 0.75 mg 12 hours later. Within 120 hours, she can take oral ulipristal acetate, 30 mg in 1 dose.

Child Safety and Protection

If there is any *reasonable suspicion* of abuse or neglect, report the case to the state child protective services (CPS) agency to address the child's safety and protection. It is not necessary to have a specific perpetrator or hypothesis in mind. In addition, the Health Insurance Portability and Accountability Act does not apply to mandated reports because communication to appropriate child protection agencies is necessary to protect the patient. Follow the state laws, which can be found on the U.S. Department of Health and Human Services Web site at www.childwelfare.gov/systemwide/laws-policies/state/.

There are more than 700 children's advocacy centers (CACs) in the United States. They function as centralized locations for victims of child maltreatment and sexual abuse. They provide coordination among community agencies and professionals, including law enforcement, CPS agencies, prosecution entities, medical organizations, victim advocacy groups, and mental health services. To find a CAC, go to www.nationalchildrensalliance.org/.

If the patient is a victim of human trafficking, ensure that the patient is not left alone. Separate the patient from their companion and call security as needed. Consult a social worker and call CPS and the National Human Trafficking Resource Center at 888/3737-888. You may also call the Homeland Security Investigations Tip Line at 866/347-2423 (24 hours a day, 7 days a week, with over 300 languages and dialects available) or submit a tip online at www.ice.gov/tips.

Indications for Consultation
- **Child protection team:** Suspected sexual abuse or genital abnormality
- **Pediatric sexual assault nurse examiner (SANE-P), if available:** Suspected sexual abuse
- **Psychiatry:** Suicidal or homicidal ideation
- **Social work:** Suspected sexual abuse
- **Pediatric gynecology:** Genital abnormality or injury

Disposition
- **Intensive care unit transfer:** Unstable vital signs or altered mental status
- **Discharge criteria:** CPS has identified a safe environment into which the child may be discharged; a follow-up plan has been established

Follow-up
- **Primary care:** 1 to 2 weeks
- **CAC:** 3 to 5 days to complete information gathering, establish care with mental health services, and screen for STIs, if indicated
- **Pediatrician who is expert in child abuse:** 3 to 4 weeks for surveillance laboratory testing and follow-up examination, if the local CAC does not have a clinical component
- **Mental health services:** 1 to 2 weeks, if not available at the nearest CAC, or referrals not provided by CAC

Pearls and Pitfalls
- The diagnosis of sexual abuse can be assigned on the basis of a clear and consistent history, such that a normal physical examination finding does not rule out sexual abuse.
- A reasonable suspicion of sexual abuse is sufficient to report the case to the local child protection authorities.
- Document observations thoroughly and clearly, using quotations when possible. Detailed notes will help inform protective agencies and law enforcement, as well as facilitate effective testimony in court.
- Use a colposcope or camera when conducting a physical examination and collecting evidence.
- Genitalia, especially female genitalia, have many variations of normal. If there is uncertainty about the findings of a physical examination, consult a child abuse expert.

Bibliography

Adams JA, Kellogg ND, Farst KJ, et al. Updated guidelines for the medical assessment and care of children who may have been sexually abused. *J Pediatr Adolesc Gynecol.* 2016;29(2):81–87

Asnes AG, Leventhal JM. Managing child abuse. *Pediatr Rev. 2010;31(2):47-55*

Centers for Disease Control and Prevention, U.S. Department of Health and Human Services. Updated guidelines for antiretroviral postexposure prophylaxis after sexual, injection drug use, or other nonoccupational exposure to HIV—United States, 2016. http://stacks.cdc.gov/view/cdc/38856. Accessed April 2016. Accessed March 1, 2017

Jenny C, Crawford-Jakubiak JE; Committee on Child Abuse and Neglect; American Academy of Pediatrics. The evaluation of children in the primary care setting when sexual abuse is suspected. Pediatrics. 2013;132(2):e558–e567

Kellogg ND; American Academy of Pediatrics Committee on Child Abuse and Neglect. Clinical report—the evaluation of sexual behaviors in children. *Pediatrics. 2009;124(3):992–998*

Workowski KA, Bolan GA; Centers for Disease Control and Prevention. Sexually transmitted diseases treatment guidelines, 2015. *MMWR Recomm Rep.* 2015; 64(RR-03):1–137

Pulmonology

Acute Asthma Exacerbation

Introduction

Asthma is a chronic respiratory disease characterized by airway inflammation and obstruction with a recurrent, reversible pattern of symptoms. The prevalence of asthma among American children is 13.5%, with significant racial, ethnic, and socioeconomic disparities. Acute asthma exacerbations (AAEs) and status asthmaticus, defined as a life-threatening asthma exacerbation with risk for respiratory failure, are among the leading causes of pediatric hospitalizations.

Clinical Presentation

History

In a patient with a known history of asthma, focus the initial history on recent asthma symptoms, medication use, and any risk factors for death (Box 104-1). Ask about fever and upper respiratory tract symptoms, which

Box 104-1. Risk Factors for Death from Asthma[a]
Asthma History
Difficulty perceiving asthma symptoms or severity of exacerbations
Hospitalization or ED visit for asthma in the past month
Lack of a written asthma action plan
Sensitivity to *Alternaria* fungi
Previous severe exacerbation (eg, intubation or intensive care unit admission for asthma)
≥3 ED visits for asthma in the past year
≥2 asthma hospitalizations in the past year
Using >2 canisters of short-acting β_2-agonist per month
Social History
Illicit drug use
Low socioeconomic status or inner-city residence
Major psychosocial problems
Comorbidities
Cardiovascular disease
Chronic psychiatric disease
Other chronic lung disease

Abbreviation: ED, emergency department.

[a] Adapted from U.S. Department of Health and Human Services; National Institutes of Health; National Heart, Lung, and Blood Institute; National Asthma Education and Prevention Program. Expert panel report 3: guidelines for the diagnosis and management of asthma. Full report 2007. Bethesda, MD: National Heart, Lung, and Blood Institute; 2007.

can suggest a viral trigger. Once the patient has been stabilized, inquire about chronic asthma symptoms (wheezing, nighttime coughing, use of short-acting β_2-agonist [SABA] rescue therapy, and limitation of activity), severity and frequency of prior exacerbations, and triggers.

Physical Examination

A patient with a moderate to severe asthma exacerbation often has decreased air movement with diffuse wheezing (classically expiratory but may be both inspiratory and expiratory), a prolonged expiratory phase, tachypnea, dyspnea, accessory muscle use, and coughing. In status asthmaticus, the respiratory examination findings can be misleading: The patient may have no wheezing because of lack of air movement ("tight" chest), so that the subsequent onset of wheezing may indicate improved air movement and response to therapy. Tachycardia is common and can be secondary to respiratory distress or dehydration or can be a medication side effect (use of SABAs).

Laboratory Workup

To assist in the assessment of the severity of an AAE, measure the oxygen saturation via pulse oximetry and peak expiratory flow, if a child 5 years and older is able to perform the technique. Otherwise, in most cases, laboratory tests and radiology examinations are not indicated. Evaluate a patient who has an atypical or prolonged disease course for potential other diagnoses (Table 104-1). When there is diagnostic uncertainty, order spirometry for a patient 5 years and older (if capable of performing the technique), because this can be particularly useful in differentiating asthma from other respiratory diseases.

Differential Diagnosis

An AAE is a diffuse process that affects the lower airways, producing wheezing and often hypoxemia. When the diagnosis is in doubt, administer a diagnostic/therapeutic trial of a SABA and monitor the patient for objective clinical improvement. No response to SABA may reflect status asthmaticus but consider other diagnoses if there is no prior history of asthma symptoms or if the disease course is unusual or prolonged (Table 104-1).

Treatment

Treat an asthma exacerbation with a SABA, supplemental oxygen as needed to maintain an oxygen (O_2) saturation level of 92% or greater, and systemic corticosteroids (Table 104-2). Many institutions use asthma clinical pathways (ie, care process models) to promote best evidence-based practices. These

Table 104-1. Differential Diagnosis of Wheezing

Acute Diagnoses	Clinical Features
Bronchiolitis	Age <2 y Often no prior history of wheezing Transmitted upper airway sounds and rales may accompany the wheezing Generally no response to SABAs
Community-acquired pneumonia	Tachypnea not responsive to SABAs Might not be hypoxic Asymmetrical breath sounds with focal crackles Chest radiographic evidence of lobar consolidation
Foreign body aspiration	May or may not have a history of aspiration Unilateral wheezing No response to SABAs Chest radiographic evidence of asymmetrical hyperinflation

Recurrent or Chronic Diagnoses	Clinical Features
Allergic bronchopulmonary aspergillosis	Recurrent infections not responsive to antibiotics May have chronic sputum production or hemoptysis Complete blood cell count demonstrates eosinophilia Chest radiographic evidence of bronchiectasis
Bronchiolitis	Age <2 y Usually no prior history of wheezing Transmitted upper airway sounds and rales may accompany the wheezing Generally no response to SABAs
Bronchopulmonary dysplasia	Age <3 y History of prematurity requiring oxygen therapy for >28 d Clinical examination findings similar to those of asthma exacerbation
Community-acquired pneumonia	Tachypnea not responsive to SABAs Usually not hypoxic Asymmetrical breath sounds with focal rales Chest radiographic evidence of lobar consolidation
Congestive heart disease	May be acute presentation Dyspnea and fatigue with feeding, as well as poor weight gain Crackles and hepatosplenomegaly Chest radiographic evidence of abnormal cardiac silhouette and pulmonary vascular markings
Cystic fibrosis	Recurrent cough, wheezing, abdominal pain, and loose stools Failure to thrive is common
Foreign body aspiration	May or may not have a history of aspiration Unilateral wheezing No response to SABAs Chest radiographic evidence of asymmetrical hyperinflation
Laryngotracheomalacia	"Noisy" breather since birth Symptoms worse when agitated, when lying flat, or with feedings No response to SABAs

Continued

Table 104-1. Differential Diagnosis of Wheezing, continued	
Recurrent or Chronic Diagnoses	**Clinical Features**
Vascular rings and slings	Chronic dysphagia, wheezing, stridor, and apnea Rare diagnosis If a high index of suspicion, obtain an esophagram
Vocal cord dysfunction	Refractory asthma symptoms with poor response to SABAs Generally no nighttime symptoms Harsh stridor noted over larynx when symptomatic Spirometry demonstrates limitation of inspiratory flow

Abbreviation: SABA, short-acting β_2-agonist.

Table 104-2. Medications for the Treatment of Asthma Exacerbation[a]		
Medication	**Dose**	**Comments**
Inhaled SABAs		
Albuterol		
MDI, 90 µg/puff	4–8 puffs every 20 min for 3 doses, then every 1–4 h; inhalation maneuver as needed; use a VHC; add a mask for a patient <6 y of age	In mild to moderate exacerbations, MDI plus VHC is as effective as nebulized therapy with appropriate administration technique and coaching by trained personnel
Nebulizer solution, 0.63 mg/3 mL 1.25 mg/3 mL 2.5 mg/3 mL 5 mg/mL	0.15 mg/kg (2.5-mg minimum) every 20 min for 3 doses, then 0.15–0.30 mg/kg (10-mg maximum) every 1–4 h as needed or 0.5 mg/kg/h via continuous nebulization	Dilute aerosols to ≥3 mL at gas flow of 6–8 L/min; use a large-volume nebulizer for continuous administration
Levalbuterol		
MDI, 45 µg/puff	See albuterol MDI dose	Indicated only for patients with unacceptable side effects from albuterol
Nebulizer solution, 0.63 mg/3 mL 1.25 mg/0.5 mL 1.25 mg/3 mL	0.075 mg/kg (1.25-mg minimum) every 20 min for 3 doses, then 0.075–0.150 mg/kg (5-mg maximum) every 1–4 h as needed	Levalbuterol administered in one-half the milligram dose of albuterol provides comparable effectiveness and safety; levalbuterol delivered via continuous nebulization has not been evaluated
Systemic Corticosteroids		
Methylprednisolone, prednisolone, prednisone		
Prednisolone (15 mg/5 mL) Prednisone (2.5-, 5-, 10-, 20-, and 50-mg tablets)	1–2 mg/kg, divided into doses administered twice a day (60-mg/d maximum)	No proven benefit of IV over oral corticosteroid. At discharge, administer 1–2 mg/kg/d (60-mg maximum) to complete a 3- to 5-d treatment course, but an extended course may be necessary Taper over several days if the patient receives steroids for >7–10 d

Table 104-2. Medications for the Treatment of Asthma Exacerbation[a], continued

Medication	Dose	Comments
Systemic Corticosteroids, continued		
Dexamethasone		
1 mg/mL	IM, IV, or oral 0.3–0.6 mg/kg doses administered once (16-mg maximum)	Limited data on dosing or benefit of 1 vs 2 doses No proven benefit over prednisolone, prednisone, or methylprednisolone
Adjunctive Therapies for Status Asthmaticus		
Magnesium sulfate		
1 g magnesium sulfate = 98.6 mg *elemental* magnesium = 8.12 mEq magnesium	50 mg/kg as IV solution (25–75 mg/kg, 2-g maximum)	Dilute to a concentration of 0.5 mEq/mL (60 mg/mL of *magnesium sulfate*); infuse over 2–4 h; do not exceed 125 mg/kg/h of magnesium sulfate Patient requires continuous monitoring, preferably in an ICU
Anticholinergics in Combination With SABAs		
Ipratropium bromide		
MDI, 18 µg/puff	4–8 puffs every 20 min as needed up to 3 h; use a VHC; add a mask for a patient <6 y of age	Use has not been shown to provide further benefit once a patient is hospitalized; do not use as first-line therapy
Nebulizer solution, 0.25 mg/mL	0.25–0.5 mg every 20 min for 3 doses, then as needed	May mix in same nebulizer with albuterol
Systemic (Injected) β₂-Agonists		
Epinephrine		
1:1,000 (1 mg/mL)	0.01 mg/kg up to 0.3–0.5 mg every 20 min for 3 doses, administered subcutaneously	No proven advantage of systemic therapy over aerosol
Terbutaline		
(1 mg/mL)	0.01 mg/kg every 20 min for 3 doses, then every 2–6 h as needed subcutaneously	No proven advantage of systemic therapy over aerosol

Abbreviations: ICU, intensive care unit; IM, intramuscular; IV, intravenous; MDI, metered dose inhaler; SABA, short-acting β₂-agonist; VHC, valved holding chamber.

[a] Adapted from U.S. Department of Health and Human Services; National Institutes of Health; National Heart, Lung, and Blood Institute; National Asthma Education and Prevention Program. Expert panel report 3: guidelines for the diagnosis and management of asthma. Full report 2007. Bethesda, MD: National Heart, Lung, and Blood Institute; 2007.

pathways have been shown to reduce cost and length of stay without increasing readmissions, while increasing adherence to best-practice techniques. The development of pathways requires a multidisciplinary team, including physicians from the inpatient setting, intensive care, pulmonology, and the emergency department, as well as respiratory therapists, pharmacists, social workers, and nurses.

Albuterol (4–8 puffs with valved holding chamber, with a mask for a child <6 years old) is the preferred SABA and method of administration because of its availability and cost. Use the patient's history and prehospital management, emergency department management, and physical examination findings to determine the initial scheduling of albuterol every 1 to 4 hours. Start with more frequent dosing, then wean the patient as tolerated. The greater the intensity of the prehospital and acute management and the more severe the physical examination findings, the more frequent the albuterol dosing.

Reassess the patient frequently—initially with each SABA administration. Check for improvement to taper the frequency of treatments or worsening that would necessitate intensifying the therapy. Assessments can also be performed by skilled members of the health care team, including respiratory therapists and nurses. A clinical scoring system may improve communication between the health care team and help standardize and facilitate the weaning process. Peak expiratory flows can also be useful to assess changes in a patient who is 5 years and older and experienced in using a peak flow meter.

Provide supplemental oxygen to correct hypoxemia (defined as an O_2 saturation level <92%) or, if the patient has acute deterioration with worsening respiratory rate, accessory muscle use and air movement, despite an O_2 saturation level of 92% or greater. As the patient improves, taper the supplemental oxygen to maintain an O_2 saturation level of 92% or greater.

Administer systemic corticosteroids, preferably orally, to any patient with an AAE. Systemic corticosteroids decrease airway inflammation, and there is no advantage to using intravenous (IV) or intramuscular steroids, unless the patient cannot tolerate oral medication. Prescribe treatment for 3 to 5 days but extend the course if the patient has prolonged symptoms that require hospitalization or recent or chronic steroid use. Taper the medication over several days if the patient receives steroids for more than 7 to 10 days to prevent rebound of respiratory symptoms. If the patient received steroids for more than 10 to 14 days, a longer taper is necessary because of the risk of adrenocortical insufficiency.

In a patient with status asthmaticus (severe respiratory distress, respiratory rate >60 breaths/min, little air movement, O_2 saturation level <92%) or an acute deterioration, give the patient nothing by mouth and begin maintenance IV fluids. Increase the SABA to continuous therapy via nebulization at 0.15 to 0.30 mg/kg/h (10–15-mg/h maximum). If a patient is receiving continuous SABA therapy for more than 24 hours, assess the electrolyte levels for hypokalemia. If there is no response after 4 to 6 hours with treatment intensification, transfer the patient to an intensive care unit (ICU), where additional therapies can be safely delivered, such as IV magnesium or heliox (70:30 helium-oxygen mixture to deliver albuterol nebulization). Additional therapies of *unproven* benefit that may be considered prior to intubation for respiratory failure include systemic IV β_2-agonists (IV or subcutaneous [SC] terbutaline or SC epinephrine), leukotriene inhibitors (montelukast), and noninvasive ventilation.

Treatments that do *not* improve outcomes for an inpatient with uncomplicated asthma exacerbations include theophylline or aminophylline, chest physiotherapy, and antibiotic therapy without a definite bacterial source. Although nebulized ipratropium bromide has been shown to decrease hospitalization rates for AAE, there is no documented benefit for its use during hospitalization for an uncomplicated AAE.

If the patient does not respond as anticipated or worsens acutely, evaluate the patient for complications, such as pneumothorax, pneumomediastinum, or secondary bacterial infections. When there is concern for impending respiratory failure, perform a complete physical examination, blood gas analysis, complete blood count, and chest radiography.

Start discharge planning at the time of admission. A critical aspect to quality inpatient asthma care is transitioning to appropriate outpatient management and facilitating a chronic asthma management plan. Ongoing discussion and communication with the family and primary care provider is essential to these goals. Several agencies, including the Centers for Medicare and Medicaid Services, have included asthma process and outcome measures as pediatric quality measures. See Table 104-3.

A discharge checklist for AAE is shown in Table 104-4. At discharge, prescribe the appropriate controller medication, as determined by classification of asthma severity. The first-line therapy for persistent asthma is an inhaled corticosteroid. Further information on classification and management of chronic asthma can be found at www.nhlbi.nih.gov/health-pro/guidelines/current/asthma-guidelines. Many institutions incorporate components of asthma teaching into an asthma education class given by a trained member of the health care team. Provide an individualized written home management plan (ie, asthma action plan), which gives families and patients simple directions for actions based on symptoms. Sample asthma action plans and other patient resources can be found at http://catalog.nhlbi.nih.gov/catalog/product/Asthma-Action-Plan/07-5251.

Table 104-3. AHRQ Dimensions of Quality Asthma Care Management (Adapted for Inpatients)

Process Measures	Measure Description
Asthma severity assessment	Assessment of asthma chronic severity
Asthma medications	Use of anti-inflammatory medications (such as inhaled corticosteroids) for patients with persistent asthma
Asthma management plan	Give patients/families a written asthma management plan; key aspects include 1. Arrangements for follow-up care 2. Environmental control and control of other triggers 3. Method and timing of rescue actions 4. Use of controllers 5. Use of relievers
Self-management support or patient education	Discuss with patients/families how to manage their asthma and avoid asthma triggers
Planned care for asthma	1. Recommend planned care visits for asthma at least every 6 mo or more frequently for more severe patients or those with comorbidities 2. Provide/recommend the influenza vaccine to patients with asthma 3. Provide smoking cessation counselling to patients with asthma
Environmental modifications	1. Advise patients/families to change things in the home, at school, or at work to reduce asthma triggers 2. Advise patients/families to avoid tobacco smoke exposure
Outcome Measures	
Daily symptom burden due to asthma in the past month	1. Review the number of days with limited activity 2. Review the number of school/work days missed 3. Review the number of days with sleeping difficulty 4. Review the number of days with (or free of) asthma symptoms 5. Review frequency of use of SABAs
Acute avoidable events due to asthma (exacerbations)	1. Review number of asthma hospitalizations 2. Review number of emergency or urgent care visits for asthma

Abbreviations: AHRQ, Agency for Healthcare Research and Quality; SABA, short-acting β_2-agonist.

Adapted from Agency for Healthcare Research and Quality. Table 4.1. Dimensions of Asthma Care Measurement. http://www.ahrq.gov/professionals/quality-patient-safety/quality-resources/tools/asthmaqual/asthmacare/table4-1.html. Reviewed October 2014. Accessed March 1, 2017.

Indications for Consultation

- **Pulmonologist or asthma specialist:** Poor response to therapy or a prolonged, recurrent, or atypical disease course
- **Tobacco dependence counselor:** Any patient who uses tobacco products or has a caretaker who uses cigarettes or electronic nicotine delivery systems (ie, electronic cigarettes)
- **Social worker:** Barriers to care, including financial or psychosocial stressors, documented history of noncompliance, and any concerns expressed by the health care team, as well as if the patient has risk factors for death

Table 104-4. Discharge Checklist[a]		
Intervention	**Dose/Timing**	**Education/Advice**
Inhaled medications (eg, MDI with VHC or spacer; nebulizer)	Select agent, dose, and frequency (eg, albuterol) Short-acting β_2-agonist: 2–6 puffs every 4–6 h for 2 d or as needed Inhaled corticosteroids: Dosing depends on the patient's chronic level of severity (generally a low to medium dose, unless an asthma specialist is involved)	Teach purpose Teach and check technique For MDIs, emphasize the importance of VHC or spacer
Oral medications	Select agent, dose, and frequency (eg, prednisone 50 mg every day for 5 d)	Teach purpose Teach side effects
Peak flow meter (PEF)	For selected patients ≥5 y and able: Measure PEF in the morning and evening and record the best of 3 tries each time	Teach purpose Teach technique Distribute a peak flow diary
Address environmental triggers, including tobacco use and tobacco smoke exposure	Ask about tobacco use and caretakers and others in the home who smoke cigarettes or use electronic nicotine delivery systems (ie, electronic cigarettes)	Provide smoking cessation counseling For more information, see http://www2.aap.org/richmondcenter/CounselingAboutSmokingCessation.html
Follow-up visit	Make appointment for follow-up care with primary clinician or asthma specialist within 1 wk	Advise patient (or caregiver) of date, time, and location of appointment within 5 d of hospital discharge
Home management plan (asthma action plan)	Before or at discharge	Instruct patient (or caregiver) on a simple plan for actions to be taken when symptoms, signs, or PEF values suggest airflow obstruction

Abbreviations: MDI, metered dose inhaler; PEF, peak expiratory flow; VHC, valved holding chamber.

[a] Adapted from U.S. Department of Health and Human Services; National Institutes of Health; National Heart, Lung, and Blood Institute; National Asthma Education and Prevention Program. Expert panel report 3: guidelines for the diagnosis and management of asthma. Full report 2007. Bethesda, MD: National Heart, Lung, and Blood Institute; 2007.

Disposition

- **ICU transfer:** No response to therapy within a 6-hour time frame or an acute deterioration
- **Discharge criteria:** No O_2 requirement, adequate oral intake, stable respiratory status with SABA inhalations no more frequent than every 4 to 6 hours, and asthma education with home management plan and follow-up appointments completed

Follow-up

- **Primary care provider:** 2 to 5 days
- **Pulmonologist, allergist, or asthma specialist:** 1 to 2 weeks if the patient has had a previous pediatric ICU admission for asthma or prior asthma admission within the past 12 months, frequent emergency department visits for asthma, or severe persistent asthma
- **Allergist:** Allergic triggers and/or atopy

Pearls and Pitfalls

- Address tobacco use or tobacco smoke exposure in 3 minutes or less by using the "2 A's and an R" (an abbreviated version of the "5 A's"): **Ask** if any caretakers smoke cigarettes or electronic cigarettes and advise them to quit, **Assist** caretakers by recommending first-line nicotine replacement therapy, and **Refer** them to the 800/QUIT-NOW line.
- Administer or recommend an influenza vaccination, unless the patient has already received it or there is a contraindication.
- Asthma clinical pathways standardize and improve inpatient asthma care.
- Asthma education and discharge planning begin at the time of admission.

Bibliography

Dexheimer JW, Borycki EM, Chiu KW, Johnson KB, Aronsky D. A systematic review of the implementation and impact of asthma protocols. *BMC Med Inform Decis Mak*. 2014;14:82

Farber HJ, Walley SC, Groner JA, Nelson KE; Section on Tobacco Control. Clinical practice policy to protect children from tobacco, nicotine, and tobacco smoke. *Pediatrics*. 2015;136(5):1008–1017

Link HW. Pediatric asthma in a nutshell. *Pediatr Rev*. 2014;35(7):287–298

National Heart, Lung, and Blood Institute. *National Asthma Education and Prevention Program 2007 Expert Panel Report 3: Guidelines for the Diagnosis and Management of Asthma*. Section 5, Managing Exacerbations of Asthma 2007. www.nhlbi.nih.gov/health-pro/guidelines/current/asthma-guidelines. Accessed March 8, 2017

Nelson KA, Zorc JJ. Asthma update. *Pediatr Clin North Am*. 2013;60(5):1035–1048

Nkoy F, Fassl B, Stone B, et al. Improving pediatric asthma care and outcomes across multiple hospitals. *Pediatrics*. 2015;136(6):e1602–e1610

Acute Respiratory Failure

Introduction

Respiratory failure may be hypercarbic or hypoxemic. One type may lead to the other, and a patient frequently has elements of both. Respiratory failure can also be acute or chronic. Acute respiratory failure (ARF) is an emergency and occurs over minutes to hours. If the body is unable to compensate, death is likely without rapid intervention.

Owing to a variety of anatomic, neuromuscular, and other considerations, infants and toddlers are particularly vulnerable to ARF. Most infants are preferential nasal breathers until 2 to 6 months of age. In addition, a younger patient has a relatively large tongue, a narrow subglottic region, small and compliant airways, fewer alveoli and poor collateral ventilation, a more compliant chest wall, easily fatigued respiratory musculature, and an immature respiratory center that results in irregular respirations or even apnea. Finally, there is a high incidence of metabolic, genetic, and developmental disorders that lead to poor airway control, chronic aspiration, severe muscle weakness, scoliosis, and restrictive lung disease.

Clinical Presentation

History

Risk factors for ARF include young age, history of prematurity, underlying disease(s), and previous respiratory problems or airway issues. The patient may initially present with fever, cough, upper respiratory infection symptoms, shock or sepsis, apnea, cyanosis, depressed mental status, or muscle weakness. Depending on the etiology, the progression can occur over minutes to days.

It is critical to learn the nature of and response to the therapies and interventions implemented at home, in the emergency department, in the outpatient setting, or in the field by emergency medical services. It is also valuable to learn what therapies and interventions have been helpful or problematic during any previous admissions.

Physical Examination

While a thorough physical examination is necessary, treatment takes priority to ensure that the patient's condition does not deteriorate. Much useful information is gained by observing the patient "from the door" and in a caregiver's arms. Ask the caregiver to expose the patient's chest and abdomen. Many children are upset by the presence of medical personnel, and this may be your only opportunity to see the child in a calm state. Note the general appearance and mental status. Irritability or anxiety suggests dyspnea, hypercarbia, hypoxemia, and more severe disease. Lethargy occurs with severe hypercarbia or hypoxemia, fatigue, and impending respiratory arrest. Extreme tachypnea and work of breathing can lead to fatigue and respiratory arrest, while bradypnea, poor air movement, and grunting are ominous findings. Stridor with poor air movement is an emergency. Hepatomegaly, facial or peripheral edema, jugular venous distention, or a gallop cardiac rhythm raises the concern for possible heart failure.

Laboratory Workup

The results of a blood gas analysis rarely help determine the best initial therapy for ARF, and the patient's distress during restraint and phlebotomy can lead to deterioration. In general, defer laboratory testing until the patient has been stabilized. In a patient with compensated chronic respiratory failure, blood gas analysis may be quite helpful, because the only sign of worsening might be increasing hypercarbia. Since oxygenation can be assessed with pulse oximetry, venous or capillary (if the patient is well perfused) blood gas samples are adequate.

Radiology Examinations

Radiographic findings are important and may help indicate a specific and potentially life-saving therapy. Obtain a chest radiograph to explicitly look for pneumonia, effusion, pneumothorax, a widened mediastinum, cardiomegaly, mass lesion, or evidence of a foreign body aspiration. Obtain an echocardiogram if a cardiac etiology is suggested by the history or examination findings.

Differential Diagnosis

Although the list is extensive (Table 105-1), the cause of a patient's acute respiratory disease rarely presents a diagnostic dilemma.

Treatment

The treatment of ARF is directed at the underlying pathophysiology. For more information, refer to other specific sections of this text.

High-flow nasal cannula oxygen (HFNCO$_2$) therapy delivers humidified, warmed oxygen at rates up to 80 L/min. HFNCO$_2$ can decrease the need for intubation in ARF and requires little technical skill. Except in small infants (<5–8 kg), positive end-expiratory pressure is not a significant component of

Table 105-1. Etiologies of Respiratory Failure	
Pathophysiology	**Diagnosis**
Nasal or other upper-airway obstruction	Adenoidal-tonsillar hypertrophy
	Choanal atresia/stenosis
	Croup
	Epiglottitis/supraglottitis
	Excessive or inspissated secretions
	Foreign body
	Neuromuscular disease and poor airway control
	Retropharyngeal abscess
Lower-airway obstruction	Asthma
	Bronchiolitis
	Bacterial tracheitis
Parenchymal lung disease	Acute respiratory distress syndrome
	Aspiration or inhalation injury
	Exacerbation of chronic lung disease
	Noncardiogenic pulmonary edema
	Pneumonia
	Pulmonary contusion
Pulmonary edema	Heart failure
Muscle weakness or paralysis	Botulism
	Guillain-Barré syndrome
	Muscular dystrophy
	Spinal cord injury
	Spinal muscular atrophy
	Transverse myelitis
	Underlying neuromuscular condition
Thoracic mass effect	Ascites
	Effusion or empyema
	Pneumothorax
	Tumor

Chapter 105: Acute Respiratory Failure

its effects. Although there is no standardized dosing for $HFNCO_2$, titrate the flow as needed. For upper limits, use 2 L/min/kg for the first 10 kg of body weight and 1 L/min/kg thereafter, up to a maximum of 40 to 80 L/min. In critical situations, these limits can be pushed further.

Heliox therapy at concentrations of 60% to 80% helium (including use with $HFNCO_2$) may provide a reduction in acute symptoms of croup, bronchiolitis, and asthma. It may "buy some time" while preparing for transfer or awaiting subspecialist consultation. However, its use can be limited by patient hypoxemia.

Nasal and Other Upper-Airway Obstruction

Treat nasal obstruction with nasal saline drops, followed by suctioning and judicious use of a topical α-agonist nasal decongestant (phenylephrine,

4 drops of 0.125% or 0.1 mL of 0.5% in each nostril, not to exceed 3 days of use to prevent a rebound). A patient with a large tongue, adenoidal-tonsillar hypertrophy, or poor airway control may find his or her own position of comfort. If not, place the patient in a lateral position, with or without a chin lift or jaw thrust. A mechanical nasal airway, such as a soft nasal trumpet or appropriately sized endotracheal tube, is usually well tolerated and can often provide significant relief. Pretreat with a topical α-agonist nasal decongestant (phenylephrine, oxymetazoline), use the largest diameter that will pass, lubricate well, and insert with gentle twisting and steady pressure to a length equal to the distance measured from the patient's nostril to the tragus. Other helpful modalities include continuous positive airway pressure (CPAP) and $HFNCO_2$.

For croup, allow the patient to assume a position of comfort, provide a calm environment, and minimize stimulation. The treatment of croup (Chapter 15) also includes corticosteroids, racemic epinephrine, and, in severe cases, heliox. Cool mist is *not* beneficial and may worsen patient distress. CPAP and $HFNCO_2$ (with heliox) may also be helpful. The patient may require endotracheal intubation, but anticipate difficulty. This is best performed with subspecialist consultation (intensivist, otolaryngologist, or anesthesiologist) if possible and usually requires an endotracheal tube that is at least one size smaller than usual for the patient.

Lower Airway Obstruction

The treatment of asthma (Chapter 104) and bronchiolitis (Chapter 109) is detailed elsewhere. If respiratory support is needed, use CPAP, bilevel positive airway pressure (BiPAP), or $HFNCO_2$. Heliox may be helpful if hypoxemia is not limiting. Intubate the patient only for refractory hypoxemia or impending respiratory arrest. Although an infant with severe bronchiolitis may need intubation, even an extreme asthma exacerbation can usually be managed without mechanical ventilation. Do not deliver bronchodilators via $HFNCO_2$, because drug delivery decreases substantially as the flow rate increases. Use traditional face mask delivery in addition to $HFNCO_2$ support.

Parenchymal Lung Disease

The mainstays of treatment are oxygen delivery, positive pressure, and, if needed, antibiotics and diuretics. Although it is worth trying $HFNCO_2$, a patient with ARF from parenchymal disease often needs CPAP, BiPAP, or intubation with mechanical ventilation. The positive pressure administered with oxygen improves airway recruitment and hypoxemia and decreases the patient's work of breathing.

Heart Failure

The treatment, including oxygen, diuretics, and inotropes, is detailed in Chapter 4, Congestive Heart Failure. Noninvasive support and mechanical ventilation improve respiratory symptoms and left-sided heart function. However, the patient is extremely fragile. Obtain subspecialist consultation early, because endotracheal intubation can worsen cardiac output and lead to cardiac arrest.

Muscle Weakness or Paralysis

Provide oxygen and mechanical support. The patient may also have upper-airway obstruction that requires treatment (see Nasal and Other Upper Airway Obstruction, as detailed earlier).

Thoracic Mass Effect

Drain or treat surgically, as indicated. Obtain appropriate subspecialist consultation (intensivist, surgeon, anesthesiologist) early, especially if sedation is required.

Indications for Consultation

- **Intensivist:** Acute respiratory failure
- **Anesthesiology:** Patient with croup that requires intubation, epiglottitis, thoracic mass effect
- **Cardiology:** ARF secondary to congestive heart failure
- **Otolaryngology:** ARF secondary to a foreign body, croup, retropharyngeal abscess, epiglottitis
- **Surgery:** Thoracic mass effect

Disposition

- **ICU transfer:** ARF
- **Discharge from ICU:** Patient maintaining oxygenation and ventilation with just the support available in the respiratory, step-down, or inpatient unit

Follow-up

- **Primary care provider:** 2 to 3 days
- **Subspecialist:** As indicated by any underlying disease

Pearls and Pitfalls

- Do not administer a muscle relaxant to a patient if the success of airway management and ventilation is uncertain. Ketamine and propofol offer satisfactory intubation conditions while allowing the patient to breathe spontaneously.
- The judicious use of sedation for a patient with extreme respiratory distress can be beneficial. However, anticipate the possibility of deterioration and the need for airway intervention and mechanical ventilation.
- Do not underestimate the importance of unobstructed nasal passages to adequate breathing in infants and other patients with poor airway control.
- Lateral positioning, with or without chin lift or jaw thrust, helps alleviate airway occlusion and may decrease sympathetic activity.
- Hypoxemia in a patient with isolated upper-airway disease (croup) is ominous and indicative of extreme hypoventilation and impending respiratory arrest.
- Heart failure is a cause of ARF that is often overlooked.

Bibliography

Finucane BT, Tsui BCH, Santora AH. Pediatric airway management. In: Finucane BT, Tsui BCH, Santora AH. *Principles of Airway Management*. 4th ed. New York, NY: Springer; 2011:415–513

Lakhanpaul M, MacFaul R, Werneke U, Armon K, Hemingway P, Stephenson T. An evidence-based guideline for children presenting with acute breathing difficulty. *Emerg Med J.* 2009;26(12):850–853

Miguel-Montanes R, Hajage D, Messika J, et al. Use of high-flow nasal cannula oxygen therapy to prevent desaturation during tracheal intubation of intensive care patients with mild-to-moderate hypoxemia. *Crit Care Med.* 2015;43(3):574–583

Milesi C, Boubal M, Jacquot A, et al. High-flow nasal cannula: recommendations for daily practice in pediatrics. *Ann Intensive Care.* 2014;4:29

Morley SL. Non-invasive ventilation in paediatric critical care. *Paediatric Respir Rev.* 2016;20:34–31

Airway Management and Respiratory Support

Introduction

Pediatric patients require ventilatory support for respiratory failure (Chapter 105), cardiac failure (Chapter 4, Congestive Heart Failure), or airway protection. Acute needs are usually rapid, dramatic, and life threatening, although chronic respiratory failure is often insidious.

Ineffective respiration occurs because of pathologic processes in at least one of the following areas:

- Lower airway or alveolar pathology: pneumonia, asthma, pneumothorax, inhalation lung injury, chronic lung disease, cystic fibrosis, scoliosis, chronic smoke exposure
- Central nervous system (CNS) loss of drive: stroke, traumatic brain injury, narcotics/toxins, posterior fossa tumor
- Peripheral nerve or muscle deficiency: muscular dystrophy, botulism, Guillain-Barré syndrome, myasthenia gravis, spinal muscular atrophy
- Restrictive: scoliosis, pneumothorax
- Upper-airway increased resistance (fixed or dynamic): palatal insufficiency, tonsil hypertrophy, croup, tracheitis, tracheomalacia, craniofacial anomaly, caustic injury, compressing mass, scoliosis

Patients with cardiac failure require respiratory support to decrease energy use and protect the airway.

Clinical Presentation

History

The determination that acute respiratory support is needed depends on the history, underlying pathologic processes, and physical examination findings. The diagnosis in patients with chronic disease requires noting changes from baseline machine settings, blood gas analysis results, and radiographs, as well as responses to previous illnesses.

Physical Examination

The most effective method to determine the level of respiratory pathologic involvement is simple observation of the respiratory pattern. Little or no respiratory effort implies a problem with respiratory drive, peripheral nerves, or muscle pathologic origins. Increased work of breathing is caused by airway resistance or alveolar pathologic processes. Auscultation of the airway from mouth to lungs will suggest both the level(s) of pathologic origin and the intervention(s) required. Note any structural anomalies that may affect treatment.

- Nose/mouth: Observe the patient for nasal flaring or open-mouth breathing. Listen behind the mandible to assess for upper-airway obstruction. If a jaw thrust reduces airway obstruction, the pathologic origin is at the level of the hypopharynx, usually caused by the tongue.
- Neck: Observe the trachea for deviation. Listen for stridor or voice changes, which indicate a pathologic origin of the larynx. Listen over the larynx to help differentiate upper-airway stridor from lung bronchospasm.
- Chest: Observe chest wall motion for asymmetry, paradoxical movement, and retractions. Listen for rales (alveolar disease), rhonchi (larger airway disease), and/or wheezing (alveolar and small airway disease).

Laboratory Workup

Pulse oximetry, capnography, and venous blood gas (VBG) analyses are the tools used most often to identify and monitor respiratory support needs.

Continuous pulse oximetry is the most useful tool to assess hypoxia, so that arterial blood gas oxygen determination is usually not needed. Important oxygen saturation (SaO_2)-arterial oxygen level correlations are

$$90\% \ SaO_2 = PaO_2 \ 60 \ mm \ Hg \ and \ 85\% \ SaO_2 = PaO_2 \ 50 \ mm \ Hg$$

Note that SaO_2 in an anemic patient can be falsely reassuring because the diminished amount of hemoglobin can be entirely saturated, while total oxygen-carrying capacity is low.

Capnography is used to measure CO_2 concentration of expired gas. End-tidal carbon dioxide ($EtCO_2$) correlates with $PaCO_2$ (usually within 5 mm Hg) in a closed respiratory system. However, in an open respiratory system (eg, mask or cannula), the correlation is less reliable. Consider correlating $EtCO_2$ with a VBG when $EtCO_2$ monitoring is initiated. If measured consistently, $EtCO_2$ is useful for trending CO_2 retention.

Serial VBGs that show increasing CO_2 (usually >50 mm Hg) over time imply respiratory fatigue, impending respiratory failure, or need to adjust existing respiratory support. VBG oxygen levels vary dramatically, depending on the sample site, and are not useful in the assessment of respiratory failure.

Other potential laboratory abnormalities include the following.

- An increased hemoglobin concentration suggests chronic hypoxemia.
- Increased serum lactate level may indicate significant tissue hypoxia.

- Increased bicarbonate level suggests chronic hypercapnia.
- Low concentrations of potassium, calcium, or phosphate can impair muscle function.

Acidosis and fever shift the oxyhemoglobin dissociation curve to the right, reducing oxygen affinity.

Radiology Examinations

Chest radiography provides additional information about pathologic processes in the vertebrae and chest wall, large and small airways, heart and blood vessels, and diaphragm. Indications for chest radiography include an acute change in respiratory status, failure to improve with interventions, or abnormal auscultatory findings. Upper-airway imaging is not indicated in croup but may help in the assessment of deep-tissue spaces.

Treatment

General Treatment

Hypoxia improves with supplemental oxygen, often with a simple nasal cannula or face mask. If respiratory drive is adequate, provide oxygen and open the upper airway with an oral or nasal airway.

Tailor treatment modalities to the patient's underlying acute and chronic pathologic findings. Apnea mandates positive-pressure ventilation initially with bag-mask ventilation via a sealed mask, oral airway, or bag-valve mask. If apnea does not resolve, place a laryngeal mask airway (LMA) or endotracheal tube (ETT). Inadequate central respiratory drive requires elimination of any offending respiratory depressant medications. Peripheral nerve or muscle deficiency improves with continuous positive airway pressure (CPAP) or bilevel positive airway pressure (BiPAP). Manage increased upper-airway resistance with insertion of an oropharyngeal or nasopharyngeal airway. If ventilation is still inadequate, add a heated high-flow nasal cannula (often effective in infants), CPAP, or BiPAP.

Laryngeal Mask Airway

LMA insertion is an expedient bridge to a more secure airway, such as an ETT. LMA insertion is simple: Place it into the mouth, direct it into the hypopharynx until resistance is met, then inflate the cuff to seal the airway. Oxygen and positive pressure can then be supplied by either a bag-valve mask or a ventilator. Ease of insertion makes LMA a useful short-term adjunct to aid in respiratory failure, especially if there is a component of hypopharyngeal obstruction (usually the tongue). Since the LMA cuff does not separate the lungs from the stomach, disadvantages include lack of airway protection (aspiration risk) and risk of stomach distention secondary to positive pressure. In addition, LMAs are not useful in patients with reduced pulmonary compliance (pneumonia, asthma).

Endotracheal Intubation

Insertion of an ETT requires muscle paralysis and laryngoscopy, because nontraumatic intubation is difficult during spontaneous breathing. Rapid sequence intubation (RSI) is a method to provide rapid tracheal intubation and general anesthesia in a patient with respiratory failure. RSI reduces the chance for pulmonary aspiration when protective airway reflexes are ablated by muscle relaxants. Have an assistant exert firm cricoid pressure to occlude the esophagus and prevent aspiration during RSI (Sellick maneuver).

Medications

Endotracheal intubation requires administration of an intravenous (IV) muscle relaxant and IV sedative, except in the situation of shock, when sedation may be contraindicated. Muscle relaxants are always required. Typical fast-acting sedatives include fentanyl, ketamine, and propofol, although many institutions limit the use of propofol to intensivists, anesthesiologists, and emergency medicine physicians. Common fast-acting muscle relaxants include rocuronium or succinylcholine. Dosages (see the following) are for IV administration and are dependent on the patient's pathophysiology and age.

Ketamine and rocuronium are commonly administered to a patient with asthma who is in respiratory failure. Avoid ketamine if there is an eye globe injury, if the patient is less than 3 years of age, or if the patient has airway problems because of laryngospasm and increased secretions.

Muscle Relaxants

- Succinylcholine: The intubating dose is 2 mg/kg (150-mg maximum), onset of action is 30 seconds, and duration is 6 to 8 minutes. Repeat with caution because of the risk of bradycardia. Do not use in a patient with a burn, trauma, rhabdomyolysis, spinal cord injury, or muscular dystrophy. There is also a U.S. Food and Drug Administration black box warning for undiagnosed skeletal muscle myopathy.
- Rocuronium: The dose is 1 mg/kg, onset of action is 1 minute, and duration is 30 minutes. No repeat doses are needed (for intubation) because of the duration of action.
- Vecuronium: The dose is 0.2 mg/kg, onset is 1 minute, and duration is 45 minutes. No repeat doses are needed (for intubation) because of duration of action.

Sedatives

- Ketamine: The dose is 0.5 to 1 mg/kg, onset of action is 1 minute, and duration is 10 minutes. One repeat dose may be administered at 5 to 15 minutes if needed. Use a lower dose (0.50–0.75 mg/kg) if propofol is also being administered.
- Fentanyl: The dose is 1 to 3 µg/kg, onset of action is 5 minutes, and duration is 30 minutes. No repeat doses are needed (for intubation) because of duration of action.
- Etomidate: The dose is 0.3 mg/kg, onset of action is 1 minute, and duration is 5 minutes. If needed, a second dose may be administered in 3 to 5 minutes. Etomidate is irritating, so avoid introducing it into small vessels.
- Propofol: The dose is 1 to 3 mg/kg, onset of action is 1 minute, and duration of action is 10 minutes. One repeat dose of 0.5 mg/kg may be administered, if needed.

Airway sizes and management strategies are provided in Tables 106-1, 106-2, and 106-3.

Table 106-1. Airway Sizes				
LMA			**ETT Size = [16 + age (y)]/4**	
Size	Patient Weight (kg)	Insufflation Volume (mL)	Patient Weight (kg)	Size
1	<5	<4	<1	2.5
1.5	5–10	<7	1–2	3.0
2	10–20	<10	2–4	3.5
3	30–50	<20	**ETT Insertion Depth**	
4	50–70	<30	Newborn Weight (kg)	Depth (cm)
5	70–100	<40	1	7
Laryngoscope blade (always use straight)			2	8
Age (y)	Size		3	9
0–1	0–1		4	10
1–2	1.0 or 1.5 (Wis-Hipple)		**Child**	
>2	2		ETT insertion depth (cm) = Age (y) + 10 Maximum depth = 20 cm	

Abbreviations: ETT, endotracheal tube; LMA, laryngeal mask airway.

Chapter 106: Airway Management and Respiratory Support

Table 106-2. Oral and Nasopharyngeal Airway Placement[a]

	OA, NPA Placement	HFNC	Nasal or Mask CPAP
Benefits	Reduces upper-airway resistance Facilitates BVM bag-valve mask ventilation	Airway stenting Reduces work of breathing	Distending pressure recruits closed alveoli
Typical indications for adjunct use	Hypotonic cerebral palsy Trisomy 21 Obese patient Postictal patient	Bronchiolitis	Bronchiolitis Upper-airway obstruction Muscle weakness
Basic procedure	**OA** Determine airway size by placing opening by corner of mouth, with tip no further than corner of the jaw Suction mouth Place OA into mouth, pointing to the palate until halfway in; then turn 180° OA will be facing tip down toward the trachea Do not secure in place **NPA** Measure from nostril to tragus of ear Can use ETT cut to size Lubricate the NPA Suction nares to ensure patency Apply neosynephrine spray to nasal mucosa Guide NPA through nare to predetermined length Secure the NPA	Use heated, humidified system Use largest size prongs/bubble possible Start flow: <1 y, 2 L/min; >1 y, 4 L/min Titrate flow to bronchiolitis respiratory score (see Chapter 109, Bronchiolitis) improvement: ↑ 1 L/min every 15 min Maximum flow <1 y: <10 kg, 4 L/min; >10 kg, 6 L/min Maximum flow >1 y: <20 kg, 6 L/min; >20 kg, 8 L/min Use blender to titrate FiO_2 to maintain appropriate oxygen saturation; maximum ~50%; if >50% FiO_2 needed, consider NCPAP Wean FiO_2 until ~40%, then ↓ flow by 1–2 L/min every 2–4 h as tolerated until: <1 y and <10 kg, 2 L/min; <1 y and >10 kg, 4 L/min; >1 y and any size, 6 L/min Then wean FiO_2 to ~30% Consider conversion to regular cannula (100% FiO_2 from wall) when at <2-L/min flow for <1 y and <3-L/min flow for >1 y	Choose correct nasal prong or mask size Nasal prongs are typically not tolerated by a patient older than a toddler Use humidified system Start at pressure of 4 cm H_2O Start FiO_2 at 30% and titrate to maintain appropriate oxygen saturation Titrate flow to ↑ pressure 1–2 cm H_2O every 20–30 min to maximum 7–8 cm H_2O (<1 y) or 10 cm H_2O (>1 y) NCPAP: Secure bonnet over patient's head to assure tight seal Mask CPAP: secure with ties Wean FiO_2 to 30%–35%, then titrate flow to ↓ pressure by 1–2 cm H_2O every 2 h as tolerated until at starting pressure Then consider change to HFNC

Table 106-2. Oral and Nasopharyngeal Airway Placement[a], continued

	OA, NPA Placement	HFNC	Nasal or Mask CPAP
Monitoring	Standard[b]	Standard[b]	Advanced[c]
Limitations	No oxygen delivery	Maximum flow 4 L (<1 y, <10 kg) or 8 L (>1 y, >20 kg) At maximum flow and 100% F_{O_2}, will provide a maximum F_{O_2} of 40% at the glottis because of entrainment of room air	Patient tolerance (may require sedation) Tight seal needed to ensure pressure provided Skilled respiratory therapist needed
Contraindications	**OA** Conscious patient will not tolerate **NPA** Coagulopathy Nasal deformity/infection Basilar skull fracture	Apnea Severe GERD Patient with CLD and respiratory acidosis Blocked nasal passages	Gastric aspiration Facial deformities Ocular injury
Complications	**OA** Gagging **NPA** Nasal erosion Epistaxis	Nasal septal erosion Epistaxis Nasal congestion (reduced by humidification of oxygen)	Pneumothorax Aspiration Skin breakdown over nasal bridge Gastric distention

Abbreviations: BVM, bag-valve mask; CLD, chronic lung disease; CPAP, continuous positive airway pressure; ETT, endotracheal tube; F_{O_2}, fraction of inspired oxygen; GERD, gastroesophageal reflux disease; HFNC, high-flow nasal cannula; NCPAP, nasal continuous positive airway pressure; NPA, nasopharyngeal airway; OA, oral airway.

[a] For all interventions, use the American Heart Association Pediatric Advanced Life Support and local standards for patient placement, respiratory therapy and other staff support, and monitoring.

[b] "Standard monitoring" is defined as oxygen saturation and cardiorespiratory monitoring.

[c] "Advanced monitoring" is defined as capnography and venous or arterial blood gas analyses, with or without invasive central line or arterial line access.

Chapter 106: Airway Management and Respiratory Support

Table 106-3. Airway Management and Adjuncts[a]

	BiPAP	LMA	ETT Airway
Delivers	Control over IPAP and EPAP delivery and rate Can synchronize with patient respirations	Positive pressure—limited Mechanical ventilation—short term Tracheal suctioning	High positive inspiratory pressure High positive end-expiratory pressure Mechanical ventilation—long term Lung isolation Tracheal suctioning
Typical patient	Neuromuscular disease Chronic lung disease	Emergent short-term respiratory failure Difficult airway	Severe tracheal injury Severe head injury Poor lung compliance
Basic procedure	Fit properly sized mask and head strap on patient Set IPAP to obtain visible chest excursion Set FiO_2 to 50% Set rate (see below) ↑ EPAP until oxygen saturations are >90%	Deflate cuff and lubricate the mask Introduce into the pharynx and advance until resistance is felt as the tube enters the hypopharynx Inflate cuff (distal opening of tube is just above the glottis) Attach breathing circuit To remove: suction airway, deflate cuff, withdraw LMA	PALS basics (position, BVM, etc) Preoxygenate 3–5 min Administer medications Cricoid pressure Perform laryngoscopy Insert ETT Verify ETT placement (auscultate lungs, stomach, check $EtCO_2$ level) Assess outcome: clinical (VS, color, aeration), blood gas, $EtCO_2$ (capnography, colorimetry best)
Ventilator settings	*(4 modes)* Set IPAP or EPAP at 4–20 cm H_2O and rate at 4–30 breaths/min Spontaneous (rate controlled by patient)	Rate: approximate for age Volume limited: Tidal volume 8–10 mL/kg; I:E start at 1:3; use a longer expiratory time for obstructive disease Pressure limited: PEEP start at 3 cm H_2O and increase as indicated; set PIP at pressure required to move chest wall (assessed by using best hand-bagging pressures)	Rate: approximate for age Volume limited: Tidal volume 8–10 mL/kg; I:E start at 1:3; use a longer expiratory time for obstructive disease Pressure limited: PEEP start at 3 cm H_2O and increase as indicated; set PIP at pressure required to move chest wall (assessed by using best hand-bagging pressures)

Table 106-3. Airway Management and Adjuncts[a], continued

	BiPAP	LMA	ETT Airway
Ventilator settings, continued	Spontaneous/timed (timed back-up rate, in case the patient's own rate drops below a specified level) Timed (rate controlled completely by machine) CPAP = 8 cm H₂O	Air leak: ≤25 cm H₂O For cuffed tube, deflate cuff, then check leak	Air leak: ≤25 cm H₂O For cuffed tube, deflate cuff, then check leak
Monitoring	Advanced[b]	Advanced[b]	Advanced[b]
Limitations	Patient tolerance Skilled respiratory therapist needed Often PICU setting	Requires sedation medications Less airway protection compared to ETT Skilled ventilator management needed PICU setting	Requires RSI or similar medications (neuromuscular blockade, sedation) Skilled ventilator management needed PICU setting
Contraindications	Absent gag/cough reflex Absent respiratory drive Upper airway obstruction	Severe GERD Laryngeal burns Decreased pulmonary compliance	Upper-airway disruption Tracheal disruption Distal tracheal stenosis
Complications	Pneumothorax Aspiration Gastric distention Facial pressure sores	Pharyngeal/laryngeal mucosal or nerve injury Aspiration	Esophageal placement Ventilator associated pneumonia

Abbreviation: BIPAP, bilevel positive airway pressure; BVM, bag-valve mask; CPAP, continuous positive airway pressure; EPAP, expiratory positive airway pressure; EtCO₂, end-tidal carbon dioxide; ETT, endotracheal tube; F₁O₂, fraction of inspired oxygen; GERD, gastroesophageal reflux disease; HFNC, high-flow nasal cannula; I:E, inspiratory-to-expiratory time ratio; IPAP, inspiratory positive airway pressure; LMA, laryngeal mask airway; PALS, Pediatric Advanced Life Support; PEEP, positive end-expiratory pressure; PICU, pediatric intensive care unit; PIP, peak inspiratory pressure; RSI, rapid sequence intubation; VS, vital signs.

[a] For all of these interventions, use the American Heart Association Pediatric Advanced Life Support and local standards for patient placement, respiratory therapy and other staff support, and monitoring.

[b] "Advanced monitoring "is defined as capnography and venous or arterial blood gas analyses, with or without invasive central line or arterial line access.

Mechanical Ventilation

Intermittent mandatory ventilation (IMV) delivers a preset number of mechanical breaths per minute. Synchronized IMV synchronizes mechanical breaths with the patient's inspiratory efforts. Pressure support ventilation provides a set positive pressure when a patient inspires. This mode of mechanical ventilation augments all spontaneous patient breaths with positive pressure. There is no set rate.

Basic Strategies

- To $\uparrow$ $Paco_2$: $\uparrow$ positive end-expiratory pressure (PEEP), mean airway pressure, inspiratory time, or fraction of inspired oxygen (Fio_2).
- To $\downarrow$ $Paco_2$: $\uparrow$ peak inspiratory pressure (PIP), rate, or tidal volume. Note that an *increased* PEEP will *increase* $Paco_2$.

Weaning Strategies

- Reduce respiratory load: Relieve bronchospasm, remove secretions, reduce pulmonary edema, and treat pulmonary infections.
- Increase muscle power (strength and endurance): Reduce hyperinflation, optimize nutrition, sprint weaning.
- Improve central drive: Avoid hypochloremic alkalosis, reduce CNS depressant medications.

Predictors of Successful Extubation

- Normal $Paco_2$
- PIP less than 14 to 16 cm H_2O
- PEEP less than 2 to 3 cm H_2O (infant) or less than 5 cm H_2O (child)
- IMV less than 2 to 4 breaths/min
- Fio_2 <40% with $Paco_2$ >70

Respiratory Adjuncts

Heliox, a low-density combination helium-oxygen mixture, improves ventilation by reducing turbulent gas flow in narrowed airways. Its use in patients with upper-airway (croup) or certain lower-airway (bronchiolitis) diseases has been associated with improved oxygenation, as well as decreased respiratory rate and work of breathing. Common mixtures are (helium/oxygen) 80/20, 70/30, and 60/40. A helium concentration less than 60% is of no benefit. Therefore, the clinical limitation to heliox use is the inability to maintain adequate oxygenation if high Fio_2 required because of parenchymal disease.

Disposition

- **Intensive care unit transfer:**
  — Fio_2 >50% necessary to maintain an oxygen saturation of $\geq$92%

— Respiratory distress accompanied by progressive fatigue
— pH level <7.2 and/or normal $Paco_2$ cannot be maintained
— Need for advanced monitoring, heliox, bilevel positive airway pressure, or intubation
— Apnea or irregular respirations
- **Tertiary center transfer:** Depends on site resources (equipment, staffing, critical care expertise)

Pearls and Pitfalls

- Recognition of respiratory failure is more important than determining the cause. Anticipate respiratory failure and prepare for it with all team members.
- Tachypnea is the first sign of respiratory distress, but bradypnea is an ominous sign of impending respiratory arrest.
- Altered mental status may indicate the presence of hypoxia and/or hypercarbia.
- Bradycardia is the ultimate sign of catastrophic respiratory compromise.
- Prevent intubation-associated bradycardia in infants with atropine premedication.
- Prevent pulmonary aspiration during ETT intubation by using an RSI protocol.
- Paralyzing agents alone are not sufficient for an intubated patient because pain can still be felt.
- For patient safety, adhere to patient care bundles to avoid complications such as skin ulcers, venous thromboembolism, and ventilator-associated pneumonia; extubate in a timely manner to avoid ventilator-associated harms; ensure adequate nutrition.

Bibliography

Amin R, Sayal A, Syed F, et al. How long does it take to initiate a child on long-term invasive ventilation? Results from a Canadian pediatric home ventilation program. *Can Respir J.* 2015;22(2):103–108

Essouri S, Martinon-Torres F. Noninvasive respiratory support in the paediatric patient. In: Rimensberger PC, ed. *Pediatric and Neonatal Mechanical Ventilation.* 3rd ed. Geneva, Switzerland: Springer; 2015:1073–1097

Freeman JF, Ciarallo C, Rappaport L, Mandt M, Bajaj L. Use of capnographs to assess quality of pediatric ventilation with 3 different airway modalities. *Am J Emerg Med.* 2016;34(1):69–74

Hull J. The value of non-invasive ventilation. *Arch Dis Child.* 2014;99(11):1050–1054

Bacterial Tracheitis

Introduction

Bacterial tracheitis is a bacterial infection that often results from a prior viral upper-respiratory infection, with an estimated mortality rate of 4% to 20%. The organisms involved most often are *Staphylococcus aureus* (methicillin-resistant *S aureus* [MRSA] is a concern), α-hemolytic *Streptococcus,* and *Streptococcus pyogenes*, while *Moraxella catarrhalis* is associated with a more severe disease course. *Klebsiella* species and *Pseudomonas* species have also been responsible in a few cases. Bacterial tracheitis tends to occur in the fall or winter months and mimics the epidemiology of croup. The mean age at diagnosis is 5 years.

The pathophysiology involves a diffuse inflammatory process of the larynx, trachea, and bronchi, with adherent or semiadherent mucopurulent membranes within the trachea. The major site of disease is at the level of the cricoid cartilage, which is the narrowest part of the trachea. Acute airway obstruction may occur secondary to subglottic edema and sloughing of the epithelial lining or accumulation of the mucopurulent membrane within the trachea.

Clinical Presentation

History

The patient initially presents with symptoms similar to those of viral croup, with rapid onset of fever, barking cough, and stridor. However, standard croup therapy is ineffective. Over the course of several days, when symptoms would typically be improving, the patient proceeds to acute respiratory decompensation.

Physical Examination

The patient is febrile and tachypneic, with a toxic appearance, stridor (can be biphasic), significant respiratory distress, retractions, dyspnea, nasal flaring, and cyanosis. Some patients will have a sore throat, odynophagia, or dysphonia. Pertinent negative findings include a lack of drooling and the patient being able to lie supine without increased respiratory distress.

Differential Diagnosis

The differential diagnosis includes persistent croup, epiglottitis, peritonsillar abscess, and retropharyngeal abscess (Table 107-1). However, a patient with bacterial tracheitis does not respond to standard croup therapy, appears toxic, and presents with acute respiratory decompensation.

Laboratory Workup

Order a bacterial culture and Gram stain of endotracheal secretions. If sepsis is a possibility, perform a complete blood count (if not done previously) and a blood culture.

Radiology Examinations

If bacterial tracheitis is suspected, obtain anteroposterior and lateral neck radiographs, which will show an irregular or "shaggy" subglottic narrowing versus the symmetrical tapering typical of croup.

Treatment

If bacterial tracheitis is suspected, immediately consult with an otolaryngologist or pulmonologist to arrange laryngotracheobronchoscopy and/or assist with emergent intubation (anesthesia may also be helpful). If these consults are not available, initiate empirical antibiotic treatment and airway stabilization as necessary, without waiting for the results of laboratory and/or radiologic studies.

Once the diagnosis is assigned, the mainstays of treatment are airway maintenance and intravenous (IV) antibiotics administered in an intensive care unit (ICU). Avoid agitating the patient. If the patient's respiratory status

Table 107-1. Differential Diagnosis of Bacterial Tracheitis	
Diagnosis	**Clinical Features**
Croup	Barking cough Nontoxic appearance Responds to inhaled epinephrine and steroids
Epiglottitis (rare)	Rapid onset Toxic appearance Drooling but no cough
Foreign body aspiration	No croup-like prodrome Acute onset of choking, gagging, coughing May have stridor or wheezing
Peritonsillar abscess	No croup-like prodrome Drooling No stridor or cough
Retropharyngeal abscess	Drooling Muffled stridor

deteriorates, it is usually secondary to movement of the membrane. Attempt bag-valve-mask ventilation, but if intubation is required, use an endotracheal tube 0.5 to 1.0 mm smaller than expected to minimize trauma in the inflamed subglottic area. Frequent suctioning and high air humidity are necessary to maintain endotracheal tube patency.

Treat with IV antibiotics. Use either cefotaxime (150 mg/kg/d, divided into doses administered every 6 hours; 8-g/d maximum) *or* ceftriaxone (100 mg/kg/d, divided into doses administered every 12 hours; 4-g/d maximum) *plus* MRSA coverage with either IV clindamycin (40 mg/kg/d, divided into doses administered every 8 hours; 4.8-g/d maximum) or vancomycin (40 mg/kg/d, divided into doses administered every 6-8 hours; 4-g/d maximum).

Indications for Consultation

- **Otolaryngology or pulmonology:** All patients (for endoscopic procedures)
- **Pediatric intensivist:** All patients

Disposition

- **ICU transfer:** All patients
- **Discharge criteria:** Patient afebrile and tolerating maintenance oral fluids, no respiratory distress

Follow-up

Primary care provider: 2 to 3 days

Pearls and Pitfalls

- Always consider bacterial tracheitis in a patient who presents with an acute, life-threatening upper-airway infection.
- Bacterial tracheitis is often misdiagnosed as severe or persistent croup.
- An acute deterioration in the patient's respiratory status is usually secondary to movement of the membrane.

Bibliography

Kuo CY, Parikh SR. Bacterial tracheitis. *Pediatr Rev.* 2014;35(11):497–499

Mandal A, Kabra SK, Lodha R. Upper airway obstruction in children. *Indian J Pediatr.* 2015;82(8):737–744

Miranda AD, Valdez TA, Pereira KD. Bacterial tracheitis: a varied entity. *Pediatr Emerg Care.* 2011;27(10):950–953

Shargorodsky J, Whittemore KR, Lee GS. Bacterial tracheitis: a therapeutic approach. *Laryngoscope.* 2010;120(12):2498–2501

Brief, Resolved, Unexplained Events (Formerly Apparent Life-Threatening Events)

Introduction

A *brief, resolved, unexplained event* (BRUE) is defined as an incident that occurs in an infant younger than 1 year of age, when the observer reports a sudden, brief, and resolved episode of one or more of the following: cyanosis or pallor; absent, decreased, or irregular breathing; marked change in tone (hyper- or hypotonia); and altered level of responsiveness. A BRUE is a diagnosis of exclusion assigned when there is no explanation for a qualifying event *after* compiling an appropriate history and conducting a physical examination.

It is important to note that, unlike the term *apparent life-threatening event* (ALTE), a BRUE does not describe a chief complaint from a caregiver prior to medical evaluation or include infants that have ongoing symptoms after the event has resolved (eg, fever or respiratory symptoms). The history and physical examination findings are critical to determine whether an event qualifies as a BRUE because most episodes that are concerning to caregivers can be explained as benign, nonrecurring, or caused by a normal physiological phenomenon, such as acrocyanosis, breath-holding spells, and periodic breathing of the newborn. Additionally, common causes like gastroesophageal reflux (GER) and oral dysphagia can be readily discerned and treated.

Even when there is no clear explanation for the event and it qualifies as a BRUE, it is unlikely that there is a serious underlying condition or risk for a serious adverse outcome. Caregivers may fear that the patient nearly died, despite the fact that BRUEs, or ALTEs, are not related to "aborted" or "near-miss" sudden infant death syndrome (SIDS). Importantly, however, a BRUE can be the manifestation of a serious, undiagnosed problem, including child maltreatment or pertussis (Table 108-1). The broad differential diagnosis, potential for a rare but serious underlying etiology, and subsequent anxiety present a unique challenge.

Table 108-1. Differential Diagnosis of Concerning Events in Infants

Diagnosis	Clinical Features
Normal in Infants	
Acrocyanosis or perioral cyanosis	Lips turn blue (not gums or face) periodically or with choking, gagging, or crying
Breath-holding spell	Crying followed by breath holding and possible brief LOC
Periodic breathing	Periodic respiratory pauses <20 s in duration Typically occurs while asleep
Startle or Moro reflex	Rapid increase in tone and flexing of extremities when startled
Common Diagnoses	
Child abuse	History of unexplained deaths in other children Inconsistent history or events witnessed by a single caretaker Bruising or petechiae on face, trunk, or extremities Patient may have failure to thrive
Oral dysphagia	Choking or gagging during or shortly after feedings Food exiting nose or mouth during or shortly after feedings
Gastroesophageal reflux	Choking or gagging after feedings Vomiting and/or regurgitation Sandifer syndrome (arching of the back) Prompt return to baseline Patient may have failure to thrive
Subclinical URI or LRI (eg, respiratory syncytial virus and pertussis)	Variable congestion, wheezing, coarse rales, tachypnea, especially if <2 mo of age
Less Common Diagnoses	
Anatomic abnormalities of the head and neck (eg, laryngomalacia or tracheomalacia, tracheoesophageal fistula, cleft)	Breathing difficulties or noisy breathing since birth Abnormal facial morphologic appearance Family history of obstructive sleep apnea Fever with or without tachycardia and hypotension
Cardiac arrhythmia	Family history: unexplained death, arrhythmia, congenital heart disease Pathologic murmur
Hypoglycemia or inborn error of metabolism	Family history of unexplained death Age <2 mo May have metabolic acidosis, failure to thrive, or seizures
Seizures	May be recurrent May be associated with focal neurologic findings and/or developmental delay May have (+) family history
Sepsis	Toxic appearance Persistent or progressive altered mental status

Abbreviations: LOC, loss of consciousness; LRI, lower respiratory infection; URI, upper respiratory infection; +, positive finding.

Clinical Presentation

History

Complete a thorough, systematic history to fully characterize what exactly occurred during the event. Attempt to distinguish concerning symptoms, such as central apnea, central cyanosis, or seizure activity, from more benign ones, like obstructive apnea, choking, pallor, "turning red," or cyanosis limited to just the perioral area or distal extremities (acrocyanosis). Understanding the temporal and contextual relationships is also important. For example, central cyanosis without a preceding event is more concerning than vomiting after a feeding, followed by gagging, choking, turning red, and hypertonia.

A careful review of symptoms (upper respiratory infection symptoms, fever), growth and development, medical history (prior BRUE or ALTE, prematurity, noisy breathing), family history (cardiac disease, apnea, and unexplained sudden death), and social history (infectious exposures, caretakers, and domestic violence) can suggest comorbid conditions, genetic predispositions, medication exposures, or social concerns.

Physical Examination

After a BRUE, the patient is asymptomatic and has negative physical examination findings. However, perform a thorough examination, focusing on the skin (bruising or petechiae, indicating child maltreatment), head and neck (anatomic abnormalities that contribute to obstructive apnea), heart (pathologic murmur), and nervous system (focality).

Risk Stratification: Lower- vs Higher-Risk BRUE

For a patient with a BRUE, use historical and physical examination features to determine if the patient is at lower risk for both BRUE recurrence and serious underlying diagnosis. Lower-risk criteria include

- Age >60 days
- Gestational age of ≥32 weeks and postconceptional age of ≥45 weeks
- Occurrence of only 1 BRUE (no prior BRUE ever and not occurring in clusters)
- Duration of BRUE <1 minute
- No cardiopulmonary resuscitation by a trained medical provider required
- No concerning historical features
- No concerning physical examination findings

Laboratory Workup

Routine laboratory testing is of minimal value in a patient who has experienced a BRUE, particularly if at lower risk (as described earlier). Do not routinely perform a complete blood cell count, sepsis evaluation, gastroesophageal reflux testing, sleep study, toxicology screening, metabolic testing, brain imaging, electroencephalography, or electrocardiography. If the infant is younger than 2 months of age or was premature, a rapid viral respiratory panel may be helpful for diagnosing a subclinical infection causing the event. Pertussis testing is indicated in areas where it is endemic, with an underimmunized population.

For a higher-risk patient, target laboratory testing based on the findings of the history and physical examination. For example, perform neuroimaging if there is a concern for child maltreatment or an electrocardiogram if there is a family history of cardiac arrhythmias or sudden, unexplained death.

Treatment

While routine admission and monitoring are unnecessary, inpatient observation may be beneficial for a higher-risk infant, especially if there have been recurrent events or if the patient is less than 60 days of age or less than 48 weeks of corrected gestational age. Inpatient observation may also be valuable to gather more information when there is concern for child maltreatment.

Specific treatment is not indicated unless there is a significant underlying diagnosis. If GER is suspected, recommend reflux precautions (small, frequent feedings; elevate the head of the bed; upright feeding). If feeding difficulties are suspected, arrange for an evaluation by a feeding expert. Most importantly, reassure the family that BRUEs are not related to SIDS. However, cardiopulmonary resuscitation training may offer additional reassurance for concerned parents.

If there are symptoms of central apneic events, obstructive apnea present since birth, or an anatomic maxillofacial abnormality, consult an otolaryngologist or pulmonologist and arrange a sleep study.

See Chapter 43, Inborn Errors of Metabolism, for the management of a suspected inborn error of metabolism. Most importantly, stop all feedings and administer an intravenous solution that contains dextrose.

The management of arrhythmias (Chapter 3), bronchiolitis (Chapter 109), child abuse (Chapter 102), seizures (Chapter 85), and sepsis (Chapter 68) is detailed elsewhere.

Indications for Consultation

- **Child abuse specialist:** Any concern or risk factor for child maltreatment
- **Gastroenterology:** Recurrent BRUE with associated GER symptoms or failure to thrive
- **Metabolic diseases:** Positive metabolic screening result, recurrent BRUE, or concerning family history
- **Neurology:** Concern for seizures or focal neurologic examination, although this can be deferred to the outpatient setting
- **Pulmonologist or sleep study specialist:** Recurrent BRUE or concern for central apnea
- **Feeding expert:** Concern for oral dysphagia

Disposition

- **Intensive care unit transfer:** Recurrent, life-threatening events that require high-intensity monitoring or medical intervention
- **Discharge criteria:** Family reassured, risk of hospitalization greater than risk of serious underlying etiology or reoccurrence

Follow-up

- **Primary care:** 1 to 2 days
- **Neurology:** 1 to 2 weeks if seizure disorder is suspected or diagnosed

Pearls and Pitfalls

- A BRUE is a diagnosis of exclusion.
- Do not use the term *ALTE*.
- Do not perform routine screening tests. Target testing and treat the patient according to risk determined from the history and physical examination features.
- Have a high index of suspicion for child abuse.

Bibliography

Tieder JS, Bonkowsky JL, Etzel RA, et al. Clinical practice guideline: brief resolved unexplained events (formerly apparent life-threatening events) and evaluation of lower-risk infants. *Pediatrics.* 2016;137(5):e20160590

CHAPTER 109

Bronchiolitis

Introduction

Bronchiolitis refers to the clinical presentation of certain viral lower respiratory tract infections in a young child, usually younger than 2 years. The typical presentation is one of obstructive lung disease caused by edema and increased mucus production involving the small airways. Respiratory syncytial virus (RSV) is the classic and most common etiologic agent, but many other viruses are implicated in bronchiolitis, including human metapneumovirus. Coinfection with more than 1 virus has also been documented.

In general, bronchiolitis is a self-limited disease, and therapy is simply supportive. Lack of effective treatments is often a source of frustration for parents and health care professionals alike. Education surrounding the typical 2-week course of illness is therefore important.

Clinical Presentation

History

Obtain a timeline of the illness. Typically, a prodromal phase of nasal congestion, often accompanied by fever, is then followed by cough and tachypnea. Obtain a birth history, because prematurity may indicate a more severe or prolonged disease course, particularly for those with chronic lung disease. Very young infants are rarely at risk of apnea, which can be the presenting symptom of bronchiolitis.

Inquire about a prior history of wheezing. Recurrent wheezing may indicate asthma rather than bronchiolitis. However, it is unclear whether recurrent, viral wheezing in an infant will become persistent asthma or requires anything more than supportive care.

Physical Examination

Observe the patient's work of breathing and respiratory rate. The patient may have a cough and increased work of breathing, characterized by retractions or visible use of accessory respiratory muscles. Periodic re-examination is helpful to assess the disease course. In a young infant who is an obligate nose breather (typically <3 months of age), an examination that follows nasal suctioning may reveal significant improvement.

Lung auscultation is usually remarkable for diffuse wheezing and/or rales and tachypnea. In more severe cases, breath sounds may be decreased because of poor air entry. It is important to distinguish the diffuse peripheral lung findings characteristic of bronchiolitis from localized findings or transmitted upper-airway sounds, which may suggest an alternate diagnosis. To evaluate the patient for upper-airway transmitted sounds, listen over the patient's nose and mouth, then "subtract" those sounds from what is heard during lung auscultation. Hypoxia is frequently encountered. Less important findings include clear rhinorrhea and middle ear effusion.

Laboratory Workup

Do not perform routine laboratory tests or imaging for a patient who presents with clinical bronchiolitis. Do not perform specific viral testing to confirm RSV, unless the patient is receiving RSV prophylaxis or testing is required for grouping patients in hospital rooms, because results will not otherwise alter care. If diagnostic uncertainty exists or if the patient is not following a predictable hospital course, obtain a chest radiograph to evaluate the patient for other pathologic conditions, including foreign body aspiration and pneumonia. However, be aware that atelectasis may be misinterpreted as pneumonia. The right upper and right middle lobes are frequently affected, and a repeat chest radiograph obtained after 24 hours will often show complete resolution of the "infiltrate" as the affected area re-expands.

There is considerable variation in the management of fever in an infant younger than 60 days (see Chapter 64) who presents with bronchiolitis. A blood culture and lumbar puncture are not routinely indicated in an otherwise well-appearing, febrile infant with clinical bronchiolitis. However, a fever that occurs later in the disease course may be an indication that the patient should be evaluated for secondary bacterial infection, such as pneumonia or otitis media.

Differential Diagnosis

Consider a differential diagnosis to include the common symptoms of wheezing/rales, tachypnea, and fever (Table 109-1). The wheezing and/or rales characteristic of bronchiolitis involve bilateral lung fields. Unilateral or upper-airway examination findings may indicate another process, such as aspiration, focal pneumonia, or laryngotracheobronchitis (croup). Other causes of diffuse wheezing and rales include pulmonary edema, perinatally acquired chlamydial infection, pertussis, or parapertussis. Distinguish between adventitial lung sounds that occur in the larger airways (rings and slings) and those that occur in the small airways (wheezing and rales).

Table 109-1. Differential Diagnosis of Bronchiolitis	
Diagnosis	**Clinical Features**
Aspiration	History is more chronic Absence of fever and rhinorrhea Possible abnormal tone and/or other neurologic signs
Chlamydia	Onset <3 mo of age Staccato cough Peripheral eosinophilia (>300/mm^3)
Croup	Inspiratory stridor Unusual in a patient <3 mo of age Wheezing less common
External airway compression	Monophasic/monophonic wheezing Central rather than peripheral wheeze
Metabolic acidosis	Tachypnea with clear lungs ↓ Bicarbonate level
Pertussis	Paroxysmal cough Wheezing is unusual Whoop may not be heard <6 mo of age
Pneumonia	Patient may have high fever Hypoxia unusual Unilateral auscultatory findings
Pulmonary edema	History of heart disease or murmur Hepatomegaly, facial or peripheral edema

Treatment

The mainstay of therapy for children with bronchiolitis is supportive care. While variation in treatment for this condition remains, the preponderance of evidence demonstrates that medications are ineffective in treating uncomplicated bronchiolitis. The American Academy of Pediatrics 2014 Clinical Practice Guideline on bronchiolitis recommends *against* the use of systemic corticosteroids, nebulized albuterol, and nebulized racemic epinephrine.

There is no proven benefit for treatment with hypertonic saline (HS). In some meta-analyses, investigators reported that use of HS reduced hospital length of stay (LOS). However, a repeat analysis of the same evidence showed significant heterogeneity among analyzed studies, which was not addressed by prior authors; when controlling for this heterogeneity, the data do not suggest that HS shortens LOS.

Hypoxia is a primary reason for inpatient admission of children with bronchiolitis. The routine use of continuous pulse oximetry monitoring and unnecessarily high target saturations may prolong hospitalization without providing other benefits. Therefore, order spot oximetry checks, unless a patient's clinical status is deteriorating. Use a target saturation of 90% as a hospitalization threshold and for weaning of supplemental oxygen.

Administration of oxygen via heated, humidified high-flow nasal cannula devices (see Chapter 106, Airway Management and Respiratory Support) is gaining popularity. Flow rates and fraction of inspired oxygen can be independently adjusted in this delivery model, and young infants who are obligate nasal breathers seem to benefit most from this modality.

Frequent nasal suctioning is beneficial, particularly before feeding attempts in the obligate nose breather (<3 months of age). However, avoid aggressive deep suctioning, which may cause edema of the nasopharynx. Also avoid chest physiotherapy, which is ineffective and potentially detrimental in bronchiolitis.

Apnea is a concern in the youngest infants with bronchiolitis, although the patients at highest risk are formerly premature patients and those with underlying neuromuscular disorders. In the absence of complicating factors, apnea may still occur in an infant younger than 2 months, although it is rare. Therefore, do not delay the discharge of an otherwise mildly ill patient solely for apnea monitoring. Treat true apnea in bronchiolitis with close monitoring and stimulation, high-flow nasal cannula oxygen, and continuous positive airway pressure and/or mechanical ventilation, if necessary.

Poor intake that leads to dehydration is a common reason for hospitalization. Closely monitor the safety of oral feeding in a patient with significant tachypnea (>60 breaths/min) and/or respiratory distress. Support hydration with nasogastric feedings or intravenous fluids as needed.

Administer or ensure appropriate administration of palivizumab, a monoclonal antibody approved for RSV prophylaxis in high-risk infants.

Indications for Consultation

Pulmonologist: Diagnosis is uncertain, patient has prolonged oxygen requirement or frequent episodes of hospitalization concerning for underlying lung disease

Disposition

- **Intensive care unit transfer:** Persistent hypoxia or respiratory distress despite increasing oxygen delivery; carbon dioxide retention despite tachypnea
- **Discharge criteria:** Improved respiratory status with decreased work of breathing, oxygen saturation >90% in room air, and adequate oral intake; there is no specific recommendation as to the amount of time that a patient must be without oxygen supplementation prior to discharge

Follow-up
Primary care: 1 to 2 days or as needed based on clinical status

Pearls and Pitfalls
- An infant with bronchiolitis often sounds much worse than their overall appearance (a "happy wheezer").
- Elevation of the minor fissure helps distinguish a radiographic opacity as right upper lobe atelectasis and associated volume loss as opposed to right upper lobe pneumonia.
- Carbon dioxide retention despite tachypnea is an ominous, though rare, sign.
- Bronchiolitis is a prolonged disease by pediatric standards, with a mean duration of symptoms (cough) of more than 2 weeks. Failure to communicate the expected course of the disease contributes to parental frustration and can result in multiple medical visits.
- To prevent readmissions, discuss discharge criteria and the expected disease course with the patient's family and primary care provider.

Bibliography
Brooks CG, Harrison WN, Ralston SL. Association between hypertonic saline and hospital length of stay in acute viral bronchiolitis: a reanalysis of 2 meta-analyses. *JAMA Pediatr.* 2016;170(6):577–584

Cunningham S, Rodriguez A, Adams T, et al. Oxygen saturation targets in infants with bronchiolitis (BIDS): a double-blind, randomised, equivalence trial. *Lancet.* 2015;386(9998):1041–1048

Meissner HC. Viral bronchiolitis in children. *N Engl J Med.* 2016;374:62–72

Ralston SL, Lieberthal AS, Meissner HC, et al. Clinical practice guideline: the diagnosis, management, and prevention of bronchiolitis. *Pediatrics.* Nov;134(5):e1474–e1502

Zhang L, Mendoza-Sassi RA, Klassen TP, Wainwright C. Nebulized hypertonic saline for acute bronchiolitis: a systematic review. *Pediatrics.* 2015;136(4):687–701

CHAPTER 110

Community-Acquired Pneumonia

Introduction

By definition, community-acquired pneumonia (CAP) occurs in a previously healthy child and is caused by an infection of the pulmonary parenchyma that has been acquired outside of the hospital. CAP can be complicated by pleural effusion, abscess, or necrosis, in which case the term *complicated pneumonia* is used. Although the etiology of CAP varies by age, about 15% of cases are bacterial in origin. However, viral infections (respiratory syncytial virus in particular, as well as influenza, parainfluenza, adenovirus) are the most common causes of pneumonia in hospitalized children with CAP.

Although the universal use of the conjugate vaccine against *Streptococcus pneumoniae* has decreased the incidence of overall infections caused by this pathogen, it remains the most common etiology of bacterial CAP in hospitalized children. The pneumococcal 13-valent vaccine (PCV13) has led to significant decreases in invasive, penicillin-resistant serotypes. However, most current pneumococcal isolates among children in the United States remain sensitive to penicillin.

In the PCV13 era, there are far fewer cases of empyema, and most pleural fluid cultures in complicated pneumonias have negative culture findings. However, polymerase chain reaction results confirm that *S pneumoniae* and *Staphylococcus aureus* are the first and second most frequent causes of complicated disease, respectively. In particular, methicillin-resistant *S aureus* (MRSA) is now a frequent cause of complicated CAP. Although group A *Streptococcus* (*Streptococcus pyogenes*) is an uncommon pathogen of pediatric CAP, it is an important cause of severe necrotizing pneumonia.

Pathogens responsible for "atypical pneumonias," such as *Mycoplasma pneumoniae* and *Chlamydophila pneumoniae*, can be found in patients across all ages, although they are more significant in children more than 5 years of age. Other bacteria, such as nontypable *Haemophilus influenzae* or *Moraxella catarrhalis*, are far less common.

Some rare causes of CAP include *Chlamydia trachomatis* (afebrile infants 1–4 months of age), *Coccidioides immitis* or San Joaquin Valley fever (desert Southwest and California), and *Histoplasma capsulatum* or spelunker's lung (central United States, Ohio River valley, lower Mississippi River).

Clinical Presentation

History

There is usually a history of a preceding upper respiratory infection, which is then followed by fever, cough, and dyspnea. A patient younger than 5 years can present with nonspecific symptoms, such as vomiting, headache, and abdominal pain. A history of dyspnea and chest pain may be elicited in a patient with complicated disease. Overall, fever is the most consistent symptom and can often be the sole complaint, as in a so-called occult pneumonia.

Physical Examination

A patient with CAP can have a range of physical findings, from just fever with or without tachypnea to significant respiratory distress and cyanosis. Tachypnea is the most sensitive sign in children. Findings such as retractions, use of accessory muscles, nasal flaring, and grunting occur with more severe pneumonias. Auscultatory findings include localized, decreased breath sounds and localized, fine, end-inspiratory rales. A patient who presents with wheezing is at low risk for having a radiographically confirmed bacterial pneumonia (especially pneumococcal). This is particularly true if the patient is afebrile. In addition, the patient may have signs of dehydration.

Laboratory Workup

Leukocytosis (white blood cell count >15,000/mm^3) with a left shift is slightly more common with a pneumococcal infection than with an atypical or viral CAP; however, a normal count can be falsely reassuring. In the pneumococcal vaccination era, a leukocytosis of 20,000/mm^3 and greater in a febrile child is associated with an "occult" pneumonia (pneumonia with radiographic evidence but no clinical signs or symptoms) in up to 9% of cases.

The yield of a blood culture is so low that it typically does not influence the clinical management. Perform a blood culture only in a case of severe or complicated disease. When available, perform testing for atypical pathogens in a patient with a higher pretest probability of having an infection with such a pathogen (>5 years of age, diffuse infiltrates on chest radiographs).

Radiology Examinations

Most patients hospitalized with CAP will have undergone chest radiography. An alveolar or lobar infiltrate is most commonly secondary to a bacterial infection. Diffuse or interstitial infiltrates suggest an atypical pathogen or a virus. However, since the radiographic findings often overlap, they have poor specificity for any specific particular pathogen. In addition, a normal chest radiographic finding does not rule out CAP. While repeat chest radiography is usually not necessary, it can be performed if there is no improvement after 24 to 48 hours of adequate treatment, if there is a worsening clinical course, or if a complication, such as an effusion or empyema, is suspected (no clinical improvement, pleuritic chest pain, percussion dullness).

Parapneumonic effusions are most commonly caused by bacteria, although viruses or atypical bacteria are sometimes implicated. Absence of "layering" on a decubitus chest radiograph is an indication of possible septations or empyema. If a complicated effusion or empyema is suspected, perform chest ultrasonography, which is more sensitive than computed tomography for evaluating the presence of septations and the nature of the pleural fluid. If pleural fluid is obtained, send it for Gram stain, culture, pH level assessment, and evaluation of lactate dehydrogenase, protein, and glucose levels. The most clinically useful finding in the pleural fluid is a pH level less than 7.2, which is associated with failure of medical management alone. In addition, a low glucose level (<40 mg/dL [<2.22 mmol/L]) and a low pH level (<7.2) are consistent with a probable empyema.

Differential Diagnosis

The presentation of pneumonia can overlap with other childhood illnesses (Table 110-1). A combination of the most common symptoms—tachypnea, fever, and cough—can be seen in pulmonary diseases (bronchiolitis), as well as nonpulmonary conditions (congestive heart failure [CHF]) or metabolic disease (diabetic ketoacidosis). Pulmonary effusion can also occur in CHF and many other extrapulmonary (pancreatitis) and neoplastic (lymphoma) illnesses.

Table 110-1. Differential Diagnosis of Community-Acquired Pneumonia	
Diagnosis	Clinical Features
Aspiration pneumonia	Chronically ill, special-needs, or technology-dependent patient
Bronchiolitis	Patient <1–2 y of age Wheezing with or without coarse rales
Foreign-body aspiration	Patient may have a history of a choking episode Recurrent pneumonia in the same site Localized hyperlucency on chest radiographs
Pertussis	Coughing paroxysms (many coughs without breathing) Whoop (>3–6 mo of age) Lymphocytosis
Tuberculosis	Presence of risk factors Ghon complex on chest radiographs Purified protein derivative (+)

"+" indicates a positive finding.

Treatment

Most current pneumococcal isolates are sensitive to penicillin, and resistance to penicillin has not been shown to affect clinical outcomes. Most treatment failures are secondary to the development of complications, such as empyema, noncompliance, and other factors not related to antibiotic susceptibility. As a result, β-lactams remain first-line treatment for suspected bacterial infections. Start treatment with oral amoxicillin (90 mg/kg/d, divided into doses administered every 8 hours; 2-g/d maximum) or intravenous (IV) ampicillin (200 mg/kg/d, divided into doses administered every 6 hours; 6-g/d maximum). Alternatives include a third-generation cephalosporin, such as IV ceftriaxone (50–100 mg/kg/d, divided into doses administered every 12–24 hours; 4-g/d maximum) or cefotaxime (150 mg/kg/d, divided into doses administered every 8 hours; 8-g/d maximum). Add IV clindamycin (40 mg/kg/d, divided into doses administered every 6–8 hours; 4.8-g/d maximum) or vancomycin (45 mg/kg/d, divided into doses administered every 8 hours; 4-g/d maximum) if the patient has severe or complicated disease in an area with a significant prevalence of MRSA. When potential penicillin allergy is a concern, administer a closely monitored trial of either cephalosporin or clindamycin (as detailed herein).

The use of antibiotics for atypical infections is controversial because there are no randomized controlled trials in children with pneumonia. Modest improvement in outcomes has been noted in adult studies. If rapid testing for an atypical pathogen yields positive results or if there is a high suspicion for an atypical infection and rapid testing is not available, add azithromycin (10 mg/kg in a single dose, followed by 5 mg/kg daily on days 2–5; maximum, 500 mg per dose). However, do not use a macrolide as monotherapy for CAP, because up to 40% of community-acquired *S pneumoniae* is resistant. While fluoroquinolones, such as oral or IV levofloxacin (10-mg/kg dose every 12 hours, 500-mg/d maximum), have activity against *S pneumoniae* and atypical pathogens, reserve them for teenagers or a patient with known severe allergies to other first- or second-line agents.

Medically treat an uncomplicated parapneumonic effusion that occupies less than 40% of the hemithorax. Medical management can also be attempted in a larger, uncomplicated parapneumonic effusion, provided the patient is not in significant respiratory distress. Features of a parapneumonic effusion that is likely to fail medical management and require drainage includes involvement of more than 40% of the hemithorax, the fluid being loculated, and the initial fluid analysis revealing an empyema (pH level <7.2). There are many choices for draining a large or complicated parapneumonic effusion, ranging from simple chest tube insertion to open thoracotomy. Early decortication with video-assisted thoracoscopic surgery (VATS) decreases length of stay, need for pain medication, and overall costs. However, chest tube insertion with instillation of fibrinolytics may be equal to VATS in terms of length of stay and superior in terms of cost. Base the choice of therapy (VATS or chest tube and fibrinolytics) on local expertise and availability.

The length of therapy for CAP caused by typical bacteria is 10 days. Initiate the transition from IV to oral therapy as soon as there is clinical improvement. There is no established duration of therapy for a patient with complicated disease. One useful strategy is to extend the duration of antibiotics until 7 to 10 days after the resolution of fever.

Indications for Consultation
- **Infectious diseases:** Unexpected pathogen identified or patient non-responsive to the appropriate initial antibiotic regimen
- **Otolaryngology:** Suspected foreign-body aspiration
- **Pulmonary:** Recurrent pneumonias or other pulmonary pathologic conditions, such as cystic fibrosis, are suspected
- **Surgery:** Drainage may be necessary (large effusion, loculations, empyema)

Disposition
- **Intensive care unit transfer:** Severe respiratory distress or signs of sepsis
- **Discharge criteria:** No oxygen requirement, defervescing or no fever, patient tolerating maintenance oral fluids, and adequate follow-up assured

Follow-up
Primary care: 2 to 3 days

Pearls and Pitfalls
- Initiation of antibiotic therapy does not mandate completing a full course if subsequent clinical or laboratory evidence suggests a viral infection.
- The initial chest radiograph can have negative findings if the patient has moderate to severe dehydration.
- A patient with complicated pneumonia can have persistent fever despite receiving adequate treatment.
- Wheezing is not consistent with a classic pneumococcal bacterial pneumonia.

Bibliography

Bradley JS, Byington CL, Shah SS, et al. Executive summary: the management of community-acquired pneumonia in infants and children older than 3 months of age: clinical practice guidelines by the Pediatric Infectious Diseases Society and the Infectious Diseases Society of America. *Clin Infect Dis*. 2011;53(7):617–630

Gardiner SJ, Gavranich JB, Chang AB. Antibiotics for community-acquired lower respiratory tract infections secondary to *Mycoplasma pneumoniae* in children. *Cochrane Database Syst Rev*. 2015;1:CD004875

Gereige RS, Laufer PM. Pneumonia. *Pediatr Rev*. 2013;34(10):438–456

Iroh Tam PY. Approach to common bacterial infections: community-acquired pneumonia. *Pediatr Clin North Am*. 2013;60(2):437–453

Jain S, Williams DJ, Arnold SR, et al; CDC EPIC Study Team. Community-acquired pneumonia requiring hospitalization among U.S. children. *N Engl J Med*. 2015;372(9):835–845

Shah VP, Tunik MG, Tsung JW. Prospective evaluation of point-of-care ultrasonography for the diagnosis of pneumonia in children and young adults. *JAMA Pediatr*. 2013;167(2):119–125

CHAPTER 111

Complications of Cystic Fibrosis

Introduction

Cystic fibrosis (CF) is a systemic disease that affects multiple organ systems, especially the respiratory and gastrointestinal tracts and the exocrine glands. Comprehensive care is usually delivered at CF centers, but a patient with a complication may present to any hospital. The most common pulmonary complications are pulmonary exacerbations, pulmonary hemorrhage/hemoptysis, and pneumothorax. The most urgent gastrointestinal concern is distal ileal obstruction syndrome (DIOS), an acute intestinal obstruction. CF-related diabetes (CFRD) is now the most common complication as a result of improved survival. If possible, always coordinate the management of a patient with CF with the staff of the CF center where the child receives routine care.

Clinical Presentation

The presentation of CF complications is summarized in Table 111-1.

Table 111-1. Presentation of CF Complications		
Complications	**Clinical Findings**	**Investigations**
Distal ileal obstruction syndrome	Abdominal pain and distention Emesis No fever	Abdominal radiograph for distal ileal obstruction
CF-related diabetes	↓ Weight or poor weight gain/growth Polydipsia/polyuria	↑ Glucose, hemoglobin A1c levels Glycosuria but no ketoacidosis Failed glucose tolerance test
Pneumothorax	Acute onset of chest pain and shortness of breath Ipsilateral ↓ or absent breath sounds	(+) Chest radiography finding
Pulmonary exacerbation	With or without fever ↑ Cough, congestion, dyspnea, and tachypnea ↑ Rhonchi and/or rales (diffuse/localized) Change in sputum viscosity or color	Worsening lung function Change in chest radiograph (↓ FEV_1)
Pulmonary hemorrhage	Pallor Cough, shortness of breath Expectoration of bright red blood	

Abbreviations: CF, cystic fibrosis; FEV1, forced expiratory volume in 1 second; +, positive finding.

History

A patient with a respiratory complication will most often complain of worsening distress, especially shortness of breath and increased respiratory rate. A pulmonary exacerbation will typically appear with increased cough and secretions at presentation, and possibly bleeding. Pneumothorax causes the acute onset of chest pain and difficulty breathing, without an increase in secretions. A patient with hemoptysis/pulmonary hemorrhage will report coughing up frank blood, with or without increased cough and worsening respiratory distress. Fever may occur with a pulmonary exacerbation but is not usually present with pneumothorax or hemoptysis. Ask about previous history of exacerbations, as well as current medications and pulmonary toilet regimen.

A patient with DIOS will complain of some combination of distended abdomen, abdominal pain, emesis, and, rarely, blood in the emesis or per rectum. The presentation of CFRD will be more insidious, with fatigue, poor energy, and possibly polydipsia and polyuria.

Physical Examination

Perform a complete physical examination, focusing on the vital signs, pulmonary findings, and abdominal examination.

Laboratory Workup

If a pulmonary complication is suspected, obtain a chest radiograph. This will allow differentiation of pneumothorax from other lung processes. With a pulmonary exacerbation, the radiograph may also demonstrate worsening infiltrates or bronchiectasis in comparison to previous images, if available. Obtain a complete blood cell count to quantify the degree of any blood loss and check for leukocytosis consistent with an acute infection. Also, if bleeding is present, order coagulation studies (activated partial thromboplastin time, international normalized ratio, fibrinogen level).

If a DIOS is suspected, obtain a plain radiograph of the abdomen, which usually has the diagnostic finding of distended, fluid-filled loops of bowel proximal to the level of obstruction. Alternatively, perform a gastrografin enema, which will confirm the diagnosis and be therapeutic. Also perform a comprehensive metabolic panel to identify any electrolyte imbalances.

The evaluation of suspected CFRD includes a comprehensive metabolic panel and a urinalysis. Typically, the blood sugar level will be high, especially postprandially, but without associated acidosis or ketosis. For a definitive diagnosis, arrange an oral glucose tolerance test.

Treatment

Always attempt to contact the primary CF provider for specific care recommendations until the patient can be transported to a CF facility.

Pulmonary Exacerbation

The mainstays of treatment are systemic antibiotics and vigorous airway clearance (every 4–6 hours) by using the best tolerated method, such as a high-frequency chest compression vest or flutter valve. Bronchodilators via metered-dose inhaler may also be of benefit and are most useful when given prior to airway clearance. In contrast, steroids and ipratropium have not been shown to be therapeutic in this situation. Inhaled antibiotics are most effective for chronic use but may be helpful during an acute exacerbation in a patient with a *Pseudomonas aeruginosa* airway infection. For mild to moderate exacerbations, order oral antibiotics directed against pathogens with which the patient is known to be infected. Reserve intravenous (IV) antibiotics for a severe exacerbation, manifesting in increased cough or sputum production, decreased exercise tolerance, increased fatigue, and absenteeism from daily activities, especially if a prior regimen of oral antibiotics has not been effective.

At accredited CF care centers, airway cultures are routinely obtained every 3 months, so information regarding the patient's airway flora will most likely be available. Typical organisms are *Haemophilus influenzae*, *Staphylococcus aureus* (methicillin-susceptible and methicillin-resistant *S aureus* [MRSA]), and *P aeruginosa*, but other gram-negative rods may be present, as well. While it is best to focus therapy on organisms known to be present in the patient's airway, if that information is not available, use a regimen that is effective against *P aeruginosa* and *S aureus,* such as tobramycin (10 mg/kg every 24 hours; adjust the dose based on serum levels) *and* an anti-pseudomonal semisynthetic penicillin (piperacillin/tazobactam, 400 mg of piperacillin component/kg/d, divided into doses administered every 6 hours; maximum, 16 g of piperacillin component/d). If MRSA is present or suspected, add vancomycin (60 mg/kg/d, divided into doses administered every 6 hours; 4-g/d maximum) to the regimen.

Pulmonary Hemorrhage/Hemoptysis

Observation and supportive care are generally sufficient until the bleeding stops. Give the patient nil per os (NPO, nothing by mouth) and administer IV fluid resuscitation with 20-mL/kg boluses of normal saline as needed. Transfuse 20 mL/kg or up to 2 units of packed red blood cells if the hemoglobin level is below 7 g/dL (<70 g/L) or if it decreases by 2 g/dL or more (≥20 g/L) over 8 hours. Bronchoscopy may be necessary when the bleeding is severe, and embolization may be indicated either acutely or after the hemorrhage has stopped. Consultation with and possible transport to a CF provider is required if embolization of the offending vessel is being considered.

Pneumothorax

If a pneumothorax measuring greater than 2 cm between the lung and chest wall is documented on a chest radiograph, consult a surgeon for chest tube placement. Since the recurrence rate is high, pleurodesis may be the preferred procedure after consultation with a CF specialist.

DIOS

Give the patient NPO, provide IV fluid resuscitation (if needed), and place a nasogastric tube (NGT) if needed. Treat with polyethylene glycol (PEG) orally (1.0–1.5 g/kg every day, 100-g/d maximum) if the obstruction is mild. Otherwise, administer the PEG orally or via continuous NGT (20–30 mL/kg/h until clear, 1-L/h maximum) if the vomiting is not severe. Alternatively, a therapeutic gastrografin enema may be necessary. However, consult a surgeon if the obstruction persists or if there is concern about a perforation (rigid abdomen, abdominal guarding, rebound tenderness, increased abdominal pain).

Diabetes

Consult an endocrinologist for dietary and insulin management guidance. Order a standard insulin bolus regimen and a high-calorie, high-fat diet.

Indications for Consultation

- **Endocrinology:** New-onset CFRD
- **Primary CF provider:** All patients
- **Surgery:** Chest tube placement, control of pulmonary hemorrhage needed, bowel obstruction

Disposition

- **Intensive care unit transfer:** Impending respiratory failure, shock, tension pneumothorax
- **Transfer to CF center:** Serious CF-related complication
- **Discharge criteria**
  — Bowel obstruction: Obstruction resolved, electrolyte imbalances corrected, patient tolerating oral maintenance fluids
  — CFRD: Blood sugar level <200 mg/dL (<11.1 mmol/L), glucosuria resolved, insulin regimen understood by patient, follow-up with CF provider or endocrinologist arranged

- Pneumothorax: Affected lung re-expanded without any reaccumulation after chest tube removal
- Pulmonary exacerbation: Patient afebrile for 48 hours with significant clinical and objective improvement in pulmonary function (to near-baseline)
- Pulmonary hemorrhage/hemoptysis: Bleeding stopped, hemoglobin level stable

Follow-up
Pulmonologist or CF center: 2 to 3 days

Pearls and Pitfalls
Have a high suspicion for complications, although they are relatively rare.

Bibliography

Colombo C, Ellemunter H, Houwen R, et al. Guidelines for the diagnosis and management of distal intestinal obstruction syndrome in cystic fibrosis patients. *J Cyst Fibros.* 2011;10(Suppl 2):S24–S28

Hurley MN, Prayle AP, Flume P. Intravenous antibiotics for pulmonary exacerbations in people with cystic fibrosis. *Cochrane Database Syst Rev.* 2015;7:CD009730

Hurt K, Simmonds NJ. Cystic fibrosis: management of haemoptysis. *Paediatr Respir Rev.* 2012;13(4):200–205

Noronha RM, Calliari LE, Damaceno N, Muramatu LH, Monte O. Update on diagnosis and monitoring of cystic fibrosis-related diabetes mellitus (CFRD). *Arq Bras Endocrinol Metabol.* 2011;55(8):613–621

Ong T, Ramsey BW. Update in cystic fibrosis 2014. *Am J Respir Crit Care Med.* 2015; 192(6):669–675

CHAPTER 112

Foreign-Body Aspiration

Introduction

Foreign-body aspiration (FBA) is potentially life threatening because of complete or partial airway obstruction. Although 80% of cases occur in children less than 3 years of age, it can occur at any age. Round foods, such as grapes, peanuts, hot dogs, and popcorn, are most commonly aspirated. Other possibilities include small toy parts, latex balloons, marbles, coins, and jewelry.

Certain foreign bodies are of particular concern because of their effects on airway tissue over time. For example, peanuts are irritating to the airway and can cause granulation tissue, while vegetable matter can absorb airway secretions and swell, leading to more severe obstruction. Button batteries can generate electrical current and erode the airway, and sharp objects can puncture the airway.

Clinical Presentation

History

The presentation of an FBA is varied, depending on what was aspirated, when, where in the respiratory tree the object lies, and the degree of obstruction. A witnessed episode of choking has the highest sensitivity for predicting FBA.

An acute, life-threatening FBA appears with choking, gagging, respiratory distress, cyanosis, and mental status change at presentation. A subacute presentation is more common, characterized by partial airway obstruction hours to days or even weeks later. Possible symptoms include choking, cough, stridor, dyspnea, wheeze, voice changes, and neck or throat pain. In some cases, there may be a history of receiving a previous diagnosis (mistakenly) of having asthma or pneumonia. Ask about hemoptysis or fever because these may be signs of airway trauma, foreign-body reaction, and/or infection.

Physical Examination

Identify any signs of respiratory distress, including tachypnea or retractions. Extrathoracic airway obstruction may appear with stridor at presentation, while intrathoracic obstruction manifests as cough, focal wheezing, and diminished lung sounds. This classic triad has high specificity but lacks sensitivity. Regional variation in lung aeration is an important clue and requires careful auscultation.

Radiology Examinations

If an FBA is suspected and the patient is stable, obtain anteroposterior and lateral radiographs of the chest. Include neck radiographs if a laryngotracheal foreign body is suspected. Organic objects may be radiolucent and not directly visible on radiographs. In such a case, obtain inspiratory and expiratory radiographs or bilateral decubitus views in a young child who cannot cooperate with inspiratory/expiratory imaging. These radiographs can increase the sensitivity of detecting a foreign body by providing indirect evidence, such as air trapping, localized hyperinflation distal to the obstruction, infiltrate, atelectasis, or mediastinal shift to the contralateral side. Normal radiographic findings do not rule out FBA. If the clinical suspicion remains high, additional diagnostic testing is required.

If radiographs are inconclusive, computed tomography (CT) is an option because it has a high negative predictive value for FBA and can be used to detect radiolucent objects. Many centers have ultrafast CT, which requires less radiation, obtains images quickly, and can generate three-dimensional images of large airways. Discuss with a radiologist the pros and cons of this modality, including availability, cost, radiation exposure, and potential delay in performing a diagnostic or therapeutic bronchoscopy.

Differential Diagnosis

The differential diagnosis of FBA is summarized in Table 112-1.

Treatment

Airway stabilization is the immediate priority. In complete airway obstruction, attempt the basic lifesaving (BLS) maneuvers for dislodging a foreign body (for patients <1 year of age, use back blows and chest thrusts; for patients >1 year of age, use abdominal thrusts or Heimlich maneuver). When BLS maneuvers fail, contact an otolaryngologist for emergent direct laryngoscopy.

Most situations are less acute because the airway is patent but FBA is certain or highly suspected. Contact an otolaryngologist or pulmonologist to perform a rigid bronchoscopy, which is the treatment of choice. There is a 95% success rate with few complications. Flexible bronchoscopy is an alternative for older children and adolescents, although the success rate is lower and it carries a risk of dislodging the object. Refer to your institutional availability and expertise with these different bronchoscopic modalities.

If the diagnosis of a foreign body is unclear, perform diagnostic flexible bronchoscopy first, and then proceed to rigid bronchoscopy for object removal.

Table 112-1. Differential Diagnosis of Foreign Body Aspiration	
Diagnosis	**Clinical Features**
Cough/dyspnea/wheezing	
Allergic reaction	Known or suspected trigger (often food)
	Dyspnea, diffuse wheezing, stridor
	Urticaria, angioedema
Asthma	Recurrent cough and wheezing with known triggers
	Bronchodilator responsive
Bronchiolitis	Upper respiratory infection prodrome
	Bilateral crackles and wheezing
Pneumonia	Fever, cough, tachypnea
	Bacterial: localized rales or decreased breath sounds
	Viral: diffuse wheezing and crackles
	Infiltrate may be seen on chest radiographs
Choking/dysphagia	
Esophageal foreign body	Drooling, dysphagia, cough
	Substernal discomfort
Mediastinal mass	Difficulty breathing and/or swallowing
	May be seen on chest radiographs (anterior mass most common)
Stridor	
Croup	Fever, barking cough, hoarse voice
Laryngotracheomalacia	Positional inspiratory stridor
	Appears early in life
Peritonsillar abscess	Fever, trismus, "hot potato" voice
	Uvula or palatal deviation
Retropharyngeal abscess	Fever, drooling
	Limited neck hyperextension
	Swelling anterior to cervical vertebrae on lateral neck radiographs

Chapter 112: Foreign-Body Aspiration

There is a subset of children in whom FBA is a consideration, but the history is equivocal and clinical suspicion is low. Such patients are asymptomatic, with normal radiographic findings. For this population, observation without bronchoscopic intervention is an appropriate option. Follow up in 1 to 2 days and arrange bronchoscopy if the symptoms persist or have progressed.

There is no evidence for routine use of antibiotics or corticosteroids after uncomplicated bronchoscopic foreign-body retrieval. On occasion, pneumonia can develop in the area of or distal to the foreign body (postobstructive pneumonia). In such a case, obtain fluid for Gram stain and culture during bronchoscopy to guide postprocedural antibiotic management.

Indications for Consultation

Pulmonology, otolaryngology, or surgery: Depends on who performs bronchoscopy at a given institution

Disposition

- **Intensive care unit transfer:** Airway instability, respiratory distress, hypoxia
- **Discharge criteria:** Foreign body removed, normal respiratory status without an oxygen requirement

Follow-up

- **Primary care**
  — Foreign body was removed: 1 to 2 weeks
  — Low suspicion for a foreign body and clinical status stable: 1 to 2 days
- **Surgical consult:** 1 week with the provider that performed the procedure

Pearls and Pitfalls

- Most airway foreign bodies are in the bronchi, the right bronchus more often than the left.
- Normal chest radiographic findings do not conclusively rule out FBA.
- Consider FBA as a diagnostic possibility in a patient with chronic cough, recurrent pneumonia on the same side, or focal wheezing.
- Accidental FBA does not typically require reporting to the local child protective services (CPS) agency. However, If FBA occurred in the context of a larger or longitudinal pattern of neglectful parenting, file the CPS report.

Bibliography

Green SS. Ingested and aspirated foreign bodies. *Pediatr Rev.* 2015;36(10):430–436

Lowe DA, Vasquez R, Maniaci V. Foreign body aspiration in children. *Clin Pediatr Emerg Med.* 2015;16(3):140–148

Mortellaro VE, Iqbal C, Fu R, Curtis H, Fike FB, St Peter SD. Predictors of radiolucent foreign body aspiration. *J Pediatr Surg.* 2013;48(9):1867–1870

Pugmire BS, Lim R, Avery LL. Review of ingested and aspirated foreign bodies in children and their clinical significance for radiologists. *RadioGraphics.* 2015;35(5):1528–1538

Rodriguez H, Passali GC, Gregori D, et al. Management of foreign bodies in the airway and oesophagus. *Int J Pediatr Otorhinolaryngol.* 2012;76(Suppl 1):S84–S91

Sink JR, Kitsko DJ, Georg MW, Winger DG, Simons JP. Predictors of foreign body aspiration in children. *Otolaryngol Head Neck Surg.* 2016;155(3):501–507

Rheumatology

Juvenile Idiopathic Arthritis

Introduction

Juvenile idiopathic arthritis (JIA) is the most common rheumatologic disease in children. JIA represents a broad spectrum of autoimmune arthritides, and systemic-onset JIA (sJIA) is the subtype most likely to be seen by the hospitalist. The peak onset is at 2 years of age, with a range between 1 and 5 years and no difference between sexes. Whereas the diagnosis of most subtypes of JIA requires a minimum of 6 weeks of arthritis in a child less than 16 years old, sJIA is a notable exception because the patient needs to be symptomatic for just 2 weeks.

Clinical Presentation

The common presentations of sJIA are summarized in Table 113-1.

Of utmost importance is recognizing macrophage activation syndrome (MAS), which is most commonly triggered by sJIA and has a mortality rate of 20% to 30%. MAS is characterized by fever, hepatosplenomegaly, lymphadenopathy, pancytopenia, consumptive coagulopathy, and liver dysfunction.

The common presentations of acute complications in a patient with sJIA are summarized in Table 113-2.

Table 113-1. Clinical Features of Systemic-Onset Juvenile Idiopathic Arthritis	
Sign/Symptom	**Clinical and Laboratory Findings**
Fever	High spiking daily (quotidian) or twice-daily fever Typically in the evenings and with associated rash
Arthritis	Nonerosive arthritis of ≥2 peripheral joints Knees, ankles, and wrists are most commonly affected May be associated with morning stiffness and gelling phenomenon
Rash	Evanescent, salmon-colored, macular rash Occurs concurrently with fevers Koebner phenomenon: identical rash appears in previously unaffected areas after being scratched or placed in hot water
Lymphadenopathy	Bilateral, symmetric in the cervical, axillary, and/or inguinal regions ↑ ESR, CRP level, and ferritin level
Splenomegaly/hepatosplenomegaly	Splenomegaly is more common than hepatomegaly ↑ Liver transaminase levels
Serositis	Pericarditis, pleuritis, sterile peritonitis

Abbreviations: CRP, C-reactive protein; ESR, erythrocyte sedimentation rate.

Table 113-2. Presentation of Acute Complications of sJIA	
Acute Complication	**Clinical Findings**
Macrophage activation syndrome	Purpura (including wet), bruising, generalized lymphadenopathy, hepatosplenomegaly, persistent fever despite improvement in arthritis ↓ WBC count, platelets, ESR, fibrinogen level, clotting factors ↑ D-dimer, triglyceride, ferritin, PT, PTT, AST, and ALT levels
Severe systemic infections (secondary to immunosuppression)	Worsening of sJIA symptoms, persistent fevers Bacterial (encapsulated organisms): *Pneumococcus, Meningococcus, Salmonella* Viral: CMV, herpes zoster Opportunistic: *Pneumocystis jirovecii, Cryptococcus*

Abbreviations: ALT, alanine aminotransferase; AST, aspartate aminotransferase; CMV, cytomegalovirus; ESR, erythrocyte sedimentation rate; PT, prothrombin time; PTT, partial thromboplastin time; sJIA, systemic-onset juvenile idiopathic arthritis; WBC, white blood cell.

History

Determine the timing, onset, duration, and intensity of symptoms. In particular, morning stiffness or "gelling" with inactivity is characteristic of JIA. The stiffness improves slowly throughout the day. The initial symptoms of a patient with sJIA at presentation may include fever and rash, without arthritis.

The fever of sJIA is typically 2 or more weeks of daily (quotidian) or twice-daily high-spiking fevers. In contrast to fevers caused by infection, the fever of sJIA predictably spikes in the evening and regresses quickly. The review of systems must include symptoms of autoinflammatory disease, including weight loss, fatigue, and hair or nail changes. Ask about a family history of autoimmune diseases.

Physical Examination

Perform a thorough physical examination. A patient with sJIA tends to look ill only during febrile periods and may develop a characteristic salmon-colored macular rash in association with fever. A detailed examination of all joints is necessary, including the sacroiliac joint, temporomandibular joint, and vertebral articulations. Perform inspection, palpation, and passive/active range of motion testing to identify effusions, warmth, mobility, and tenderness and compare both sides of the body, when appropriate. Also examine all tendons for signs of enthesitis (inflammation at tendon insertions), including warmth, tenderness, and swelling. Check the fingers for rheumatoid nodules and contractures.

In addition, look for lymphadenopathy, splenomegaly, or hepatomegaly, which are all supportive of sJIA. The lymphadenopathy of sJIA is typically bilateral and symmetric and affects the cervical, axillary, or inguinal lymph nodes. An ophthalmologic examination should be performed to look for uveitis.

Laboratory Workup

The International League of Associations for Rheumatology criteria for the diagnosis of sJIA does not include laboratory values, as no test results are diagnostic for sJIA. However, erythrocyte sedimentation rate (ESR), C-reactive protein (CRP) level, and ferritin level are typically increased, while rheumatoid factor results are usually negative, and antinuclear antibody results are rarely positive. There may be other nonspecific laboratory abnormalities, including anemia, thrombocytosis, leukocytosis, and increased liver enzyme levels.

About 5% of children with sJIA meet criteria for MAS. If MAS is suspected, obtain a complete blood cell count, liver panel, prothrombin time and partial thromboplastin time, and D-dimer, fibrinogen, lactate dehydrogenase, triglyceride, and ferritin levels. Progression to MAS leads to high serum ferritin levels, up to 10,000 µg/L. In addition, consumptive coagulopathy depletes fibrinogen. Bone marrow biopsy is indicated to exclude malignancy and hemophagocytic lymphohistiocytosis (HLH).

Differential Diagnosis

Maintain a high level of suspicion for sJIA. The diagnosis requires arthritis, 2 or more weeks of fever, and 1 or more of the following: rash, lymphadenopathy, splenomegaly/hepatosplenomegaly, or serositis. A patient with undiagnosed sJIA may have fever and rash, fever, or arthritis and is therefore admitted with a concern for infection (especially in the setting of fever of unknown origin), malignancy, or other autoimmune/autoinflammatory diseases.

The differential diagnosis of sJIA is summarized in Table 113-3.

Treatment

Because of the side-effect profile of immunomodulators, consultation with a rheumatologist is essential. Treatment of the early, systemic phase of sJIA depends on the severity of disease, and the therapies may be additive as disease severity increases. Early and aggressive treatment of sJIA most effectively treats chronic arthritis, the long-term sequela of sJIA. Nonsteroidal anti-inflammatory drugs and corticosteroids are now used as bridge or adjunctive therapy to immunomodulators.

Treatment of MAS must be comanaged by a rheumatologist. Initial treatment typically consists of high-dose methylprednisolone, cyclosporine, and anakinra.

Table 113-3. Differential Diagnosis of Systemic-Onset Juvenile Idiopathic Arthritis

Categories of Disease	Suggestive Features
Rheumatologic	
Reactive arthritis	Recent gonorrheal, chlamydial, or enteric infection Conjunctivitis, urethritis, oral ulcers, rash
Acute rheumatic fever	Evidence of a recent streptococcal infection Migratory/asymmetric arthritis Carditis with a prolonged PR interval Uncommon: erythema marginatum, subcutaneous nodules, chorea
Serum sickness	Exposure to new medication or immunization High fever, pruritic rash Arthralgia and occasional arthritis Improvement within 48 h of removal of offending agent
Systemic lupus erythematosus	Malar or discoid rash Oral or nasopharyngeal ulcerations Pericarditis, pleuritis, arthritis (+) ANA, anti-Smith antibodies, anti-DNA antibodies
Inflammatory bowel disease	Weight loss, abdominal pain Diarrhea, bloody stools, rectal fissure
Infectious	
Septic arthritis	Synovial fluid WBC with >100,000 WBC/mm^3 Neutrophil predominance
Subacute bacterial endocarditis	Low-grade fevers, myalgia, weight loss, fatigue, murmur Splinter hemorrhages, Janeway lesions, Osler nodes, Roth spots, (+) blood cultures
Tick-borne diseases	Possible vector exposure Fever, petechial rash, headache, photophobia, myalgia Lyme disease: knee arthritis without erythema
Other	
Malignancy: leukemia, osteosarcoma, neuroblastoma, HLH	Leukopenia, anemia, thrombocytopenia Hepatosplenomegaly, bone pain

Abbreviations: ANA, antinuclear antibody; CRP, C-reactive protein; ESR, erythrocyte sedimentation rate; HLH, hemophagocytic lymphohistiocytosis; PT, prothrombin time; PTT, partial thromboplastin time; WBC, white blood cell, +, positive finding.

Indications for Consultation

- **Rheumatology**: All patients suspected of having sJIA or admitted for a complication
- **Oncology**: As needed for bone marrow biopsy to exclude primary HLH
- **Infectious diseases**: As needed to diagnose and treat severe, systemic infections

Disposition

- **Transfer to a center with a rheumatologist:** Any patient with suspected MAS or new-onset sJIA
- **Intensive care unit transfer**: Progressive MAS, shock, sepsis
- **Discharge criteria**: Patient afebrile with improvement of clinical symptoms and decreasing systemic inflammation

Follow-up

- **Primary care:** 1 to 4 days
- **Rheumatology:** 1 to 4 weeks

Pearls and Pitfalls

- The arthritis of sJIA may not manifest during the initial febrile illness.
- sJIA can appear with MAS at presentation, which is the most severe complication of sJIA and carries a 20% to 30% mortality rate.
- In MAS, the ESR decreases paradoxically (because of consumption of fibrinogen) while the CRP level continues to increase.
- Patients with sJIA who are taking corticosteroids or biological therapies are at increased risk of severe, systemic infections.

Bibliography

Correll CK, Binstadt BA. Advances in the pathogenesis and treatment of systemic juvenile idiopathic arthritis. *Pediatr Res.* 2014;75(1–2):176–183

Espinosa M, Gottlieb BS. Juvenile idiopathic arthritis. *Pediatr Rev.* 2012;33(7):303–313

Hay AD, Ilowite NT. Systemic juvenile idiopathic arthritis: a review. *Pediatr Ann.* 2012; 41(11):1–6

Petty RE, Southwood TR, Manners P, et al. International League of Associations for Rheumatology classification of juvenile idiopathic arthritis: second revision. *J Rheumatol.* 2004;31(2):390–392

Ravelli A, Davì S, Minoia F, Martini A, Cron RQ. Macrophage activation syndrome. *Hematol Oncol Clin North Am.* 2015;29(5):927–941

Stoll ML, Cron RQ. Treatment of juvenile idiopathic arthritis: a revolution in care. *Pediatric Rheumatol.* 2014;12(13):1–10

Systemic Lupus Erythematosus

Introduction

Systemic lupus erythematosus (SLE) is a multisystem, chronic autoimmune disease characterized by periods of increased disease activity, or "flares," that are associated with systemic inflammation. Fifteen percent of SLE cases appear before 18 years of age, but onset before 5 years of age is rare. SLE has a female predominance that increases during puberty (3:1 before puberty; 9:1 after puberty). Childhood-onset SLE carries higher morbidity and mortality rates, because most children develop renal and/or neuropsychiatric complications within the first 2 years of diagnosis. The most common SLE complications are disease flares and systemic infections, but other serious complications include progressive glomerulonephritis/renal failure, thrombotic events, and macrophage activation syndrome (MAS).

Clinical Presentation

The common clinical features of SLE are summarized in Table 114-1.

The presentation of acute SLE complications is summarized in Table 114-2.

Table 114-1. Clinical Features of SLE According to Organ System	
Organ System	**Clinical Findings/Laboratory Studies**
Constitutional	Fever, generalized lymphadenopathy, anorexia, weight loss, fatigue Pain amplification
Immunologic	**Antinuclear antibody abnormal titer** (in the absence of drugs known to induce a SLE-like syndrome) **Anti-dsDNA** **Anti-Smith antibody**
Mucocutaneous	**Malar (butterfly) rash** **Discoid rash** **Photosensitivity** rash after sun exposure **Oral** (hard palate) or **nasal septal ulcers,** usually painless Alopecia (temporal thinning)
Musculoskeletal	**Nonerosive arthritis** of >2 joints (small or large) Arthralgia (morning stiffness)
Cardiopulmonary	**Serositis** (pericarditis or pleuritis) Myocarditis or noninfective endocarditis (Libman-Sacks) Interstitial pneumonitis, pulmonary hemorrhage, or pulmonary hypertension
Renal	**Persistent proteinuria** (>0.5 g/d) or **cellular casts** (RBC, granular, tubular, or mixed) Severe hypertension Peripheral edema

Continued

Table 114-1. Clinical Features of SLE According to Organ System, continued

Organ System	Clinical Findings/Laboratory Studies
Hematologic	Leukopenia (<4,000/mm^3 on ≥2 occasions) or Lymphopenia (<1,500/mm^3 on ≥2 occasions) or Hemolytic anemia with reticulocytosis or Thrombocytopenia (<100,000/mm^3 in the absence of offending drugs)
Neuropsychiatric	**Psychosis, delirium,** or **seizures** (in the absence of drugs or metabolic derangements)
Vascular	Antiphospholipid antibody syndrome Vasospasm (livedo reticularis, Raynaud phenomenon) Nail fold capillary changes, periungual erythema Cutaneous vasculitis, retinal vasculitis, small-vessel CNS vasculitis Thrombotic microangiopathies

Abbreviations: anti-dsDNA, anti–double-stranded DNA; CNS, central nervous system; RBC, red blood cell; SLE, systemic lupus erythematosus.

Items listed in **bold** are the 11 diagnostic criteria as defined by the American College of Rheumatology. Most patients who receive a diagnosis of SLE meet 4 or more of the 11 criteria (often not concurrently).

Table 114-2. Complications of SLE

Complications	Clinical Findings/Laboratory Studies
Disease flares	Worsening or return of initial SLE symptoms ↑ ESR
Systemic infections	Worsening of SLE symptoms, fever ↑ CRP level
Progressive glomerulonephritis Renal failure	↑ Blood urea nitrogen, creatinine, and urine protein levels Severe hypertension, dependent edema Oliguria, anuria, or high urine output
Thrombotic events	Severe headache (cerebral vein thrombosis) Thrombosis or inflammation of any-size vessel (DVT, PE) Thrombotic thrombocytopenic purpura (thrombotic microangiopathy) ↑ Risk with (+) anticardiolipin antibodies and SLE anticoagulants
Macrophage activation syndrome	See Chapter 113, Juvenile Idiopathic Arthritis

Abbreviations: CRP, C-reactive protein; DVT, deep venous thrombosis; ESR, erythrocyte sedimentation rate; PE, pulmonary embolism; SLE, systemic lupus erythematosus; +, positive finding.

History

Each patient with SLE will present with a different profile of symptoms, the most common being fatigue, fever, weight loss, anorexia, arthritis, and malar or discoid rash, which are diagnostically discriminating. Given the periodicity of the illness, an incomplete review of systems may lead to delays in diagnosis. In a child with known SLE, key questions to ask include the similarities between the present and previous disease flares and current medication usage (including compliance and adverse effects). Family history may reveal others with SLE and/or autoimmune disease.

Physical Examination

Perform a complete physical examination and focus on the patient's general appearance and the cutaneous, musculoskeletal, lymphatic, and abdominal findings. Check for fever, which suggests infection or hypertension secondary to renal disease. Typical skin findings include pallor, malar rash, and temporal alopecia. A malar (butterfly) rash appears raised (or flat), is nonpruritic and nonscarring, spares the nasolabial folds, and is sometimes photosensitive. A discoid rash is typically a raised rash over the forehead and scalp, with adherent scaling, atrophic scarring, and follicular plugging, but it is rare in childhood-onset SLE. Painless oral or nasal ulcers may be identified. A careful examination of the retinas and nail beds may demonstrate vascular changes.

The arthritis of SLE is painful, polyarticular, and frequently symmetric and may cause deformities. Small and large joints can be involved with effusions, limited range of motion, and stiffness.

Decreased or abnormal breath sounds or a cardiac rub may suggest pleural effusion, pneumonitis, interstitial lung disease, or pericardial effusion. Lower-extremity edema can be seen with renal involvement or malnutrition. Generalized lymphadenopathy and/or hepatosplenomegaly are common findings in new-onset childhood SLE and disease flares. Abnormal mental status and/or neurologic examination findings occur with SLE neuro-psychiatric involvement.

Laboratory Workup

Laboratory studies serve a dual purpose in SLE: to aid in diagnosis and to monitor disease activity. Two of the 11 diagnostic criteria are immunologic, and laboratory values play a key role in diagnosing renal and hematologic-coagulation manifestations of SLE.

Immunologic tests include testing for antinuclear antibodies (ANA) (most sensitive), anti-Smith antibodies (most specific and associated with more severe disease), anti–double-stranded DNA (more specific and associated with renal disease), anti-ribonuclear protein antibodies, anti-Ro antibodies (associated with neonatal lupus in children of affected mothers), and anti-La antibodies. Hypocomplementemia (complement component 3 [C3] and 4 [C4]) supports the diagnosis of SLE, and testing is indicated during initial diagnosis, as well as flares.

In terms of renal tests, proteinuria, hematuria, and/or casts at urinalysis suggest lupus nephritis. Spot urine protein to creatinine ratios can be used to monitor response to therapy in lupus nephritis. Hypoalbuminemia and/or increased creatinine levels also suggest lupus nephritis.

Hematologic/coagulation tests can be used during initial diagnosis and flares. Obtain a complete blood count to evaluate the presence of cytopenias, coagulation studies (D-dimer level, activated partial thromboplastin time, international normalized ratio, fibrinogen level), and antiphospholipid antibody levels to assess hypercoagulability.

The erythrocyte sedimentation rate (ESR) is typically increased, while the C-reactive protein (CRP) level remains normal or minimally increased in SLE, except in the setting of serositis or MAS. A liver panel often reveals transaminitis, which occurs in association with corticosteroid therapy, adverse drug reactions, or SLE flares.

Maintaining a high index of suspicion for opportunistic infections is important, especially for patients taking systemic steroids or immunomodulators. For suspicion of MAS, look for ferritinemia, cytopenias, transaminitis, and increasing CRP level with decreasing ESR (because of consumption of fibrinogen).

Differential Diagnosis

The differential diagnosis of the initial presentation of SLE complications is summarized in Table 114-3.

The differential diagnosis of an acute SLE flare includes antiphospholipid syndrome, hemophagocytic lymphohistiocytosis, mixed connective tissue disease, sarcoidosis, and systemic vasculitis, as well as any infectious cause of fever of unknown origin.

Treatment

The treatment of SLE involves a multidisciplinary approach that includes at least a pediatric rheumatologist, who will tailor treatment to disease severity and manifestations. All of the medications used in the treatment of SLE have potential serious side effects, so weigh the treatment options with a discussion of risk-benefit ratio. Aspirin and prednisone are approved by the U.S. Food and Drug Administration (FDA) for use in SLE, but most other therapies are "off-label." Belimumab, a B-lymphocyte stimulator-specific inhibitor, is an FDA-approved SLE therapy; trials in children are underway.

Disease Flares

The mainstays of treatment are systemic corticosteroids, the route, dose, frequency, and duration of which are dependent on the severity of disease. In the case of renal or neurologic complications or for use as a steroid-sparing agent, use immunosuppressive agents (azathioprine or mycophenolate mofetil) in consultation with a rheumatologist. For patients with severe arthritis or

Table 114-3. Differential Diagnosis of the Initial Presentation of Systemic Lupus Erythematosus	
Diagnosis	**Clinical Features**
Acute rheumatic fever	Fever, new murmur, rash Migratory polyarthritis, subcutaneous nodules
Antiphospholipid syndrome	Livedo reticularis, headaches, blood clots
Crohn disease	Abdominal pain, diarrhea, weight loss, anemia Erythema nodosum, oral/anal ulcers
Hemolytic uremic syndrome	Oliguria, hypertension, uremia Anemia, thrombocytopenia
Hemophagocytic lymphohistiocytosis	Fever, jaundice, hepatosplenomegaly, lymphadenopathy, rash Pancytopenia, ↑ ferritin level
Infectious cause of fever of unknown origin	See Table 66-1: Differential Diagnosis of Fever of Unknown Origin
Juvenile dermatomyositis	Heliotrope (pinkish-purple) rash of face, eyelids, hands, elbows Calcinosis, muscle weakness/contractures
Langerhans cell histiocytosis	Fever, weight loss, bone lesions, rash Enlarged liver, spleen, and/or lymph nodes
Leukemia or lymphoma	Fever, weight loss, bleeding, bruising, pallor, lymphadenopathy Anemia, high or low WBC count
Mixed connective tissue disease	Malaise, joint and muscle pain/swelling Raynaud syndrome, sclerodactyly
Neuroblastoma	Fatigue, loss of appetite, pallor Fever, abdominal swelling
Sarcoidosis	Fatigue, shortness of breath, cough, weight loss Lymphadenopathy, erythema nodosum
Sjögren syndrome	Dry eyes, dry mouth, conjunctivitis Gastroesophageal reflux
Systemic juvenile idiopathic arthritis	Fever, arthritis, and a salmon-pink rash Arthritis
Systemic vasculitis	Headache, weight loss, myalgia Rash, ulcers, aneurysms

Abbreviation: WBC, white blood cell.

serositis, use nonsteroidal anti-inflammatory drugs. Treat mild symptoms of arthritis and/or rash with antimalarials (hydroxychloroquine and chloroquine) or methotrexate.

Systemic Infections

Consider patients with SLE to be functionally asplenic and immunocompromised. Conduct a thorough workup to find the source of infection and start broad-spectrum antibiotics and possibly antivirals, pending the results of that workup. Give special consideration to encapsulated bacterial organisms, systemic cytomegalovirus, herpes zoster, and *Pneumocystis jirovecii* or

Cryptococcus, because patients with SLE are particularly at risk for infection with these organisms. Avoid the use of sulfonamides in a patient with SLE because they can precipitate a disease flare.

Progressive Glomerulonephritis/Renal Failure

Consult a nephrologist for possible biopsy and management. Aggressively treat hypertension and/or proteinuria with angiotensin-converting enzyme (ACE) inhibitors, targeting a normal blood pressure. Review all nephrotoxic medications, dose appropriately, and order a renal diet, with strict monitoring of intake and output. Mycophenolate mofetil (oral) or cyclophosphamide (intravenous [IV]) are often used for induction of remission and maintenance therapy in more severe lupus nephritis.

Thrombotic Events

Use heparin or low–molecular weight heparin to treat or prevent thrombosis. Low-dose aspirin is also useful for decreasing risk of thrombotic events. Screen patients with SLE who are positive for SLE-anticoagulant and/or anticardiolipin antibodies for other deficiencies of antithrombin III, protein C, or protein S.

Macrophage Activation Syndrome

Rapid recognition is key to MAS treatment. Once identified, treat with high-dose corticosteroids and escalate care accordingly. In severe cases, adjunctive therapies include IV immunoglobulin and cyclosporine.

Indications for Consultation

- **Rheumatology:** All patients
- **Nephrology:** Renal complications/involvement
- **Adolescent medicine, cardiology, dermatology, neurology, psychiatry, psychology:** Based on organ system involvement

Disposition

- **Transfer to a center with a rheumatologist:** Serious SLE-related complication
- **Intensive care unit transfer:** Sepsis, shock, progressive MAS, renal failure
- **Discharge criteria:**
  — Appropriate follow-up with a rheumatologist is scheduled
  — Disease flares: symptoms improving, medication regimen established
  — Systemic infections: clinical improvement with targeted antibacterial or antiviral therapy

— Renal insufficiency/failure: creatinine level stable or improving, adequate urine output, outpatient renal follow-up available
— Thrombotic events: clinical improvement with stable anticoagulant dosing
— MAS: clinical improvement, declining ferritin level

Follow-up

- **Primary Care:** 1 to 5 days
- **Rheumatologist:** 2 to 3 days
- **Nephrologist:** 2 to 3 days as needed
- **Various subspecialties:** 2 to 3 days as needed

Pearls and Pitfalls

- Suspect SLE in an adolescent female patient with constitutional symptoms (fever, lymphadenopathy, weight loss), malar or discoid rash, and arthritis/arthralgia.
- Childhood-onset SLE is more severe than adult-onset SLE, with higher morbidity and mortality rates.
- Disease flares often appear with signs and symptoms similar to those at the initial presentation.
- Glomerulonephritis and neuropsychiatric symptoms are common in the first 2 years after diagnosis.
- Immunize the patient for influenza, but do not use any live-attenuated immunizations.

Bibliography

Barsalou J, Levy DM, Silverman ED. An update on childhood-onset systemic lupus erythamatosus. *Curr Opin Rheumatol.* 2013;25(5):616–622

Borgia RE, Silverman ED. Childhood-onset systemic lupus erythematosus: an update. *Curr Opin Rheumatol.* 2015;27(5):483–492

Levy DM, Kamphuis S. Systemic lupus erythematosus in children and adolescents. *Pediatr Clin North Am.* 2012;59(2):345–364

Lo MS. Childhood-onset systemic lupus erythematosus. In: Tsokos G, ed. *Systemic Lupus Erythematosus: Basic, Applied and Clinical Aspects.* London, United Kingdom: Elsevier; 2016:467–470

Weiss J. Pediatric systemic lupus erythematosus: more than a positive antinuclear antibody. *Pediatr Rev.* 2012;33(2):62–74

Sedation and Analgesia

Pain Management

Introduction

The International Association for the Study of Pain defines *pain* as an unpleasant sensory and emotional experience that arises from actual or potential tissue damage. Historically, pediatric pain is underrecognized and undertreated. Traditional barriers to providing good pain control to children include a lack of knowledge of pain recognition and treatment, as well as a fear of adverse effects, such as respiratory depression or addiction.

Creating an "Ouchless" Environment

According to the American Academy of Pediatrics Clinical Report on Relief of Pain and Anxiety in Pediatric Patients in Emergency Medical Systems, posttraumatic stress symptoms can occur after procedures or stressful medical experiences that were not accompanied by appropriate pain control or sedation, and this can lead to adverse reactions to subsequent procedures. Efforts to decrease anxiety and pain in children have paved the way for creation of "ouchless" environments. This can include hiding "scary" medical equipment, developing a child-friendly décor, and employing child life specialists to comfort children during procedures and serve as liaisons between providers and families. In addition, routine practices are changing, with greater use of topical, transmucosal, and oral pain medications, rather than injectable ones.

Pain Assessment

The best way to assess pediatric pain is by asking the patient, if possible. Ask the parents as an alternative if the child is unable to communicate. Increased pulse and blood pressure may suggest that a nonverbal child is in pain, while the absence of altered vital signs does not preclude the child being in pain, especially if the pain is chronic. Another option is to provide the patient with pain medication and then reassess their pain level. However, there are many reasons why a child might deny feeling pain. These include being told to be brave, concern about medication side effects or taste, anxiety that pain means they are getting sicker, inadequate understanding that pain can be treated, worry that pain will prevent discharge home, a desire to protect their parents, or fear of injection site pain associated with intramuscular (IM) or subcutaneous pain control.

The American Academy of Pediatrics recognizes that children's pain is underestimated because of the underuse of appropriate assessment tools and the failure to account for the wide range of children's developmental stages. In a neonate, infant, or nonverbal or neurodevelopmentally disabled patient, assessing pain can present a challenge. As an aid, there are many pain scales available that combine both physiological and behavioral parameters, such as the Neonatal Infant Pain Scale and the Face, Legs, Activity, Cry, Consolability scale (Table 115-1).

Children 3 to 8 years of age are able to articulate that they have pain and may be able to localize it. They might use different words to express pain, such as "hurt" or "ouch," although they are less capable of describing the quality or intensity of the pain. In this age group, use a child pain scale that includes color or a faces-based scale like the Wong-Baker FACES Pain Rating Scale (Figure 115-1). Assess a patient older than 8 years (or cognitively >8 years) with the standard visual pain scale that is used for adults (Figure 115-2). Keep in mind that following a trend in pain score is more helpful than an individual pain score in assessing the response to your intervention.

Treatment

There are a number of basic principles in pediatric pain management.

- Pediatric pain practices may not be evidence based, because most medications are used off-label and rely on extrapolation of adult study data.
- Complementary modalities, such as relaxation and breathing exercises, hypnosis, guided imagery, Reiki, biofeedback, massage, acupuncture/acupressure, or distraction (eg, art, pet, play, or music therapy), can greatly reduce the need for pharmacologic management of pain in a child.
- With the assistance of a child life specialist—who is one of the few professionals that is not directly involved with causing emotional stress or physical pain—treat anxiety, sadness, and fear as components of suffering that increase the child's perception of pain.
- Strive to use the most painless (oral, transdermal, topical) route of administration, while avoiding IM and rectal medications.
- For an infant, start at a low dose but titrate up quickly as needed.
- Reassess the patient frequently for continuing pain and the effectiveness of treatment.
- Less medication is required to prevent pain than to eliminate it. Therefore, initially use as much medication as necessary to achieve pain control and then dose as frequently as needed to maintain adequate analgesia.

Table 115-1. FLACC Scale[a]			
Category	**Scoring**		
	0	**1**	**2**
Face	No particular expression or smile	Occasional grimaces or frowns; withdrawn, disinterested	Frequent to constant frown, clenched jaw, quivering chin
Legs	Normal position or relaxed	Uneasy, restless, tense	Kicking or legs drawn up
Activity	Lying quietly Normal position Moves easily	Squirming Shifting back and forth Tense	Arched, rigid, or jerking
Cry	No cry (awake or asleep)	Moans or whimpers, occasional complaint	Crying steadily Screams or sobs Frequent complaints
Consolability	Content Relaxed	Reassured by occasional touching, hugging, or "talking to" Distractible	Difficult to console or comfort

Abbreviation: FLACC, face, legs, activity, cry, consolability.

[a] From Merkel SI, Voepel-Lewis T, Shayevitz JR, Malviya S. The FLACC: a behavioral scale for scoring postoperative pain in young children. *Pediatr Nurs.* 1997;23(3):293–297. Printed with permission of the regent of the University of Michigan.

Figure 115-1. FACES Pain Scale

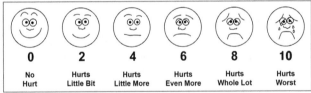

From Wong-Baker FACES Foundation (2016). Wong-Baker FACES® Pain Rating Scale. Retrieved July 31, 2017 with permission from http://www. WongBakerFACES.org. Originally published in Whaley & Wong's Nursing Care of Infants and Children. © Elsevier Inc.

Figure 115-2. Visual Analogue Pain Scale

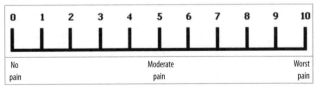

- A patient with advanced cancer or sickle cell pain often requires far higher doses of analgesics and adjuncts to achieve adequate pain control.
- Attempt to achieve control of long-term pain with scheduled or long-acting medications and provide immediate-release medications for incidental or "breakthrough" pain episodes.

Medications

Acetaminophen

Acetaminophen is a mild analgesic and antipyretic that is available in oral, rectal, and intravenous (IV) forms. The onset of action occurs within 30 minutes after oral administration and 10 minutes of IV administration. It is primarily metabolized in the liver and may therefore be contraindicated in hepatic failure. Also, because of a risk of chronic liver toxicity, limit the duration of around-the-clock therapy to 3 days.

Oral or rectal dosage:

- 10 days to ≤12 years of age: 10 to 15 mg/kg per dose every 4 to 6 hours (75 mg/kg/d or 4,000-mg/d maximum)
- 12 years and older: 325 to 650 mg every 4 to 6 hours or 1,000 mg per dose, 2 to 3 times a day (4,000-mg/d maximum)

IV dosage:

- <13 years of age or weight <50 kg: 12.5 mg/kg every 4 hours or 15 mg/kg every 6 hours (750 mg per dose or 75-mg/kg/d maximum, up to 3,750 mg)
- >13 years of age or weight >50 kg: 650 mg every 4 hours or 1,000 mg every 6 hours (4,000-mg/d maximum)

Nonsteroidal Anti-Inflammatory Drugs

Nonsteroidal anti-inflammatory drugs (NSAIDs) have analgesic, anti-inflammatory, and antipyretic effects. Side effects include gastritis, nephropathy, and bleeding from platelet anti-aggregation.

Ibuprofen

The dose of ibuprofen is 10 mg/kg per dose every 6 hours (child) or 400 to 600 mg every 6 hours up to 800 mg every 8 hours (adolescent). The onset of action occurs in 30 to 60 minutes.

Ketorolac

Ketorolac is available in both oral and IV forms. The IV dose is 0.5 mg/kg every 6 hours (maximum, 30 mg per dose) and is particularly useful as a parenteral agent when trying to avoid opioids. The onset of action is 30 minutes. Ketorolac shares the same side-effect profile as the other NSAIDs in terms of bleeding risk and potential effect on renal function, with a higher risk in patients with baseline renal impairment or gastric disease. Do not use ketorolac for more than 5 days because of an increased risk of side effects.

Opioids

Opioids are available in multiple forms, including IV, oral, rectal, and transdermal. They are most effective when administered around the clock (ie, on a schedule) for chronic or persistent pain, with additional (pro re nata [PRN]) doses indicated every 3 to 4 hours for breakthrough pain. Start with a PRN dose that is equal to 10% to 15% of the total daily maintenance dose, but if more than 4 to 6 PRN doses are required, increase the daily maintenance dose by 50%. If there are side effects, such as severe nausea or sleepiness, decrease the maintenance dose by 25%. Tapering is usually necessary if opioids are administered for more than 1 week.

When attempting to rapidly achieve pain control with opioids, it is helpful to do a rapid IV titration by using morphine, hydromorphone, or, occasionally, fentanyl. This process may take several hours and requires close attention to the patient's response to each dose. To treat pain in a patient who is already receiving opioids, increase the dose by 25% to 50% for mild to moderate pain and 50% to 100% for severe pain. Although this approach requires additional physician and nurse presence, the pain relief can be achieved much more effectively with a direct, hands-on approach.

Anticipate and treat opioid side effects, the most serious of which is respiratory depression. Treat with naloxone, 0.1 mg/kg per dose (2-mg maximum). Manage nausea in patients over 1 month of age with IV or oral ondansetron (0.05–0.10 mg/kg every 6 hours PRN; maximum, 4 mg per dose). Treat pruritus with either diphenhydramine (5 mg/kg/d, divided into doses administered every 6 hours; 300-mg/d maximum) or hydroxyzine (2 mg/kg/d, divided into doses administered every 8 hours; <6 years of age, 50-mg/d maximum; >6 years of age, 600-mg/d maximum). Always start a bowel regimen if multiple doses or prolonged use of opioids is anticipated. Reactions to one opioid are not predictive of reactions to another, so if side effects such as pruritus occur, change to another opioid. In general, the more potent the opioid (from weaker to more potent: morphine < oxycodone < hydromorphone < fentanyl), the less histamine release.

Morphine

Morphine can be administered orally (immediate or sustained release), sublingually, subcutaneously, intravenously, and rectally. It is indicated for moderate to severe pain. Use with caution in a patient with renal failure.

The IV morphine dose is 0.05 to 0.30 mg/kg every 3 to 4 hours (maximum, 10 mg per dose). The onset of action is 5 to 10 minutes. The oral dose for immediate-release morphine is 0.15 to 0.30 mg/kg per dose (initial dose of 0.3 mg/kg for severe pain) every 3 to 4 hours. The oral dose is 3 times the IV dose (0.3 mg/kg [oral] vs 0.1 mg/kg [IV]). The onset of action of the oral dose is 30 minutes.

In a child who has not been given opioids previously, begin at the lower dose and titrate up as needed. However, if the patient has chronic pain management requirements, convert to a long-acting, orally administered opioid once the daily requirement has been established (via either IV or oral administration).

One of the most common side effects is pruritus, either at the injection site or diffusely. This is not an allergic reaction and is therefore not a contraindication to continuing the drug. Order diphenhydramine or hydroxyzine (dosing as detailed earlier). However, treat urticaria that develops at a site remote from the injection site as an allergic reaction.

Morphine Patient-Controlled Analgesia

Patient-controlled analgesia (PCA) is administered with a programmable pump that allows the patient to control IV analgesia by choosing when to deliver a dose of opioid for quick relief, in addition to facilitating titration to pain needs. The lockout interval for the bolus dose is related to the onset and peak action of the opioid. The patient must be mature enough to understand how and when to push the demand button for boluses.

PCA is now universally accepted as the safest technique for IV opioid (morphine, fentanyl, or hydromorphone) administration in the treatment of acute postoperative pain. When administered by himself or herself, the patient will not request further boluses if sedated and sleeping and therefore cannot self-overdose. Continuous infusion may reduce the safety of PCA, because it is administered independently of the patient's sedation level. A continuous background opioid infusion in conjunction with PCA does not have any advantages over PCA-only postoperative analgesia. A PCA with continuous infusion is useful when analgesia is required for vaso-occlusive crises in a patient with sickle cell disease, postoperative pain, or cancer pain and when goals of care have transitioned to primarily palliative.

Begin a morphine PCA regimen with a loading dose of 0.05 to 0.10 mg/kg per dose. Then start the PCA at a basal (continuous) rate of typically 0.01 to 0.03 mg/kg/h. Order a demand dose of 0.01 to 0.03 mg/kg per dose with a lockout period of 8 to 10 minutes. Therefore, for a 25-kg patient, the continuous rate is 0.3 to 0.8 mg/h with 0.25-mg PCA demand doses (up to 10 in 1 hour, if the patient is still in pain). Increase the basal rate by 10% if the patient requires more than 3 boluses per hour and decrease it by the same amount if more than 3 boluses per hour are requested. A continuous infusion dose should be around 50% of the estimated daily demand.

Close monitoring by trained pediatric personnel is required for any patient undergoing the initiation of PCA or IV opioid treatment. Consult with a pain specialist or the palliative care service when more complex pain management is needed.

Oxycodone

Oxycodone is available in oral form and is indicated for mild to moderate pain. If the patient will be receiving other acetaminophen-containing preparations, do not use oxycodone preparations that also contain acetaminophen (due to the risk of acetaminophen overdose). The dose is 0.05 to 0.20 mg/kg every 4 to 6 hours (5-mg maximum).

Fentanyl

Fentanyl can be administered intravenously, with a buccal tab or lozenge, intranasally, or by transdermal patch. It is indicated for severe pain, but reserve the transdermal patch for an opioid-tolerant patient and pain of anticipated long duration. Fentanyl administered intravenously, intranasally, and by the buccal route has rapid onset with a relatively brief duration of action, so if a longer period of analgesia is necessary, use a continuous infusion or transdermal preparation. The dose is 0.5 to1.0 µg/kg per dose every 1 to 2 hours as needed and 1.5 µg/kg for intranasal dosing. Side effects of rapid administration in some patients are glottic and chest wall rigidity. Therefore, follow a careful monitoring protocol and have resuscitation equipment available when administering the drug via infusion. Nonallergic facial pruritus can occur as with morphine (see the details given earlier), but histamine release is far less common than with morphine or hydromorphone. Because of its high lipophilicity, fentanyl tends to accumulate in fatty tissues, leading to a prolonged elimination in patients receiving long-term treatment. Discontinuation of fentanyl after as few as 3 days of use has been associated with abstinence syndrome, necessitating close observation and consideration for weaning in patients receiving long-term treatment.

Hydromorphone

Hydromorphone is 5 to 7 times more potent than IV morphine. It is available in oral or IV form. The IV dose is 0.015 mg/kg per dose every 4 to 6 hours as needed (1.2-mg maximum). The oral dose is 0.04 to 0.08 mg/kg per dose every 6 hours as needed. It may also be used via PCA in place of morphine or in a regimen of planned opioid rotation. Consultation with a pain or palliative care service is helpful in planning a rotation of opioids.

Methadone

Methadone is available in oral and IV forms and may be given subcutaneously, as well. The IV and oral dose for children is 0.1 mg/kg per dose every 4 hours for 2 to 3 doses, then every 6 to 12 hours as needed, with a maximum dose of 10 mg. The oral elixir is 60% to 90% bioavailable and is therefore highly effective. It has a long half-life with a slow peak and long steady state, so it is optimal for patients who require chronic analgesia. It accumulates slowly with high partitioning to the fatty tissues, so it can take 5 to 7 days to reach a steady state. Thus, the dose of methadone that produces good analgesia acutely may lead to excess sedation within 3 to 5 days of chronic usage. When pain management is no longer required, do not stop the medication abruptly. Reduce the dose by 10% to 20% every 48 hours to prevent withdrawal.

Opioid Tolerance

Opioid tolerance is the development of the need to increase the dose of the medication to achieve the same sedative or analgesic effect. Cross-tolerance among all opioids occurs, but not on a 1:1 basis. Therefore, in conversion to another opioid, it is best to administer a percentage of the equianalgesic dose (80% for a short-acting medication) and then titrate up. Every child is different, and dosage must be individualized. However, to minimize tolerance, rotate narcotics or—in severe cases—use adjuncts such as a ketamine infusion, which enhances the response to opioids. In such complex pain management situations, consult with a pain specialist or the palliative care service.

Weaning

The goal of weaning is to prevent withdrawal symptoms (abstinence syndrome), which can occur within 24 hours of abrupt cessation of the medication or immediately if the patient is given naloxone. The symptoms peak within 72 hours of cessation and include cramping, vomiting, diarrhea, tachycardia, hypertension, diaphoresis, restlessness, insomnia, movement disorders, and seizures.

Begin the weaning process when the patient is receiving 0.025 mg/kg/h or less of morphine (basal rate plus bolus). The initial step is to convert from continuous IV to around-the-clock bolus treatment. Continue the bolus treatments for 48 hours prior to weaning the dose by no more than 20% per day. Discontinue IV analgesia only when the patient is tolerating an oral regimen. Criteria for transitioning to oral analgesia are normal gastrointestinal function (patient tolerating oral intake and passing gas) and pain typically quantified as 6 or lower on a scale of 10. Begin oral analgesia when the morphine equivalent is 10 to 20 µg/kg/h.

When transitioning from PCA to oral medication, administer a dose of the oral analgesic first, then discontinue the basal infusion 30 to 60 minutes later. Concurrently, reduce the IV bolus dose by 25% to 50%. Then discontinue the PCA if the patient has not required a bolus dose in more than 6 hours. If the patient requires 1 to 3 bolus doses over a 6-hour period and is in persistent pain after evaluation, increase the oral analgesic dose by 25% to 50%. Increase by 50% to 100% if 3 to 6 boluses are required over a 6-hour period or add an oral adjuvant, such as acetaminophen. However, always assess whether there are other, psychologically based motivations why the patient continues to push the button.

In some institutions, the preference may be to convert the patient to oral methadone to permit continued weaning after discharge. It generally takes several days to achieve complete conversion after the parenteral opioids have been weaned to an acceptably low level, as described earlier. The availability of methadone for outpatient use may limit this approach in some communities.

Naloxone

Naloxone, an opioid antagonist, is indicated when a patient receiving narcotics is unresponsive to physical stimulation and has shallow respirations (<8 breaths/min and at risk for intubation) and pinpoint pupils. If the patient is hypoxemic or hypoventilating or if there is hemodynamic compromise, discontinue the opioid and provide face-mask oxygen. For life-threatening opiate overdose, the initial dose of naloxone is 0.1 mg/kg (maximum, 2 mg per dose), which can be repeated every 2 to 3 minutes until a response is seen. If no response is seen after a total of 10 mg, consider other causes of respiratory depression. Administering higher doses may precipitate acute abstinence syndrome in patients receiving longstanding opioids, with adverse physical and psychological consequences. Cardiac decompensation may also occur when fully reversing opiates acutely. Administer the naloxone slowly, and monitor the patient closely for a response. The onset of IV action is about 2 minutes. Discontinue the naloxone as soon as the patient responds, but continue to monitor the patient because the effective duration of action of naloxone is about 30 minutes, which is frequently shorter than the opiate, necessitating additional doses of naloxone. The patient will then require nonopioid pain relief. However, once the patient is easily arousable with a respiratory rate greater than 9 breaths/min, restart the opioid at half of the previous dose.

A continuous, low-dose naloxone infusion may be useful in patients receiving PCA morphine or epidural analgesia. It reduces systemic side effects and may reduce the speed of tolerance development. The pain service or anesthesiology must be consulted prior to initiating.

Special Considerations in Opioid Dosing

For infants, morphine clearance is delayed in the first 1 to 2 months of life. Prescribe a starting dose that is one-third to one-half that used for an older child. In addition, an infant is more sensitive to the respiratory depressant effects of opioids, so close monitoring is needed. Additionally, children with central nervous system (CNS) disease (ie, perinatal asphyxia, metabolic disease affecting the CNS) may be more sensitive to the depressant effects of opioids and may require lower doses.

For children 2 to 6 years of age, since there is an increased liver mass compared with adults, use more frequent dosing, although concomitant acetaminophen (oral or IV) or NSAIDs reduces opiate need. Do not administer codeine because of its variable metabolism, which leads to unpredictable effectiveness.

Epidural and Regional Anesthesia

Regional anesthesia is becoming routine in many pediatric institutions. In particular, epidural anesthesia with opiates and bupivacaine can provide both postoperative pain management and pain control for complex pain conditions. Regional blocks for both limb pain and intercostal blocks for pain associated with rib fractures, chest tubes, and chest wall pain are easily performed at the bedside with ultrasonographic guidance by pediatric pain specialists. Such approaches reduce the need for systemic medications and avoid many of the adverse effects of systemic agents, including more rapid weaning of analgesia when no longer required. Consultation with the pediatric pain service or anesthesiology is necessary for these modalities. Avoid systemic opioids as adjuncts to epidural anesthesia.

Specific Analgesia Recommendations

Postoperative Pain

Initially manage postoperative pain with around-the-clock analgesics, then taper the medication, as tolerated, to PRN dosing. If the patient underwent abdominal surgery or cannot tolerate oral medications, IV morphine administered every 3 to 4 hours or via PCA is useful, with appropriate monitoring.

Sickle Cell Pain

Manage vaso-occlusive crisis pain aggressively and ask the patient/parents what has worked well in the past. Depending on the patient's age and the severity of the pain and disease, it may be best to start with morphine PCA. If the patient is too young to use a PCA, order around-the-clock IV morphine. For a patient of any age, ketorolac may also be necessary (after confirmation of normal serum creatinine level) (see Chapter 50, Sickle Cell Disease). Be aware of the potential need to use higher doses of opioids than required in other pain syndromes.

Orthopedic Pain

The proper management of orthopedic pain permits earlier mobilization, which can lead to decreased morbidity and shortened hospital stay. Around-the-clock opioids, such as IV morphine, provide optimal analgesia, which can then be tapered accordingly. Ensure that adequate analgesia is given prior to mobilization or physical therapy.

Pearls and Pitfalls

- When managing pediatric pain, do it "by the child, by the mouth, and by the clock." That is, individualize an analgesia regimen for a specific patient that is administered around the clock (every 3–6 hours) and is ideally delivered orally (painless administration).
- Do not undertreat pain because of fear of adverse effects. Consult with a pain specialist when the pain severity requires you to practice outside your comfort zone.
- Do not overlook the benefit of nonpharmacologic techniques to aid in relief of both pain and anxiety (ie, using child life specialists, creating an "ouchless" environment).
- When choosing a pain assessment tool, keep in mind the child's physical, social, and emotional development. Remember that a trend in pain score is more helpful than an individual score. The trend in score will aid in assessing the response to your intervention.

Bibliography

Ali S, Drendel AL, Kircher J, Beno S. Pain management of musculoskeletal injuries in children: current state and future directions. *Pediatr Emerg Care.* 2010;26(7):518–524

American Academy of Pediatrics Committee on Fetus and Newborn and Section on Anesthesiology and Pain Medicine. Prevention and management of procedural pain in the neonate: an update. *Pediatrics.* 2016;137(2):1–13

Anand KJ, Willson DF, Berger J, et al. Tolerance and withdrawal from prolonged opioid use in critically ill children. *Pediatrics.* 2010;125(5):e1208–e1225

Chou R, Gordon DB, de Leon-Casasola OA, et al. Management of postoperative pain: a clinical practice guideline from the American Pain Society, the American Society of Regional Anesthesia and Pain Medicine, and the American Society of Anesthesiologists' Committee on Regional Anesthesia, Executive Committee, and Administrative Council. *J Pain.* 2016;17(2):131–157

Fein JA, Zempsky WT, Cravero JP, et al. Clinical report: relief of pain and anxiety in pediatric patients in emergency medical systems. *Pediatrics.* 2012;130(5):e1391–e1405

George JA, Lin EE, Hanna MN, et al. The effect of intravenous opioid patient-controlled analgesia with and without background infusion on respiratory depression: a meta-analysis. *J Opioid Manag.* 2010;6(1):47–54

Klick JC, Hauer J. Pediatric palliative care. *Curr Probl Pediatr Adolesc Health Care.* 2010;40(6):120–151

Sedation

Introduction

The goal of pediatric sedation is to allow diagnostic and therapeutic procedures to be performed as safely, comfortably, and efficiently as possible. Consider each situation on an individual basis to determine the appropriate level of sedation needed and to address the individual patient's needs regarding control of pain, anxiety, memory, and motion during the procedure.

Definitions

The level of drug-induced sedation is divided into 4 different states.

Minimal Sedation/Anxiolysis

The patient can respond normally to verbal commands. Although cognitive function and coordination may be impaired, ventilatory and cardiovascular functions are maintained.

Moderate Sedation

The patient can respond purposefully to verbal commands, either alone or accompanied by light to moderate tactile stimulation. No interventions are required to maintain a patent airway; adequate spontaneous ventilation and cardiovascular functions are usually maintained.

Deep Sedation

The patient cannot be easily aroused but responds purposefully to repeated verbal or painful stimulation. Ventilatory function and protective airway reflexes may be impaired, and the patient may require assistance in maintaining a patent airway and/or require positive-pressure ventilation. Cardiovascular function is usually maintained.

General Anesthesia

The patient cannot be aroused, even by painful stimulation. Ventilatory function is often impaired, and the patient will often require assistance in maintaining a patent airway. Positive-pressure ventilation may be needed because of depressed spontaneous ventilation or neuromuscular function. Cardiovascular function may also be impaired.

Principles

The guiding principles for safe and effective sedation are

1. Maximize patient comfort and minimize pain and distress.
2. Use nonpharmacologic interventions as an adjunct. Whenever possible, supplement sedation with other pain-reducing modalities, such as topical analgesia and nerve blocks, as well as nonpharmacologic techniques, such as involving a child life specialist.
3. Prepare the child and family.
4. Ensure health provider competency in performing procedures and sedation.
5. Use appropriate monitoring to ensure safety.

Training

Each institution must develop a specific training and certification program, ideally in conjunction with the institution's department of anesthesiology. This will help ensure the competence of medical providers in performing safe sedation techniques and will also clearly delineate hospitalist roles and limitations. Specific guidelines must include the medications that may be used, American Society of Anesthesiologists (ASA) physical status classes that may be sedated (see Table 116-1), and the timing and location of hospitalist-run sedations. The training program must also ensure that the hospitalist is comfortable with and prepared to manage contraindications, common side effects and complications, and basic rescue mechanisms, including airway management.

Table 116-1. American Society of Anesthesiologists Physical Status Classification		
Class	**Disease State**	**Examples**
I	No organic, physiological, biochemical, or psychiatric disturbance	
II	Mild to moderate systemic disturbance	Mild asthma Controlled diabetes or seizures
III	Severe systemic disturbance	Moderate-severe asthma Poorly controlled diabetes or seizures
IV	Severe systemic disturbance that is life threatening	Sepsis Bronchopulmonary dysplasia Advanced cardiac, endocrine, hepatic, pulmonary, or renal disease
V	Moribund patient with little chance of survival	Septic shock Severe trauma

Each patient's responses to different medications can vary, so be prepared to manage deeper levels of sedation than what was planned. For example, if moderate sedation is intended, be qualified and prepared to manage a patient who is deeply sedated. Become familiar with a small number of anesthetic agents to be able to simplify sedation plans and maximize safety and efficiency. For example, ketamine is useful for painful procedures, while dexmedetomidine or pentobarbital are reasonable options for imaging procedures that require a motionless state.

Institutional needs and resources will dictate what levels of training are available for hospitalists, and a tiered system may be appropriate in some cases. For example, a first tier of hospitalists may be approved to sedate ASA class I–II patients in the emergency unit where multiple resources are available, while a second tier may be approved to sedate ASA class I–III patients in specified specialty units during daytime hours when anesthesia is available for backup, and a third tier may be approved to use a wider variety of agents or sedate patients after hours.

Presedation Evaluation

Perform a screening evaluation prior to the induction of sedation. Include a focused history, guided by the mnemonic "SAMPLE" (Box 116-1). At physical examination, pay particular attention to airway, respiratory, and cardiovascular status. Screen the patient for a personal or family history of complications from sedation or anesthesia; a history of snoring, wheezing, or stridor; recent illnesses; obesity; and anatomic abnormalities (small jaw, short neck, large tongue) that may make airway obstruction more likely and rescue procedures more difficult. Evaluate the patient's ASA physical status (Table 116-1) and arrange an anesthesia consultation prior to sedation if the ASA class is III, IV, or V.

Box 116-1. SAMPLE Mnemonic for Patient History	
S:	Signs and symptoms
A:	Allergies to medications, food, or latex
M:	Medications used regularly or recently
P:	Past medical and surgical history, including history of sedations
L:	Last liquid and solid intake
E:	Events leading to current illness, injury, or need for procedure

As with any procedure, observe and document a time-out before sedation is initiated. Encourage the presence of the family, provided they can tolerate the procedure and understand that they cannot interfere with the medical care.

Presedation Fasting

It is generally believed that fasting decreases the likelihood of aspiration. Therefore, follow the ASA recommendations for nil per os (nothing by mouth) times (Table 116-2) for all elective procedural sedations. For emergent sedations, carefully balance the risks of sedation with the benefits of completing the procedure quickly. In an emergent case, when the fasting interval is insufficient, use the lightest effective sedation.

Presedation Preparation

To optimize patient safety, ensure the presence of a medical provider with advanced resuscitation skills at all times during sedation. This person may also perform the procedure during moderate sedations, provided there is an assistant present who can closely monitor the patient and record vital signs data. Ideally, this assistant will have skills for the recognition and rescue of airway obstruction. During deep sedations, the sedation provider may offer brief, interruptible assistance to a separate proceduralist if it does not interfere with the ability to closely monitor the patient at all times.

Before beginning sedation, confirm that all potentially needed rescue equipment (see the article of Coté et al in the Bibliography) and medications are easily accessible. Keep a crash cart nearby, with precalculated doses of common rescue medications, as well as airway rescue equipment, such as laryngoscopes with appropriately sized blades, endotracheal tubes, stylettes, and laryngeal mask airways. Have an anesthesia or continuous positive airway pressure bag readily available and connected to an oxygen source with an appropriately sized face mask attached. Connect a large-bore suction catheter to wall suction in case of emesis. The "SOAPME" mnemonic is useful for patient care during sedation: Suction, Oxygen, Airway, Poisitioning, Monitoring, End-tidal carbon dioxide.

Table 116-2. Nil Per Os Guidelines for Elective Sedations	
Food or Liquid	**No. of Nil Per Os Hours**
Medications with a sip of water	Any time
Clear liquids[a]	2 h
Breast milk	4 h
Infant formula	6 h
All other food and liquid	6 h

[a] Clear liquids include water, clear soda, clear tea, and clear fruit juice with no pulp.

Sedation and Recovery Monitoring

During minimal and moderate sedations and recovery, continuously monitor the patient's heart rate, ventilation (auscultation), and pulse oximetry data. Also monitor end-tidal carbon dioxide ($EtCO_2$) level when the sedation practitioner is at a distance and cannot directly observe the patient (eg, during magnetic resonance imaging). Reassess blood pressure and respiratory rate every 5 minutes once a stable level of sedation has been achieved. Obtain intravenous (IV) access for moderate or deeper sedation.

For deep sedation and recovery, monitor the patient as detailed earlier, always with IV access. Monitor $EtCO_2$ level during the sedation and recovery period if feasible, since ventilatory function is often compromised before oxygenation. Perform deep sedation only in an area that is both familiar to the sedation provider and properly supplied with all necessary equipment. Do not perform deep sedation in a routine inpatient bed.

In addition to the above-mentioned monitoring, directly observe the patient during sedation, paying particular attention to the level of consciousness, color, airway patency, ventilatory effort and adequacy, and perfusion. Continue to monitor the patient after sedation and ensure that the institutional recovery criteria are met before the patient is discharged or returned to the inpatient floor. Follow the specific hospital's protocols for appropriate documentation of patient monitoring data during both sedation and recovery, specifically noting in the medical record all vital signs and patient information mentioned earlier.

Discharge Criteria

The patient may be discharged from monitoring 30 minutes after the final medication administration, if all of the following discharge criteria are met:

- Patent airway without respiratory depression
- Return to baseline vital signs, motor function, and level of consciousness
- Adequate hydration and no spontaneous vomiting, although nausea may be expected
- Adequate pain control

Billing and Coding

Billing anesthesia codes vary across the United States, sometimes on a state-by-state or local basis. This becomes an important factor in determining the level of funding available for pediatric hospital sedation programs. The Centers for Medicare & Medicaid Services requires that sedation services be overseen by a hospital's anesthesiology division or department, which necessitates a close working relationship between the anesthesia group and others who provide moderate and deep sedation. Anesthesia codes can be used appropriately by nonanesthesiologists when the level of care provided meets the standard of those codes, with reimbursement being most successful when both teams within an institution agree on the appropriate use of these codes. In contrast, it can be difficult to obtain reimbursement when there is disagreement about these codes among various hospital departments.

Bibliography

American Academy of Pediatrics; American Academy of Pediatric Dentistry, Coté CJ, Wilson S; Work Group on Sedation. Guidelines for monitoring and management of pediatric patients during and after sedation for diagnostic and therapeutic procedures: an update. *Pediatrics.* 2006;118(6):2587–2602

American Society of Anesthesiologists Committee. Practice guidelines for preoperative fasting and the use of pharmacologic agents to reduce the risk of pulmonary aspiration: application to healthy patients undergoing elective procedures: an updated report by the American Society of Anesthesiologists Committee on Standards and Practice Parameters. *Anesthesiology.* 2011;114(3):495–511

Coté C, Wilson S, American Academy of Pediatrics, American Academy of Pediatric Dentistry. Guidelines for monitoring and management of pediatric patients before, during, and after sedation for diagnostic and therapeutic procedures: update 2016. *Pediatrics.* 2016;138(1):e1–e31

Doctor K, Roback MG, Teach SJ. An update on pediatric hospital-based sedation. *Curr Opin Pediatr.* 2013;25(3):310–316

Pacheco GS, Ferayorni A. Pediatric procedural sedation and analgesia. *Emerg Med Clin North Am.* 2013;31(3):831–852

Srinivasan M, Bhaskar S, Carlson DW. Variation in procedural sedation practices among children's hospitals. *Hosp Pediatr.* 2015;5(3):148–153

Thomas A, Miller JL, Couloures K, Johnson PN. Non-intravenous sedatives and analgesics for procedural sedation for imaging procedures in pediatric patients. *J Pediatr Pharmacol Ther.* 2015;20(6):418–430

Surgery

Abdominal Masses

Introduction

Abdominal masses may be caused by a range of conditions, from benign (eg, constipation) to life threatening (eg, neuroblastoma), and many are found incidentally by a parent or health care provider. Masses can be associated with solid organs, the mesentery, or the bowel. A mass may also represent organomegaly, which may suggest an infiltrative disorder. The initial hospitalization is usually focused on the diagnostic evaluation, with imaging (often ultrasonography [US]) findings as the mainstay of diagnosis.

Clinical Presentation

History

Presenting symptoms will vary, based on the size and location of the mass. These may include abdominal pain (localized or diffuse), abdominal distention, early satiety, anorexia, vomiting, constipation, fever or night sweats, hematuria, and weight loss or failure to thrive. Significant distention can limit diaphragmatic excursion, resulting in respiratory distress. Ask about any systemic symptoms, such as fever and lethargy. Some masses are secondary to genetic conditions, so the family history may be important.

Physical Examination

Superficial venous distention suggests impingement on deep venous drainage by a large mass. Similarly, a large mass may cause lower-extremity edema and scrotal or labial swelling. Hypertension is a common finding when a primary kidney tumor (most commonly Wilms tumor) or a suprarenal mass (most commonly neuroblastoma) results in compression of the kidney(s) and/or renal vasculature. A mass involving the liver may appear with jaundice and edema or signs of a coagulopathy at presentation, if synthetic function is affected. The presence of cutaneous hemangiomas in an infant may be associated with an occult infantile hepatic hemangioma. When these infantile hepatic hemangiomas are large and symptomatic, they may cause high-output heart failure.

Laboratory Workup

If a malignancy is suspected, obtain a complete blood cell count with differential, as well as lactate dehydrogenase, uric acid, and electrolyte levels. Then choose laboratory tests based on the location of the mass and the patient's associated symptoms (Table 117-1). Always perform a urine pregnancy test early in the workup of a postmenarchal female subject (and prior to imaging).

Radiology Examinations

Imaging is essential to the diagnosis of an abdominal mass. Often, abdominal radiographic findings will have confirmed the presence of a mass, or mass effect, prior to hospital admission. However, the key test is abdominal US, which is highly effective in the differentiation of cystic from solid masses when narrowing the differential diagnosis. Generally, US is useful for imaging the liver, biliary tract, kidneys, pylorus, and female reproductive organs. However, image quality is dependent on the skill of the sonographer and may be limited by obesity or excessive bowel gas. Computed tomography (CT), magnetic resonance imaging, or nuclear medicine can subsequently be performed to further characterize the mass and extent of disease. CT of the chest, abdomen, and pelvis is indicated in the evaluation of malignancy to clearly define margins and assess the patient for distal metastases. If possible, discuss the clinical concerns and examination findings with a radiologist to determine the most appropriate imaging study. A summary of imaging modalities is included in Table 117-2.

Differential Diagnosis

The differential diagnosis is, to some extent, age dependent. For example, a liver mass in an infant is most likely infantile hemangioendothelioma; in a young child, it is likely a mesenchymal hamartoma or hepatoblastoma; and in an adolescent (especially a teenage female subject using oral contraceptives), it is likely a hepatic adenoma. The most common masses palpated in children involve the kidney, with hydronephrosis or multicystic dysplastic kidney being

Table 117-1. Initial Laboratory Tests in the Evaluation of an Abdominal Mass

Type or Source of Mass	Initial Laboratory Tests
Liver	Liver function tests, including albumin level PT/PTT AFP level
Kidney/adrenal	BUN and creatinine levels Urinalysis, urine HVA/VMA levels
Ovary	AFP level Quantitative β-HCG level
Pancreas	Amylase and lipase levels

Abbreviations: AFP, α-fetoprotein; BUN, blood urea nitrogen; HCG, human chorionic gonadotropin; HVA, homovanillic acid; PT, prothrombin time; PTT, partial thromboplastin time; VMA, vanillylmandelic acid.

Table 117-2. Choice of Imaging Modality for Evaluation of Abdominal Masses

Imaging Modality	Indications	Limitations
Abdominal radiography	May confirm presence of mass May help rule out acute obstruction or perforation	Limited ability to demonstrate exact anatomic location and structure of mass

Ultrasonography	Initial evaluation of most abdominal masses
	Particularly useful for:
	  Renal and adrenal masses
	  Vascular malformations
		Dependent on skill of sonographer
		Imaging may be limited by obesity or bowel gas

Computed tomography (with contrast material)	Suspect malignancy (also obtain pelvic and chest images) Suspect teratoma Suspect focal hepatic lesion Suspect infection/abscess	Radiation exposure (decreased with newer technology)
Magnetic resonance imaging (with and without contrast material)	Evaluate hepatobiliary masses Suspect Kasabach-Merritt syndrome	Potential need for sedation or anesthesia

frequent diagnoses. Hydronephrosis has many potential underlying etiologies, but consider ureteropelvic obstruction, ureterovesicular obstruction, vesicoureteral reflux, and renal duplication. Wilms tumor is the most common renal malignancy in children and occurs mostly between 2 and 8 years of age. Other relatively common solid tumors in young children include neuroblastoma and rhabdomyosarcoma, both of which may appear with an abdominal mass at presentation. Hepatosplenomegaly may be caused by a diffuse infiltrative process, which may be oncologic (ie, leukemia), metabolic (ie, glycogen storage disease), or infectious (ie, viral or fungal disease). Table 117-3 includes common diagnoses to consider in children who present with an abdominal mass.

Treatment

Treatment is highly dependent on the etiology of the mass. Consult hematology/oncology if a malignancy is suspected. Consult surgery if a biopsy is needed for diagnosis or if total resection is the treatment of choice. If the mass is associated with a solid organ, refer the patient to the relevant specialist (ie, a pediatric gastroenterologist or nephrologist). Begin venous thromboembolism prophylaxis if the patient has signs of venous obstruction and/or other risk factors for thrombosis (see Chapter 5, Deep Venous Thrombosis). Treat an abscess with intravenous (IV) meropenem (20–40 mg/kg every 8 hours, 6-g/d maximum) or IV piperacillin/tazobactam (100 mg/kg every 6 hours, 12-g/d maximum).

Organ System	Most Likely Diagnoses		
	Infant	Child	Adolescent
Adrenal	Adrenal hemorrhage Congenital neuroblastoma	Neuroblastoma	
Bowel	Duplication cyst Intussusception Pyloric stenosis Volvulus	Appendicitis Constipation Intussusception	Appendicitis Constipation
Genitourinary	Germ cell tumor Teratoma	Germ cell tumor Rhabdomyosarcoma Teratoma	Germ cell tumor Ovarian cyst Pregnancy Rhabdomyosarcoma
Hepatobiliary	Choledochal cyst Hamartoma Hemangioma Hepatoblastoma	Hamartoma Hepatoblastoma Hepatomegaly Sarcoma	Focal nodular hyperplasia Hepatocellular adenoma Hepatocellular carcinoma
Kidney	Congenital mesoblastic nephroma Hydronephrosis Multicystic dysplastic kidney Polycystic kidney disease	Multilocular cystic nephroma Renal abscess Pyelonephritis Renal vein thrombosis Wilms tumor	Renal abscess Renal vein thrombosis Pyelonephritis
Mesentery	Meconium pseudocyst	Mesenteric cyst	Non-Hodgkin lymphoma
Pancreas	Congenital pancreatic cyst	Pancreatoblastoma Pancreatic pseudocyst	Pancreatic pseudocyst
Spleen	Congenital splenic cyst	Posttraumatic cyst Splenic abscess Splenomegaly	Posttraumatic cyst Splenic abscess Splenomegaly

Table 117-3. Differential Diagnosis of an Abdominal Mass

Disposition
- **Intensive care unit transfer:** Shock, toxic appearance, respiratory compromise secondary to distention
- **Discharge criteria:** Definitive diagnosis with treatment underway or planned, presenting symptoms managed effectively, adequate oral intake

Follow-Up
- **Primary care:** 1 to 3 days
- **Surgery (if patient underwent a procedure or one is to be scheduled):** 1 to 2 weeks
- **Subspecialist:** Per subspecialist recommendations

Pearls and Pitfalls

- *Do not administer corticosteroids* if there is any possibility that the patient has a malignancy.
- To avoid radiation exposure and the need for sedation, perform plain radiography and/or abdominal US as the initial imaging examination, especially in a patient younger than 4 years old.
- Masses complicating abdominal trauma, such as pancreatic or splenic pseudocysts, can appear weeks after the trauma.

Bibliography

Clayton KM. Pediatric abdominal imaging. *Pediatr Rev*. 2010;31(12):506–510

Crane GL, Hernanz-Schulman M. Current imaging assessment of congenital abdominal masses in pediatric patients. *Semin Roentgenol*. 2012;47(1):32–44

Ladino-Torres MF, Strouse PJ. Gastrointestinal tumors in children. *Radiol Clin North Am*. 2011;499(4):665–677

Malkan AD, Loh A, Bahrami A, et al. An approach to renal masses in pediatrics. *Pediatrics*. 2015;135(1):142–158

Pai DR, Ladino-Torres MF. Magnetic resonance imaging of pediatric pelvic masses. *Magn Reson Imaging Clin N Am*. 2013;21(4):751–772

Acute Abdomen

Introduction

Acute abdomen, also known as "surgical abdomen," appears with the acute onset of abdominal pain, peritoneal signs, and evidence of obstruction at presentation. Since a true "acute abdomen" is a surgical emergency, it is imperative to identify this diagnosis early. However, this can be a difficult task, given the wide range of etiologies and the variation in presentations, especially among young children.

Appendicitis is the most common surgical cause of pediatric acute abdomen, but the differential diagnosis includes nonsurgical entities, such as constipation. Age is a major determinant of the diagnoses to consider (Box 118-1). For example, the most common causes of acute abdomen in infants include intussusception and incarcerated inguinal hernia.

Clinical Presentation

History

The symptoms associated with acute abdomen typically evolve over hours. The description of the pain, along with the associated signs and symptoms, help to differentiate among potential surgical and medical causes. For example, recent

Box 118-1. Common Etiologies of Abdominal Pain[a]			
Infant	Toddler/Child	Adolescent	
AGE	AGE	AGE	Appendicitis
Constipation	Appendicitis	Constipation	Dysmenorrhea
Hirschsprung disease	Constipation	Ectopic pregnancy	IBD/IBS
Intussusception	HSP	Mittelschmerz	Ovarian torsion
Incarcerated hernia	Strep throat	Pancreatitis	PID
Nonaccidental trauma	Pneumonia	Pneumonia	Strep throat
UTI	Trauma[b]	UTI	Trauma[b]
Volvulus	UTI		

Abbreviations: AGE, acute gastroenteritis; HSP, Henoch-Schönlein purpura; IBD, irritable bowel disease; IBS, irritable bowel syndrome; PID, pelvic inflammatory disease; UTI, urinary tract infection.
[a] This Table is a guide to the most common causes and is not a comprehensive list.
[b] Includes nonaccidental trauma.

contact with sick persons who had a similar illness would make infectious conditions, such as acute gastroenteritis (AGE), more likely.

It is important to develop the pain history. Pain location can suggest a potential cause, such as appendicitis (initially periumbilical then migrating to the right lower quadrant) or biliary disease (right upper quadrant). However, being able to localize pain is a developmental milestone, so younger children may not be capable of doing it. The pain time course can also be helpful. For example, appendicitis pain tends to be constant and made worse with movement. Alternatively, the pain of intussusception, nephrolithiasis, and intermittent volvulus is episodic or colicky. In general, younger patients are more likely to have an atypical presentation of surgical diagnoses.

Physical Examination

Abdominal pain can be focal or generalized, and it is typically made worse with movement. The patient may refuse to walk or walk hunched over, splinting from the pain. Bowel sounds may be present or diminished. Typically, there are peritoneal signs, such as rebound tenderness. Later, as with appendiceal rupture, there can be signs of generalized peritonitis, including abdominal distention and rigidity. Bloody stool is a late finding of ischemia and necrosis that can occur in conditions such as intussusception and volvulus, although this is also seen in nonsurgical conditions such as AGE.

Depending on the child's age and level of cooperation with the examination, it may be necessary to try several different approaches to evaluate peritoneal signs, such as bumping into the bed, asking the child to jump, and distracting the child with a stethoscope. The absence of rebound tenderness suggests that appendicitis is much less likely.

A patient with appendicitis tends to find a position of comfort and lie still. In contrast, episodes of intense pain and movements aimed at finding a comfortable position suggest other etiologies, such as nephrolithiasis or ischemia (ovarian torsion, intussusception, volvulus, incarcerated hernia). A patient with retrocecal appendicitis may not have rebound tenderness, because the overlying distended cecum protects the appendix and results in less pain. To determine if there is retroperitoneal inflammation, look for the psoas and obturator signs. The psoas sign is elicited via passive hip hyperextension. The obturator sign involves passive internal rotation of the hip while the hip is flexed.

As the utility and reliability of radiologic studies continue to evolve, there is less reliance on the digital rectal examination (DRE). For example, DRE pain is not a reliable sign of appendicitis, and DRE is no longer recommended in the evaluation of constipation. However, DRE can provide insight into alternative diagnoses, such as helping to determine when diarrhea is more likely caused by encopresis rather than gastroenteritis.

Laboratory Workup

There is no universal standard for the laboratory evaluation of possible acute surgical abdomen. The diagnosis remains a clinical one, although younger children often have an atypical presentation, which makes this difficult. Some laboratory testing is usually required to eliminate important diagnoses, such as pregnancy or a urinary tract infection (UTI).

In general, if surgical abdomen is possible, obtain blood for a complete blood cell count (CBC); evaluation of C-reactive protein (CRP) level and/or erythrocyte sedimentation rate, electrolyte levels, and lipase level; and liver function tests. Obtain urine for urinalysis. A pregnancy test is a priority for any female subject who is postmenarchal or over 11 years of age.

The absence of leukocytosis and a left shift do not conclusively rule out appendicitis but make it much less likely, especially when coupled with a low index of suspicion based on history and physical examination findings. However, initial laboratory findings can sometimes be misleading. For example, an inflamed appendix or abscess in contact with the bladder can cause pyuria and/or hematuria.

Radiology Examinations

Appropriate radiologic studies depend on local preference and overall clinical suspicion. Ultrasonography (US) is emerging as a screening tool for appendicitis, although its accuracy is dependent on the skill of the operator and it is notably less sensitive among children who are overweight. US is the preferred imaging modality for gynecologic diagnoses, especially for possible ovarian torsion.

Classic appendicitis is a clinical diagnosis that can be assigned solely on the basis of physical examination findings, without the use of imaging. If the physical examination findings and laboratory evaluation results are not diagnostic, perform US if local expertise is present. However, when the clinical picture is unclear and US is not available, computed tomography (CT) may be indicated. Local preference dictates the choice of contrast material (intravenous [IV], oral, and/or rectal). The only finding that rules out appendicitis is visualization of a normal appendix. When there is enough clinical suspicion to perform an imaging study, the lack of seeing a normal appendix is an indication for surgical intervention.

It is difficult to quantify the radiation exposure from abdominal CT because of the many variables involved, including patient size and scanner technology.

However, because of increasing concern over radiation exposure and risks from CT, magnetic resonance (MR) imaging with contrast material is becoming more popular. The primary limitations to MR imaging use are acceptance by local radiology and surgical specialists, availability, and potential need for sedation.

With the exception of chest radiography when there are notable respiratory symptoms, plain films are not very helpful. Although abdominal radiography is often performed to look for obstruction, free air, or other gross abnormalities, up to half of abdominal radiographic findings can be normal in appendicitis, while less than 10% have a diagnostic appendicolith. Obtaining prone and supine radiographs to look for air distribution throughout the large colon can be helpful when considering intussusception, because a lack of air suggests the diagnosis. See Table 118-1 for radiologic testing suggestions based on clinical suspicion.

Differential Diagnosis

Nonsurgical conditions, such as AGE, severe constipation, strep throat, and lower-lobe pneumonia, can all cause severe abdominal pain and mimic acute abdomen.

The likelihood of appendicitis increases with each additional component of the classic picture: initially periumbilical pain that migrates to the right lower quadrant, increased white blood cell (WBC) count, increased neutrophil percentage (left shift), and increased CRP level. However, a normal WBC count and CRP level do not rule out appendicitis. These classic criteria are represented in appendicitis scores, such as the Alvarado score, which can help

Table 118-1. Radiologic Tests Based on Clinical Suspicion	
Suspected Diagnosis	**Radiologic Study**
Appendicitis	US (preferred) or CT with IV, oral, and/or rectal contrast material MR imaging if available and sedation not required
Constipation	Left lateral decubitus and supine radiography or KUB radiography
Ileus	Left lateral decubitus and supine radiography or KUB radiography
Intussusception	US (diagnostic only) Air (or contrast-enhanced) enema (diagnostic and therapeutic)
Malrotation Volvulus	Emergent UGI study or CT with IV contrast material
Ovarian torsion	US with Doppler
Pneumonia	PA and lateral chest radiography
Renal stone	CT without contrast material

Abbreviations: CT, computed tomography; IV, intravenous; KUB, kidney, ureter, bladder; MR, magnetic resonance; PA, posteroanterior; UGI, upper gastrointestinal; US, ultrasonography.

identify patients with appendicitis. However, these scoring rubrics are confounded by atypical presentations, which are especially common in younger patients. Furthermore, many other serious entities, such as volvulus and intussusception, can have normal laboratory evaluation findings. The differential diagnosis of acute abdomen is summarized in Table 118-2.

There are associations of symptoms and history that are consistent with certain diagnostic considerations. Bilious emesis suggests intestinal obstruction, ileus, or volvulus. These are emergencies that require prompt surgical consultation. Bloody stool is most commonly associated with bacterial gastroenteritis but can be a late finding of intussusception or other bowel ischemia. Consider ovarian torsion, ovulatory pain (mittelschmerz), imperforate hymen, pelvic inflammatory disease, and pregnancy in a postmenarchal female subject. Prior abdominal surgery can increase the risk of adhesions and bowel obstruction. Food intake typically decreases the pain in ulcer disease and gastritis but worsens the discomfort in pancreatitis and biliary disease. At presentation, Henoch-Schönlein purpura can appear with severe abdominal pain that precedes the typical purpuric rash and can sometimes be associated with intussusception and/or gastrointestinal (GI) bleeding. Meckel diverticulum is commonly described as appearing with painless GI bleeding, but 30% of patients can have obstruction or perforation that results in pain, vomiting, and distention.

Functional abdominal pain often involves underlying dysmotility issues, such as gastroparesis, in the context of an amplified pain response, often along with anxiety and other psychological factors. Typically, the patient has recurrent bouts of periumbilical abdominal pain without fever, vomiting, or diarrhea. However, this is a diagnosis of exclusion that requires an extensive evaluation of other possible causes.

Treatment

When the symptoms are consistent with acute abdomen, give the patient nil per os (NPO, nothing by mouth), request surgical consultation, and start antibiotics with piperacillin/tazobactam (350 mg/kg/d, divided into doses administered every 6 hours; 12-g/d maximum) *or* IV meropenem (20 mg/kg every 8 hours, 6-g/d maximum) *or* cefoxitin (30 mg/kg every 6 hours, 12-g/d maximum) *or* cefotetan (30 mg/kg every 12 hours, 6-g/d maximum).

If the patient is nontoxic with a presentation inconsistent with acute abdomen, conduct serial abdominal examinations and repeat the laboratory studies (CBC count, CRP level) as dictated by the degree of clinical suspicion. It is often prudent to give the patient NPO and defer starting antibiotics until the diagnosis is more certain. For example, a patient with isolated nonbilious

Table 118-2. Differential Diagnosis of Acute Abdomen

Diagnosis	Clinical Features
Abdominal migraine	Moderate–severe abdominal pain Nausea, vomiting, anorexia Recurs every 3–4 wk, episodes last 18 h on average
Acute gastroenteritis	Fever, nausea, vomiting, diarrhea Pain may be relieved by vomiting Contact with sick persons, travel, contact with certain animals
Appendicitis	Anorexia and fever (most patients) Patient remains still for comfort Pain precedes vomiting (nonbilious) Pain migration periumbilical, moving to right lower quadrant
Constipation	History of infrequent, painful stools Patient febrile Pain does not migrate Hard stool in the ampulla
Intussusception	Episodic pain with drawing up of the legs or intermittent lethargy Patient afebrile Bloody stool or frank blood (late finding) Lead point more likely in patients >2 y of age
Irritable bowel disease Malignancy (uncommon)	Weight loss Recurrent episodes of abdominal pain Bloody stools
Nephrolithiasis	Episodic severe pain radiates to flank or groin Patient afebrile Hematuria
Ovarian torsion	Episodic and unilateral lower quadrant pain (can be generalized) Patient afebrile Associated nausea and vomiting
Pancreatitis	Epigastric pain that may radiate to the patient's back Pain relieved by leaning forward ↑ Amylase/lipase levels
Pelvic inflammatory disease	Sexually active female subject Vaginal discharge, fever Cervical motion tenderness
Pneumonia	Fever, tachypnea, cough, chest pain Auscultation: rales or ↓ breath sounds
Small-bowel obstruction	Anorexia, bilious vomiting Crampy periumbilical pain without migration Peritoneal signs Air-fluid levels on abdominal radiographs
Urinary tract infection	Dysuria, urgency, frequency May have costovertebral angle tenderness Pyuria, bacteriuria
Volvulus	Episodic pain Patient afebrile Bilious emesis

emesis, anorexia, generalized abdominal pain, fever, and increased WBC count could have AGE, appendicitis, or a UTI. In such a case, it is useful to observe the patient for changes in symptoms (such as the onset of diarrhea), physical examination findings, fever curve, CRP level, and possibly abdominal radiography findings, depending on the level of concern.

If appendicitis is likely, start antibiotic treatment (as detailed herein for perforation), because it is becoming increasingly common to defer surgery until the next morning, when the patient and hospital staff are better prepared.

About one-quarter of patients with appendicitis, particularly those younger than 5 years of age, will have a ruptured appendix before presentation, and this typically occurs within 72 hours of the start of symptoms. There is continuing controversy over the best treatment of a patient with a ruptured appendix. After consultation with surgery, one approach is to treat with parenteral antibiotics until there is clinical improvement (patient afebrile >24 hours, patient tolerating maintenance oral intake, and decreased inflammatory markers), then transition to an oral regimen. Specific drug regimens vary by institution, but one approach is to add IV metronidazole (7.5 mg/kg every 6 hours, 4-g/d maximum) to one of the antibiotics detailed earlier. At discharge, change to amoxicillin/clavulanate (90 mg/kg/d of amoxicillin, divided into doses administered twice a day; 4-g/d maximum) with or without metronidazole (oral dose same as the IV dose herein). Interval appendectomy may be scheduled after about 6 weeks per surgical preference, especially if there was a fecalith.

There is no reason to withhold analgesia. Although pain medication can change some aspects of examination, this does not increase the likelihood of a misdiagnosis of surgical candidates and may actually facilitate a more thorough examination. Administer IV morphine (0.05–0.20 mg/kg every 2–4 hours; maximum, 8 mg per dose) as needed for pain.

There is no evidence to support the routine use of antiemetics for the patient with abdominal pain, outside of the diagnosis of acute gastroenteritis.

Indications for Consultation

- **Gynecology or pediatric surgery:** Possible ovarian torsion
- **Surgery:** Rebound tenderness, abdominal rigidity, bilious emesis, or presence of other findings of acute abdomen

Disposition

- **Intensive care unit transfer:** Shock, toxic appearance
- **Discharge criteria:** Definitive diagnosis, treatment, and recovery have occurred and the patient is tolerating adequate oral intake and medications, if needed

Follow-up

- **Primary care:** 1 to 3 days
- **Surgery (if patient underwent a procedure or if one is to be scheduled):** 1 to 2 weeks

Pearls and Pitfalls

- Laboratory tests and radiographs alone cannot be used to rule out the diagnosis of acute abdomen.
- The younger the child, the less likely the symptoms will conform to the classic presentation of appendicitis.
- Do not withhold pain medication.
- Not all cases of acute abdomen require immediate surgery. A perforated appendix may be treated medically, with or without interval appendectomy.
- Be circumspect of assigning the diagnosis of AGE when nausea and vomiting are not accompanied by diarrhea.

Bibliography

Hennelly KE, Bachur R. Appendicitis update. *Curr Opin Pediatr*. 2011;23(3):281–285

Kulik DM, Uleryk EM, Maguire JL. Does this child have appendicitis? A systematic review of clinical prediction rules for children with acute abdominal pain. *J Clin Epidemiol*. 2013;66(1):95–104

Lavine EK, Saul T, Frasure SE, Lewiss RE. Point-of-care ultrasound in a patient with perforated appendicitis. *Pediatr Emerg Care*. 2014;30(9):665–667

Pogorelić Z, Rak S, Mrklić I, Jurić I. Prospective validation of Alvarado score and Pediatric Appendicitis Score for the diagnosis of acute appendicitis in children. *Pediatr Emerg Care*. 2015;31(3):164–168

Saito JM. Beyond appendicitis: evaluation and surgical treatment of pediatric acute abdominal pain. *Curr Opin Pediatr*. 2012;24(3):357–364

Pyloric Stenosis

Introduction

Pyloric stenosis is the most common cause of upper gastrointestinal obstruction in infancy, with an incidence of 2 to 4 per 1,000 live births. Male infants are 4 to 6 times more likely to be affected, with 30% of patients being first-born male subjects. With prompt diagnosis and intervention, pyloromyotomy can prevent complications such as significant metabolic derangements, failure to thrive (FTT), shock, and death.

Clinical Presentation

History

The patient typically presents at 10 days to 8 weeks of life with progressively forceful, nonbilious emesis after feedings. The vomiting may be described as projectile or fountainlike and is almost always nonbilious and nonbloody.

Depending on the duration of symptoms, the patient may have a range of presentations, from vigorous and ravenous (especially immediately after vomiting) with adequate weight gain to listless and emaciated with profound FTT. Other complaints may include irritability, colic, and constipation.

Physical Examination

The physical examination findings may be completely normal. However, if symptoms have progressed over several weeks, the patient may appear dehydrated with significant weight loss or inadequate weight gain. Focus on assessing the degree of dehydration.

The classic finding is a palpable "olive," which is the hypertrophied pylorus, in the epigastric region or right upper quadrant. To appreciate the mass, place the patient supine with the hips flexed. Examine from the patient's left side and attempt to "slip" a hand under the edge of the right rectus muscle. The presence of the olive is pathognomonic; however, its absence does not exclude the diagnosis. Another unique finding is a visible abdominal peristaltic wave seen while the infant is sucking.

Laboratory Workup

Obtain serum electrolyte levels. An infant with pyloric stenosis characteristically develops a hypochloremic, hypokalemic, metabolic alkalosis (bicarbonate level >24 mEq/L [>24 mmol/L]). Note that a normal bicarbonate level in this age group is 18 mEq/L (18 mmol/L). However, early in the disease course, electrolyte levels may be normal.

Radiology Examinations

Abdominal ultrasonography (US) has replaced contrast-enhanced studies as the modality of choice for diagnosing pyloric stenosis. However, if US is unavailable, classic findings of an upper gastrointestinal (UGI) series are the "string sign" (pyloric channel filled with a thin stream of barium) or the "shoulder sign" (extrinsic compression of the stomach by a hypertrophied pylorus) in the presence of significant stenosis.

Pyloric US will allow measurements of both canal length and thickness. Pyloric stenosis is confirmed if the muscle width on a cross-sectional image is greater than 3 mm, while 2 to 3 mm is equivocal and less than 2 mm is a negative finding; and pyloric stenosis is also confirmed if the pyloric length is longer than 14 to 15 mm. However, pyloric stenosis is a progressive process, so a negative or equivocal pyloric US finding may be seen during the early stages of disease. If symptoms persist, arrange a repeat study in 1 week.

Differential Diagnosis

Pyloric stenosis causes unopposed (ie, no diarrhea) nonbilious vomiting. A number of conditions, ranging from mild (gastroesophageal reflux) to life threatening (acute adrenal insufficiency), can appear with unopposed vomiting (Table 119-1).

Other causes of hypochloremic metabolic alkalosis in an infant include Bartter syndrome, diuretic use, cystic fibrosis, exogenous alkali ingestion, and a chloride-deficient diet.

Treatment

Preoperative

Consult a surgeon to arrange a pyloromyotomy. However, this is not an emergent procedure. The priority is correcting dehydration and any electrolyte abnormalities. Generally, the anesthesiologist will defer surgery until the bicarbonate level is below 30 mEq/L (<30 mmol/L) and the chloride level is above 100 mEq/L (>100 mmol/L).

Treat significant dehydration ($\geq$10%) with a normal saline (NS) bolus (or boluses) to restore intravascular volume. If renal function is normal and the patient remains alkalotic, administer 5% dextrose one-half NS with 2 mEq (2 mmol) KCl/100 mL at 150% of the maintenance rate until urine output is adequate. This will help correct the alkalosis, which is "chloride responsive."

Table 119-1. Differential Diagnosis of Pyloric Stenosis	
Diagnosis	**Clinical Features**
Antral web	Similar presentation
Congenital adrenal hyperplasia Adrenal insufficiency/crisis	Clitoromegaly or hyperpigmented scrotum Hyperkalemia, hyponatremia No alkalosis
Gastroenteritis	Patient may have fever Diarrhea Patient not ravenous after vomiting
Gastroesophageal reflux	Lower-volume vomitus Nonprojectile emesis May be positional
↑ Intracranial pressure	Bulging fontanelle Sunsetting eyes Cranial nerve VI palsy
Overfeeding	Good/robust weight gain Nonprojectile emesis Normal electrolyte levels
Sepsis	Fever, lethargy Acidosis ↑ or ↓ White blood cell count
Volvulus	Bilious spit-up or nonprojectile vomiting No alkalosis

Once the patient's hydration status and electrolyte levels have normalized, switch to a maintenance intravenous solution and rate. It is not necessary to give the patient nil per os (nothing by mouth) until the appropriate time has arrived for preoperative fasting.

Surgical

Depending on individual preference, a laparoscopic or traditional open pyloromyotomy will be performed.

Postoperative

There is a range of approaches to the reinstitution of feeding. Findings of recent studies suggest withholding feedings for 4 hours postoperatively, then advancing to ad libitum feedings without stepwise volume acceleration.

Regurgitation after surgery occurs in most patients. This may be secondary to anesthesia, gastritis, irritation from the longstanding obstruction, residual inflammation after the pyloromyotomy, or an incomplete repair. If the infant continues to vomit for more than 5 days after surgery, repeat abdominal US examination and contact the surgeon, who may want to perform a UGI series. Consult the surgeon if fever with abdominal distention occurs within the first

24 hours, because this may be caused by an unsuspected perforation.
Acetaminophen usually suffices for postoperative analgesia.

Disposition
- **Interinstitutional transfer:** Pediatric surgeon not available
- **Discharge criteria:** Adequate oral intake without vomiting

Follow-up
- **Primary care:** 1 week
- **Surgeon:** 1 to 2 weeks

Pearls and Pitfalls
- Always consider pyloric stenosis in a young infant with unopposed vomiting.
- Pyloric stenosis is not an emergency. Correct any electrolyte abnormalities before surgery.

Bibliography

Graham KA, Laituri CA, Markel TA, Ladd AP. A review of postoperative feeding regimens in infantile hypertrophic pyloric stenosis. *J Pediatr Surg.* 2013:48(10):2175–2179

Hernanz-Schulman M. Pyloric stenosis: role of imaging. *Pediatr Radiol.* 2009;39(Suppl 2): S134–S139

Kamata M, Cartabuke RS, Tobias JD. Perioperative care of infants with pyloric stenosis. *Pediatr Anaesth.* 2015;25(12):1193–1206

Pandya S, Heiss K. Pyloric stenosis in pediatric surgery: an evidence-based review. *Surg Clin North Am.* 2012;92(3):527–539

Ranells JD, Carver JD, Kirby RS. Infantile hypertrophic pyloric stenosis: epidemiology, genetics, and clinical update. *Adv Pediatr.* 2011;58(1):195–206

Index

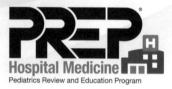

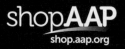